Approaches to Chronic Kidney Disease

Jerry McCauley
Seyed Mehrdad Hamrahian • Omar H. Maarouf
Editors

Approaches to Chronic Kidney Disease

A Guide for Primary Care Providers and Non-Nephrologists

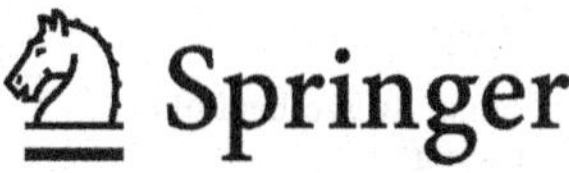 Springer

Editors
Jerry McCauley
Thomas Jefferson University
Philadelphia, PA
USA

Omar H. Maarouf
Division of Nephrology
Department of Medicine
Thomas Jefferson University
Philadelphia, PA
USA

Seyed Mehrdad Hamrahian
Department of Medicine
Division of Nephrology
Sidney Kimmel School of Medicine
Thomas Jefferson University
Philadelphia, PA
USA

ISBN 978-3-030-83084-7   ISBN 978-3-030-83082-3   (eBook)
https://doi.org/10.1007/978-3-030-83082-3

This Springer imprint is published by the registered company Springer Nature Switzerland AG
The registered company address is: Gewerbestrasse 11, 6330 Cham, Switzerland

Preface

Chronic kidney disease (CKD) is a major public health problem worldwide, affecting alone in the United States nearly one in seven adults. It is a disease process that integrates chronic illness at several levels leading to a progressive condition complicated by several comorbidities including cardiovascular disease. Respectively, the annual mortality rate for patients with CKD is twice that of patients without the disease. The spending cost on the care of patients with CKD including for those who progress to end-stage renal disease (ESRD) requiring dialysis or kidney transplantation is in billions of US dollars, imposing a tremendous economic burden on the health care system.

Early interventions and referral to nephrology will not only improve the quality of life of the individual with the disease, but can also slow the progression to ESRD or delay clinical complications including cardiovascular disease and death. Primary healthcare provider's awareness of basic CKD clinical guidelines, ability to predict the progression of the disease, and accurate timing of referral could increase the likelihood of preemptive kidney transplantation and improve the transition to renal replacement therapy including starting hemodialysis with a permanent vascular access rather than a tunneled dialysis catheter if peritoneal dialysis is opt out reducing the associated health care costs.

This textbook provides a comprehensive, current state-of-the-art review of this field and will serve as a valuable resource for non-nephrology clinicians – especially in underserved rural areas with limited resources who care for patients with CKD. The book addresses the epidemiology and risk factors for the disease. It also discusses CKD comorbidities and preparation for an inevitable need for renal replacement therapy, including renal transplant.

Philadelphia, PA, USAJerry McCauley
Philadelphia, PA, USASeyed Mehrdad Hamrahian
Philadelphia, PA, USAOmar H. Maarouf

Acknowledgments

We would like to thank all our patients, who have been the best mentors to us over all these practicing years. We are especially thankful to all the authors for the contributed time and effort to produce this valuable book. Finally, we would like to thank our families for being supportive through this long process despite all the challenges we have experienced in the COVID -19 pandemic.

Mehrdad Hamrahian
Jerry McCauley
Omar H. Maarouf

Contents

Contributors

Hasan Arif, MD Medicine-Nephrology, Sidney Kimmel Medical College at Thomas Jefferson University, Philadelphia, PA, USA

Lea Borgi, MD Brigham and Women's Hospital, Boston, MA, USA

Yasmin Brahmbhatt, MD, FASN AstraZeneca, Philadelphia, PA, USA

William Dennis Coffey, MD Department of Radiology, Thomas Jefferson University, Philadelphia, PA, USA

Xiaoying Deng, MD, PhD, FACP and MBA Department of Medicine, Division of Nephrology, Sanford Clinic North, North Fargo, ND, USA

Bonita Falkner, MD Thomas Jefferson University, Philadelphia, PA, USA

Department of Medicine, Nephrology, Philadelphia, PA, USA

Jesse M. Goldman, MD, FASN, FAHA Division of Nephrology, Department of Medicine, Sidney Kimmel School of Medicine, Thomas Jefferson University, Philadelphia, PA, USA

Maitreyee M. Gupta, MD Department of Medicine, Division of Nephrology, Thomas Jefferson University, Philadelphia, PA, USA

Fitsum Hailemariam, MD Department of Medicine, Division of Nephrology, Thomas Jefferson University, Philadelphia, PA, USA

Seyed Mehrdad Hamrahian, MD Department of Medicine, Division of Nephrology, Sidney Kimmel School of Medicine, Thomas Jefferson University, Philadelphia, PA, USA

Harald Jüppner, MD Endocrine Unit, Department of Medicine, Massachusetts General Hospital, Harvard Medical School, Boston, MA, USA

Pediatric Nephrology Unit, Massachusetts General Hospital, Harvard Medical School, Boston, MA, USA

Goni Katz-Greenberg, MD Division of Nephrology, Department of Medicine, Duke University School of Medicine, Durham, NC, USA

Gurwant Kaur, MD, FASN Department of Medicine, Division of Nephrology at PennState Hershey Medical Center, Hershey, PA, USA

Penn State Milton S. Hershey Medical Centre, Department of Medicine (Nephrology), Hershey, PA, USA

Omar H. Maarouf, MD Division of Nephrology, Department of Medicine, Thomas Jefferson University, Philadelphia, PA, USA

Olivia Marchionda, PharmD, BCCCP Department of Pharmacy, Thomas Jefferson University Hospital, Philadelphia, PA, USA

Maria P. Martinez Cantarin, MD Medicine-Nephrology, Sidney Kimmel Medical College at Thomas Jefferson University, Philadelphia, PA, USA

Ubaldo E. Martinez Outschoorn, MD Medical Oncology, Sidney Kimmel Medical College at Thomas Jefferson University, Philadelphia, PA, USA

T. Conor McKee, MD Department of Radiology, Thomas Jefferson University Hospital, Philadelphia, PA, USA

Christina Mejia, MD Medicine-Nephrology, Johns Hopkins University, Baltimore, MD, USA

Andrew Moyer, PharmD, BCCCP Department of Pharmacy, Augusta Health, Fishersville, VA, USA

Sagar U. Nigwekar, MD, MMSc Division of Nephrology, Department of Medicine, Massachusetts General Hospital, Harvard Medical School, Boston, MA, USA

Vikram Patney, MD, MS, MBA BJC Medical Group Belleville, Belleville, IL, USA

Kelsey Pawson, M.S. in Nutrition Friedman School of Nutrition Science and Policy, Tufts University, Dietetic Intern, Frances Stern Nutrition Center, Tufts Medical Center, Boston, MA, USA

Ignacio A. Portales-Castillo, MD Division of Nephrology, Department of Medicine, Massachusetts General Hospital, Harvard Medical School, Boston, MA, USA

Monica Salas, M.S. in Nutrition Friedman School of Nutrition Science and Policy, Tufts University, Dietetic Intern, Frances Stern Nutrition Center, Tufts Medical Center, Boston, MA, USA

Pooja Sanghi, MD Department of Medicine, Division of Nephrology, Geisinger Medical Center, Geisinger, PA, USA

Colette Shaw, MB, BCh, BAO Department of Radiology, Thomas Jefferson University Hospital, Philadelphia, PA, USA

Pooja Singh, MD Division of Nephrology, Department of Medicine, Thomas Jefferson University Hospital, Philadelphia, PA, USA

Hannah Roni Troutman, DO Department of Nephrology, Thomas Jefferson University, Sidney Kimmel Medical College, Philadelphia, PA, USA

Anju Yadav, MD, FASN Division of Nephrology, Hypertension and Transplantation, Thomas Jefferson University Hospital, Philadelphia, PA, USA

Elaine W. Yu, MD Endocrine Unit, Department of Medicine, Massachusetts General Hospital, Harvard Medical School, Boston, MA, USA

Jingjing Zhang, MD Department of Medicine, Division of Nephrology, Thomas Jefferson University Hospital, Philadelphia, PA, USA

Chapter 1
Renal Physiology for Primary Care Clinicians

Fitsum Hailemariam and Bonita Falkner

Introduction

The function of the kidney is to maintain fluid and chemical homeostasis and to contribute to hemodynamic stability. The kidneys have an enormous capacity for filtering plasma and for reabsorbing the plasma filtrate. For example, the normal glomerular filtration rate is around 125 ml/min per 1.73 m². At the normal rate of filtration for an average 70 kg person, 180 l of filtrate will be produced in 24 hours. This daily glomerular filtrate will contain over 1 kg of sodium chloride and other plasma constituents in similar large amounts [1, 2]. Because daily urine output is approximately 1–2 l, over 98% of the glomerular filtrate is reabsorbed by the renal tubules [2]. In addition to reabsorbing sodium and chloride, other filtered substances, including glucose, bicarbonate, and amino acids, must also be reabsorbed. At certain tubular sites, some substances, in particular potassium and hydrogen ion, will be secreted and added to the filtrate [1]. This chapter will review the anatomy and physiology of the kidneys. The chapter will also address several clinical conditions that are relevant to renal physiology.

The size of each kidney is dependent on age, sex, and height. In an adult, the average length is approximately 10–12 cm, and the right kidney may be slightly smaller than the left kidney [3].

Although there is considerable variability, the average human kidney is composed of approximately one million individual functioning nephrons, each

F. Hailemariam
Department of Medicine, Division of Nephrology, Thomas Jefferson University, Philadelphia, PA, USA
e-mail: Fitsum.Hailemariam@jefferson.edu

B. Falkner (✉)
Thomas Jefferson University, Philadelphia, PA, USA

Department of Medicine, Nephrology, Philadelphia, PA, USA
e-mail: Bonita.Falkner@jefferson.edu

© Springer Nature Switzerland AG 2022
J. McCauley et al. (eds.), *Approaches to Chronic Kidney Disease*,
https://doi.org/10.1007/978-3-030-83082-3_1

containing a single glomerulus or filtering unit [4]. While the function of each nephron varies somewhat depending on its regional location, all nephrons are considered collectively in the clinical determination of renal function. The overall concept of renal function is that of a steady filtering of body water through rapid recycling of plasma fluid. This is accomplished by three major components of nephron activity: (1) glomerular filtration, (2) tubular reabsorption, and (3) tubular secretion. These functional components respond to a variety of other factors including renal blood flow, neuroendocrine effects, and the fluid and nutrient supply to the body.

Vascular Structure of the Kidney

Under resting conditions, the kidneys are perfused with 1.2 l of blood per minute which represents about 25% of the cardiac output. Relative to other vascular beds, vascular resistance in the kidneys is low [5]. The organizational pattern of the vascular supply to the kidney is related to varying components of renal function. The basic pattern of blood flow into the kidney is depicted in Fig. 1.1. From the abdominal aorta, the main renal artery carries blood into the kidney and then branches segmental arteries followed by branching to interlobar arteries. Next there is branching to arcuate arteries, followed by branching to interlobular arteries, and final branching to afferent arterioles. The afferent arterioles subdivide and extend into a capillary network which forms the glomerular tuft. The confluence of the glomerular capillary network forms the efferent arteriole. The vasa recta emerge from the efferent arteriole (not shown) and are vascular bundles which extend deep into the medulla [6].

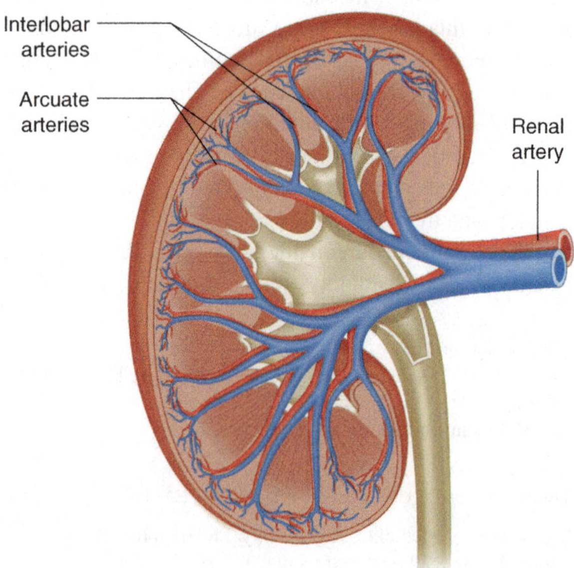

Fig. 1.1 Vascular structure of the kidney

Blood flow into the kidney from the main renal artery does not have a uniform distribution throughout the kidney. Ninety percent of the total renal blood flow (RBF) goes to the renal cortex which comprises 75% of the renal mass. The rate of cortical blood flow is about 500 ml/min per 100 g of kidney. The rate of medullary flow is about 100 ml/min per 100 g of kidney in the outer zone and 25 ml/min per 100 g in the inner zone. With this distribution, detectable changes in RBF will largely reflect changes in the cortex [7].

Differences between blood flow between the renal cortex and the medulla also play a significant role in the regulation of tubular osmolality. High blood flow through the peritubular capillaries in the cortex maintains an interstitial osmolarity that is similar to plasma. However, the interstitial osmolarity is higher in the medulla. This difference maintains the medullary osmotic gradient that is necessary for water reabsorption and sodium excretion [8].

Factors which control renal blood flow (RBF) are (1) systemic arterial pressure, (2) circulating blood volume, and (3) renal vascular resistance. Renal vascular resistance in the kidney is regulated by the arterioles. These vessels respond to extrinsic nervous and hormonal mechanisms.

For example, in clinical situations where blood pressure is very low or circulating volume is low due to hemorrhagic shock or dehydration, renal vascular resistance is increased by efferent arteriole constriction, and the tubular filtrate is maximumly reabsorbed to conserve plasma volume and glomerular filtration. There is also an intrinsic autonomous mechanism that contributes to renal vascular resistance designated "renal autoregulation." The mediators involved in renal autoregulation include a response to glomerular tubular feedback, in which chloride uptake by the macula densa segment of the distal tubule signals a myogenic vascular response in afferent and efferent arterioles [9].

Clinical conditions involving the renal vascular system are renal artery stenosis. Renal artery stenosis is generally associated with significant hypertension. In a younger patient, renal artery stenosis is usually due to fibromuscular dysplasia of the main renal artery or segmental arteries, whereas, in an older patient, renal artery stenosis is usually due to atherosclerotic lesions.

Glomerular Filtration Rate (GFR)

The filtering function of the kidney resides in the glomerulus, which is a specialized capillary network interposed between the afferent and efferent arterioles (see Fig. 1.2). Filtration occurs from the intracapillary space across the capillary wall into the urinary space of the glomerular capsule.

The permeability of the glomerular capillary wall is far greater than that of other capillaries in the body due to the increased number and size of pores in the endothelial cells on the inner lumen and also the specialized structure of the capillary basement membrane (i.e., glomerular basement membrane)

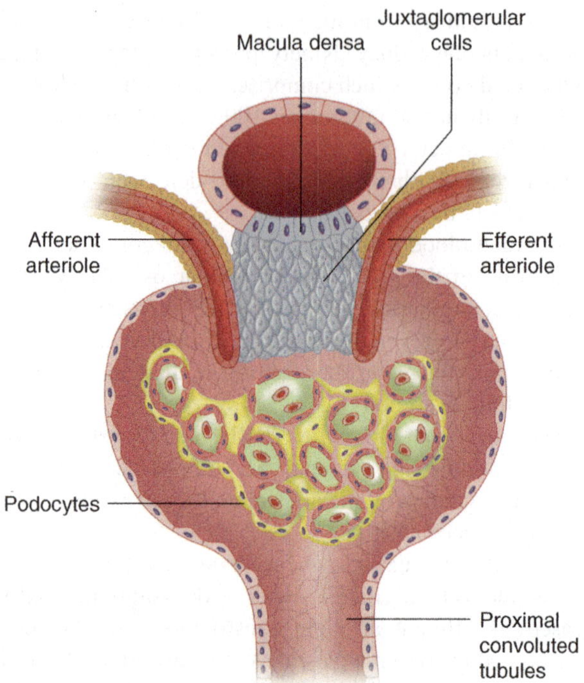

Fig. 1.2 The structure of the renal corpuscle

At the vascular pole of the glomerulus, the afferent and efferent arterioles and their relationship to the macula densa and juxtaglomerular cells are shown. The capsule is lined by parietal epithelial cells, and it continues into the cells of the proximal tubule at the urinary pole. The visceral epithelium (podocytes) is also shown covering the glomerular basement membrane and the fenestrated endothelial cells (picture used with permission from Dr. Tinsae Alemayehu).

Factors which regulate GFR include (1) permeability of the glomerular basement membrane; (2) capillary blood pressure; (3) intracapsular hydrostatic pressure; and (4) colloid osmotic pressure.

The intracapillary hydrostatic pressure is the major variable in the regulation of GFR and is dependent on systemic arterial pressure and resistance of the glomerular afferent and efferent arterioles. Thus:

(a) Afferent arteriole constriction decreases intracapillary hydrostatic pressure.
(b) Afferent arteriole dilation increases intracapillary hydrostatic pressure.
(c) Efferent arteriole constriction increases intracapillary hydrostatic pressure.
(d) Efferent arteriole dilation decreases intracapillary hydrostatic pressure

Both neural and hormonal factors affect arteriole constriction and dilation.

Intracapsular hydrostatic pressure is the pressure created by the volume of filtrate in the capsule of the glomerulus. This represents a force opposing filtration. Under normal conditions this pressure is slight. However, under conditions of a massive solute diuresis, the volume of fluid in the capsule increases and raises the intracapsular hydrostatic pressure.

Colloid osmotic pressure is a force opposing filtration and is created by the osmotic effect of plasma proteins. The plasma protein concentration is relatively stable under usual physiological conditions. Colloid osmotic pressure is probably not significant in altering GFR except in situations in which the intracapillary hydrostatic pressure falls to very low levels (in which case GFR would decrease markedly)

Chronic glomerulonephritis and diabetic nephropathy are common renal disorders that impair glomerular function from chronic inflammation. Reduction in functioning nephrons with compensatory hyperfiltration remaining nephrons leads to further glomerular injury. In these conditions, angiotensin-converting enzyme inhibitors (ACE-I) can provide glomerular protection by blocking vasoconstriction of efferent arteries to decrease intracapillary hydrostatic pressure and reducing hyperfiltration [10].

Renal Tubular Function

Two populations of nephrons exist. The cortical nephrons reside more peripherally in the outer cortex and have relatively short loops of Henle. The juxtamedullary nephrons reside in the inner cortex. These nephrons have very long loops of Henle which extend deep into the renal medulla. Due to their extension into the medullary regions of high tonicity, the tubules of the juxtamedullary nephrons have a more powerful concentrating capacity [11].

The tubules are divided anatomically and functionally into four basic segments: (1) proximal convoluted tubule; (2) loop of Henle; (3) distal convoluted tubule; and (4) collecting tubule. (Fig. 1.3) Transport mechanisms, which affect the movement of water and solutes from the tubular lumen to the extracellular fluid compartment, vary at the different tubular sites.

Transport of solutes and water follow one of two basic pathways. Active transport consists of a transcellular pathway in which the ion moves into the epithelial cell. Movement across the luminal epithelial surface is governed by an established concentration or electrochemical gradient. The substance is then pumped into the interstitium by an active transport mechanism. The other course of movement is the paracellular pathway. Solutes and water move across the intercellular spaces in a passive manner. The passive movement occurs down gradients created by active transport. The rate of passive movement is also contingent on the relative permeability of the intercellular junctions [1].

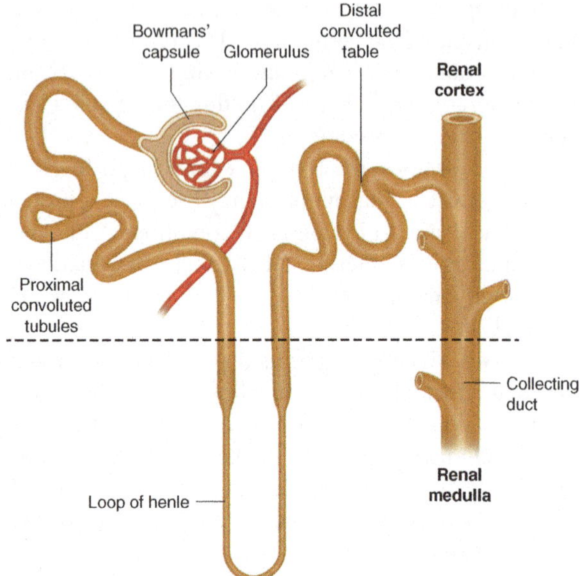

Fig. 1.3 This is a diagram of a long juxtamedullary nephron with all different segments labeled and the collecting duct (picture used with permission from Dr.T Alemayehu MD PedsID)

Proximal Tubular Segments

At least 60–70% of the glomerular filtrate is reabsorbed in the proximal tubular segments.

Proximal tubules contribute to fluid, electrolyte, and nutrient homeostasis by also reabsorbing a greater proportion of $NaHCO_3$ and nearly all of the nutrients in the ultrafiltrate [12]. The transport process is isosmotic, with movement across the tubular lumen directed by electrical potential gradients [1].

The first phase of proximal reabsorption affects the preferential reabsorption of essential nutrients including sugars, amino acids, bicarbonate, and organic metabolites. These are sodium-coupled transport processes. The transport mechanism for glucose is the Na-glucose cotransporter. This is notable because a new class of antidiabetic drugs, the SGLT2 inhibitors block the activity of the Na-glucose cotransporter resulting in glucosuria and greater Na delivery to distal tubules [1]. Water transport follows solute transport and is driven passively by a small osmotic gradient.

The second phase of proximal tubule reabsorption affects sodium and chloride reabsorption. New gradients are created by the preceding reabsorption of bicarbonate, sodium, and organic solutes. Chloride and sodium move from the tubular lumen into the tubular cell and then are actively pumped into the interstitium, with some further passive water transport.

Organic ions and many drugs are removed from the plasma by secretion from the proximal tubular cells into the lumen. In addition to solute reabsorption and secretion, proximal tubule cells also have metabolic activity. 25-Hydroxy-vitamin D is converted to 1,250dihydroxy-vitamin D by proximal tubule cells [12].

Loop of Henle

The loop of Henle consists of the thin descending limb and the thin ascending limb. These segments have unique permeability characteristics which govern their role in urinary concentration and dilution [13].

Tubular fluid entering the thin descending limb is isomotic relative to plasma with a concentration of about 300 milliosmoles. This segment is very permeable to water and relatively impermeable to solutes. Therefore, as the tubular fluid is exposed to the progressively hypertonic medullary interstitium, water moves from the tubular lumen to the interstitium [14].

At the bend of Henle's loop, the thin ascending limb begins. This portion of the loop is water impermeable and highly permeable to NaCl. The tubular fluid then flows along a course of gradually decreasing interstitial osmolarity. Sodium and chloride move out of the tubular lumen, rendering the tubular fluid progressively less concentrated. The absence of any significant water permeability permits the tubular epithelium to maintain the osmotic gradients [13, 14].

Distal Tubular Segments

The distal tubular segments consist of the thick ascending limb and the distal convoluted tubule. The transition point between the two segments is the area of the macula densa [15].

The macula densa separates the thick ascending limbs from the distal convoluted tubule. This portion of the distal nephron is in contact with the afferent arteriole entering the glomerulus and the efferent arteriole exiting the glomerulus. Together these tubular and vascular structures make up the juxtaglomerular (JG) apparatus. Granular cells in the afferent arteriole secrete renin, the enzyme essential for the generation of angiotensin II. The JG apparatus, which consists of tubular and vascular cells, act as a syncytium. When sodium concentration is low, or tubular volume is low, renin release is activated, ultimately resulting in stimulation of aldosterone secretion and enhanced sodium conservation [16].

The bumetanide-sensitive Na^+-K^+-$2Cl^-$ cotransportor (NKCC2) in the thick ascending limb is another major site for Na reabsorption, accounting for 25–30% of Na reabsorption. The loop diuretics act on NKCC2 to block sodium reabsorption in the thick ascending limb to effect diuresis and sodium excretion [17].

Tubular fluid emerging from the thick ascending limb and entering the distal convoluted tubule is hypotonic relative to plasma. The distal tubule is very impermeable to water.

Further dilution of tubular fluid occurs by active transport of sodium with further NaCl reabsorption in the absence of water movement. The Na^+Cl^- cotransporter (NCC) contributes another 4% of Na reabsorption under normal conditions [17]. The activity of NCC is regulated by the Na^+ delivery to the distal tubule and also by aldosterone [1]. The distal convoluted tubule is the main segment for transcellular calcium reabsorption, regulated by parathyroid hormone, calcitriol, and other factors. NCC in the distal tubule is the site of action for thiazide-like diuretics; and thiazide diuretics are also known to increase calcium reabsorption through their effect on NCC [18].

Collecting Tubules

The first portions of the collecting tubules are designated connecting tubule and initial cortical collecting tubule. Following these segments, the collecting tubules begin to join. The progressive confluence of nephrons results in an increasing collecting tubule diameter. The collecting tubule segments are the sites for the final regulation of sodium, potassium, hydrogen ion, and water composition. The collecting tubules are composed of different cell types which regulate these various transport functions. Most of the filtered potassium is reabsorbed before the tubular fluid reaches the collecting tubule. Cells of the collecting tubule are capable of both potassium reabsorption and potassium secretion, depending on dietary intake.

The epithelial Na^+ channel (EnaC) in the principal cells is the main mechanism for Na^+ reabsorption and is regulated by aldosterone. EnaC-mediated Na^+ reabsorption follows an electrochemical gradient and contributes to K^+ secretion in principal cells and H^+ secretion by intercalated cells [19]. The active transport mechanisms are efficient enough to produce urine with a sodium concentration of 1 meq/L during conditions of sodium deprivation.

The collecting tubules are the sites of hormonal regulation. Parathormone and calcitonin affect calcium secretion and act at the initial portion of the collecting tubules. Aldosterone stimulates sodium reabsorption, potassium secretion, and hydrogen ion secretion. The regulation of systemic water and osmotic balance is maintained through the hypothalamic-pituitary-renal axis. In response to thirst (hypothalamus), vasopressin (pituitary antidiuretic hormone: ADH) is secreted, and water is reabsorbed in the final portion of the collecting tubules. This is the mechanism by which the final concentration of the tubular fluid (i.e., urine) is achieved.

References

1. Christov M, Alper SL. Tubular transport: core curriculum. Am J Kidney Dis. 2010;56(6):1202–17.
2. Weisberg LS, Zanger R. Minerals in dialysis therapy: an introduction. Semin Dial. 2010;23:547–8.
3. Glodny B, Unterholzner V, Taferner B, et al. Normal kidney size and its influencing factors – a 64-slice MDCT study of 1.040 asymptomatic patients. BMC Urol. 2009;9:19. Published 2009 Dec 23.
4. Pollak MR, Quaggin SE, Hoenig MP, Dworkin LD. The glomerulus: the sphere of influence. Clin J Am Soc Nephrol. 2014;9(8):1461–9. https://doi.org/10.2215/Cjn.09400913.

5. Kaufman DP, Basit H, Knohl SJ. Physiology, glomerular filtration rate (Gfr). Statpearls Publishing. Last Update: April 25, 2019.
6. Leslie SW, Sajjad H. Anatomy, abdomen and pelvis, renal artery. Statpearls Publishing. Updated 2019 Oct 21.
7. Young LS, Regan MC, Barry MK, et al. Methods of renal blood flow measurement. Urol Res. 1996;24:149–60.
8. Dalal R, Bruss ZS, Sehdev JS. Physiology, renal blood flow and filtration. Statpearls Publishing. Updated 2019 May 15.
9. Burke M, Pabbidi MR, Farley J, Roman RJ. Molecular mechanisms of renal blood flow autoregulation. Curr Vasc Pharmacol. 2014;12(6):845–58.
10. Hostetter TH, Rennke HG, Brenner BM. The case for intrarenal hypertension in the initiation and progression of diabetic and other glomerulopathies. Am J Med. 1982;72(3):375–80.
11. Jamison RL. Short and long looped nephrons. Kidney Int. 1987;31:597–605.
12. Curthoys NP, Moe OW. Proximal tubule function and response to acidosis. Clin J Am Soc Nephrol. 2014;9(9):1627–38.
13. Dantzler WH, Layton AT, Layton HE, Pannabecker TL. Urine-concentrating mechanism in the inner medulla: function of the thin limbs of the loops of Henle. Clin J Am Soc Nephrol. 2014;9(10):1781–9.
14. Sands JM, Layton HE. The physiology of urinary concentration: an update. Semin Nephrol. 2009;29(3):178–95.
15. Mount DB. Thick ascending limb of the loop of Henle. Clin J Am Soc Nephrol. 2014;9(11):1974–86.
16. János P, Raymond H. Macula densa sensing and signaling mechanisms of renin release. J Am Soc Nephrol. 2010;21(7):1093–6.
17. Layton A, Laghmani K, Vallon V, Edwards A. Solute transport and oxygen consumption along the nephrons: effects of Na+ transport inhibitors. Am J Physiol Renal Physiol. 2016;311(6):F1217–29.
18. Subramanya AR, Ellison DH. Distal convoluted tubule. Clin J Am Soc Nephrol. 2014;9(12):2147–63.
19. Pearce D, Soundararajan R, Trimpert C, Kashlan OB, Deen PMT, Kohan DE. Collecting duct principal cell transport processes and their regulation. Clin J Am Soc Nephrol. 2015;10(1):135–46.

Chapter 2
State of the Care, Definition, and Epidemiology of Chronic Kidney Disease

Jingjing Zhang

Definition of Chronic Kidney Disease

Chronic kidney disease (CKD) is a global health issue. The adverse outcomes of CKD lead to high mortality and social economic burdens but can be prevented through early detection and intervention. To detect early-stage CKD through routine laboratory measurements universally, the National Kidney Foundation Kidney Disease Outcomes Quality Initiative (NKF KDOQI) first published a definition of CKD to standardize disease diagnosis criteria and disease staging in 2002.

According to KDOQI-CKD guideline, all individuals with a glomerular filtration rate (GFR) <60 mL/min/1.73 m^2 for longer than 3 months are classified as having CKD, irrespective of the presence or absence of kidney damage. All individuals with kidney damage are classified as having CKD, irrespective of the GFR level. Notably, a stable GFR must be present for longer than 3 months before CKD stage classification in patients (Table 2.1) [1]. Kidney damage is defined as microscopic hematuria, proteinuria, or anatomic abnormalities of the kidneys. Patients who are classified as having stage 5 CKD, who are on dialysis are considered to have an end-stage renal disease (ESRD). In 2012, after realizing the importance of albuminuria in CKD progression, cardiovascular death, acute kidney injury, and all-cause death, the International Society of Nephrology and *Kidney Disease: Improving Global outcomes (KDIGO)* modified the KDOQI-CKD staging system, adding the level of albuminuria to the five stages into a heat map (Table 2.2) [2]. The heat map divides each CKD stage into three subgroups according to the level of albuminuria. The patients with high proteinuria levels progress to ESRD faster than those with low

J. Zhang (✉)
Department of Medicine, Division of Nephrology, Thomas Jefferson University Hospital, Philadelphia, PA, USA
e-mail: Jingjing.zhang@jefferson.edu

© Springer Nature Switzerland AG 2022
J. McCauley et al. (eds.), *Approaches to Chronic Kidney Disease*,
https://doi.org/10.1007/978-3-030-83082-3_2

Table 2.1 Definition and stages of CKD

GFR (ml/min/1.73 m^2)	With kidney damage[a]	Without kidney damage
≥90	1	
60–89	2	
30–59	3	3
15–29	4	4
<15 (or dialysis)	5	5

[a]Kidney damage is defined as pathologic abnormalities or markers of damage, including abnormalities in the blood, urine tests, or imaging studies. (Table modified from Ref. [1])

Table 2.2 Prognosis of CKD according to GFR and albuminuria levels

Prognosis of CKD by GFR and Albuminuria Categories: KDIGO 2012			Persistent albuminuria categories Description and range		
			A1 Normal to mildly increased <30 mg/g <3 mg/mmol	**A2** Moderately increased 30-300 mg/g 3-30 mg/mmol	**A3** Severely increased >300 mg/g >30 mg/mmol
GFR categories (ml/ min/ 1.73 m^2) Description and range	G1	Normal or high	≥90	Green	Yellow	Orange
	G2	Mildly decreased	60-89	Green	Yellow	Orange
	G3a	Mildly to moderately decreased	45-59	Yellow	Orange	Red
	G3b	Moderately to severely decreased	30-44	Orange	Red	Red
	G4	Severely decreased	15-29	Red	Red	Red
	G5	Kidney failure	<15	Red	Red	Red

Derived from KDIGO: Chapter 1, definition and classification of CKD. Kidney International Supplements (2013) [2]. (With permission from KDIGO Team)

Green, low risk (if no other markers of kidney disease, no CKD); yellow, moderately increased risk; orange, gray, high risk; red, very high risk

CKD chronic kidney disease, *GFR* glomerular filtration rate, *KDIGO* Kidney Disease: Improving Global Outcomes

levels. Subsequently, KDIGO recommended that CKD should be classified based on the cause (C), GFR category (G), and albuminuria (A) level; this CGA system addressed the importance of reversible risk factors for CKD and serves as an indicator of rapid progression [2].

Significance of Chronic Kidney Disease

In 2010, CKD was ranked 18th on the list of causes of the total number of global deaths(annual death rate 16.3 per 100,000); in 1990, it was 27th [3]. In England, from 2006 to 2008, 28.7–38.2% of ESRD patients died within 3 years [4]. CKD is also a major public health problem in the USA. According to the most recent US Renal Data System (USRDS) data, 726,331 Americans had ESRD in 2016, and the crude prevalence was 2160.7 per one million population. Within the ESRD population, 63.1% were receiving maintenance hemodialysis (HD), 7% were doing peritoneal dialysis (PD), and 29.6% had functional transplanted kidneys. In 2016 alone, 124,675 new cases of ESRD were reported, and the crude incidence rate was 373.4 per million [5].

Even though the mortality rate in patients with ESRD had greatly improved from that 15 years ago, only 2/3 and 4/5 of the patients on receiving HD and PD will still be alive 2 years after initiation of dialysis according to USRDS data [5]; this is an astonishingly high mortality rate. The high mortality not only affects patients with ESRD, but also affects patients with CKD independent of dialysis. One study of 28,000 patients found that only 3.1% of patients with stage 2 CKD to stage 4 CKD progressed to needing renal replacement therapy, while 24.5% passed away during the 5 and half year observation period [6]. Another study showed that among 1,120,295 adults who had their kidney function measured, the mortality rate was 20% higher in patients with stage 3 CKD than in patients with stage 2 CKD, and 80% higher in patients with stage 4 CKD than in patients with stage 2 CKD after a follow-up period of 2.84 years. The worst is of course stage 5 CKD [7]; the mortality rate is 3.2 times higher than that for stage 2 CKD. In addition to high mortality in patients with CKD, other events, such as cardiovascular events and hospitalization, were also associated with CKD in a large community-based population. Cardiovascular disease is the leading cause of mortality in CKD patients [8, 9], and even mild reductions in the GFR are associated with high cardiovascular risk [6].

Economic Burden of Chronic Kidney Disease

Patients with ESRD suffer physically and emotionally, and the expenses incurred by ESRD patients cause an economic burden to the whole society. In the USA, ESRD patients constituted less than 1% of Medicare beneficiaries but accounted for 5% of Medicare program expenditures. In 1999, approximately 350,000 people in the USA suffered from ESRD, resulting in a cost of $12.7 billion to the Medicare ESRD program [10]. These costs were expected to increase to $28 billion per year by 2010 [11]. By 2015, $34 billion was spent for beneficiaries with ESRD according to a USRDS report [12].

The costs associated with CKD without dialysis and transplant are also tremendous. The higher the CKD stage, the higher the expenditure. The Medicare per-person cost for stage 1–2 CKD was $17,969, for stage 3 CKD was $19,392, for stages 4–5 CKD was $25,623, and for ESRD was $65,142 in 2012 [13]. This analysis laid the foundation for the vision that identifying and slowing the progression of CKD early will decrease medical expenditures. In 2015, the total expenditure for Medicare beneficiaries with kidney disease alone was nearly $100 billion. This included over $64 billion for all Medicare beneficiaries who had only CKD and not ESRD. In 2019, approximately 20% of dollars in the traditional Medicare program are spent on Americans with kidney disease. To increase the efficacy of spending for patients with kidney diseases, Health and Human Services launch the president's "advancing American Kidney Health" initiative in July 2019 [14].

Common Causes of ESRD

Prevention strategies for CKD and ESRD need to focus on the causes that lead to kidney disease. The primary diagnosis of ESRD has been reported in the USRDS database since 1988. In 2009, the USRDS reported that the primary causes of ESRD were diabetes mellitus (DM) (38%); hypertension (HTN) (24%); glomerulonephritis (15%); cystic kidney disease (5%); urologic diseases, including stones (2%); and unknown causes (16%) [15]. In 2016, the primary causes of ESRD were reported to be DM (48%), HTN (29%), glomerulonephritis (8%), cystic kidney disease (3%), and unknown causes (13%) [5]. Despite the variable percentages of contributions of original diseases to ESRD, DM, HTN, and glomerulonephritis are still the most common etiologies (Fig. 2.1). The primary diseases leading to ESRD are also the most common causes of CKD without dialysis.

Epidemiology/Prevalence of Chronic Kidney Disease

Both CKD and ESRD cause heavy economic burdens to society. Almost all cases of ESRD are preceded by CKD [16]. Given its natural history, an antecedent change in CKD epidemiology would be expected before a substantial change in ESRD epidemiology.

Several studies have shown the epidemiological characteristics of CKD have changed in the past three decades in the USA along with new definition, and biomarkers were established using National Health and Nutrition Examination Survey (NHANES) data. Hsu and colleagues estimated that between the NHANES II (1976–1980) and NHANES III (1988–1994), the overall prevalence of CKD (defined in that study as an estimated (e)GFR <60 mL/min/1.73 m^2) increased by 1.7% per year among persons aged 20–74 years [17]. Coresh and associates reported a 3.5% annual increase in stage 1 to 4 CKD between the NHANES III(1988–1994) and NHANES 1999–2004 using a serum creatinine–based eGFR [18], and Grams

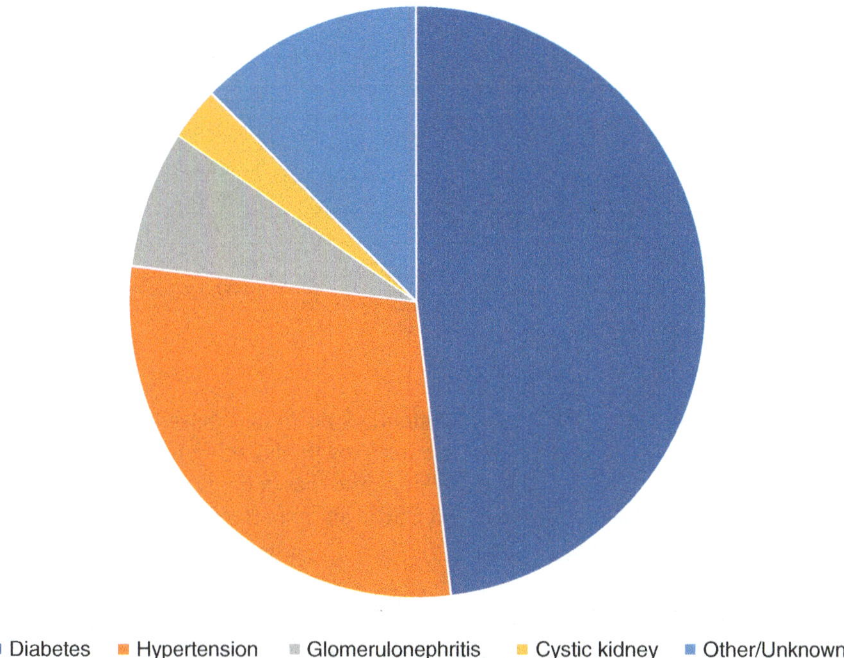

Fig. 2.1 The distributive causes of ESRD in 2016, data from the USRDS 2018 report. (Modified from Ref. [5])

and coworkers reported a yearly increase in stage 3 to 4 CKD of up to 5.0% from the NHANES III (1988–1994) to NHANES 1999–2002 using cystatin C –based eGFR [19].

Another study showed that the prevalence of CKD in the USA increased from 10.0 to 13.1% between 1988–1994 and 1999–2004; the aging population and increases in the prevalence of DM, HTN, and obesity seem to partly account for this increase.

Finally, temporal trends have shown that the increase in CKD prevalence has slowed down since the early 2000s. In most subgroups stratified by age, sex, race/ethnicity, and DM status [20], all ethnicities reached a CKD prevalence plateau, except non-Hispanic blacks, who are still experiencing an increasing trend. According to the USRDS, the ESRD incidence rate in the USA (adjusted for age, sex, and race/ethnicity) was 386 cases per million persons per year in 2003, and 356, 352, and 351 cases per million persons per year in 2011, 2012, and 2013, respectively; these values demonstrate a plateau approximately a decade later.

The prevalence of early stage of CKD, while relatively stable at 14.8%, implies that an estimated 30 million American adults have CKD and millions of others have an increased risk. Among the early stages of CKD, stage 3 CKD comprises the majority of the CKD population, followed by stage 2 CKD, and CKD4 accounts for less than 0.5% of the population (Table 2.3).

Table 2.3 Prevalence of CKD Stages in US adults aged 20 years or older based on the NHANES 1988–1994 and NHANES 1999–2004

CKD stage	Prevalence, % (95% CI)	
	NHANES 1988–1994	NHANES 1999–2004
1	1.71(1.28–2.18)	1.78(1.35–2.25)
2	2.70(2.17–3.24)	3.24(2.61–3.88)
3	5.42(4.89–5.95)	7.69(7.02–8.36)
4	0.21(0.15–0.27)	0.35(0.25–0.45)
5	NA	NA
Total	10.03(9.16–10.91)	13.07(12.04–14.10)

Modified from the Ref. [19]

The global burden of CKD is substantial, as death and disability due to CKD have increased, largely driven by population growth and aging [21] until the early twenty-first century. The global trend is similar to that in the USA.

Trends in the prevalence of CKD and ESRD are important for health care policy development and planning.

Risk Factors for CKD and CKD Prevalence

CKD is associated with the prevalence of HTN, DM, and obesity in the USA and worldwide. In recent years, there has been an overrepresentation of DM and HTN in US minority populations and many Asian countries. While HTN and DM are the leading causes of CKD in many developing countries, infectious diseases, environmental pollution, pesticides, water, analgesic abuse, and herbal medications are also common causes of CKD in these regions [22].

To prevent CKD, controlling risk factors for CKD is key. Diabetes, HTN, and obesity are the major preventable causes of CKD in the USA, unless the patients are immigrants from developing countries.

Investigating evidence of the association between DM and CKD will require standardized diagnostic criteria. Using hemoglobin A1C (HbA1c) levels for the diagnosis of DM was formally recommended by an International Expert Committee convened by the American Diabetes Association (ADA) in 2009 [23] and endorsed by the World Health Organization (WHO) in 2011 [24], with the criterion of HbA1c $\geq 6.5\%$ as a diagnostic criterion for DM. By this definition, according to the NHANES data, between 1988–1994 and 2011–2012, the prevalence of DM increased in the overall population and in all subgroups evaluated more rapidly than in the period of 1988–1994 [25]. The estimated prevalence of DM was 12–14% among US adults in 2011–2012, with the highest prevalence in participants who were non-Hispanic black, non-Hispanic Asian, and Hispanic.

Worldwide, the WHO and the International Diabetes Federation (IDF) have estimated the increase in DM worldwide since 1998. One estimate suggested that there were 171 million people with DM in 2000 and predicted that this figure would rise to 366 million by 2030 [26], a number that was already surpassed in 2013 [27].

As another major risk factor for CKD, the prevalence of HTN is well studied. According to JNC 8 update [28], blood pressure higher than 140/90 mmHg is a criterion for HTN, and the prevalence of HTN was 30.5% among men and 28.5% among women in 2009 and 2010 [29]. After the Systolic Blood Pressure Intervention Trial (SPRINT) study was published in 2015 [30], the American Heart Association (AHA) updated the HTN guideline, considering 130/80 as the cut-off for HTN [31], meaning that 46% of the population in the USA meets the criteria for the diagnosis of HTN [32]. During the SPRINT study, which included patients at high risk for cardiovascular events but without DM, targeting a blood pressure value of less than 120 mm Hg compared with less than 140 mmHg via intensive control resulted in lower rates of fatal and nonfatal major cardiovascular events and death from any cause. The study was terminated during the interim analysis stage due to the obvious benefits of intense blood pressure control. To control HTN, awareness of HTN is important. Using data from eight sets of NHANES, the prevalence and temporal trends, awareness, treatment, and control of HTN among US young adults aged 18–39 years were compared with other adult age groups during the years 1999–2014. Overall awareness, treatment, and control among adults with HTN improved during the study interval, and the prevalence is stabilized, but young adult men aged 18–39 had the lowest awareness and lowest rate of treatment and control and thus need additional education from medical providers, especially primary physicians [33].

Even though glomerulonephritis is the third most common cause of ESRD, clinical and pathological diagnoses are complex, and glomerulonephritis is generally not preventable. Therefore, DM and HTN are the primary risk factors for the development of CKD, and obesity, a condition that can be prevented, is also highly associated with CKD.

Obesity accelerates death risk and has been associated with many comorbidities, such as cardiovascular disease; type 2 diabetes; HTN; dyslipidemia; obstructive sleep apnea; fatty liver and biliary disease; osteoarthritis; various malignancies, including kidney cancer and neuropsychiatric complications; and impaired health-related quality of life.

A growing body of evidence from the USA and other countries indicate that obesity is a potent risk factor for the development of de novo CKD and ESRD independent of DM and HTN [34].

In one study of a cohort of 11,104 healthy participants, 1377 participants (12.4%) had developed CKD (defined as a GFR <60 mL/min/1.73 m^2) after 14 years of follow-up. A high body mass index (BMI) at the beginning of the study was shown to be a risk factor for the development of CKD. Participants whose BMI increased by more than 10% during the follow-up period had a significant increase in their risk of developing CKD (OR 1.27) [35].

The relationship between obesity and proteinuria was first discovered more than four decades ago, when the first study in which a minority of obese patients developed proteinuria was published [36]. Focal segmental glomerulosclerosis (FSGS) is the most frequently encountered histologic lesion in the renal biopsies of these patients [37]. Proteinuria is a risk factor for cardiovascular disease and the rapid progression of CKD. A prospective and randomized study showed the influence of weight loss on inducing a reduction in proteinuria in patients with different protein-uric nephropathies [38]. Whether weight loss is beneficial for kidney function is still unclear, but one study involving an adolescent population showed a benefit. In that study, following bariatric surgery, the eGFR increased by 3.9 mL/min/1.73 m^2 for each 10-unit BMI decrease after adjustment in obese children. Early kidney abnormalities improved in adolescents with evidence of preoperative kidney disease [39].

However, obesity is still prevalent in the USA. One meta-analysis in 2008 estimated that 24.2% and 33.9% of American men and women are obese, respectively. In industrialized countries, 13.8% of CKD in men and 24.9% of CKD in women could be related to overweight and obesity. Obesity increases the risk for CKD in the general population, and the association appears to be stronger in women than in men [36]. In the USA, between 2007–2008 and 2015–2016, increases in obesity and severe obesity prevalence rates persisted among adults; however, there were no overall significant trends among youth [37]. The prevalence of obesity in adults may eventually decrease as youth grow up.

A worldwide a study was conducted by assembling data from 195 countries to model trends in overweight and obesity and related morbidity and mortality. The result showed that the prevalence of obesity has more than doubled from 1980 to 2017. In 2017, the prevalence of obesity was 5% in children and 12% in adults [38]. Interestingly, Asians will have more complications from obesity than African Americans.

Obesity should be always evaluated and addressed at primary physician visits. Early weight reduction education can help prevent the development of CKD.

Awareness of CKD

To prevent CKD and slow CKD progression, patients and primary physicians should be aware of the diagnosis. Most published reports support the importance of early CKD awareness. Late CKD detection and nephrology referrals have been associated with adverse outcomes. Among patients with CKD who initiated dialysis, late referral was unsurprisingly associated with a higher risk of death within 1 year than early referral [39].

Worldwide, only 6% of the general population and 10% of the high-risk population are aware of their CKD status [40]. In the USA, the NHANES 1999–2000 data showed that 8.2% of participants with stage 3 CKD self-reported a history of renal disease [41]. Additional studies confirmed that less than 10% of those with stage 3 CKD knew that they had the disease but the awareness increased approximately 40% in those with stage 4 CKD [42].

There are different reasons causing the late evaluation of patients with CKD by a nephrologist. Late evaluation by a nephrologist has been shown to be associated with black ethnicity and a lack of health insurance. This will obviously lead to increased burdens and severities of comorbid diseases, and mortality [43].

Late evaluation for CKD by a nephrologist is also partially due to denial by the patients or the unalertness of providers. Low awareness among healthcare providers has been reported in several studies. Fewer than 10% of individuals with moderately decreased kidney function (stage 3 CKD) reported ever being told that they had weak or failing kidneys in 2005 in the USA [41]. These data showed that CKD is underdiagnosed and undertreated by a range of medical providers. In Europe, similar results have been reported. In a nationwide audit of 451,548 adults followed by general practitioners in Italy [44], only 17% had undergone serum creatinine testing, of whom 16% had an eGFR lower than 60 mL/min per 1.73 m^2. Among these adults, CKD had been correctly diagnosed in only 15%. In another study from Italy, of 39,525 hypertensive patients, 23% had CKD, but general practitioners diagnosed it correctly in only 3.9% [45]. The situation may be even worse in developing countries, especially in countries in which renal replacement therapy (RRT) cannot always be provided. A study from India showed that an incorrect diagnosis resulted in delayed referrals to nephrologists, leading to missed opportunities to implement strategies for slowing disease progression, increasing cardiovascular protection, and preparing for RRT [46].

Given that late CKD detection and nephrology referral have been associated with adverse outcomes, programs, such as the Kidney Disease Outcomes Quality Initiative staging system, National Institutes of Health National Kidney Disease Education Program(NIH NKDEP) [47], and National Kidney Foundation Kidney Early Evaluation Program, (NKF-KEEP) [1], were developed to promote CKD awareness. The NKF-KEEP is the first national health screening program to target adult populations at high risk for CKD and promote awareness [48].

Prevention and Screening

ESRD usually results from CKD, and the early stages of CKD can be detected through routine laboratory measurements. Adverse outcomes of CKD can also be prevented or delayed through early detection and treatment.

Screening

Diagnostic testing for CKD may be necessary in several groups of patients who seek medical attention for other reasons [49], especially those with DM, HTN, cardiovascular disease, structural renal-tract disease, autoimmune diseases with a potential of kidney involvement, and a family history of CKD or hereditary kidney disease [49, 50].

Strategies for the early identification and treatment of people with CKD, who are at risk of cardiovascular events and progression to ESRD, are needed worldwide, especially in countries where RRT is not readily available.

The best way to screen people to identify who will benefit most from preventive measures is disputed. Current recommendations suggest screening individuals with DM, HTN, cardiovascular disease, structural diseases of the renal tract, auto-immune diseases with a potential of kidney involvement, and family history of kidney disease, during routine primary health encounters. Some studies have shown that screening for CKD is cost effective, especially for DM patients. In patients with DM, statistical models have shown that the addition of screening for proteinuria followed by the use of angiotensin-converting enzyme inhibitors in people with abnormal proteinuria values reduced costs and the cumulative incidence of ESRD and improved life expectancy [51]. Similar findings were found in an economic assessment of the reduction in endpoints in the angiotensin antagonist losartan study [52]. Over 3.5 years, treatment with losartan in patients with type 2 DM and nephropathy not only reduced the incidence of ESRD by 33.6 days per patient but also resulted in substantial cost savings, with a net savings of $3522 per patient.

Another study by Palmer showed that screening for nephropathy in patients with type 2 DM who are hypertensive can improve clinical outcomes substantially and save costs after 2 years. Sensitivity analysis demonstrated the robustness of the results—screening and optimal treatment always led to improved patient outcomes, had excellent value monetarily, and even led to overall cost savings in some circumstances. Financial concerns should not be a barrier to the implementation of screening for nephropathy in this group of patients [51].

The cost-effectiveness of screening for CKD in the general population, however, is unclear.

Slowing the Progression of CKD

Effective strategies can slow the progression of CKD and reduce the risk of cardiovascular mortality and ESRD. The primary strategies are blood pressure control, preferably with agents that block the renin-angiotensin-aldosterone pathway and good glycemic control. Weight reduction also requires attention at each annual check-up. Lipid-lowering therapies, irrespective of the starting cholesterol concentration, reduce the incidence of major atherosclerotic events in patients with CKD [53], although no evidence supports the use of statins to slow the loss of renal function. The correction of acidosis is thought to slow declining in GFRs, countering acidosis in the early CKD is called for attention now [54]. An inexpensive and easily applicable approach is to achieve the optimum intake of salt and protein. Finally, self-management and support groups can improve lifestyle and dietary habits, knowledge of the disease, and adherence to treatment and might improve anthropometric indices and glycemic and blood pressure control [55]. The cost-effectiveness of a self-management-based intervention for people with stage 3 CKD is currently being investigated in a randomized clinical trial [56]. A multidisciplinary approach is needed to implement treatment strategies.

Targeting the renin-angiotensin-aldosterone system (RAAS) blockade was the only treatment option to slow down the progression of CKD until recently. Eighteen years after The Reduction of Endpoints in NIDDM with the Angiotensin II Antagonist Losartan (RENAAL) trial was published [57], a new categorical medication, a sodium-glucose cotransport-2 inhibitor (SGLT2 inhibitor), was shown to be effective in slowing the progression of CKD in patients with DM; it also confers cardiovascular protection [58]. The 2019 American Diabetes Association (ADA) guidelines recommend SGLT2 inhibitors as the preferred class of agents to be added after metformin in patients with type2 DM and a history of heart failure or CKD [59]. Endocrinologists, cardiologists, nephrologists, and even primary physicians need to be aware of the new era of the SGLT2 inhibitor and prescribe the medication to eligible patients. We should see the change in CKD epidemiology in the next decade.

Summary

CKD epidemiology alone has received much attention over the past 2 decades and has been incorporated into nationwide health promotion programs and disease prevention goals, for example, the Healthy People 2020 initiative of the USA. Department of Health and Human Services has set a target of a 10% proportional reduction in CKD prevalence in the US population by 2020 [60].

In July 2019, Health and Human Services launch another kidney initiative: the President's "Advancing American Kidney Health" initiative, with three goals: (1) to reduce the number of Americans who develop ESRD by 25% by 2030; (2) have 80 %t of new ESRD patients in 2025 either receive dialysis at home or undergo a transplant; and (3) double the number of kidneys available for transplant by 2030 [14].

All the efforts made by all the medical providers will increase awareness of CKD, slow the progression of CKD, reduce mortality due to CKD and ESRD, and decrease the economic burden of CKD.

References

1. Levey AS, Coresh J, Bolton K, et al. K/DOQI clinical practice guidelines for chronic kidney disease: evaluation, classification, and stratification. Am J Kidney Dis. 2002;39:S1–266.
2. Chapter 1: definition and classification of CKD. Kidney Int Suppl. 2013;3:19–62. https://doi.org/10.1038/kisup.2012.64.
3. Lozano R, Naghavi M, Foreman K, et al. Global and regional mortality from 235 causes of death for 20 age groups in 1990 and 2010: a systematic analysis for the Global Burden of Disease Study 2010. Lancet. 2012;380:2095–128. https://doi.org/10.1016/S0140-6736(12)61728-0.

4. Storey BC, Staplin N, Harper CH, et al. Declining comorbidity-adjusted mortality rates in English patients receiving maintenance renal replacement therapy. Kidney Int. 2018;93:1165–74.
5. 2018 USRDS annual report data, ESRD in United State. Mortality. USRDS.
6. Keith DS, Nichols GA, Gullion CM, et al. Longitudinal follow-up and outcomes among a population with chronic kidney disease in a large managed care organization. Arch Intern Med. 2004;164:659–63.
7. Go A, Chertow G, Fan D, et al. Chronic kidney disease and the risks of death, cardiovascular events, and hospitalization. NEJM. 2004;351:1296–305.
8. Garg AX, Clark WF, Haynes RB, House AA. Moderate renal insufficiency and the risk of cardiovascular mortality: results from the NHANES I. Kidney Int. 2002;61:1486–94.
9. Weiner DE. Chronic kidney disease as a risk factor for cardiovascular disease and all-cause mortality: a pooled analysis of community-based studies. J Am Soc Nephrol. 2004;15:1307–15. https://doi.org/10.1097/01.ASN.0000123691.46138.E2.
10. 2001 USRDS annual report. Economic costs of ESRD.
11. Joyce AT, Iacoviello JM, Nag S, et al. End-stage renal disease-associated managed care costs among patients with and without diabetes. Diabetes Care. 2004;27:2829–35. https://doi.org/10.2337/diacare.27.12.2829.
12. Saran R, Robinson B, Abbott KC, et al. US renal data system 2017 annual data report: epidemiology of kidney disease in the United States. Am J Kidney Dis. 2018;71:A7. https://doi.org/10.1053/j.ajkd.2018.01.002.
13. Wang V, Vilme H, Maciejewski ML, Boulware LE. The economic burden of chronic kidney disease and end-stage renal disease. Semin Nephrol. Elsevier. 2016;36:319–30.
14. Division N. HHS launches President Trump's 'Advancing American Kidney Health' initiative. In: HHS.gov. https://www.hhs.gov/about/news/2019/07/10/hhs-launches-president-trump-advancing-american-kidney-health-initiative.html. 2019. Accessed 30 Nov 2019.
15. Incidence, prevalence, patient characteristics, and treatment modalities. Am J Kidney Dis. 2012;59:e183–94. https://doi.org/10.1053/j.ajkd.2011.10.027.
16. El Nahas AM, Bello AK. Chronic kidney disease: the global challenge. Lancet. 2005;365:331–40.
17. Hsu C, Vittinghoff E, Lin F, Shlipak MG. The incidence of end-stage renal disease is increasing faster than the prevalence of chronic renal insufficiency. Ann Intern Med. 2004;141:95. https://doi.org/10.7326/0003-4819-141-2-200407200-00007.
18. Coresh J, Selvin E, Stevens L, et al. Prevalence of chronic kidney disease in the United States. JAMA. 2007;298:2038–47.
19. Grams ME, Juraschek SP, Selvin E, et al. Trends in the prevalence of reduced GFR in the United States: a comparison of Creatinine- and Cystatin C–based estimates. Am J Kidney Dis. 2013;62:253–60. https://doi.org/10.1053/j.ajkd.2013.03.013.
20. Murphy D, McCulloch CE, Lin F, et al. Trends in prevalence of chronic kidney disease in the United States. Ann Intern Med. 2016;165:473. https://doi.org/10.7326/M16-0273.
21. Xie Y, Bowe B, Mokdad AH, et al. Analysis of the Global Burden of Disease study highlights the global, regional, and national trends of chronic kidney disease epidemiology from 1990 to 2016. Kidney Int. 2018;94:567–81.
22. Hsiao L-L. Raising awareness, screening and prevention of chronic kidney disease: it takes more than a village. Nephrology. 2018;23:107–11. https://doi.org/10.1111/nep.13459.
23. Kilpatrick ES, Bloomgarden ZT, Zimmet PZ. International Expert Committee report on the role of the A1C assay in the diagnosis of diabetes: response to the International Expert Committee. Diabetes Care. 2009;32:e159.
24. Organization WH. Use of glycated haemoglobin (HbA1c) in diagnosis of diabetes mellitus: abbreviated report of a WHO consultation. Geneva: World Health Organization; 2011.
25. Menke A, Casagrande S, Geiss L, Cowie CC. Prevalence of and trends in diabetes among adults in the United States, 1988–2012. JAMA. 2015;314:1021–9.

26. Wild S, Roglic G, Green A, et al. Global prevalence of diabetes: estimates for the year 2000 and projections for 2030. Diabetes Care. 2004;27:1047–53.
27. Guariguata L, Whiting DR, Hambleton I, et al. Global estimates of diabetes prevalence for 2013 and projections for 2035. Diabetes Res Clin Pract. 2014;103:137–49.
28. James PA, Oparil S, Carter BL, et al. 2014 Evidence-based guideline for the management of high blood pressure in adults: report from the panel members appointed to the Eighth Joint National Committee (JNC 8). JAMA. 2014;311:507. https://doi.org/10.1001/jama.2013.284427.
29. Guo F, He D, Zhang W, Walton RG. Trends in prevalence, awareness, management, and control of hypertension among United States adults, 1999 to 2010. J Am Coll Cardiol. 2012;60:599–606.
30. The SPRINT Research Group. A randomized trial of intensive versus standard blood-pressure control. N Engl J Med. 2015;373:2103–16. https://doi.org/10.1056/NEJMoa1511939.
31. Lloyd-Jones DM, Morris PB, Ballantyne CM, et al. 2017 focused update of the 2016 ACC expert consensus decision pathway on the role of non-statin therapies for LDL-cholesterol lowering in the management of atherosclerotic cardiovascular disease risk. J Am Coll Cardiol. 2017;70:1785–822. https://doi.org/10.1016/j.jacc.2017.07.745.
32. Muntner P, Carey RM, Gidding S, et al. Potential US population impact of the 2017 ACC/AHA high blood pressure guideline. J Am Coll Cardiol. 2018;71:109–18.
33. Zhang Y, Moran AE. Trends in the prevalence, awareness, treatment, and control of hypertension among young adults in the United States, 1999 to 2014. Hypertension. 2017;70:736–42. https://doi.org/10.1161/HYPERTENSIONAHA.117.09801.
34. Rhee CM, Ahmadi S-F, Kalantar-Zadeh K. The dual roles of obesity in chronic kidney disease: a review of the current literature. Curr Opin Nephrol Hypertens. 2016;25:208–16. https://doi.org/10.1097/MNH.0000000000000212.
35. Gelber RP, Kurth T, Kausz AT, et al. Association between body mass index and CKD in apparently healthy men. Am J Kidney Dis. 2005;46:871–80. https://doi.org/10.1053/j.ajkd.2005.08.015.
36. Wang Y, Chen X, Song Y, et al. Association between obesity and kidney disease: a systematic review and meta-analysis. Kidney Int. 2008;73:19–33. https://doi.org/10.1038/sj.ki.5002586.
37. Hales CM, Fryar CD, Carroll MD, et al. Trends in obesity and severe obesity prevalence in US youth and adults by sex and age, 2007–2008 to 2015–2016. JAMA. 2018;319:1723. https://doi.org/10.1001/jama.2018.3060.
38. Gregg EW, Shaw JE. Global health effects of overweight and obesity. N Engl J Med. 2017;377:80–1. https://doi.org/10.1056/NEJMe1706095.
39. Kazmi WH, Obrador GT, Khan SS, et al. Late nephrology referral and mortality among patients with end-stage renal disease: a propensity score analysis. Nephrol Dial Transplant. 2004;19:1808–14.
40. Ene-Iordache B, Perico N, Bikbov B, et al. Chronic kidney disease and cardiovascular risk in six regions of the world (ISN-KDDC): a cross-sectional study. Lancet Glob Health. 2016;4:e307–19.
41. Coresh J, Byrd-Holt D, Astor BC, et al. Chronic kidney disease awareness, prevalence, and trends among US adults, 1999 to 2000. J Am Soc Nephrol. 2005;16:180–8.
42. Plantinga LC, Boulware LE, Coresh J, et al. Patient awareness of chronic kidney disease: trends and predictors. Arch Intern Med. 2008;168:2268–75.
43. Kinchen KS, Sadler J, Fink N, et al. The timing of specialist evaluation in chronic kidney disease and mortality. Ann Intern Med. 2002;137:479. https://doi.org/10.7326/0003-4819-137-6-200209170-00007.
44. Minutolo R, De Nicola L, Mazzaglia G, et al. Detection and awareness of moderate to advanced CKD by primary care practitioners: a cross-sectional study from Italy. Am J Kidney Dis. 2008;52:444–53.
45. Ravera M, Noberasco G, Weiss U, et al. CKD awareness and blood pressure control in the primary care hypertensive population. Am J Kidney Dis. 2011;57:71–7.

46. Parameswaran S, Geda SB, Rathi M, et al. Referral pattern of patients with end-stage renal disease at a public sector hospital and its impact on outcome. Natl Med J India. 2011;24:7.
47. National Kidney Disease Education Program, National Institutes of Health. Improving the understanding, detection and management of kidney disease. [Cited 2 Apr 2012]. Available from URL: http://www.nkdep.hih.gov/ – Google Search. https://www.google.com/search?q=National+Kidney+Disease+Education+Program%2C+National+Institutes+of+Health.+Improving+the+Understanding%2C+Detection+and+Management+of+Kidney+Disease.+%5BCited+2+Apr+2012.%5D+Available+from+URL%3A+http%3A%2F%2F+www.nkdep.hih.gov%2F&rlz=1C1GGRV_enUS748US749&oq=National+Kidney+Disease+Education+Program%2C+National+Institutes+of+Health.+Improving+the+Understanding%2C+Detection+and+Management+of+Kidney+Disease.+%5BCited+2+Apr+2012.%5D+Available+from+URL%3A+http%3A%2F%2F+www.nkdep.hih.gov%2F&aqs=chrome..69i57.507j0j8&sourceid=chrome&ie=UTF-8. Accessed 9 Jan 2020.
48. Saab G, Whaley-Connell AT, McCullough PA, Bakris GL. CKD awareness in the United States: the Kidney Early Evaluation Program (KEEP). Am J Kidney Dis. 2008;52:382–3. https://doi.org/10.1053/j.ajkd.2008.05.026.
49. Powe NR, Boulware LE. Population-based screening for CKD. Am J Kidney Dis. 2009;53:S64–70. https://doi.org/10.1053/j.ajkd.2008.07.050.
50. Levey AS, Atkins R, Coresh J, et al. Chronic kidney disease as a global public health problem: approaches and initiatives – a position statement from Kidney Disease Improving Global Outcomes. Kidney Int. 2007;72:247–59. https://doi.org/10.1038/sj.ki.5002343.
51. Palmer AJ, Valentine WJ, Chen R, et al. A health economic analysis of screening and optimal treatment of nephropathy in patients with type 2 diabetes and hypertension in the USA. Nephrol Dial Transplant. 2008;23:1216–23.
52. Herman WH, Shahinfar S, Carides GW, et al. Losartan reduces the costs associated with diabetic end-stage renal disease: the RENAAL study economic evaluation. Diabetes Care. 2003;26:683–7.
53. Baigent C, Landray MJ, Reith C, et al. The effects of lowering LDL cholesterol with simvastatin plus ezetimibe in patients with chronic kidney disease (Study of Heart and Renal Protection): a randomised placebo-controlled trial. Lancet. 2011;377:2181–92.
54. Madias NE. Metabolic acidosis and CKD progression. Clin J Am Soc Nephrol. 2020. https://doi.org/10.2215/CJN.07990520.
55. Cueto-Manzano AM, Martinez-Ramirez HR, Cortés-Sanabria L. Management of chronic kidney disease: primary health-care setting, self-care and multidisciplinary approach. Clin Nephrol. 2010;74:S99–104.
56. Blickem C, Blakeman T, Kennedy A, et al. The clinical and cost-effectiveness of the BRinging Information and Guided Help Together (BRIGHT) intervention for the self-management support of people with stage 3 chronic kidney disease in primary care: study protocol for a randomized controlled trial. Trials. 2013;14:28.
57. Brenner BM, Cooper ME, de Zeeuw D, et al. Effects of losartan on renal and cardiovascular outcomes in patients with type 2 diabetes and nephropathy. N Engl J Med. 2001;345(12):861–9.
58. Perkovic V, Jardine MJ, Neal B, et al. Canagliflozin and renal outcomes in type 2 diabetes and nephropathy. N Engl J Med. 2019;380:2295–306. https://doi.org/10.1056/NEJMoa1811744.
59. American Diabetes Association. 11. Microvascular complications and foot care: *standards of medical care in diabetes—2019*. Diabetes Care. 2019;42:S124–38. https://doi.org/10.2337/dc19-S011.
60. Chronic Kidney Disease | Healthy People 2020. https://www.healthypeople.gov/2020/topics-objectives/topic/chronic-kidney-disease/objectives. Accessed 30 Nov 2019.

Chapter 3
Screening Tests for CKD Detection

Maitreyee M. Gupta and William Dennis Coffey

Introduction

Chronic kidney disease (CKD) is defined as abnormalities of kidney structure or function, present for >3 months, with implications on health [1]. This specifically includes either a decline in GFR < 60 ml/min/1.73 m^2 or the presence of one or more markers of kidney damage (albuminuria >30 mg/g, urine sediment abnormalities, electrolyte, and other abnormalities due to tubular disorders, structural abnormalities detected by imaging, those detected by histology, and history of kidney transplantation) present for >3 months. This chapter presents a discussion on screening tests for CKD detection, their utility, and interpretation in CKD. The most important test in our armory to detect and assess kidney disease is, first and foremost, a simple urinalysis. Next is glomerular filtration rate (GFR), which not only defines CKD but also allows us to stage the severity. Beyond GFR, proteinuria and hematuria are very important in assessing CKD, and this is touched upon next in this chapter. Subsequent discussion is on radiological studies, another useful tool to evaluate kidney disease. Lastly, we conclude with kidney biopsy, which remains the gold standard for diagnosing the etiology of CKD. The goal of using screening tests is to identify, evaluate CKD early, address the cause, and retard the progression of kidney disease.

M. M. Gupta (✉)
Department of Medicine, Division of Nephrology, Thomas Jefferson University, Philadelphia, PA, USA
e-mail: Maitreyee.gupta@jefferson.edu

W. D. Coffey
Department of Radiology, Thomas Jefferson University, Philadelphia, PA, USA

© Springer Nature Switzerland AG 2022
J. McCauley et al. (eds.), *Approaches to Chronic Kidney Disease*,
https://doi.org/10.1007/978-3-030-83082-3_3

Urinalysis

Urinalysis is a basic diagnostic test to evaluate kidney function and urinary tract disease. It is easy to perform in an ambulatory and hospital setting. A complete urinalysis should be performed in a patient with a reduction in glomerular filtration rate or suspected kidney disease on the basis of clinical findings (new onset edema, hematuria) or when other diseases are associated with the kidney function (systemic lupus erythematosus, small vessel vasculitis, and diabetes mellitus).

A complete urinalysis consists of three components: gross evaluation, dipstick analysis, and microscopic examination of urinary sediment which are discussed in the ensuing sections [2].

Urine Specimen Collection

The patient must be asked to clean the external genitalia and midstream specimen collected after the first portion is discarded [3]. Strenuous physical exercise must be avoided in the preceding 72 hours to avoid exercise-induced proteinuria and hematuria. In women, urinalysis is best avoided during menstruation to avoid contamination. Urine can also be obtained from an indwelling catheter, using a freshly produced sample. Note that the catheter may cause hematuria.

The specimen should be examined at room temperature within 2 hours of retrieval. Refrigeration of specimen at +2 to +8°C assists preservation for later analysis.

Gross Examination

1. Turbidity – Turbid urine is seen in infection, or precipitated crystals, or chyluria.
2. Color – The color of urine is lighter when urine is dilute and darker when concentrated. The conditions that can cause color changes of the urine are hematuria, hemoglobinuria, or myoglobinuria (pink, red, brown urine); jaundice (dark yellow, brown urine); drugs like rifampin and phenytoin (orange-red urine); methylene blue (blue urine); chyluria and phosphate crystals (white urine); alkaptonuria, ochronosis, myoglobinuria, and hemoglobinuria (black urine); and bacteriuria in patients with urinary catheters (purple urine).
3. Red-Brown Color Urine – To differentiate between the variety of conditions that cause this, the first step is centrifugation of urine to see if the red color is urine sediment (has hematuria) or the supernatant (has hemoglobinuria, myoglobinuria, or other causes like certain drugs).
4. Hemoglobinuria and myoglobinuria:

   - Hemoglobinuria is the presence of free hemoglobin in urine. This happens in conditions which release hemoglobin from inside of intact red blood cells, such as intravascular hemolysis, acute transfusion reaction, and severe malaria treated with medication, also associated with reduced haptoglobin levels in serum. It gives red-brown "cola color" urine.

- Myoglobin, nonprotein bound, is rapidly filtered and excreted and occurs when there is skeletal muscle breakdown (rhabdomyolysis), also associated with creatinine kinase elevation in serum.

Urine Dipstick

This provides a rapid semiquantitative assessment of urinary characteristics on test pads embedded on a reagent strip. The following urine parameters can be detected: pH, heme, leukocyte esterase, nitrite, albumin, specific gravity, and glucose:

1. Heme – It is detected by its pseudoperoxidase activity, which causes the reaction of peroxide and chromogen to produce a color change. A positive test does not establish the presence of red blood cells, and confirmation with microscopy is required. A positive test, in the absence of red cells, is from free hemoglobin or myoglobin in urine and a high concentration of bacteria with pseudoperoxidase activity. False-negative results are mainly due to ascorbic acid in excess vitamin C ingestion.
2. Protein – Physiologic proteinuria does not exceed 150 mg/24 hours in adults. Three approaches can be used to evaluate proteinuria:

   - Urine dipstick: The changes in dipstick color rely on property that protein in buffer changes pH proportional to its concentration. It is most sensitive for albumin but important limitations to know are that it does not detect moderate albuminuria (formerly called "microalbuminuria") of 30–300 mg/day range and that the semiquantitative categories of albuminuria reported (trace, 1+, 2+, 3+) are not necessarily accurate.
   - 24-hour protein excretion: Remains gold standard. It also measures total protein, rather than albumin alone, and hence can detect light chains in myeloma.
   - Protein-creatinine ratio: It is a practical alternative to a 24-hour protein excretion. There is a correlation between the protein-creatinine ratio in a random urine sample and 24-hour protein excretion. It is not influenced by water intake variation and has become part of chronic kidney disease staging and prognostication [4].
   - Detection of non-albumin protein: Specifically, immunoglobulin light chains can be screened by sulfosalicylic acid. A quantitative analysis of urine protein can be performed by electrophoresis on cellulose acetate or agarose gel.

3. Leukocyte esterase – This is released by macrophages and is a marker for the presence of white blood cells. False-negative results can happen from high glucosuria or proteinuria.
4. Nitrites – This detects bacteria that reduce nitrates to nitrites, such as most gram negatives in urine (*Enterobacteriaceae*). Those that do not reduce nitrates

(*Pseudomonas, Enterococcus*) often are implicated in complicated urinary tract infection. The sensitivity of the test is low, especially when urine dwell time in the bladder is short.

5. pH – Urine pH ranges from 4.5 to 8, depending upon systemic acid-base balance.
6. Glucose – Glucose catalyzes peroxidase, leading to chromogen oxidation. False-negative can occur with ascorbic acid and infection. The foremost and obvious cause of glucosuria is uncontrolled diabetes mellitus. Glucosuria, with normal plasma glucose, occurs in patients with proximal renal tubular defect, which is also accompanied with phosphaturia, uricosuria, and renal tubular acidosis. Glucosuria is also seen in those receiving sodium-glucose cotransporter 2 inhibitors.

Urine Sediment

The microscopic examination of urine sediment is an essential part of urinalysis and allows evaluation of etiology and disease activity in CKD through the study of cells, casts, and crystals shed in the urine. Red cell casts are pathognomonic of glomerulonephritis. White cells and white cell casts are seen in pyelonephritis, interstitial nephritis, and other tubulointerstitial disorders. Broad casts or waxy casts form in tubules that have become dilated and atrophic due to chronic parenchymal disease.

The method to spin the urine is simple and can be performed in an ambulatory office. A 10 ml of urine is centrifuged at 3000 rpm for 5 minutes. After discarding supernatant, the pellet is resuspended with gentle shaking, and a drop is pipetted on the glass slide and covered with a coverslip and evaluated under low (X100) and high (X400) power of the microscope.

Varying patterns of urine sediment findings bear emphasis in delineating the etiology of CKD. These are discussed below [5, 6].

1. Nephritic and Nephrotic Sediment: Nephritic syndrome is defined by active urine sediment, proteinuria, hypertension, and decreased glomerular filtration rate. Urine sediment is characterized by a large number of red blood cells (RBC) and RBC casts:

   - Red blood cells and RBC casts: Isomorphic RBCs (appear similar to RBC on blood smear) are not specific for glomerular cause. They can be seen with any extraglomerular causes also such as nephrolithiasis, urinary tract infections, excessive anticoagulation, and urologic malignancies. Dysmorphic RBCs are more specific for glomerular injury, being formed likely as they pass through gaps in the injured glomerular basement membrane (Fig. 3.1a).

   Nephrotic syndrome is characterized by edema, hypoalbuminemia, high-grade proteinuria (protein excretion >3.5 g), and hypercholesterolemia. The urine sediment, in general, is bland (acellular). Urine sediment may have findings of lipiduria and lipid casts.

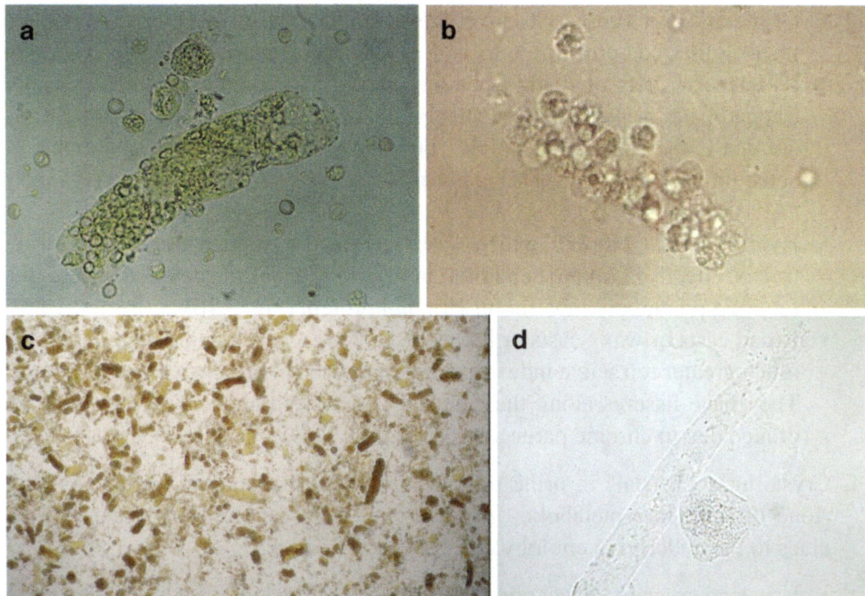

Fig. 3.1 (**a**) RBC cast – Red cell casts is composed of a matrix containing red blood cells in various stages of degeneration and characteristics. (**b**) WBC casts – White cell casts with polymorphonuclear leukocytes identifiable by their lobulated nucleus. (**c**) Granular casts – Muddy brown, fine, or coarse granular casts. (**d**) Hyaline cast – Hyaline casts appear pale and slightly refractile in the urine and are common findings in the urine

2. Interstitial Nephritis: Often the clue is elevated creatinine and abnormalities in urine. Urinalysis may show positive leukocyte esterase with negative urine culture result, low-grade proteinuria:

   - White blood cells and WBC casts: Urine sediment may show white blood cells (WBC) and WBC casts. WBC are larger than red cells, are smaller than RTECs, and have a multilobed structure. WBC casts are also seen in pyelonephritis (Fig. 3.1b).

3. Acute Kidney Injury: A series of acute kidney injury episodes will result in chronic scarring in the kidney and CKD.

   Along with the rise in creatinine, acutely or chronically, the urine sediment will have variable numbers of renal tubular epithelial cells, hyaline casts (in prerenal injury), and granular casts in (acute tubular necrosis, ischemic injury). Massive crystalluria can also be seen in acute kidney injury due to intratubular obstruction (acute uric acid nephropathy, ethylene glycol poisoning, drugs):

   - Renal tubular epithelial cells: These cells are exfoliated tubular epithelium from various nephron segments and are large (twice the size of red blood cell), with round or polygonal shapes.

- Granular casts: These casts are composed of degraded cell lysosomes trapped in ultra-filtered serum protein and glycoprotein matrix, called uromodulin secreted by cells of thick ascending Henle's loop (fine granular casts) or trapped cells in the matrix (coarse granular casts). When the granular casts are dense, they are called "muddy brown casts." They are pathognomonic of acute tubular necrosis (ATN) in hospitalized patients with acute kidney injury (AKI) (Fig. 3.1c).
- Hyaline casts: Colorless, with low refractive index, seen in prerenal AKI from true or effective volume depletion, in which urine is concentrated and acidic, favoring precipitation of Tamm-Horsfall protein (Fig. 3.1d).
- Broad casts or waxy casts or broad casts are made of hyaline material with a much greater refractive index than hyaline casts, hence the waxy appearance. They have fissures along the edges. They form in atrophic tubules that are dilated due to chronic parenchymal disease.

4. Crystalluria: Crystals in urine provide important information in patients with stone disease, rare metabolic disorders, and drug nephrotoxicity and provide clues to the underlying etiology of CKD (Fig. 3.2a–c):

- Uric acid crystals – They precipitate in acidic urine pH < 5.8 and have a wide range of the appearance including rhomboids.
- Calcium oxalate – Not dependent on urine pH and may appear in monohydrate form with "dumbbell" shape or dihydrate form as envelope shape.
- Calcium phosphate – Form in relatively alkaline urine, pH > 7.0, and have a coffin-like structure.

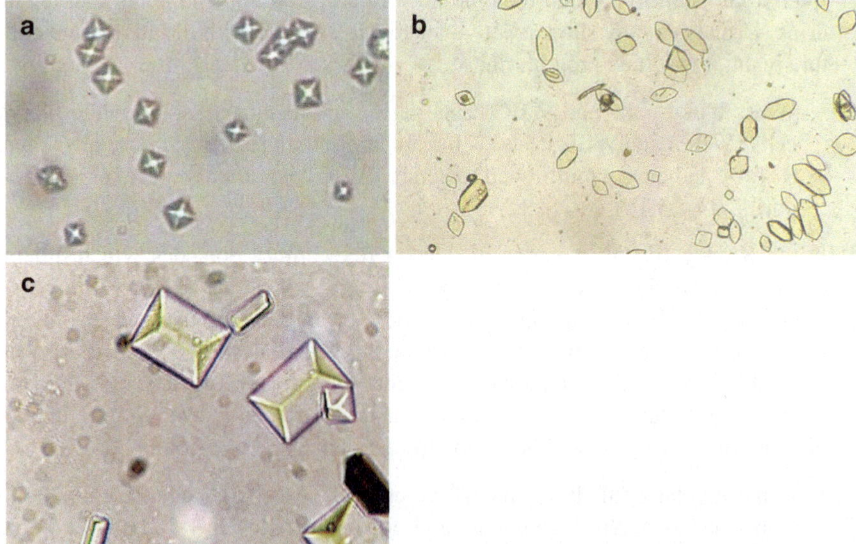

Fig. 3.2 (a) Calcium oxalate crystals. (b) Uric acid crystals. (c) Triple phosphate crystals

- Cystine crystals – Have a hexagonal shape, diagnostic of cystinuria.
- Triple phosphate crystals – Composed of magnesium ammonium phosphate and are found in alkaline urine. They occur in urine infected with urease-producing microorganisms such as ureaplasma urealyticum.
- Crystal due to drugs – Low urinary pH, volume depletion, precipitate drug crystallization. Examples include sulfonamides, ciprofloxacin, acyclovir, methotrexate, atazanavir, intravenous vitamin C (calcium oxalate), ethylene glycol, and intoxication (calcium oxalate crystals).

Glomerular Filtration Rate and Its Assessment

When kidney disease is discovered, the most important initial information regarding the presence and degree of kidney dysfunction is achieved by estimation of glomerular filtration rate (GFR).

The GFR is the product of average filtration rate of each single nephron and the number of nephrons in both kidneys. The normal value of GFR is approximately 130 ml/min per 1.73 m^2 for men and women respectively, with considerable variation based on age, sex, and body size [7].

Assessment of GFR

Measurement of GFR is complex and time-consuming in everyday clinical practice, and hence GFR is estimated from serum markers, using estimation equations.

Measurement of GFR

GFR cannot be measured directly. Instead, it is measured as the urinary clearance of an ideal filtration marker [2].

Clearance of a substance, C_x, is defined as the volume of plasma cleared of a marker by excretion per unit of time:

$$C_x = \left(U_x \times V \right) / P_x$$

where P_x is the filtered load, U_x is the urinary concentration of x, and V is the urine flow rate.

An ideal filtration marker is one which is freely filtered at the glomerulus, neither secreted nor reabsorbed in the tubules, and not changed during its excretion by the kidney. Thus, filtered load (GFR $\times P_x$) is the same as the rate of urinary excretion ($U_x \times V$):

$$GFR \times P_x = \left(U_x \times V \right)$$

By substitution in the first equation:

$$GFR = C_x$$

Plasma clearance is an alternative to urinary clearance for GFR measurement, and it avoids the need for timed urine collections. It is performed by timed plasma measurements after administering a bolus of IV injection of an exogenous filtration marker; the clearance equation is:

$$C_x = A_x \, / \, P_x$$

where A_x is the amount of marker administered and P_x is the plasma concentration computed area under the curve of plasma concentration disappearance vs time.

The ideal filtration marker is freely filtered at the glomerulus and neither secreted, reabsorbed, or synthesized or metabolized in the body. Thus, the amount filtered by glomerulus is the amount excreted in urine. The gold standard for exogenous filtration marker is inulin but is expensive and more cumbersome. Alternative filtration markers (such as radioactive or nonradioactive iothalamate, DTPA, or EDTA) are used for research studies or where an accurate assessment of GFR is needed, such as dosing toxic medications with a narrow therapeutic index and prior to kidney donation [8, 9].

Estimation of GFR

The most common methods to estimate GFR in clinical practice use endogenous filtration marker, serum creatinine.

These include measurement of creatinine clearance and estimation equations based upon serum creatinine such as the Cockcroft-Gault equation, the Modification of Diet in Renal Disease (MDRD) study equation, and the Chronic Kidney Disease Epidemiology Collaboration (CKD-EPI) equation.

Endogenous filtration markers can only be used to estimate GFR with stable kidney function. As with rapidly changing kidney function, there has not been enough time for accumulation of the endogenous marker, say creatinine, to reflect the degree of kidney disease severity.

Creatinine as a Marker to Estimate GFR

Creatinine is derived from muscle catabolism and dietary meat intake. Creatinine generation is proportional to muscle mass, which can be estimated from age, gender, race, and body size. Creatinine is freely filtered, and not reabsorbed, and therefore is used as a marker of kidney function. It is secreted in the proximal tubules, and 10–40% of urinary creatinine is derived from this.

Advantages of using creatinine as a marker for GFR estimation include its ease of measurement, widespread availability of assays, and low cost. Disadvantages include the large number of non-GFR determinants (Table 3.1) leading to a wide range of GFR for a given plasma creatinine level.

Serum creatinine values are lower in women and higher in the black race, reflecting lesser and greater, respectively, muscle mass and creatinine.

In addition, creatinine is contained in intestinal secretions and degraded by bacteria. If GFR is reduced, the amount of creatinine eliminated through the extrarenal route is increased. Hence, antibiotics can raise serum creatinine by reducing gut flora.

Clinically, it is difficult to distinguish the cause of the rise in serum creatinine concentration due to inhibition of creatinine secretion or extrarenal elimination, but processes other than a decline in GFR should be suspected if serum urea concentration remains unchanged despite a significant change in serum creatinine concentration in a patient with an initially reduced estimated GFR (eGFR).

Creatinine Clearance

Creatinine clearance is calculated from the creatinine excretion in a 24-hour urine collection and a single measurement of serum creatinine in the steady state. The following is an example:

In a 60-kg lady, the following results are obtained: SCr = 1.3 mg/dL; UCr = 100 mg/dL

$$V = 1.5\,L\,/\,day$$

$$\text{Thus, CrCl} = \left[100 \times 1.3\right] / 1.5 = 87\,L\,/\,day.$$

Table 3.1 Factors affecting serum creatinine concentration

	Condition/mechanism	Effect on serum creatinine
Factors affecting creatinine production	Dietary intake (vegan)	Decrease
	Reduction in Muscle mass (amputation, malnutrition, muscle wasting)	Decrease
Factors affecting tubular creatinine secretion	Nephrotic syndrome, sickle cell disease (increased tubular creatinine secretion)	Decrease
	Drugs such as trimethoprim, cimetidine, fenofibrated (increased tubular creatinine secretion)	Increase
Interference with alkaline picrate creatinine assay	Keto acids and cephalosporins	Increase

To convert to mL/min, the value is multiplied by 1000 convert to mL and then divided by 1440 (number of minutes in a day).

$$CrCl = [87 \times 1000] / 1440 = 60 \, mL / min$$

Inaccurate collection is a major limitation to using this method. In a complete collection, excretion of creatinine should be approximately 20–25 ml/kg per day and 15–20 ml/kg per day in healthy young men and women, respectively.

Creatinine clearance overestimates GFR because of tubular secretion. At low values of GFR, the amount of creatinine excreted by tubular secretion may exceed the amount filtered [10].

Equations for Estimating GFR from Serum Creatinine

GFR can be estimated from serum creatinine by equations that use age, sex, race, and body size as surrogates for creatinine generation. They are reasonably accurate to follow GFR changes over time. They are not accurate in setting where kidney function is changing rapidly [10].

Cockcroft-Gault Formula

It estimates creatinine clearance from serum creatinine, age, sex, and body weight.

$$CrCl\,(ml/min) = \left[(140 - Age) \times Lean\ body\ weight\,(kg) / Cr\,(mg/dL) \right]$$
$$/[Cr\,(mg/dL) \times 72$$

The formula accounts for age-related decreased creatinine production and higher creatinine with greater weight, although in the current era of obesity, a higher weight may not mean greater muscle mass. The equation is not adjusted for body surface area, and it was developed prior to the use of standardized creatinine assays.

MDRD Study Equation

This was developed in 1999. It uses standardized SCr, age, sex, and race to estimate GFR for BSA (ml/min/ 1.73 m^2). The revised four-variable equation has been re-expressed for use with standardized serum creatinine values (SCr).

$$GFR\,(ml/min/1.73m^2) = 175 \times SCr^{-1.154} \times age^{-0.203} \times 0.742\,(if\ female)$$
$$\times 1.210\,(if\ black)$$

It is reasonably accurate in nonhospitalized patients, with CKD, regardless of diagnosis. It is imprecise at higher GFR, and hence the eGFR >60 ml/min/1.73 m^2 computed using the MDRD study equation is not reported as a numeric value [11, 12].

CKD-EPI Equation

The CKD-EPI equation was developed in 2009 and uses the same four variables as the MDRD study equation. It was developed to provide a more accurate estimate of GFR among these with normal or mildly reduced GFR (i.e., above 60 mL/min per 1.73 m^2) [12, 13]. At this time, large commercial clinical laboratories in the US have changed from using the MDRD study equation to the CKD EPI equation for eGFR reporting. The CKD EPI performs better at higher levels of GFR; and in subgroups defined by sex, race, diabetes, and transplant status, in older adults; and at higher levels of BMI. By contrast, MDRD study equation performs better at lower levels of GFR [14].

In multiple studies, with varied populations, the use of CKD-EPI equations results in a lower prevalence estimate of CKD and more accurate risk prediction for adverse outcomes compared with MDRD equations [15, 16].

The three estimation equations are affected by factors that affect serum creatinine, as they all inherently make use of serum creatinine. Variation in creatinine production and handling in certain patient groups will make these equations less accurate, such as in diabetics, pregnant women, specific race groups (Asians), and those with extremes of body mass or habitus.

Alternative confirmatory tests such as a 24-hour urine sample for creatinine clearance, estimated GFR from cystatin C or creatinine-cystatin estimating equation, and measurement of an exogenous filtration marker will allow accurate assessment of GFR than from creatinine alone.

Urea as a Marker for GFR

The blood urea nitrogen (BUN) has a limited value as an estimate of GFR, as a large number of widely variable non-GFR determinants affect it, mainly urea generation and tubular reabsorption.

Urea is the end product of protein catabolism in the liver. The rate of urea generation increases with a high-protein diet (hyperalimentation), corticosteroid administration, and absorption of blood after gastrointestinal hemorrhage. Catabolic states like chemotherapy, severe malnutrition, and liver disease decrease urea generation.

Thus, liver disease may be associated with a near-normal BUN (due to decreased urea production) and serum creatinine (due to muscle wasting) despite a relatively large reduction in GFR [17].

Urea is freely filtered in the glomerulus, and 40–50% is passively reabsorbed, mostly in the proximal tubule. Volume depletion leads to enhanced proximal sodium and urea reabsorption, resulting in a rise in BUN disproportionately with change in GFR and serum creatinine. This elevation in BUN/serum creatinine ratio is indicative of decreased renal perfusion, as the cause of renal insufficiency.

Urea clearance measurement is useful in advanced kidney disease patients. Owing to tubular reabsorption, the urinary clearance of urea underestimates the GFR and creatinine clearance overestimates the GFR (tubular secretion); one method to estimate the GFR in patients with advanced kidney disease is to average both the clearances.

$$\text{Estimated GFR} = \left(\text{Clearance of Creatinine} + \text{Clearance of Urea}\right)/2$$

Serum Cystatin C

Recently, there has been considerable interest in using cystatin C as an alternative or complementary marker to creatinine for estimation of GFR and maybe particularly advantageous in patients with higher GFR levels. Cystatin C is a 122 amino acid protein that is a member of the cysteine protease inhibitors. It is produced at a constant rate by a gene expressed in all nucleated cells. It is freely filtered at the glomerulus and not reabsorbed. It is metabolized in the tubules and hence cannot be used directly to measure clearance. Its rate of production has been thought to be relatively constant, and not affected by changes in diet. Although cystatin C was believed to be unaffected by gender, age, and muscle mass, higher cystatin C levels have now been associated with males, greater height and weight, lean body mass, fat mass, diabetes, markers of inflammation, and rising age [18]. Substantial variation in cystatin C assay has been observed, even with the same test. International standardization is in process. The assays are more expensive than serum creatinine determination.

The combination of serum creatinine and cystatin C in a single equation has been shown to consistently provide more accurate eGFR than equations using ether marker alone [19, 20].

GFR estimated based upon cystatin C is recommended as a confirmatory test. The prognostic advantage of cystatin C is most apparent in individuals with GFR >45 ml/min/m^2. It can be used as a confirmation of the diagnosis of CKD in a patient with estimated GFR 45–60 ml/min/m^{2}and no other evidence of kidney disease, such as albuminuria or radiographic abnormalities [1].

GFR Assessment in Circumstances Requiring High Degree of Accuracy

Kidney Donor Evaluation

Requires a clearance measurement, such as 24-hour urine for creatinine clearance or urinary/plasma clearance of an exogenous filtration marker.

Drug Dosing

Historically Cockcroft-Gault equation was used to develop drug dosing guidelines. Studies have shown greater concordance between the MDRD study equation and measured GFR than the Cockcroft-Gault equation and measure GFR [21]. Thus, for most patients MDRD and CKD-EPI equations can be used for drug dosing decisions. In patients with changes in creatinine production or secretion such as extremes of muscle mass and unusual diet, limiting the accuracy of creatinine-based estimation equations, dosing decisions can be made by using cystatin- or creatinine-cystatin C-based equations, measured creatinine clearance, or measured GFR using exogenous filtration markers, especially for drugs with narrow therapeutic window [22].

Assessing Kidney Function Beyond eGFR

The assessment of renal function by estimation of the glomerular filtration rate (GFR) and urinalysis was discussed in the previous section. Beyond GFR, the evaluation of patients also includes history and physical examination and serologic evaluation for systemic diseases which are implicated in CKD. Proteinuria and hematuria are the key parameters in the clinical assessment of CKD, hence discussed in greater depth next. Radiologic imaging of the kidneys and kidney biopsy for tissue diagnosis are discussed subsequently.

Disease Duration

The assessment of disease duration is best performed by comparing current urinalysis and creatinine with previous trends. Imaging showing small-sized kidneys is a characteristic finding of chronicity. Increased renal parenchymal echogenicity on ultrasound suggests nonspecific renal disease. Increased echogenicity, combined with small-sized kidney, supports the diagnosis of CKD.

Anemia due to erythropoietin deficiency, hyperphosphatemia, and hypoalbuminemia are common findings in advanced CKD, but are not specific.

Major Causes and Classification of Kidney Disease

Has been categorized as prerenal (decreased renal perfusion), intrinsic renal (glomerular/tubular or interstitial pathology), or post renal (obstructive) based on the cause and location of kidney damage [1].

A. Prerenal disease: Occurs in ongoing heart failure and cirrhosis, with persistently decreased renal perfusion.
B. Postrenal (obstructive) disease: Chronic obstruction due to any etiology (prostatic, abdominal/pelvic tumor compressing ureters, retroperitoneal fibrosis), if untreated, leads to irreversible retroperitoneal fibrosis.
C. Intrinsic renal disease: Vascular disease such as nephrosclerosis damaging blood vessels. Intrinsic glomerular disease can present with a nephritic or nephrotic pattern. A nephritic pattern is suggested by microscopic hematuria abnormal urine microscopy with red cell casts and dysmorphic red cells. A nephrotic pattern is associated with proteinuria (>3.5 g) and an inactive urine microscopy with few cells and casts. Proteinuria and hematuria are discussed here further.

Proteinuria

Proteinuria is one of the most important parameters in the clinical evaluation of chronic kidney disease for several reasons. Firstly, it may be the only sign of early kidney disease, even when the GFR is normal, and serum creatinine has not risen; a classic example of this is diabetic nephropathy. Persistent proteinuria is diagnostic of CKD regardless of GFR. Secondly, proteinuria is also the single most important risk factor for future loss of kidney function and progression of CKD. Interventions that reduce proteinuria, such as blood pressure and diabetes control, also retard progression of CKD. Thirdly, proteinuria is an independent and important risk factor for cardiovascular mortality.

Proteinuria may reflect an abnormal loss of plasma proteins due to (A) increased glomerular permeability to large molecular proteins (albuminuria or glomerular proteinuria), (B) incomplete tubular reabsorption of normally filtered proteins (tubular proteinuria), or (C) increase plasma concentration of low molecular weight proteins (overproduction proteinuria, such as immunoglobulin light chains).

Albuminuria

It is a type of plasma protein found in normal subjects and in large quantities in patients with kidney disease. Albuminuria, rather than proteinuria has become more in use clinically, and guidelines classify kidney disease by level of albuminuria. Recent epidemiologic data demonstrate a strong graded relationship of albuminuria with cardiovascular risk [23]. It is the earliest marker of glomerular diseases, prior to fall in GFR, including diabetic glomerulosclerosis. It is often associated with underlying hypertension, obesity, and vascular disease, where underlying renal pathology is not known.

Amounts of albuminuria: Normal rate of albumin excretion is <20 mg/day. Persistent albuminuria is between 30 and 300 mg/day, formerly called "microalbuminuria."

Measurement of Total Urine Protein Excretion

The semiquantitative urine dipstick measurement was discussed earlier in urinalysis. A 24-hour urine collection is the gold standard for quantitative measurement of total protein excretion, with a normal value being <150 mg/day. It is used to make initial treatment decisions. It is cumbersome for patients and often collected incorrectly. Protein/creatinine ratio (UPCR) and albumin/creatinine ratio (UACR) in a spot first morning specimen are used to estimate a 24-hour excretion and to follow treatment effects in CKD patients [1, 24].

Approach to Patient with Proteinuria

Transient proteinuria is diagnosed if a repeat qualitative test no longer shows proteinuria. It can occur with fever and exercise and urinary tract infection, especially in young adults [25]. Orthostatic proteinuria is also a benign condition in adolescents, characterized by increased protein excretion in an upright position but normal excretion when supine. A normal UPCR in the first voided urine specimen, or a normal supine UPCR in 24-hour split urine collection confirms the diagnosis [25].A thorough evaluation is warranted for persistent proteinuria including measurement of creatinine, serum and urine immunofixation, other serological work-up, radiology, and kidney biopsy.Screening for proteinuria is not recommended in individuals with no signs of kidney disease or risk factors such as diabetes, hypertension.Nephrotic range proteinuria (>3.5 g/day) is associated with poorer outcomes in patients with a primary and secondary glomerular disease and treatments to reduce proteinuria are reno-protective. Isolated, non-nephrotic proteinuria may have a more indolent course.

Hematuria

Hematuria may be macroscopic (visible to the naked eye) or microscopic (presence of three or more RBC per high power field in spun urine sediment. Microscopic hematuria is common in glomerular diseases and should be considered if dysmorphic RBC, RBC casts, and proteinuria are associated with it. A thorough history and urine culture to exclude infection should be done. Renal imaging (CT with and without contrast, also called CT urography) helps to exclude polycystic kidney disease, stones, and tumor. If glomerular cause investigation is nondiagnostic, a renal biopsy should be performed. In those >35 years of age with persistent isolated microscopic hematuria, without glomerular etiology, cystoscopy is mandatory to exclude urothelial malignancy.

Macroscopic hematuria is noted with red or brown urine. A positive dipstick for blood and red or brown color in the supernatant suggests myoglobinuria or hemoglobinuria. Other causes of hematuria include Ig A nephropathy (episodic frank hematuria within a day of upper respiratory infection), loin pain groin syndrome, thin membrane disease. Macroscopic hematuria requires urologic evaluation including cystoscopy at any age unless the history is characteristic of glomerular hematuria.

Screening for hematuria with routine urinalysis in patients who have no symptoms suggestive of urinary tract disease is not recommended.

Radiologic Assessment in Renal Disease

Many radiologic studies are used to evaluate patients with renal disease. With the growing range of imaging methods available, the selection of the optimal method to provide accurate diagnosis is sometimes not obvious. The American College of Radiology has published Appropriateness Criteria guidelines that suggest the choice of imaging to provide a rapid answer to a clinical situation while minimizing cost and potential adverse effects to the patient such as radiation exposure and contrast-induced nephropathy [26].

The commonly used imaging studies are listed below and discussed in greater depth in this topic:

1. Ultrasound
2. Computed tomography (CT)
3. Magnetic resonance imaging (MRI)
4. Plain radiography
5. Renal angiography
6. Radionuclide studies
7. Retrograde or antegrade pyelography

Ultrasound

It is the preferred and most common radiologic study in patients presenting with renal disease. It is inexpensive and provides a rapid way to assess kidney size and parenchymal thickness (echogenicity) (Fig. 3.3a). The combination of increased echogenicity and kidney length < 10 cm almost always indicates untreatable disease. This is a very important decision factor in the management of chronic kidney disease in etiologies such as glomerulonephritis [27] (Fig. 3.3b).

Ultrasound image of a normal right kidney in the longitudinal plane. Normal adult kidney size is 9–12 cm in length. Note the normal echogenicity of the renal cortex, which is slightly hypoechoic compared to the adjacent liver (open white arrow). The medullary pyramids are more hypoechoic compared to the cortex in

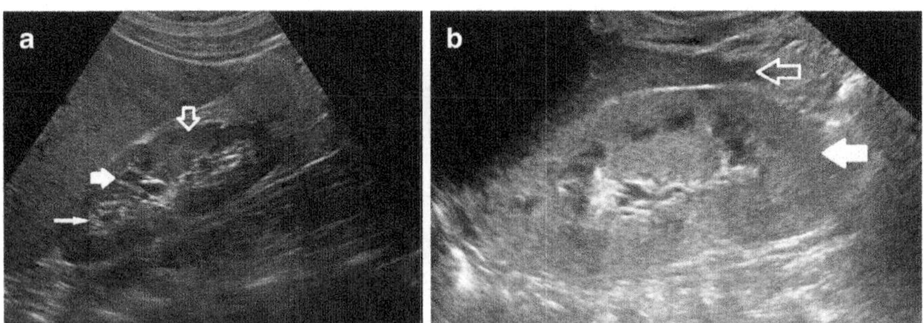

Fig. 3.3 (**a**) Renal ultrasound: normal kidneys. (**b**) Renal ultrasound: echogenic kidneys

adults (thick white arrow). The renal sinus is echogenic due to the presence of fat (thin white arrow).

Ultrasound image of an echogenic right kidney in the longitudinal plane. The renal cortex (solid white arrow) is more echogenic than the adjacent liver (open white arrow), a nonspecific finding but one that can be seen in medical renal disease.

Ultrasound also identifies hydronephrosis, level of urinary tract obstruction, and stones. Sensitivity for visualization of renal calculus depends on the size of the calculus. A unilateral enlarged kidney is often due to obstruction. One has to note that obstruction without dilation can occur in retroperitoneal fibrosis. Also, dilated collecting system can be present without necessarily having functional obstruction. In such a case, a nuclear isotope MAG 3 scan can be used to differentiate between the two.

Ultrasound is able to differentiate solid from simple renal cystic lesions. Further delineating solid and complex cystic lesions may require CT or MRI.

The urinary bladder wall and bladder contents, as well as bilateral urine jets, can be seen well. In individuals with prostatic enlargement chronically, bladder with trabeculated walls and increased post-void residual volume (normal <50 ml) can be demonstrated by ultrasound.

Doppler US is performed to evaluate blood flow in kidney vessels. The resistive index is a parameter used to evaluate vascular compliance and resistance. In adult patients a value >0.7 is considered abnormal. While it is commonly reported on transplanted kidneys, it is an insensitive and nonspecific indicator of rejection [28]. The morphology of doppler waveforms can be indicative of renal artery stenosis. However, be cautioned that renal artery stenosis screening by ultrasound is a technically challenging study and is reliable only in high volume centers when performed by experienced radiologists. A unilateral small, scarred kidney can be seen in chronic renal artery stenosis.

Computed Tomography (CT)

CT examination of kidneys helps evaluate structural causes of CKD such as renal calculi (Fig. 3.4a, b) and renal mass (Fig. 3.4c) and locate ectopic kidneys, retroperitoneal masses, complex cysts, and masses.

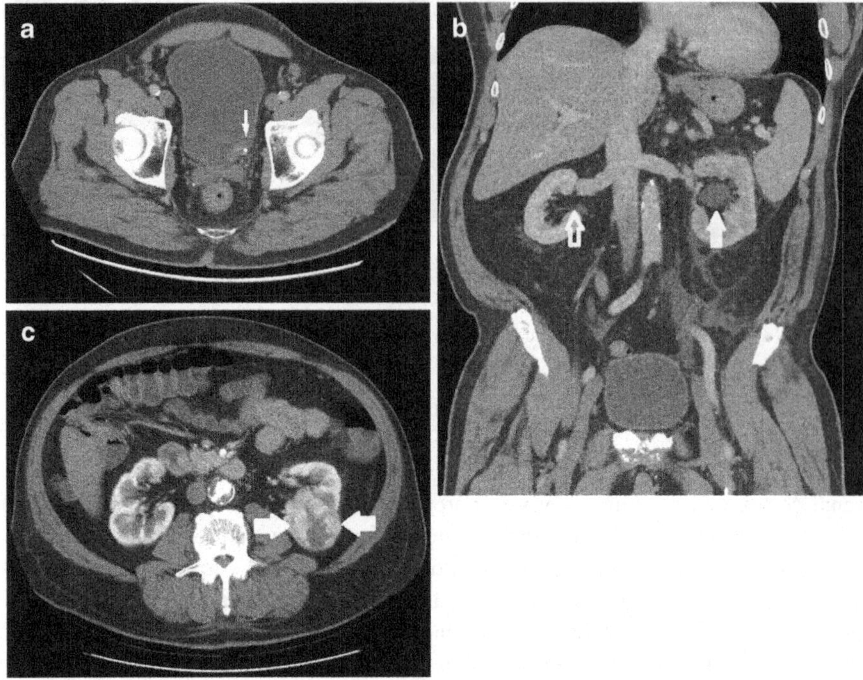

Fig. 3.4 (**a**) CT Calculus. (**b**) Hydronephrosis and stone. (**c**) CT renal mass

Axial slice from a CT demonstrates a 4 mm obstructing stone at the ureterovesical junction (white arrow).

A coronal slice of a contrast-enhanced CT of the abdomen and pelvis in the same patient shows mild left hydronephrosis (solid white arrow). Note the nondilated collecting system on the right (open white arrow).

Axial slice of a contrast-enhanced CT of the abdomen and pelvis demonstrates a 5 cm mass in the midpole left kidney (solid white arrows). The mass exhibits peripheral enhancement with a central region of low density compatible with necrosis. Findings are suspicious for renal cell carcinoma.

Episodes of acute renal colic and obstruction eventually lead to chronic scarring and loss of kidney function. Noncontrast CT scan is sensitive for detection of small parenchymal and ureteral stones, not detected by renal ultrasound or plain films of the abdomen. It is the gold standard for the evaluation of stones.

CT is also for the staging of renal tumors and for diagnosing renal vein thrombosis. It also has higher sensitivity for detection of adult polycystic disease in younger patients, than a screening ultrasound.

CT angiography (CTA) allows visualization of both arterial wall and lumen, which helps in the planning of the renal artery revascularization procedures (Fig. 3.5). A good delineation of the renal vasculature and iliac vessels is a crucial step in kidney transplantation in both donors and recipients.

To minimize contrast nephropathy, contrast material should not be given to patients with GFR below 30 ml/min without careful risk assessment and should be

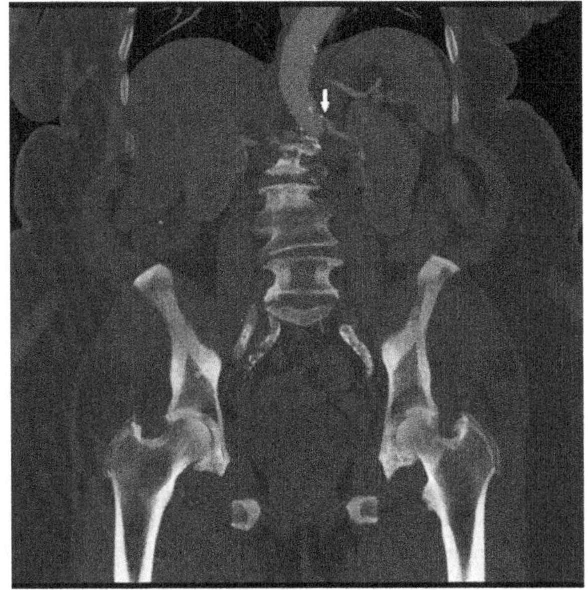

Fig. 3.5 CT angiogram (coronal slice). Coronal slice of a CT angiogram using maximum intensity projection algorithm demonstrates moderate narrowing at the origin of the left renal artery (arrow). Note the small atherosclerotic calcification at the origin of the left renal artery

used with caution with GFR of 30–60 ml/min [29]. It should be noted that patients who have end-stage renal disease (ESRD), established on hemodialysis, can get intravenous iodinated radiocontrast, without worrying about timing and affecting eGFR or creatinine. The residual renal function, however, in those ESRD patients who are on peritoneal dialysis, should be preserved, as they rely heavily on it. Intravenous iodinated radiocontrast should be avoided in these patients.

Magnetic Resonance Imaging

MRI is typically used as an adjunct to another imaging modality and is rarely the first modality.

MRA is used in evaluating for renovascular hypertension and is less invasive than catheter angiography. However, the administration of gadolinium during MRI was strongly linked to a severe disease called nephrogenic systemic fibrosis (NSF) among patients with reduced estimated glomerular rate, especially those on dialysis. This thinking is now changed. Recent studies have shown that newer Group II gadolinium agents have a very low risk, if any, of NSF development, regardless of renal function or dialysis status [30].

The US Food and Drug Administration (FDA) recommended that gadolinium-based imaging be avoided, if possible, in patients with an eGFR <30 ml/min/1.73 m^2. However, it acknowledges since the risk of NSF may be minimal with newer gadolinium agents, discussion with a radiologist is advised [31, 32].

MRI, along with renal venography and CT scanning, is considered the gold standard for the diagnosis of renal vein thrombosis. MRI is helpful in distinguishing complex solid and cystic masses. It is a helpful adjunct when ultrasonography and CT are nondiagnostic, and radiocontrast media cannot be administered due to allergy or reduced renal function.

Abdominal Radiography

It is not commonly performed to evaluate renal disease. A plain film of the abdomen will identify stones such as calcium-containing ones, struvite and cysteine stones, but will miss radiolucent uric acid stones. It will also miss small stones that may be overlying bony structures (Fig. 3.6a, b).

The abdominal radiograph shows several calculi overlying the lower pole left kidney (open arrow). The outline of the left kidney can be seen due to the interface between the perirenal fat and renal parenchyma (solid arrows).

Coronal slice CT of the same patient confirms the presence of nephrolithiasis in the lower pole left kidney (solid arrow). Additionally, there is mild prominence of the left renal pelvis and calyces (open arrow) due to mild ureteropelvic junction stenosis (not seen on this image slice).

Renal Arteriography

The conventional angiogram is performed often after CTA or MRA when there is a plan for intervention. Renal arteriography is used less frequently in work-up of CKD because of the availability of noninvasive tests such as CT and MR angiography. It remains suitable in clinical settings such as suspected polyarteritis nodosa.

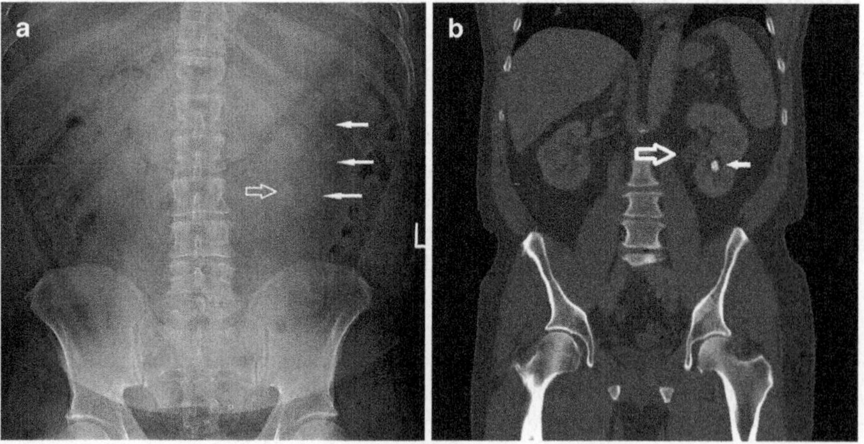

Fig. 3.6 (**a**) Plain KUB film showing stone. (**b**) KUBstonecorrelate.jpeg

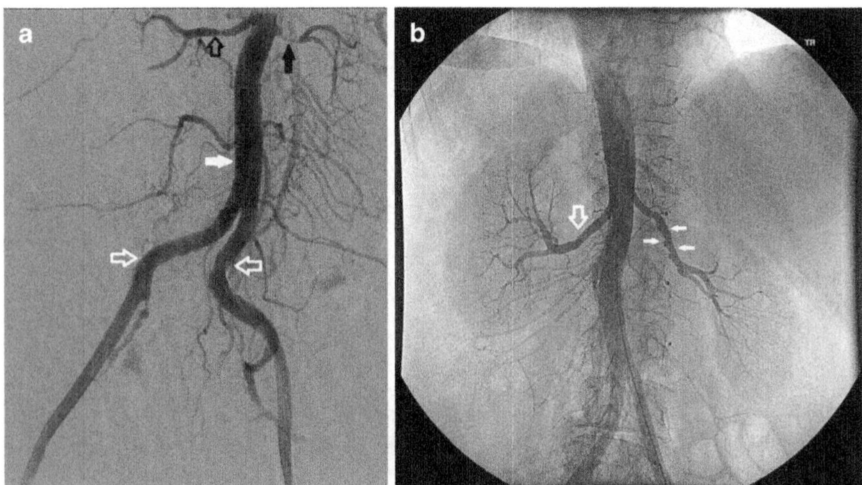

Fig. 3.7 (**a**) Renal arteriography (renal artery stenosis): Arteriography of the abdominal aorta and its major branches shows diffuse severe stenosis of the left renal artery (solid black arrow). Right renal artery (open black arrow), abdominal aorta (solid white arrow), and common iliac arteries (open white arrows). (**b**) Renal arteriography (fibromuscular dysplasia): renal arteriography demonstrates multifocal areas of relative stenoses alternating with small fusiform aneurysms in the right renal artery, referred to as the string-of-bead appearance (solid arrows). The left renal artery is normal (open arrow)

Besides, being invasive and associated with the risk of contrast-induced nephropathy, it also has a risk of cholesterol embolization (Fig. 3.7a, b).

Radionuclide Studies

Renal scans provide both functional and anatomic renal assessment. It is the study of choice for differentiating between obstructive and nonobstructive hydronephrosis (pelivectasis) and also identifies differential function between the two kidneys. It is the study of choice for evaluation of renal transplant donor measured GFR evaluation at many transplant centers in the USA [33].

Agents with different mechanisms of actions are available to image kidneys. Technetium Tc 99m-labeled diethylenetriaminepentaacetic acid (^{99} Tc-DTPA) is a common glomerular agent used for imaging and GFR calculation. In patients with poor renal function, renal imaging with tubular secretion agents such as mercaptoacetyltriglycine (^{99}Tc-MAG3) is superior to DTPA (Fig. 3.8). Tubular retention agents include 99m Tc-labeled dimercaptosuccinate (DMSA), provide excellent cortical imaging, and can be used in suspected renal scarring or infarction and pyelonephritis (bind with high affinity to sulfhydryl groups in proximal tubule).

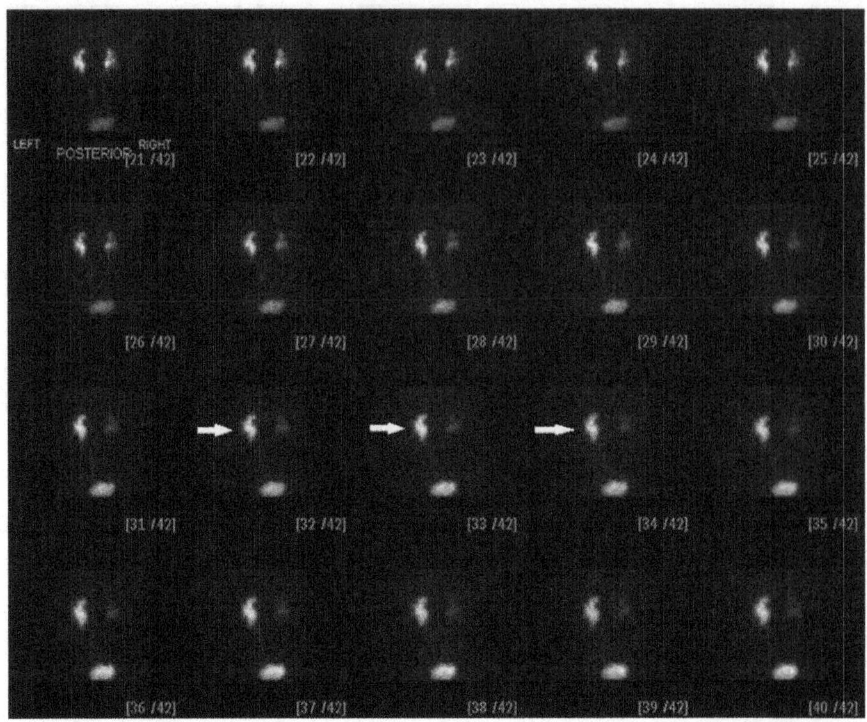

Fig. 3.8 Nuclear medicine scan (Mag scan) showing delayed clearance of tracer to suggest obstruction: Following the intravenous administration of radiopharmaceutical, both kidneys show normal perfusion and function. However, after administration of Lasix, there is delayed clearance of tracer from the left kidney (white arrows) in keeping with obstructed collecting system

Retrograde or Anterograde Pyelography

Retrograde and anterograde pyelography is performed by interventional radiologists and urologists often during interventions when ureters are poorly visualized on other imaging studies. It allows visualization of the renal pelvis and ureter and can be used for cytologic sampling. Ileal conduits can be evaluated by a retrograde (loop-o-gram) or an antegrade study.

Renal Biopsy

A percutaneous renal biopsy is an important tool in diagnosing the exact etiology of kidney disease and also ascertaining the degree of active (reversible) and chronic scarring (irreversible) changes, allowing prognostication of the disease and response to treatment. The routine evaluation of biopsy specimen involves light microscopy, immunofluorescence, and electron microscopy.

Indications of Renal Biopsy

Analysis of renal biopsy should identify a specific diagnosis, reflect disease activity and chronicity, and provide information to direct the treatment plan.

The following reviews the clinical situations in which renal biopsy is indicated or not [34, 35].

Nephrotic syndrome: Renal biopsy will be pursued when the etiology of nephrotic syndrome is not known. Likely one of the three causes is present: minimal change disease, focal segmental glomerulosclerosis, or membranous nephropathy (anti PLA2R blood test is now used to distinguish primary from secondary membranous). Other diagnoses, such as amyloidosis, membranous nephropathy with underlying lupus, and membranoproliferative glomerulonephritis, may be present without typical serologic markers. It may not be needed in patients with nephrotic proteinuria due to conditions where the patient has diabetes for many years, with retinopathy; massive obesity (with slowly increasing proteinuria, secondary FSGS related to obesity); and overt malignancy (membranous nephropathy associated with solid tumors, melts away with treatment of malignancy).

Acute nephritic syndrome: hematuria, cellular casts, proteinuria, hypertension, and renal insufficiency are often caused by a systemic disease that requires a renal biopsy, such as microscopic polyangiitis, granulomatosis with polyangiitis, anti-GBM disease, lupus, hepatitis B- or C-related renal disease, in which therapy and intensity of treatment will be determined by biopsy findings.

Unexplained acute on chronic renal kidney disease such as in drug-related acute interstitial nephritis, obstruction, prerenal disease, and acute tubular necrosis can be diagnosed without the need for biopsy. Small kidneys, or slowly progressive chronic renal failure, are not usually biopsied, since less likely to find treatable disease, unless urine findings have changed significantly and dictate otherwise.

Isolated glomerular hematuria: If not associated with proteinuria and has a normal renal function, then a biopsy will not change the treatment. Generally, the most common diagnoses are thin basement membrane disease, Ig A nephropathy, and Alport's syndrome. Without proteinuria, they have a good long-term prognosis, and no specific treatment needs to be instituted besides angiotensin-converting enzyme inhibitor. Ongoing follow-up monitoring for disease progression and development of proteinuria is required.

Isolated non-nephrotic proteinuria: Renal biopsy is generally not indicated with low-grade proteinuria 500–1000 mg/day. Some of these patients have primary focal segmental glomerulosclerosis, Ig A nephropathy, or membranous nephropathy. Immunosuppressive therapy will not be indicated in these.

Contraindications

Below are the contraindications to the procedure:

- Small hyperechoic kidneys (<9 cm) generally indicative of chronic irreversible disease
- Multiple cysts
- Solitary kidney
- Hydronephrosis
- Uncontrolled bleeding diathesis
- Uncontrolled hypertension
- Active urinary tract infection

Absolute contraindications for percutaneous biopsy include severe hypertension, uncontrolled bleeding diathesis, uncooperative patient, and solitary native kidney [36].

Pre-biopsy Work-Up

Basic work-up prior to a percutaneous kidney biopsy includes, a history, physical examination, and selected lab tests including complete biochemical profile, complete blood count, platelet count, prothrombin time, partial thromboplastin time, and the bleeding time to evaluate if the patient is at increased risk for bleeding [37]. Patients who are taking antiplatelet or antithrombotic agents (e.g., aspirin, omega 3 fatty acids, glycoprotein IIb/IIIa inhibitors, dipyridamole, and nonsteroidal anti-inflammatory drugs should ideally discontinue these medications at least 1 week prior to a scheduled percutaneous renal biopsy and remain off for at least 1 week after [38, 40].

Thrombocytopenia <140,000/µL has been linked to increased bleeding after renal biopsy. The risk of symptomatic hematoma is highest (40 percent) in patients with platelet count <100,000/µL [40].

Complications

Bleeding is the major complication of renal biopsy. The biopsy of the kidney has the highest bleeding risk among that of any other organ (1.2%). Bleeding can occur in collecting system, leading to gross hematuria; into perinephric space, leading to hematoma and falling hematocrit; or underneath renal capsule leading to pressure tamponade [41, 42]. Other potential complications include pain at the site, gross hematuria, arteriovenous fistula formation, and soft tissue infection. Observation for 24 hours is often done, and major complications are identified in this period, with vitals and hematocrit monitoring.

References

1. KDIGO 2012.
2. Floege J, Johnson RL, Feehally J. Comprehensive clinical nephrology. 4th ed. Missouri: Elsevier Saunders; 2010.
3. Kouri T, Fogazzi G, Gant V, et al. European urinalysis guidelines. Scand J Clin Lab Med. 2000;60(Suppl 231):1–96.
4. Tangri N, Stevens LA, Griffith J, et al. A predictive model for progression of chronic kidney disease to kidney failure. JAMA. 2011;305:1553.
5. Perazella MA. The urine sediment as a biomarker of kidney disease. Am J Kidney Dis. 2015;66(5):748–55.
6. Cavanaugh C, Perazella MA. Urine sediment examination in the diagnosis and management of kidney disease: core curriculum. Am J Kidney Dis. 2019;73(2):258–72.
7. Stevens LA, Coresh J, Levey AS. Assessing kidney function-measured and estimated glomerular filtration rate. N Engl J Med. 2006;354:2473.
8. Stevens LA, Levey AS. Measured GFR as a confirmatory test for estimated GFR. J Am Soc Nephrol. 2009;20:2305.
9. Stevens LA, Levey AS. Measurement of renal function in chronic renal disease. Kidney Int. 1990;38:167–84.
10. Rowe C, Stitch AJ, Barrat J, et al. Biological variation of measured and estimated glomerular filtration rate in patients with chronic kidney disease. Kidney Int. 2019;96:429.
11. KDIGO 2012 Clinical practice guideline for the evaluation and management of chronic kidney disease. Kidney Int Suppl. 2013;3:19–62.
12. Levey AS, Bosch JP, Lewis JB, et al. A more accurate method to estimate glomerular filtration rate from serum creatinine a new prediction equation. Modification of diet in Renal Disease Study Group. Ann Intern Med. 1999;130:461.
13. Levey AS, Stevens LA, Schmid CH, et al. A new equation to estimate glomerular filtration rate. Ann Intern Med. 2009;150:604.
14. Stevens LA, Schmid CH, Greene T, et al. Comparative performance of the CKD Epidemiology Collaboration (CKD-EPI) and modification of diet in renal disease (MDRD) study equations for estimating GFR levels above 60 ml/min/1.73m2. Am J Kidney Dis. 2010;56:486.
15. Matsushita L, Mahmoodi BK, Woodward M, et al. Comparison of risk prediction using the CKD-EPI and the MDRD study equation for estimated glomerular filtration rate. JAMA. 2012;307:1941.
16. Levey AS, Stevens LA. Estimating GRF using CKD epidemiology collaboration (CKD-EPI) creatinine equation: more accurate GFR estimates, lower CKD prevalence estimates, better risk predictions. Am J Kidney Dis. 2010;55:622.
17. Florencia IA, Magdalena B, Fernanada M, et al. How to evaluate renal function in stable cirrhotic patients. Postgrad Med. 2017;129(8):866–71.
18. Knight EL, Verhave JC, Spiegelman D, et al. Factors influencing serum cystatin C levels other that renal function and impact on renal function measurement. Kidney Int. 2004;65:1416.
19. Ma YC, Zuo L, Chen JH, et al. Improved GFR estimation by combined creatinine and cystatin C measurements. Kidney Int. 2007;72:1535.
20. Inker LA, Schmid CH, Tighiouart H, et al. Estimating glomerular filtration rate from serum creatinine and cystatin C. N Engl J Med. 2012;367:20.
21. Stevens LA, Nolin TD, Richardson MM, et al. Comparison of dosing recommendations based on measured GFR and kidney function estimating equations. Am J Kidney Dis. 2009;54:33.
22. Matzke GR, Aronoff GR, Atkinson AJ Jr, et al. Drug dosing consideration in patients with acute and chronic kidney disease- a clinical update from kidney disease: improving global outcomes (KDIGO). Kidney Int. 2011;80:1122.
23. Mok Y, Ballew S, Sang Y, et al. Albuminuria as a predictor of cardiovascular outcomes in patients with acute myocardial infarction. J Am Heart Assoc. 2019;8:e010546. https://doi.org/10.1161/JAHA.118.010546.

24. Lamb EJ, MacKenzie F, Stevens P. How should proteinuria be detected and measured? Ann Clin Biochem. 2009;46:206–17.
25. Robinson RR. Isolated proteinuria in asymptomatic patients. Kidney Int. 1980;18:395.
26. ACR appropriateness criteria. Available at: https://acsearch.acr.org.
27. Moghazi S, Jones E, Schroepple J, et al. Correlation of renal histopathology with sonographic findings. Kidney Int. 2005;67:1515.
28. Lubas A, Grzegorz K, Niemczyk S. Renal resistive index as a marker of vascular damage in cardiovascular diseases. Int Urol Nephrol. 2014;46:395–402.
29. Bahrainwala JZ, Leonberg-Yoo AK, Rudnick MR. Use of radiocontrast agents in CKD and ESRD. Semin Dial. 2017;30:290–304. Weisbord S, Gallagher M, Jneid H, et al. N Engl J Med. 2018;378:603–14.
30. ACR manual on contrast media. https://www.acr.org/-/media/ACR/Files/Clinical-Resources/Contrast_Media.pdf.
31. Schieda N, Blaichman J, Costa AF, et al. Gadolinium-based contrast agents in kidney disease: comprehensive review and clinical practice guideline issued by Canadian Association of Radiologists. Can Assoc Radiol J. 2018;69(2):136–50.
32. Endrikat J, Dohanish S, Schleyer N. 10 years of nephrogenic systemic fibrosis: a comprehensive analysis of nephrogenic systemic fibrosis reports received by a pharmaceutical company from 2006–2016. Investig Radiol. 2018;53(9):541–50.
33. Levy AS, Inker LA. GFR evaluation in living kidney donor candidates. J Am Soc Nephrol. 2017;28(4):1062–71. https://doi.org/10.1681/ASN.2016070790.
34. Feehally J, Appel GB. Renal biopsy: how effective, what technique, and how safe. J Nephrol. 1993;6:4.
35. Whittier WL, Korbet SM. Renal biopsy: update. Curr Opin Nephrol. 2004;13:661.
36. Clinical competence in percutaneous renal biopsy. Health and public policy committee. American College of Physicians. Ann Intern Med. 1988;108:301.
37. Korbet SM. Percutaneous renal biopsy. Semin Nephrol. 2002;22:254.
38. Manno C, Strippoli GF, Arnesano L, et al. Predictors of bleeding complications in percutaneous ultrasound-guided renal biopsy. Kidney Int. 2004;66:1570.
39. Hogan JJ, Mocanu M, Berns JS. The native kidney biopsy: update and evidence for best practice. Clin J Am Soc Nephrol. 2016;11:354.
40. Simard-Meilleur MC, Troyanov S, Roy L, et al. Risk factors and timing of native kidney biopsy complications. Nephron Extra. 2014;4:42.
41. Whittier WL, Korbet SM. Timing of complications in percutaneous biopsy. J Am Soc Nephrol. 2004;15:142.
42. Corapi KM, Chen JL, Balk EM, Gordon CE. Bleeding complications of native kidney biopsy: a systematic review and metanalysis. Am J Kidney Dis. 2012;60:62.

Chapter 4
Slowing Chronic Kidney Disease Progression

Pooja Sanghi and Yasmin Brahmbhatt

Introduction

Chronic kidney disease (CKD) is defined as glomerular filtration rate (GFR) < 60 ml/min or markers of kidney damage, or both, of at least 3 months of duration. CKD is linked with adverse clinical outcomes, poor quality of life, and high healthcare costs. CKD can progress to end-stage renal disease (ESRD), a condition that requires renal replacement therapy with dialysis, until patients are able to receive a kidney transplant.

Many chronic kidney diseases independent of the underlying etiology lead to renal fibrosis. It is well accepted that renal fibrosis is not only a static "scar" but a dynamic process involving complex cellular events which provoke the development of fibrogenesis. Prevention of fibrogenesis or slowing the fibrogenesis process is key to preventing CKD progression.

The four main interventions that reduce CKD progression are blood pressure control <140/90 mm Hg and the use of angiotensin-converting enzyme inhibitors (ACEI or angiotensin receptor blockers (ARBs) for albuminuria and hypertension, diabetes control, and correction of metabolic acidosis. Statin-based therapies reduce vascular events in CKD. Nephrology referral for advanced CKD is associated with improved outcomes. Optimizing control of other CKD risk factors like hyperlipidemia and smoking can also reduce CKD progression.

P. Sanghi
Department of Medicine, Division of Nephrology, Geisinger Medical Center, Geisinger, PA, USA
e-mail: psanghi@geisinger.edu

Y. Brahmbhatt (✉)
AstraZeneca, Philadelphia, PA, USA
e-mail: Yasmin.Brahmbhatt@astrazeneca.com

© Springer Nature Switzerland AG 2022
J. McCauley et al. (eds.), *Approaches to Chronic Kidney Disease*,
https://doi.org/10.1007/978-3-030-83082-3_4

CKD Detection

Expert panels have identified insufficient evidence to support general population-based testing for CKD. The KDOQI and KDIGO guidelines have recommended targeted testing for CKD among high-risk populations with diabetes and/or hypertension. In practice, detection of CKD often occurs during routine care because serum creatinine testing is included in ubiquitous basic and comprehensive metabolic panels. Early detection of CKD offers an opportunity to avert complications before symptoms occur.

Detection of CKD based on estimated glomerular filtration rate (eGFR) is a more accurate assessment of kidney function than serum creatinine alone. Quantification of albuminuria has been less widely adopted in clinical practice than the assessment of eGFR, but it is crucial to evaluating prognosis. A spot urine albumin creatinine ratio is more sensitive and specific than a spot urine protein-creatinine ratio although both are predictive of clinical outcomes (Fig. 4.1).

Among patients without a CKD diagnosis but with risk factors for CKD like hypertension and diabetes mellitus, only 43.2% of Medicare beneficiaries had urine albumin testing in 2017, a relatively low rate of testing given that this is a high-risk population [2].

Prognosis of CKD by GFR and Albuminuria Categories: KDIGO 2012			Persistent albuminuria categories Description and range		
			A1	**A2**	**A3**
			Normal to mildly increased	Moderately increased	Severely increased
			<30 mg/g <3 mg/mmol	30-300 mg/g 3-30 mg/mmol	>300 mg/g >30 mg/mmol
GFR categories (ml/ min/ 1.73 m^2) Description and range	G1	Normal or high	≥90		
	G2	Mildly decreased	60-89		
	G3a	Mildly to moderately decreased	45-59		
	G3b	Moderately to severely decreased	30-44		
	G4	Severely decreased	15-29		
	G5	Kidney failure	<15		

Fig. 4.1 Progression of CKD by GFR and albuminuria categories: KDIGO 2012. (Green, low risk (if no other markers of kidney disease, no CKD); yellow, moderately increased risk; orange, high risk; red, very high risk [1])

Slowing CKD Progression by Optimizing Hypertension Control

Hypertension (HTN) is a modifiable risk factor for cardiovascular morbidity and mortality, and reduction of elevated blood pressure (BP) is an important intervention for slowing kidney disease progression. Over the past 10 years, the optimal BP target has been an area of intense research and debate and is discussed elsewhere. Currently, in patients with CKD, the KDIGO 2012 HTN guidelines recommend aiming for systolic blood pressure less than 130 mmHg and diastolic blood pressure less than 80 mmHg in all patients with CKD regardless of the degree of proteinuria.

ACE inhibitors (ACEI) and ARBs are the mainstays of HTN treatment in CKD. ACE inhibitors block the conversion of angiotensin I to the potent vasoconstrictor peptide angiotensin II, whereas ARBs competitively block the angiotensin II receptors. This blockade has the effect of reducing aldosterone secretion and reducing peripheral vascular resistance, effectively reducing systemic BP. Importantly, the blockade of angiotensin II also results in dilation of the efferent arteriole of the glomerulus, which reduces intraglomerular pressure and is the putative mechanism for the renoprotective effects of these agents. The use of ACEI and ARBs is now well established for the treatment of proteinuric CKD and is therefore part of the AHA/ACC 2017 HTN guidelines. There is uncertainty regarding the benefits of ACEI or ARB's in HTN with CKD without proteinuria as the evidence is mixed. However, in practice this dilemma is less fraught as patients are commonly not labeled as having CKD unless they have proteinuria or a serum creatinine high enough to merit a diagnosis of CKD stage 3. In addition, the majority of such patients with HTN require multiple agents to achieve adequate control which very often includes an ACE inhibitor or ARB. A mineralocorticoid receptor antagonist can be used as a fourth or fifth agent if a high aldosterone state has been confirmed by laboratory measurements. KDOQI guidelines recommend that all patients with CKD and HTN should receive an ACEI or an ARB as these agents have been shown to slow the GFR decline independent of their blood pressure lowering effects [3]. There is good evidence to continue with an ACE inhibitor or ARB therapy in advanced CKD as well unless there is concern that these agents are contributing to GFR decline or in the presence of hyperkalemia [4]. In earlier stages of CKD (CKD stage 1 to CKD stage 3b), these agents are usually up-titrated to minimize proteinuria, as lower degrees of proteinuria are associated with slower GFR decline. Once a medication is adjusted, the provider should ideally evaluate the response to therapy in 4 weeks.

A high-salt diet blunts the effectiveness of ACEI, and sodium reduction enhances the anti-proteinuric effect of ARBs. In fact, recent data reveal that a high-salt diet (>14 g/day) is associated with an increased risk of ESRD (independent of BP) in patients with proteinuric CKD [5]. Ingestion of a diet rich in fruits and vegetables with close monitoring of the potassium levels in the setting of advanced CKD reduces SBP and DBP compared to a usual diet [6]. Individualization of treatment and patient-centered medical therapy should be emphasized. Avoidance of complex dosing regimens and high out-of-pocket costs improves patient adherence. Careful evaluation and avoidance of side effects will improve compliance to medications as well. Identification and discontinuation of substances which can increase blood pressure, like NSAIDs and combined oral contraceptive pills, is paramount [7].

In many cases it is difficult to assess whether the HTN caused CKD or vice versa. Aortic stiffening induces renal damage through hemodynamic (flow and pressure) mechanisms. Specifically, aortic stiffening widens aortic pulsatile pressure, which is transmitted deep into the vulnerable microvasculature in high-flow organs such as the kidney and the brain. The resultant increase in pulsatile tensile stress can cause microvascular damage as well as endothelial dysfunction, oxidative stress, and chronic inflammation. Renal tissue often reveals inflammatory changes around the microvasculature, glomeruli, or tubules not only in accelerated hypertension but also milder hypertension [8] and, therefore, can lead to CKD progression.

Atherosclerosis and arteriosclerosis are evident in most CKD patients. Atherosclerosis is a progressive occlusive damage secondary to lipid-laden plaques forming along the vessel walls resulting in diffuse intimal calcification. The CKD environment leads to arteriosclerosis, defined as a diffuse arterial vascular remodeling and eventual loss of vessel elasticity occurring as a result of medial calcification of arteries secondary to abnormal calcium phosphate homeostasis and osteogenic differentiation. Poorly controlled mild-moderate hypertension can contribute to arteriolar nephrosclerosis, a vascular lesion in the preglomerular arterioles that leads to glomerular ischemia and subsequent CKD progression. "Hypertensive nephrosclerosis" is a nonspecific clinical diagnosis applied to nondiabetic patients, often those with recent African ancestry, who present with CKD, low-level proteinuria, and elevated blood pressure. Patients who lack an obvious cause of nephropathy are often labeled as having "hypertensive nephrosclerosis" after a cursory evaluation. Genetic breakthroughs (the presence of two apolipoprotein L1 gene (APOL1) renal-risk variants) demonstrate that inherited forms of glomerulosclerosis can present in a similar fashion to arteriolar nephrosclerosis, and these renal-limited disorders secondarily elevate blood pressure [9]. This genetic discovery explains to a certain extent why specific ethnicities are at greater risk of CKD. In addition, many patients with these genetic variants may not be diagnosed with CKD until they have elevated blood pressure, at which point, significant CKD progression may have already occurred. Hence, population health measures that focus on early screening and detection of CKD in these high-risk populations may help with reducing CKD progression.

Slowing CKD Progression by Reducing Proteinuria

CKD progression is most likely multifactorial but proteinuria and HTN may worsen kidney function decline [10]. RAAS (renin-angiotensin-aldosterone system) blockade reduces the risk of CKD progression mainly by reducing blood pressure. Drugs that inhibit angiotensin-converting enzymes reduce glomerular-capillary permeability to protein, thus reducing proteinuria and preventing the development of glomerulosclersosis [11]. The beneficial effects of RAAS blockade on slowing CKD progression increase with increasing amounts of proteinuria. The Modification of Diet in Renal Disease (MDRD) study showed that patients with higher baseline proteinuria had a faster rate of GFR decline. This study showed that lower blood pressure significantly reduced proteinuria and GFR decline. They suggested that patients with over 1 g proteinuria should aim for a BP < 125/75 and patients with 0.25–1 g/day proteinuria a blood pressure of <130/80 should be targeted [12].

Other landmark studies with ACEIs and angiotensin receptor blockers (ARBs) [13] both in diabetics and nondiabetics [3, 14] have consistently been shown to slow proteinuric CKD progression. The beneficial effect of ACE inhibitors was mediated by factors in addition to reducing blood pressure and urinary protein excretion. The Ramipril Efficacy in Nephropathy (REIN) study a1 [15] was the first to demonstrate that the ACE inhibitor, ramipril, had a kidney-protective effect in slowing declining GFR in nondiabetic CKD patients with a proteinuria of 3 g/24 hour.

Another major trial with type 2 diabetics, Reduction in Endpoints in Non-insulin-Dependent Diabetes Mellitus with the Angiotensin II Antagonist Losartan (RENAAL), showed that with ARB therapy, every 50% reduction in albuminuria in the first 6 months was associated with a reduction in risk of 36% for the renal end-point (defined as doubling of the serum creatinine) and 45% for ESRD during later follow-up [16]. In addition, the AASK trial which looked at the benefits of ACE inhibitors in African Americans without diabetic kidney disease revealed an equal benefit to slowing CKD progression and reducing the risk of ESRD, even at lower levels of proteinuria. Another major trial found that dual blockade with ACE inhibitor and ARB was associated with increased adverse effects of hypotension and renal dysfunction [17].

An abundance of literature reveals that ACEIs or ARBs are first-line agents in CKD with HTN with/without proteinuria to prevent CKD progression. Current KDOQI guidelines state that patients with CKD and HTN should be on an ACE inhibitor or an ARB.

There are other medications and lifestyle measures that have been shown to reduce proteinuria. A recent meta-analysis of over 78,000 patients confirmed that a 30% reduction in albuminuria confers a 23.7% reduction in risk of progression to ESRD, irrespective of drug class [18]. Non-dihydropyridine CCBs significantly reduced proteinuria independent of BP changes when compared with dihydropyridine CCBs due to their preferential dilation of the efferent arteriole [19].

A systematic review and meta-analysis [20] demonstrated beneficial effects on reducing blood pressure and urinary protein excretion in CKD with the addition of the mineralocorticoid receptor antagonist (spironolactone) to ACE inhibitor or ARB therapy. However, these benefits may be offset by the increased risk of hyperkalemia or decline in renal function. In addition, this study did not look at GFR decline or ESRD as an end-point. Another meta-analysis [21] of RCTs in patients with CKD stages 1–4 showed significant benefits of dietary sodium restriction in reduction of blood pressure as well as albuminuria. Low-salt decreased 24-hour proteinuria and albuminuria by 0.39 g/day and 0.05 g/day, respectively, with respect to higher salt intake. Changes in proteinuria were linearly associated with changes in systolic BP, suggesting that the anti-proteinuric effect of sodium restriction may be dependent on BP reduction. One small randomized study showed that moderate weight loss showed significant improvement in proteinuria in patients with proteinuric CKD [22].

Overall, it is well established that ACE inhibitors and ARBs reduce proteinuria and retard CKD progression. Non-dihydropyridine calcium channel blockers and mineralocorticoid antagonists can be used as additional therapy. Careful up-titration of the ACEI or ARBs to reduce proteinuria to less than 500 mg/day can slow CKD progression and must be done with close monitoring of electrolytes and blood pressure. All patients should be educated on the importance of a low-salt diet.

Slowing Diabetic Kidney Disease

The natural progressive course of diabetic kidney disease (DKD) was changed dramatically in the early 1990s after the landmark trial by E. Lewis et al. [23] showed that ACE inhibitors protect against deterioration in renal function in insulin-dependent diabetic nephropathy, independent of its effects on blood pressure. Since then numerous studies have shown benefits from ACE inhibitors and ARB therapy in slowing the progression of DKD in patients with type I and insulin-dependent and insulin-independent type II diabetes. The mechanism of nephroprotection with ACEI and ARBs is mentioned above. Current KDIGO guidelines recommend all patients with CKD and albuminuria should receive ACE inhibitors or ARB treatment in addition to targeting BP < 130/80 to delay DKD progression. However, combination therapy (ACE inhibitors and ARBs) should be avoided due to the risks of complications with acute kidney injury and hyperkalemia. Worsening proteinuria is a sign of CKD progression, and ACE inhibitor or ARB therapy should be up-titrated to reduce proteinuria if electrolytes, renal function, and blood pressure allow. The prevention of DKD in type I and type II DM also involves intensive glucose control from early in the course of diabetes. In patients with type I DM, intensive glucose control targeting a HbA1c level less than or equal to 7% reduced the 9-year risk of developing microalbuminuria and macroalbuminuria by 34% and 56%, respectively, compared with standard care [24]. KDIGO guidelines recommend a target HbA1c of close to 7% to prevent or delay the progression of the microvascular complications of diabetes. However, patients with hypoglycemia, such as those with diabetes and CKD, should not be treated to a HbA1C target of less than 7%. The recent CREDENCE trial [25] showed that patients with type 2 diabetes and albuminuric chronic kidney disease with eGFR over 30 ml/min, who received the sodium-glucose cotransporter (SGLT2) inhibitor, Canagliflozin, had a 30% lower risk of kidney failure and cardiovascular events. Patients received canagliflozin 100 mg daily in conjunction with ACE inhibitors or ARBs. There were no adverse side effects or complications compared to the placebo group.

Sodium-glucose cotransporter type 2 in the renal proximal tubule reabsorbs approximately 90% of filtered glucose. In type 2 diabetes, the maladaptive upregulation of sodium-glucose cotransporter type 2 contributes to the maintenance of hyperglycemia. Inhibiting these transporters has been shown to effectively improve glycemic control through inducing glycosuria and is generally well tolerated. The SGLT-2 inhibitors also reduce blood pressure and urate and induce a diuresis. The early hyperfiltration injury that occurs in DKD is reversed with SGLT2inh and is thought to be the main mechanism for slowing CKD progression. At the time of therapy initiation, we typically reduce concomitant diuretic dosage by 50% and monitor electrolytes closely. There can be a small rise in serum creatinine for a few weeks (similar to ACE inhibitor or ARB therapy) which stabilizes with time. This class of drug is not approved for kidney transplant patients at the time of this writing. This new therapy has changed the landscape of DKD management.

Population-based approaches to reducing DKD cannot be emphasized enough. A recent study revealed that implementation of guidelines for the treatment of hypertension and diabetes, regular albuminuria testing, the use of ACE-inhibitors and ARBs, multidisciplinary care with primary care providers, and additional services to support nutrition, physical activity, and diabetes education reduced diabetes-related kidney failure by 54% [26].

Slowing CKD Progression in Cardiovascular Disease

Cardiovascular disease (CVD) remains the leading cause of death in patients worldwide accounting for 41% of deaths in patients on dialysis and being 20 times higher than the general population [27]. Among patients with CKD, death from CVD is far more common than progression to ESKD [28]. Patients with CVD and CKD may be at higher risk for CKD progression due to shared risk factors (such as diabetes, hypertension, hyperlipidemia, smoking, etc.), atherosclerosis affecting the renal vasculature, homeostatic changes that decrease renal perfusion in the setting of heart failure, and exposure to contrast dye and atheroemboli from diagnostic procedures [29]. The chronic renal insufficiency cohort (CRIC) study revealed that self-reported heart failure was an independent risk factor for ESKD or a 50% decline in GFR [30]. Additionally, Elsayad et al. [31] show that cardiovascular disease was independently associated with kidney function decline and the development of kidney disease. Therefore, optimizing therapy for CVD is paramount not only to reduce mortality but also to reduce GFR decline. The main hemodynamic mechanisms include salt and water retention leading to fluid overload, which results in cardiac and renal venous congestion. Renal venous congestion might be key for the acceleration of renal dysfunction in this clinical context ultimately leading to renal fibrogenesis and CKD progression [32]. Careful attention to volume status and maintaining euvolemia is key to preventing CKD progression. Further effects of CVD on the kidney can be found elsewhere in this book.

Slowing CKD Progression by Optimizing Metabolic Acidosis

In CKD, the capacity of the kidneys to excrete the daily acid load as ammonium and titratable acid is impaired, resulting in acid retention and metabolic acidosis (MA). The prevalence of MA increases with declining GFR. Untreated chronic metabolic acidosis often leads to an accelerated reduction in GFR in patients with CKD. This is due to intra-kidney paracrine hormones including angiotensin II, aldosterone, and endothelin-1 that mediate increased acid excretion, but their chronic upregulation promotes inflammation and fibrosis [33]. Chronic MA also stimulates ammoniagenesis that increases acid excretion but also leads to ammonia-induced complement activation and deposition of C3 and C5b-9 that can cause tubule-interstitial damage, further worsening CKD progression. All these effects along with acid accumulation in kidney tissue combine to accelerate the progression of kidney disease. In addition to GFR decline, metabolic acidosis is also associated with bone demineralization, skeletal muscle catabolism, and mortality.

KDIGO guidelines recommend treating metabolic acidosis with oral alkali therapy if serum HCO3 is less than 22 meq/dL and aim to keep it in the normal range if there are no contraindications [1]. However, large clinic trials to determine the efficacy and safety of correction of MA with oral alkali in CKD patients have yet to be conducted. Small studies support the notion that treating MA preserves kidney function [34].

Nutritional alkali therapy with fruits and vegetables is probably warranted in most individuals with CKD as long as serum potassium concentration allows and is monitored. One study in patients with hypertensive CKD showed that fruits and vegetables in advanced CKD were just as effective as oral alkali therapy at GFR preservation without inducing hyperkalemia [35]. However, if nutritional therapy is contraindicated due to hyperkalemia or lack of patient adherence, pharmacological treatment can be considered.

The decision to initiate pharmacologic treatment should consider these factors: severity of MA, blood pressure, and volume status. Hyperkalemia along with metabolic acidosis is probably the most important reason to start alkali therapy because this can help reduce serum potassium concentration and allowing continued RAAS blockade. If patients have persistent MA with serum HCO3 less than 18 meq/L, it is reasonable to initiate alkali therapy assuming there is no short-term condition that might account for the low bicarbonate concentration. The primary concern with sodium-based alkali therapy is fluid retention, elevation of blood pressure, and peripheral and pulmonary edema. To date, results from small studies in CKD showed that differences in blood pressure, weight, and hospitalizations for heart failure were not significantly different between sodium bicarbonate-/citrate-treated patients and controls. This is not entirely unexpected because sodium-related fluid retention is more substantial when sodium is accompanied by the chloride anion and not with other anions. Although the mechanisms for this are complex and multifactorial, hyperchloremia induces renal vasoconstriction through tubuloglomerular feedback. The reduction in GFR leads to increased sodium and water reabsorption.

Alkali therapy may also cause hypokalemia if bicarbonaturia occurs. Hence, close monitoring of potassium is warranted. Some patients have gastrointestinal side effects with sodium bicarbonate. Bloating and burping are common gastrointestinal side effects, and switching to sodium citrate should be considered if these limit adherence.

Although pharmacological therapy appears to be safe, there are potential risks that require monitoring. Large-scale trials to determine whether alkali therapy is beneficial and safe are well overdue.

Hyperlipidemia

Data on whether lipid-lowering therapy slows CKD progression is less clear, and there are currently no recommendations on prescribing these medications to slow CKD progression.

However, several large trials examining lipid-lowering therapies in patients with CKD have been published in the last 10 years [36, 37], and a metanalysis [38] revealed that lipid-lowering therapy decreases cardiac death and atherosclerosis-mediated cardiovascular events in persons with CKD. The KDIGO 2014 lipid therapy in CKD guidelines recommend that all non-dialysis patients over the age of 50 years with CKD should be prescribed statin therapy to reduce overall CVD risk [39]. Although dyslipidemia is a major modifiable risk factor for CVD and is common in patients with CKD, only about 50% of these patients who also have elevated low-density lipoprotein (LDL) cholesterol levels receive lipid-lowering therapy [40]. On the contrary, patients with lower baseline LDL-C concentrations, including those with CKD, have an increased risk of intracerebral hemorrhage (ICH) which may be exacerbated by lipid-lowering therapy. Many studies have not been powered to detect differences for this particular outcome and do not report complications (including ICH) stratified according to LDL-C concentrations at baseline and during follow-up [41].

Other lipid-lowering agents, specifically the fibric acid derivatives are commonly used in CKD and can increase the serum creatinine level. Interestingly, despite the rise in creatinine, studies do not show an increased risk of ESRD [42].

Hyperuricemia

Uric acid has emerged as a possible modifiable risk factor for the development and progression of CKD. Hyperuricemia is defined as a serum urate concentration > 7 mg/dL and is common among patients with CKD. It increases with the deterioration of kidney function due to decreased renal clearance. Whether hyperuricemia contributes to CKD progression has been debated for decades. Recent evidence [43] suggests that hyperuricemia contributes to the development of hypertension. Animal studies reveal that hyperuricemia induces HTN by activating vasoactive and inflammatory processes that favor sodium retention, vascular constriction, and elevated blood pressure. Uric acid is a potent activator of the renin-angiotensin-aldosterone system (RAAS). It activates prorenin receptors in the proximal tubular cells of the kidney that stimulate the intrarenal RAAS, as well as increasing renal renin expression, plasma renin activity, serum aldosterone levels, and intracellular angiotensin II levels [44]. Sato et al. [44] describe the pro-inflammatory effects of uric acid in detail and how this may increase kidney interstitial inflammation. Subsequently, numerous studies investigating the effects of uric acid lowering have shown benefit in slowing CKD progression, but many other studies have not. Two large metanalyses in 2014 and 2018 [45, 46] concluded that urate-lowering therapies may slow CKD progression but that larger randomized controlled trials were needed to assess the impact of uric acid-lowering therapy on CKD progression. Two more recent randomized controlled trials [47, 48] revealed that allopurinol did not slow GFR decline despite lowering urate. Therefore, due to inconclusive evidence, urate-lowering therapy is not recommended to slow CKD progression in patients with asymptomatic hyperuricemia, although this is occasionally done in practice on a case-by-case basis. Additionally, safety of uric acid lowering therapies is also a cause for concern. A recent randomized double-blind controlled trial compared febuxostat (a nonpurine xanthin oxidase inhibitor) with allopurinol (a purine base analog xanthin oxidase inhibitor) in patients with gout and cardiovascular disease. The study found that febuxostat was noninferior to allopurinol with respect to rates of adverse cardiovascular events but all-cause mortality and cardiovascular mortality were higher with febuxostat than with allopurinol [49]. In addition, although allopurinol is very effective at reducing uric acid levels, in some patients it can induce severe cutaneous adverse reactions (SCARs). HLA-B*5801 is a very strong marker for allopurinol-induced SCARs. HLA-B*5801 carrier frequency is reported to be 2–4% in Africans, 1–6% in Caucasians, 3–15% in Asian Indians, and 8.8–10.9% in Chinese patients [50]. A recent study [50] found that the incidence of allopurinol-induced SCARs was considerably high in CKD patients with HLA-B58 and that the presence of HLA-B58 may increase the risk of allopurinol-induced SCARs. Given this evidence, serum HLA-B58 testing should ideally be done in high-risk populations if allopurinol is being considered. If HLA-B58 testing is positive, consider another medication. Certainly, this screening can aid management, increase prescribing safety, and prevent withholding allopurinol from patients that may benefit.

Obesity and CKD Progression

Obesity is a risk factor for CVD and death in people without CKD, but the effect of obesity in people with CKD is uncertain. Many studies have shown that obesity is associated with the development of incident CKD [51].

The exact mechanisms whereby obesity may worsen or cause CKD remain unclear. All obese patients do not end up with CKD. The deleterious renal consequences of obesity may be mediated by comorbid conditions such as diabetes mellitus or hypertension which are the classic risk factors for CKD and CVD, but there are also direct effects of adiposity on the kidney by the production of endocrine factors called adipokines. These lead to oxidative stress and modification of the intestinal flora along with increased production of insulin and insulin resistance predisposing to the generation of uremic toxins and propagating decline in kidney function. The inflammatory milieu harvested by an obese diabetic patient predisposes to the development of glomerulosclerosis and tubulointerstitial atrophy. Obesity-related glomerulopathy (ORG) is a distinct entity characterized by glomerulomegaly, progressive glomerulosclerosis, and renal functional decline. Obesity has been associated with focal segmental glomerulosclerosis for several decades. In addition, increased insulin resistance, increased fat tissue, and increased adipokines lead to overactivation of the renin-angiotensin-aldosterone system (RAAS) which can lead to glomerular hyperfiltration, increased GFR, sodium, and water reabsorption. This can lead to hypertension with associated proteinuria which can subsequently lead to CKD progression. Higher BMI is also associated with an increased prevalence of nephrolithiasis by promoting insulin resistance, low urinary pH, and increased urinary oxalate excretion [52].

Considering the overwhelming deleterious effects of obesity on various disease processes, it is seemingly counterintuitive that obesity has been consistently associated with lower mortality rates in patients with advanced CKD and ESRD. Epidemiologic studies show an inverse paradoxical relationship between BMI and survival in patients with non-dialysis dependent CKD (NDD-CKD), such that BMI in the overweight or obese range is associated with a survival benefit. Patients with NDD-CKD and a BMI between 25 and 30 had fewer atherosclerotic events compared to NDD-CKD patients with BMI between 20 and 25 kg/m^2. However, there was no significant difference in atherosclerotic events in NDD-CKD patients with a BMI over 30 compared to a BMI of 20–25 [53]. This suggests that higher BMI may be protective against cardiovascular events in patients with CKD but this conclusion must be taken with caution. It is possible that the seemingly protective effect of a high BMI is the result of the imperfection of BMI as a measure of obesity, as it does not differentiate the effects of adiposity from those of higher non-adipose tissue. Studies that separated the effects of a higher waist circumference from those of higher BMI showed a reversal of the inverse association with mortality [54]. Higher muscle mass has also been shown to explain at least some of the positive effects attributed to elevated BMI. Although BMI is easy to calculate and used in many nutritional guidelines, this metric is a poor estimate of fat mass distribution, especially in CKD. In addition, many studies show improvement in GFR after weight loss and bariatric surgery reflecting improved HTN and DM control [55], which subsequently can reduce CKD progression.

In overweight or obese diabetic patients, lifestyle interventions including caloric restriction and increased physical activity compared with a standard follow-up based on education and support to sustain diabetes treatment reduced the risk for incident CKD by 30%. No safety concerns regarding kidney-related adverse effects were seen [56]. CKD risk increases with a waist circumference and a waist/hip ratio of more than 102 cm and 0.9, respectively, for men, and more than 88 cm and 0.8, respectively, for women. Obesity is a major component of metabolic syndrome. Several studies have shown that metabolic syndrome is associated with incident CKD development [[57–59]. Recent studies have identified a unique subtype of obesity called "metabolically healthy obesity" which has distinct features of low metabolic burden such as better lipid and inflammatory profiles, lower insulin resistance, and lower blood pressure than traditional obesity. A recent observational Korean study found that both metabolic abnormality and obesity are associated with a significantly increased risk for CKD progression. Even obese patients without metabolic abnormality had an elevated risk for CKD progression [60]. Despite weight loss leading to overall decreased mortality and morbidity in obese patients, there is little data to show GFR preservation or slower CKD progression with weight loss in the nondiabetic population.

Due to the overall lack of evidence, there are currently no recommendations on weight loss to prevent CKD progression. Lifestyle recommendations to reduce body weight in obese people at risk of CKD and in those with early CKD appear justified, particularly recommendations for the control of diabetes and HTN. As the independent effect of obesity control on the incidence and progression of CKD is difficult to disentangle from the effects of HTN and type II DM, recommendation of weight loss in the minority of metabolically healthy, non-hypertensive obese patients remains unwarranted.

Smoking

Smoking was first described as a risk factor for CKD in individuals with diabetes, and more recent evidence has shown it is a risk factor for the development of CKD in the general population [61]. Observational studies show that smoking adversely affects kidney function, but the biological mechanisms through which this occurs remain incompletely understood. Both hemodynamic and non-hemodynamic-mediated changes may cause kidney damage in smokers. Proposed non-hemodynamic-mediated mechanisms through which smoking causes kidney damage include oxidative stress, decreased bioavailability of nitric oxide, increased endothelin 1 concentration, tubular cell damage, and increased vasopressin secretion [62]. A heightened inflammatory state has also been shown to result from cigarette smoking and to be associated with declining kidney function [63]. The hemodynamic-mediated changes include a transient but significant increase in blood pressure from smoking initiation. These transient increases in systemic blood pressure have been associated with kidney disease progression [64]. CKD is interwoven with cardiovascular disease (CVD) and smoking [65]. Several studies have documented that the prevalence of unilateral and bilateral atherosclerotic renal artery stenosis is higher in smokers and therefore it is likely that smoking accelerates the course of renal failure [66]. This assumption is based on the consideration that apart from luminal narrowing of the renal artery, a combination of arteriolar and atheroembolic damage (i.e., cholesterol microembolism) is thought to contribute to progressive loss of renal function. Smoking is also a known risk factor for cholesterol embolization which can lead to kidney function decline.

Smoking can also cause structural alterations to the glomerulus. Nasr et al. [67] describe a large case series of patients who were current heavy smokers or had a history of smoking who developed idiopathic nodular glomerulosclerosis (ING). These patients were predominantly elderly and white and had a mean cumulative 15-year duration of smoking. The majority of these patients presented with renal failure and proteinuria. Nephrotic syndrome was present in over 20% of patients. All renal biopsies described diffuse and nodular mesangial sclerosis and arteriosclerosis. The median time from biopsy to ESRD was only 26 months. Continuation of smoking and lack of angiotensin II blockade had a negative impact on renal survival.

Multiple earlier studies [68, 69] have shown that smoking increases the risk of ESRD, including a marked increased risk of macroalbuminuria which is associated with the male gender and number of cigarettes smoked. Halimi et al. [70] studied volunteers from the general population and found that current smokers had a higher risk (adjusted RR 3.26 and 2.69, respectively) for macroalbuminuria than former smokers (adjusted RR 3.26 and 2.69, respectively) indicating nonreversible kidney damage related to smoking. A community-based Japanese study [71] and multiple others have highlighted high cumulative smoking exposure (lifetime cigarette exposure of 25 pack-years) as an independent risk factor for CKD both in men and women. Additionally a more recent metanalysis [72] suggested evidence for cigarette smoking as an independent risk factor for incident CKD.

Despite the lack of randomized control data, there is good evidence that smoking cessation retards proteinuria and slows progression to ESRD in patients with CKD and diabetes [73–75]. It is reasonable to assume that the benefits of smoking cessation (i.e., decreased mortality, reduced rates of cardiovascular disease, and cancer) that hold for the general population are also applicable to individuals with CKD.

A relatively small number of observational studies have examined the risk of mortality, CKD progression, and vascular events associated with smoking among patients with CKD. Two multicenter prospective cohort studies [53, 76] indicated that smoking adversely affects mortality and cardiovascular events in patients with CKD. However, there is significant heterogeneity between the studies, and the association of smoking with CKD progression remains unclear.

While more evidence regarding the outcomes of smokers with CKD is warranted, KDOQI guidelines recommend all patients with CKD and ESRD should be counseled on smoking cessation to slow CKD progression and reduce cardiovascular risk. Fourmanek et al. [77] have described a combination of pharmacologic therapy and motivational interviewing/behavioral techniques which have the best success rates at smoking cessation.

New Therapies Targeting Renal Fibrosis to Slow CKD Progression

Renal fibrosis is the common outcome of many chronic kidney diseases independent of the underlying etiology. It is well accepted that renal fibrosis is not only a static "scar" but a dynamic process involving a complexity of cellular events which provoke the development of fibrotic stages. Fibrogenesis is characterized by several events namely increase of matrix production, inhibition of matrix degradation, mesangial and fibroblast activation, tubular epithelial to mesenchymal cell transition, myofibroblast activation, and cell apoptosis [78]. Bardoxolone methyl has been studied to prevent renal fibrosis. The main mechanism of action is the upregulation of transcription factors involved in the upregulation of cytoprotective genes which ultimately lead to anti-inflammatory effects. Studies involving humans [79] in patients with type II DM and CKD stage 3b or stage 4 CKD have shown that bardoxolone methyl can reduce the serum creatinine for up to 52 weeks. However, a later trial [80] which was aimed at investigating outcomes of ESRD or death from cardiovascular causes with bardoxolone methyl found that there was no reduction in the risk of ESRD or death from cardiovascular causes. In addition, a higher rate of cardiovascular events with this drug prompted early termination of the trial.

The challenges regarding drug efficacy and safety are attributed to both the diversity of molecular mechanisms identified in CKD as well as the complexity of kidney structure. In addition, due to the fact that the tubular and glomerular functions are affected in CKD and fibrosis, the administered drug concentration most of the time cannot be efficiently distributed to the renal target cell in addition to other challenges. However, there are currently over 20 clinical trials investigating gene therapies which mainly involve using miRNA or small interfering RNA (siRNA)-based drugs that ameliorate various pathologies in correlation with impaired expression of particular target genes.

Conclusion

Slowing CKD progression is key to improving patient outcomes. This chapter highlights current evidence-based therapies and national guidelines to reduce CVS risk in CKD and slow CKD progression. However, despite these guidelines, current evidence shows that there are major gaps in healthcare delivery. A recent nationwide study [81] found a high prevalence of uncontrolled HTN, a decrease in ACE-inhibitor/ARB usage over the last 15 years, and a low percentage of patients prescribed statins. Further studies focused on achieving sustainable high-quality healthcare delivery for CKD patients should be explored.

References

1. Levin A, Stevens PE. Summary of KDIGO 2012 CKD Guideline: behind the scenes, need for guidance, and a framework for moving forward. Kidney Int. 2014;85(1):49–61.
2. Saran R, et al. US renal data system 2019 annual data report: epidemiology of kidney disease in the United States. Am J Kidney Dis. 2020;75(1 Suppl 1):A6–a7.
3. Jafar TH, et al. Angiotensin-converting enzyme inhibitors and progression of nondiabetic renal disease. A meta-analysis of patient-level data. Ann Intern Med. 2001;135(2):73–87.
4. Hsu TW, et al. Renoprotective effect of renin-angiotensin-aldosterone system blockade in patients with predialysis advanced chronic kidney disease, hypertension, and anemia. JAMA Intern Med. 2014;174(3):347–54.
5. Vegter S, et al. Sodium intake, ACE inhibition, and progression to ESRD. J Am Soc Nephrol. 2012;23(1):165–73.
6. Appel LJ, et al. A clinical trial of the effects of dietary patterns on blood pressure. DASH Collaborative Research Group. N Engl J Med. 1997;336(16):1117–24.
7. Brahmbhatt Y, Gupta M, Hamrahian S. Hypertension in premenopausal and postmenopausal women. Curr Hypertens Rep. 2019;21(10):74.
8. Hashimoto J, O'Rourke MF. Inflammation and arterial stiffness in chronic kidney disease: cause or consequence? Am J Hypertens. 2017;30(4):350–2.
9. Freedman BI, Cohen AH. Hypertension-attributed nephropathy: what's in a name? Nat Rev Nephrol. 2016;12(1):27–36.
10. Jafar TH, et al. Progression of chronic kidney disease: the role of blood pressure control, proteinuria, and angiotensin-converting enzyme inhibition: a patient-level meta-analysis. Ann Intern Med. 2003;139(4):244–52.
11. Ruggenenti P, Perna A, Remuzzi G. Retarding progression of chronic renal disease: the neglected issue of residual proteinuria. Kidney Int. 2003;63(6):2254–61.
12. Peterson JC, et al. Blood pressure control, proteinuria, and the progression of renal disease. The Modification of Diet in Renal Disease Study. Ann Intern Med. 1995;123(10):754–62.
13. Strippoli GF, Craig M, Craig JC. Antihypertensive agents for preventing diabetic kidney disease. Cochrane Database Syst Rev. 2005;(4):Cd004136.
14. Maschio G, et al. Effect of the angiotensin-converting-enzyme inhibitor benazepril on the progression of chronic renal insufficiency. The Angiotensin-Converting-Enzyme Inhibition in Progressive Renal Insufficiency Study Group. N Engl J Med. 1996;334(15):939–45.
15. Randomised placebo-controlled trial of effect of ramipril on decline in glomerular filtration rate and risk of terminal renal failure in proteinuric, non-diabetic nephropathy. The GISEN Group (Gruppo Italiano di Studi Epidemiologici in Nefrologia). Lancet. 1997;349(9069):1857–63.
16. de Zeeuw D, et al. Proteinuria, a target for renoprotection in patients with type 2 diabetic nephropathy: lessons from RENAAL. Kidney Int. 2004;65(6):2309–20.
17. Yusuf S, et al. Telmisartan, ramipril, or both in patients at high risk for vascular events. N Engl J Med. 2008;358(15):1547–59.
18. Heerspink HJ, et al. Drug-induced reduction in albuminuria is associated with subsequent renoprotection: a meta-analysis. J Am Soc Nephrol. 2015;26(8):2055–64.
19. Bakris GL, et al. Differential effects of calcium antagonist subclasses on markers of nephropathy progression. Kidney Int. 2004;65(6):1991–2002.
20. Currie G, et al. Effect of mineralocorticoid receptor antagonists on proteinuria and progression of chronic kidney disease: a systematic review and meta-analysis. BMC Nephrol. 2016;17(1):127.
21. Garofalo C, et al. Dietary salt restriction in chronic kidney disease: a meta-analysis of randomized clinical trials. Nutrients. 2018;10(6):732.
22. Morales E, et al. Beneficial effects of weight loss in overweight patients with chronic proteinuric nephropathies. Am J Kidney Dis. 2003;41(2):319–27.

23. Lewis EJ, et al. The effect of angiotensin-converting-enzyme inhibition on diabetic nephropathy. The Collaborative Study Group. N Engl J Med. 1993;329(20):1456–62.
24. Barnett AH, et al. Efficacy and safety of empagliflozin added to existing antidiabetes treatment in patients with type 2 diabetes and chronic kidney disease: a randomised, double-blind, placebo-controlled trial. Lancet Diabetes Endocrinol. 2014;2(5):369–84.
25. Perkovic V, et al. Canagliflozin and renal outcomes in type 2 diabetes and nephropathy. N Engl J Med. 2019;380(24):2295–306.
26. Bullock A, et al. Vital signs: decrease in incidence of diabetes-related end-stage renal disease among American Indians/Alaska Natives – United States, 1996–2013. MMWR Morb Mortal Wkly Rep. 2017;66(1):26–32.
27. Cozzolino M, et al. Cardiovascular disease in dialysis patients. Nephrol Dial Transplant. 2018;33(Suppl_3):iii28–34.
28. Gargiulo R, Suhail F, Lerma EV. Cardiovascular disease and chronic kidney disease. Dis Mon. 2015;61(9):403–13.
29. Fox CS, et al. Predictors of new-onset kidney disease in a community-based population. JAMA. 2004;291(7):844–50.
30. Rahman M, et al. Association between chronic kidney disease progression and cardiovascular disease: results from the CRIC study. Am J Nephrol. 2014;40(5):399–407.
31. Elsayed EF, et al. Cardiovascular disease and subsequent kidney disease. Arch Intern Med. 2007;167(11):1130–6.
32. Schefold JC, et al. Heart failure and kidney dysfunction: epidemiology, mechanisms and management. Nat Rev Nephrol. 2016;12(10):610–23.
33. Wesson DE, Buysse JM, Bushinsky DA. Mechanisms of metabolic acidosis-induced kidney injury in chronic kidney disease. J Am Soc Nephrol. 2020;31(3):469–82.
34. de Brito-Ashurst I, et al. Bicarbonate supplementation slows progression of CKD and improves nutritional status. J Am Soc Nephrol. 2009;20(9):2075–84.
35. Goraya N, et al. A comparison of treating metabolic acidosis in CKD stage 4 hypertensive kidney disease with fruits and vegetables or sodium bicarbonate. Clin J Am Soc Nephrol. 2013;8(3):371–81.
36. Palmer SC, et al. HMG CoA reductase inhibitors (statins) for people with chronic kidney disease not requiring dialysis. Cochrane Database Syst Rev. 2014;(5):Cd007784.
37. Baigent C, et al. The effects of lowering LDL cholesterol with simvastatin plus ezetimibe in patients with chronic kidney disease (Study of Heart and Renal Protection): a randomised placebo-controlled trial. Lancet. 2011;377(9784):2181–92.
38. Upadhyay A, et al. Lipid-lowering therapy in persons with chronic kidney disease: a systematic review and meta-analysis. Ann Intern Med. 2012;157(4):251–62.
39. Wanner C, Tonelli M. KDIGO Clinical practice guideline for lipid management in CKD: summary of recommendation statements and clinical approach to the patient. Kidney Int. 2014;85(6):1303–9.
40. Parikh NI, et al. Cardiovascular disease risk factors in chronic kidney disease: overall burden and rates of treatment and control. Arch Intern Med. 2006;166(17):1884–91.
41. Van Laecke S. Lipid lowering and risk of haemorrhagic stroke in CKD. Nat Rev Nephrol. 2019;15(11):667–9.
42. Jun M, et al. Effects of fibrates in kidney disease: a systematic review and meta-analysis. J Am Coll Cardiol. 2012;60(20):2061–71.
43. Feig DI, et al. Uric acid and the origins of hypertension. J Pediatr. 2013;162(5):896–902.
44. Sato Y, et al. The case for uric acid-lowering treatment in patients with hyperuricaemia and CKD. Nat Rev Nephrol. 2019;15(12):767–75.
45. Liu X, et al. Effects of uric acid-lowering therapy on the progression of chronic kidney disease: a systematic review and meta-analysis. Ren Fail. 2018;40(1):289–97.
46. Bose B, et al. Effects of uric acid-lowering therapy on renal outcomes: a systematic review and meta-analysis. Nephrol Dial Transplant. 2014;29(2):406–13.

47. Doria A, et al. Serum urate lowering with allopurinol and kidney function in type 1 diabetes. N Engl J Med. 2020;382(26):2493–503.
48. Badve SV, et al. Effects of allopurinol on the progression of chronic kidney disease. N Engl J Med. 2020;382(26):2504–13.
49. White WB, et al. Cardiovascular safety of febuxostat or allopurinol in patients with gout. N Engl J Med. 2018;378(13):1200–10.
50. Chung WH, Hung SI, Chen YT. Human leukocyte antigens and drug hypersensitivity. Curr Opin Allergy Clin Immunol. 2007;7(4):317–23.
51. Kramer H, et al. Obesity and prevalent and incident CKD: the hypertension detection and follow-up program. Am J Kidney Dis. 2005;46(4):587–94.
52. Kovesdy CP, Furth S, Zoccali C. Obesity and kidney disease: hidden consequences of the epidemic. Physiol Int. 2017;104(1):1–14.
53. Ricardo AC, et al. Healthy lifestyle and risk of kidney disease progression, atherosclerotic events, and death in CKD: findings from the Chronic Renal Insufficiency Cohort (CRIC) study. Am J Kidney Dis. 2015;65(3):412–24.
54. Postorino M, et al. Abdominal obesity and all-cause and cardiovascular mortality in end-stage renal disease. J Am Coll Cardiol. 2009;53(15):1265–72.
55. Stenvinkel P, Zoccali C, Ikizler TA. Obesity in CKD--what should nephrologists know? J Am Soc Nephrol. 2013;24(11):1727–36.
56. Wing RR, et al. Cardiovascular effects of intensive lifestyle intervention in type 2 diabetes. N Engl J Med. 2013;369(2):145–54.
57. Huh JH, et al. An association of metabolic syndrome and chronic kidney disease from a 10-year prospective cohort study. Metabolism. 2017;67:54–61.
58. Lucove J, et al. Metabolic syndrome and the development of CKD in American Indians: the Strong Heart Study. Am J Kidney Dis. 2008;51(1):21–8.
59. Kurella M, Lo JC, Chertow GM. Metabolic syndrome and the risk for chronic kidney disease among nondiabetic adults. J Am Soc Nephrol. 2005;16(7):2134–40.
60. Yun HR, et al. Obesity, metabolic abnormality, and progression of CKD. Am J Kidney Dis. 2018;72(3):400–10.
61. Briganti EM, et al. Smoking is associated with renal impairment and proteinuria in the normal population: the AusDiab kidney study. Australian Diabetes, Obesity and Lifestyle Study. Am J Kidney Dis. 2002;40(4):704–12.
62. Orth SR. Smoking--a renal risk factor. Nephron. 2000;86(1):12–26.
63. Pecoits-Filho R, et al. Associations between circulating inflammatory markers and residual renal function in CRF patients. Am J Kidney Dis. 2003;41(6):1212–8.
64. Orth SR. Effects of smoking on systemic and intrarenal hemodynamics: influence on renal function. J Am Soc Nephrol. 2004;15(Suppl 1):S58–63.
65. White SL, et al. Chronic kidney disease in the general population. Adv Chronic Kidney Dis. 2005;12(1):5–13.
66. Orth SR. Smoking and the kidney. J Am Soc Nephrol. 2002;13(6):1663–72.
67. Nasr SH, D'Agati VD. Nodular glomerulosclerosis in the nondiabetic smoker. J Am Soc Nephrol. 2007;18(7):2032–6.
68. Klag MJ, et al. Blood pressure and end-stage renal disease in men. N Engl J Med. 1996;334(1):13–8.
69. Pinto-Sietsma SJ, et al. Smoking is related to albuminuria and abnormal renal function in nondiabetic persons. Ann Intern Med. 2000;133(8):585–91.
70. Halimi JM, et al. Effects of current smoking and smoking discontinuation on renal function and proteinuria in the general population. Kidney Int. 2000;58(3):1285–92.
71. Yamagata K, et al. Risk factors for chronic kidney disease in a community-based population: a 10-year follow-up study. Kidney Int. 2007;71(2):159–66.
72. Xia J, et al. Cigarette smoking and chronic kidney disease in the general population: a systematic review and meta-analysis of prospective cohort studies. Nephrol Dial Transplant. 2017;32(3):475–87.

73. Chase HP, et al. Cigarette smoking increases the risk of albuminuria among subjects with type I diabetes. JAMA. 1991;265(5):614–7.
74. Orth SR. Cigarette smoking: an important renal risk factor – far beyond carcinogenesis. Tob Induc Dis. 2002;1(2):137–55.
75. Chuahirun T, et al. Cigarette smoking exacerbates and its cessation ameliorates renal injury in type 2 diabetes. Am J Med Sci. 2004;327(2):57–67.
76. Staplin N, et al. Smoking and adverse outcomes in patients with CKD: the Study of Heart and Renal Protection (SHARP). Am J Kidney Dis. 2016;68(3):371–80.
77. Formanek P, Salisbury-Afshar E, Afshar M. Helping patients with ESRD and earlier stages of CKD to quit smoking. Am J Kidney Dis. 2018;72(2):255–66.
78. Nastase MV, et al. Targeting renal fibrosis: mechanisms and drug delivery systems. Adv Drug Deliv Rev. 2018;129:295–307.
79. Pergola PE, et al. Bardoxolone methyl and kidney function in CKD with type 2 diabetes. N Engl J Med. 2011;365(4):327–36.
80. de Zeeuw D, et al. Bardoxolone methyl in type 2 diabetes and stage 4 chronic kidney disease. N Engl J Med. 2013;369(26):2492–503.
81. Tummalapalli SL, Powe NR, Keyhani S. Trends in quality of care for patients with CKD in the United States. Clin J Am Soc Nephrol. 2019;14(8):1142–50.

Chapter 5
Progression of CKD and Uremic Symptoms

Gurwant Kaur and Vikram Patney

Definition of Chronic Kidney Disease (CKD)

CKD is defined as below [1]:

1. GFR is <60 ml/min/1.73 m^2 (present for more than 3 months).
2. Markers of kidney damage (one or more present for more than 3 months):

   (a) Albuminuria: urine albumin $\geq$30 mg per 24 hours or urine albumin-to-creatinine ratio (ACR) $\geq$ 30 mg/g
   (b) Urinary sediment abnormalities
   (c) Markers of kidney damage such as hematuria or structural abnormalities of kidneys as per images
   (d) Renal tubular disorders
   (e) History of kidney transplantation

Clinical Presentation

Patients are asymptomatic in the early chronic kidney disease (CKD). This brings the importance of early education, intervention, and prevention of factors contributing to the progression of CKD. Subtle clues may include feeling tired, presence of

G. Kaur (✉)
Department of Medicine, Division of Nephrology at PennState Hershey Medical Center, Hershey, PA, USA

Penn State Milton S. Hershey Medical Centre, Department of Medicine (Nephrology), Hershey, PA, USA
e-mail: gkaur1@pennstatehealth.psu.edu

V. Patney
BJC Medical Group Belleville, Belleville, IL, USA

© Springer Nature Switzerland AG 2022
J. McCauley et al. (eds.), *Approaches to Chronic Kidney Disease*,
https://doi.org/10.1007/978-3-030-83082-3_5

anemia, and/or urine abnormalities. Many times routine investigations done on visits with primary care physicians detect abnormalities as mentioned in the definition of CKD and lead to diagnosis of CKD. It is very important to have the findings consistent for more than 3 months to make diagnose of CKD; timeline helps to differentiate it from acute kidney injury (AKI).

Things to Include in Routine History and Physical in a Patient with CKD

1. Asking patients if they have ever heard of CKD or if they ever have been diagnosed with CKD is important to get an idea about their baseline understanding of the disease process.
2. Inquiring about the use of nonsteroidal anti-inflammatory drugs (NSAID) and the duration of intake (weeks to months or years) is crucial. Getting history about chronic pains to help get to the history of use of such drugs would be helpful (e.g., chronic headaches, back or joint pains, or severe pain during menstruation in females).
3. Getting details regarding any prior episodes of AKI is vital along with details of dialysis if it was needed.
4. Any significant history of repeated urinary tract infections (UTIs) since birth or early childhood.

Making Use of Existing Laboratory Data and Imaging Studies

1. Many patients, when evaluated in the clinic, have prior laboratory data available. Comparing the current estimated GFR (eGFR) to the previously known values is vital to get a meaningful insight into the patient's disease and its trajectory.
2. The results of previous urinalysis (UA) could provide many clues to give an idea of the abnormalities in the kidney function which might not be obvious otherwise:

    (a) Careful interpretation of UA is important to detect positivity for blood. It is important to pay attention if there were corresponding red blood cells (RBC) listed as well on UA or not. It is important to be careful in female patients to make sure they were not on their menstruation period at the time of collection of a urine sample.
    (b) Lower specific gravity can give clues regarding poor concentration ability of kidneys, which can happen with CKD and with advanced age.
    (c) Assess for proteinuria on UA and see if quantification is available, either as urine albumin-to-creatinine ratio (ACR) or urine protein-to-creatinine (UPC) ratio.
    (d) The presence of any crystals would aid in defining the etiology in certain cases for CKD.

3. A dedicated ultrasound of kidneys or any other imaging (e.g., computed tomography of the abdomen), done for some unrelated health problem in the past, could be used to evaluate the anatomy of kidneys. A plan abdominal x-ray can help to detect calcification of kidney parenchyma (nephrocalcinosis) or a stone in the urinary system (nephrolithiasis).

CKD and Its Risk Factors

Patients with any of the following risk factors [1] are at higher risk of CKD and should be followed closely:

- Diabetes mellitus (DM)
- Hypertension
- AKI
- Cardiovascular disease (chronic heart failure, post heart transplant, cerebral vascular disease, peripheral vascular disease, ischemic heart disease)
- Presence of hematuria or proteinuria
- Obesity
- Smoking
- Ethnic minority status
- Family history of CKD, ESRD, or any hereditary kidney disease
- Kidney stones, renal tract structural changes, or prostate hypertrophy
- Systemic diseases, e.g., systemic lupus nephritis (SLE), and multiple myeloma (MM), etc.

Etiology of CKD

- Diabetes and hypertension have been the leading causes of CKD globally
- Glomerulonephritis
- Tubulointerstitial and vascular diseases (renal artery/vein thrombosis)
- Multiple and recurrent AKIs
- NSAIDS and contrast exposure
- Infections (e.g., human immunodeficiency virus (HIV), hepatitis especially hepatitis B virus and hepatitis C virus)
- Environmental exposures nephropathy, herbal remedies, and pesticides as proposed in Mesoamerican nephropathy
- CKD in presence of other systemic diseases (e.g., in the heart, liver disorders, and chronic rheumatological disorders)
- Any congenital (congenital aplasia or absence of one kidney, polycystic kidney disease) or acquired loss of nephron mass (resection for renal cell carcinoma)

Stages of CKD and Its Progression

CKD is categorized into five different stages based on eGFR; it is classified as G1 when eGFR is ≥90 mL/min/1.73 m^2), G2 when eGFR is between 60 and 89 mL/min/1.73 m^2), G3a when eGFR is between 45 and 59 mL/min/1.73 m^2, G3b when eGFR is between 30 and 44 mL/min/1.73 m^2, G4 when eGFR is between 15 and 29 mL/min/1.73 m^2, and G5 when eGFR is <15 mL/min/1.73 m^2 as given in Fig. 5.1. Albuminuria staging is classified as A1 when urine ACR <30 mg/g, A2 when ACR is between 30 and 300 mg/g, and A3 when it is >300 mg/g as shown in Fig. 5.2.

Based on the above classification, if a patient has eGFR of 38 ml/min/1.73 m^2 and albuminuria of 280 mg/g for more than 3 months, the patient will be categorized as CKD3bA2. In order to assess for progression, these need to be followed up closely over a period of time.

CKD and Its Progression

During a discussion with the patients, the most valuable question to answer is regarding the progression of CKD. Identifying the risk factors and trying to delineate the etiology of CKD is highly important as well. In this chapter, we will discuss the factors that help determine the progression of CKD. The answer is very broad. It really depends on the cause of CKD and nature of the comorbidities that we are dealing with.

Stage		Description	eGFR(ml/min/1.73m2)
G1		Normal or high	≥ 90
G2		Mild decrease	60-89
G3	G3a	Mild - moderate	45-59
	G3b	Moderate - severe	30-44
G4		Severe decrease	15-29
G5		Kidney Failure	<15

Fig. 5.1 Stages of chronic kidney disease; eGFR indicates glomerular filtration rate [1]. (Modified) KDIGO: Kidney Disease Improving Global Outcomes (2012)

Urine albumin/creatinine ratio (mg/gm)		
A1	<30	Normal – mild increase
A2	30-300	Moderate increase
A3	>300	Severe increase

Fig. 5.2 Categorization of chronic kidney disease as per albuminuria [1]. (Modified) KDIGO: Kidney Disease Improving Global Outcomes (2012)

Definition of CKD Progression and Its Assessment

The main determinant of the progression is the cause of CKD; and its progression is assessed by values of eGFR and albuminuria:

- A clear definition of CKD progression, which is reliable and reproducible is lacking. Rapid progression may be used based on the outcomes considered, such as kidney failure versus death [2].
- CKD progression is inevitable [3]. The natural course of CKD is its progression as evident by the decline in eGFR, eventually leading to ESRD. eGFR and albuminuria are checked to assess its rate of progression [4]. The reduction in the decline in renal function leads to significant benefits, in terms of delaying CKD progression to its natural course to ESRD and delaying or reducing the needs of dialysis.
- The rate of CKD progression varies based on the presence of risk factors and co-morbidities among individuals with the same cause of CKD or a similar degree of functional impairment.
- Close monitoring of CKD is required based on individual risk profile and overall clinical context. All patients with CKD do not require intense monitoring [5].
- As the kidney function declines, it would need more frequent clinical assessment with history taking to get details of symptoms and physical examination. Close monitoring of metabolic picture to assess the trends in eGFR, serum creatinine along with serum electrolytes, and urine studies for proteinuria is required. The expertise and clinical judgment of the treating physicians are the key features of the care.

Disclosing to Patients

Disclosing a diagnosis of CKD can be very distressing and uncomfortable on the part of the treating physician as well as on the patient. Lower kidney function may not be abnormal in advanced age in an asymptomatic patient. The word "chronic" can be very stress-provoking and can give rise to a chain of thoughts of "seriousness," and the word "kidney disease" immediately makes them to start thinking on lines of dialysis or a transplant. It might be more appropriate to determine if the decline in eGFR is age appropriate or its age inappropriate to have a better acceptance from patients' perspective [6].

Referral to a Nephrologist

Patients should be referred to a nephrologist when eGFR falls below 30 mL/min/1.73 m^2, to discuss and plan for RRT. Late referral to the nephrologist can happen due to asymptomatic CKD presenting in an advanced stage, patient's refusal to seek help until symptomatic, AKI leading to ESRD, socioeconomic barriers, referral bias among the physicians, and health system variabilities. Based on the geography of the practice, wait time for referrals may vary from place to place. It is always a good idea to be familiar with the specialists available in your area. Urgent referrals for symptomatic and advanced CKD patients are accepted on a priority basis in most practices.

Natural History of Renal Disease

After an insult to the kidneys, the clinical manifestations can vary from being asymptomatic to long-term sequel and need of renal replacement therapy. As an adaptive process to the injury, the nephrons undergo change to maintain the filtration rate. This involves increasing the filtration rate by remaining nephrons and is called adaptive hyperfiltration. This process is beneficial initially; however, it can result in long-term damage in the nephrons and their glomeruli. It manifests as proteinuria and advancement in renal failure. It sets the chronic changes including atrophy of tubules, interstitial fibrosis, and glomerulosclerosis.

Among the patients with CKD, the rate of decline in kidney function is nonlinear. It varies among the individuals depending upon the underlying etiology of CKD, extent of the comorbidities, socioeconomic status, individual genetic variations, ethnicity, and other factors. Episodes of AKI may add to the additional progression of CKD and eventually leading to ESRD [7].

With aging, there are structural and functional changes that happen in the body organs. Similarly, kidneys undergo senescence changes. Changes in kidney volume and the appearance of renal cysts constitute the macroanatomic changes. Cortical thinning with loss of nephrons, glomerulosclerosis along with tubular atrophy (TA) and interstitial fibrosis (IF) constitute the microanatomic changes. Loss of GFR is the functional change. The distinction between normal aging processes vs. pathological decline in GFR from a preventable or treatable disease process is important. However, the current classification of CKD doesn't account for age. It is also important to note that there are no therapies available till date to prevent age-related decline in GFR. Lower nephron reserve in older individuals makes them more prone to the risk of AKI.

Pathophysiology of CKD and Its Progression

Chronic changes in tubules and interstitial tissue as TA and IF, respectively, are the dominant pathological findings in CKD. Repeated, frequent, and are the result of especially severe AKIs are emerging as a significant cause of CKD and its progression to ESRD. These are the result of maladaptive repair after initial AKI and involves inflammatory mediators along with individual factors such as age, gender, genetics, and chronic comorbid conditions [8]. This interrelationship between AKI, CKD, and ESRD is depicted in Fig. 5.3. Even a single episode of AKI would raise the risk of CKD [9]. The severity of CKD and its progression will depend on the remaining functioning nephrons and the extent of scarring in the interstitium. Drugs such as NSAIDS, antibiotics, etc. can affect the healthy renal parenchyma with interstitial inflammation and can lead to IF. Vascular damage as in conditions such as vasculitis, chronic ischemia as part of cardiovascular disorders or as part of system diseases such as DM and SLE, etc. can affect the vasculature and glomerular capillary endothelium and sets the overwhelming inflammation that leads the pathways to TA and IF as a result. CKD is a state of chronic inflammation. Activation of RAAS plays a significant role in the progression of CKD. The presence of an angiotensin-converting enzyme (ACE) in the brush border membrane of the proximal tubule [10] sets a local activation of RAAS. ACE has also been detected

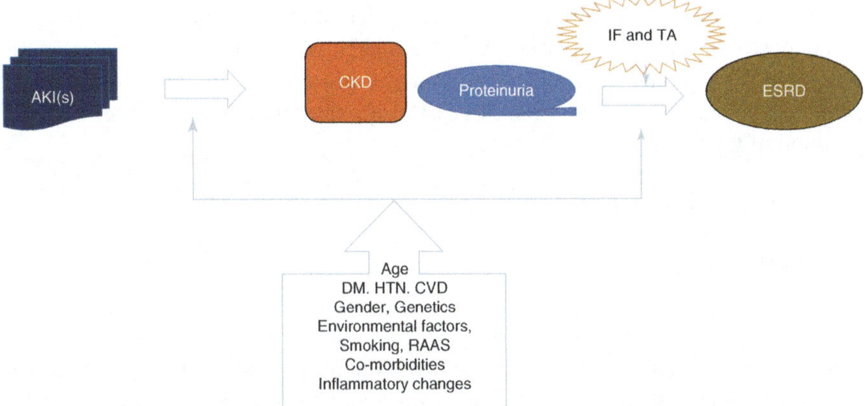

Fig. 5.3 The relationship between AKI, CKD, and ESRD and contributing factors. (AKI, acute kidney injury; CKD, chronic kidney disease; ESRD, end-stage renal disease; DM, diabetes mellitus; HTN, hypertension; CVD, cardiovascular disease; RAAS, renin-angiotensin-aldosterone system; IF, interstitial fibrosis; TA, tubular atrophy)

in a tubular fluid of distal tubules. Angiotensin II also drives the fibrosis in renal tissue.

Factors to Predict the Progression of CKD

Many factors have been identified that are associated with the rapid loss of kidney function. These include the adaptive hyperfiltration including intraglomerular hypertension and glomerular hypertrophy, albuminuria, uncontrolled HTN, hyperglycemia, and black race.

Intraglomerular Hypertension and Glomerular Hypertrophy

As a compensatory response to lost nephrons, the remaining nephrons attempt to increase glomerular pressure to maintain GFR. The fall in GFR is minimized by renal vasodilation, increasing the intraglomerular pressure and glomerular size. However, these adaptations happen at a cost by reduced flow to the macula densa and leading to activation of tubuloglomerular feedback. This disturbs the physiological autoregulation of glomerular pressure in the kidneys. The RAAS regulates the vascular tone of the renal vasculature and maintains salt and water balance along with controlling the tissue growth in the kidney [11]. Prolonged RAAS activation leads to systemic and glomerular capillary hypertension that results in vascular endothelial damage. Increased wall stress may lead to detachment of glomerular epithelial cells (podocytes) from the glomerular capillary wall. Kidney injury is also aided by increased strain on the mesangial cells. Mesangial cell stretch leads to expansion of the mesangium and glomerulosclerosis by stimulating the synthesis and deposition of extracellular matrix (ECM) [12]. Additionally, kidney damage is promoted by angiotensin II and aldosterone by pro-fibrotic and pro-inflammatory actions. This makes the inhibition of RAAS an important target to reduce the progression of CKD.

Proteinuria

Proteinuria has been identified as a pathogen for the progression of renal disease. Lowering the proteinuria shields kidney from the progression of CKD both in diabetic and in non-diabetic patients. The presence of proteinuria increases the cardiovascular and overall mortality [13] in CKD patients. This is also the best predictor of CKD progression in nondiabetics with proteinuria [14]. Among diabetic patients, the absence of albuminuria or proteinuria carried a much lower rate of CKD progression compared with those with these abnormalities [15]. Multiple factors can contribute to kidney damage from albuminuria, including toxicity to mesangial cells, tubular overload, and their hyperplasia. Specific filtered substances, e.g., iron/transferrin and albumin-bound fatty acids, can induce toxicity as well. Blood pressure control is an important element to limit the proteinuria. Glomerular epithelial cell (podocyte) injury leads to albuminuria, and cell injury may play a significant role in setting the glomerulosclerosis changes.

Tubulointerstitial Fibrosis

Tubular cell thinning and atrophy, dilatation of the tubular lumen, and fibrotic changes in the interstitium mark the chronic and irreversible damage to kidney tissue. These changes are a predictor of long-term prognosis and GFR in chronic progressive kidney diseases.

Diabetes Mellitus and CKD

DM is one of the leading causes of CKD. Diabetic nephropathy (DN) is one of the commonly encountered the complication of DM. Diabetic kidney disease is discussed in detail in this book in Chapter 4a. Diabetics have a rapid decline in GFR than nondiabetics [16]. Disturbed glomerular hemodynamics, adaptive glomerular hyperfiltration along with oxidative stress and inflammation from advanced glycation end products (AGE), and impaired tubuloglomerular feedback play a major role in the pathogenesis of CKD in diabetic patients. Glomerular hypertrophy (mesangial cell hypertrophy and ECM accumulation), TA, and IF are the dominant pathological findings.

Metabolic Acidosis

With progressive damage and reduction in the total number of functioning nephrons, the remaining nephrons adapt to excrete more acid. Acid is excreted mainly as ammonium (H^+ are excreted as NH_4Cl). The accumulation of ammonia activates the complement system and leads to tubulointerstitial damage. Limiting the ammonia production by the use of alkali therapy helps prevent the progression of renal injury.

Uric Acid

Uric acid being a small filterable molecule has an inverse relationship with GFR. High uric acid levels could result from lower clearance in advanced CKD. Baseline high uric acid levels when renal function is preserved have more relevance for kidney failure than at advanced CKD with lower GFR. Data is inconsistent regarding the routine use of uric acid-lowering medications and their impact on CKD progression. It is shown to have a J-shaped curve in relation to all-cause mortality [17].

Use of Smoking and Illicit Drugs

The use of illicit drugs (cocaine, marijuana, and heroin) and tobacco anytime in life was associated with a higher risk of CKD progression and all-cause mortality [18].

Interaction with Healthcare Professionals

Poor patient experience in their interactions with primary care physicians (PCP) was associated in an observational study with a higher risk of hospital admissions among Hispanic patients with CKD, but not with death or ESRD incidence [19].

Taking a Charge of Own Health

Individual engagement in CKD self-management behaviors is shown to be associated with clinical outcomes. Poor outcomes have resulted in those who do not participate in recommended behaviors. Better engagement could be protective in the progression of CKD, especially in diabetics. It is to be noted that emotional problems and cognitive dysfunction play an important role to prevent adherence to recommended self-management [20]. Higher medication nonadherence as self-reported by patients of CKD was found to be associated with a higher decline in GFR [21].

Socioeconomic Impact

After controlling for sociodemographic and clinical aspects, individuals with lower education status have more albuminuria and decreased GFR. The odds of lower kidney function was 11% lower among college graduates comparing with individuals not graduating high school [22]. Among both blacks and whites, neighborhood poverty was strongly associated with a higher incidence of ESRD [23]. Language barrier, literacy level, lack of transportation to medical professionals, health insurance coverage, out-of-pocket cost, and personal beliefs shape the complex interplay between socioeconomic, cultural, and psychosocial factors when looking in CKD and its progression.

APOL1 Genotype in African Americans (AA)

Apolipoprotein L-1 (APOL1) gene includes:

I. G1 allele (substitutions of serine for glycine and isoleucine for methionine, at positions 342 and 384, respectively).
II. G2 allele (deletion of the two amino acids asparagine and tyrosine from positions 388 and 389).

It is important to mention that in the AA population, in order to develop CKD from these genetic variations, it requires a "second hit" in form of another risk factor or health event, which in the presence of these underlying genetic changes leads to increased risk of CKD.

High-risk genotypes, e.g., homozygous (G1/G1, G2/G2) or compound heterozygote (G1/G2), presents with an increased risk of renal issues [24]. 13% of AA are found to have two of the APOL1 high-risk alleles; only 20% of AA with high-risk genotype develop ESRD [25]. This leads to a twofold increase in the risk of CKD; seven- to tenfolds increase the risk of nondiabetic ESRD and increased risk of kidney transplant failure [26–28]. Grafts from kidney donors who had variants presented worse survival [24]. High-risk genotypes are associated with a 17-fold increased risk of primary focal segmental glomerulosclerosis (FSGS), 29-fold increased risk of HIV-associated nephropathy, 7-fold increased risk of hypertensive nephrosclerosis, and 3-fold increased risk of lupus nephritis in AA patients as compared to non-African American patients [29, 30]. Interestingly, these genetic variations provide protection from a parasitic disease from *trypanosomiasis* in the endemic regions.

Managing Progression of CKD Details on the prevention of progression of CKD are discussed in Chapter 3b in this book. Overall, it includes:

1. Blood pressure control
2. Diabetes control
3. Control of proteinuria
4. Weight reduction
5. Smoking cessation
6. Stability of co-morbidities (e.g., cardiac and liver function in cardiorenal and hepatorenal, respectively)
7. Treatment of infections (hepatitis B and C virus, HIV, etc.)

8. Stopping any offending agents (e.g., NSAIDs)
9. Minimizing and reserving contrast exposure to indications when no alternatives are available. Exposure to contrast agents needs to be assessed on an individual basis if it would change the management.

In order to understand ways to stop progression of CKD, it is highly important to understand the risk factors as mentioned before in this chapter and the underlying pathophysiology of CKD.

CKD Manifestations and Their Management

Progression of CKD has the following clinical and biochemical changes:

(a) Metabolic: hyperkalemia
(b) Acid-base: metabolic acidosis
(c) Anemia
(d) Bone and mineral disorders, secondary hyperparathyroidism
(e) Volume status/blood pressure
(f) Uremic symptoms

Uremia

The term uremia or uremic syndrome refers to the symptoms and signs that occur in kidney failure that cannot be explained by volume overload, abnormal inorganic ion concentrations, or lack of hormones like erythropoietin that are secreted by normally functioning kidneys. Uremia is thought to be caused by nitrogenous and other organic waste accumulation in the body due to kidney failure [31]. The definition of uremia has changed over time due to an improved understanding of the pathogenesis of conditions like tetany, hyperkalemia, acidosis, hypertension, and anemia that are commonly associated with kidney failure and with the advent of renal replacement modalities like dialysis and renal transplantation.

Pathogenesis of Uremia

The symptoms due to uremia are thought to be due to the retention of organic solutes due to kidney failure. These retained solutes cause direct toxic effects, as well as post translational protein modifications that lead to atherogenesis, insulin resistance, increased free radical production, apoptosis, and disruption of normal cellular function [32]. While urea is quantitatively the most important organic solute that accumulates in the blood of patients with kidney failure, multiple retained organic solutes are thought to be responsible for the symptoms of uremia [33]. Many researchers including the European Uremic Toxin Work Group have identified more than 100 solutes that are retained in kidney failure [34]. Due to the retention of multiple solutes and the variety and subtlety of uremic symptoms, it is difficult to identify the responsible solutes. The failure to identify the solutes that are toxic limits our ability to tailor our therapy towards the removal of these solutes with dialysis or other modalities [35]. Urea is the organic solute that is excreted out by the kidneys in the largest quantities and is easy to measure. For convenience, urea is used as a "representative" solute to measure the adequacy of dialysis in removing uremic toxins. However, it is well-known that the dialysis as currently prescribed is effective at removing smaller solutes like urea as compared to larger solutes like beta 2 -microglobulin and myoglobin. This may result in the persistence of some uremic symptoms even in patients with kidney failure who are on dialysis. This has been named the residual syndrome by Depner and consists of inadequately treated uremia and effects due to dialysis-induced shifts in extracellular volume as well as inorganic ion disturbances [36].

Signs and Symptoms of Uremia

The symptoms of uremia have an insidious onset and may start appearing in varying severity as GFR drops below 60 ml/min/1.73 m^2. Early symptoms of uremia-like fatigue are nonspecific and easy to overlook. These symptoms are easier to identify in advanced stages of chronic kidney disease when the GFR is in the 10–15 ml/min/1.73 m^2. These can include the following [31]:

- Fatigue
- Altered mental status
- Seizures
- Coma
- Sleep disturbances
- Restless legs
- Peripheral neuropathy
- Anorexia
- Nausea
- Altered taste and smell
- Itching
- Cramps
- Hiccups
- Amenorrhea and sexual dysfunction
- Muscle wasting
- Serositis (includes pericarditis)
- Growth retardation in children
- Intrauterine growth retardation in the fetus

Uremia can lead to the following metabolic effects including:

- Insulin resistance
- Reduced resting energy expenditure
- Reduced body temperature
- Increased oxidant levels
- Albumin oxidation

The cellular effects from uremia may include:

- Platelet dysfunction
- Granulocyte and lymphocyte dysfunction
- Shortened erythrocyte survival

It is important to recognize the relationship between uremia and the co-occurrence of malnutrition, inflammation, and atherosclerosis (malnutrition-inflammation-atherosclerosis syndrome or the MIA syndrome) in patients with advanced CKD and ESRD. Malnutrition is associated with increased mortality in patients on dialysis. Uremic toxins cause increased oxidative stress, insulin resistance, endothelial dysfunction, and worsening atherosclerosis that increases cardiovascular mortality in these patients. In addition, the sense of well-being and the ability to function productively in daily life are impaired in patients with advanced chronic kidney disease [37]. It is likely that the symptoms of uremia have a dominant role in the poor quality of life experienced by these patients. Hence, it is important to recognize symptoms of uremia in patients with advanced CKD and to plan treatment before the patient becomes severely malnourished, starts losing weight, or becomes debilitated before start of dialysis or transplantation.

Approach to Management of Uremia

The initiation of dialysis (hemodialysis or peritoneal dialysis) is the dominant treatment modality for the management of uremia and other complications of ESRD. The indications to start dialysis due to uremia include the occurrence of weight loss due to anorexia, altered taste, nausea, and vomiting. It also includes uremic pericarditis, bleeding, and encephalopathy. Other indications to start dialysis include hyperkalemia, volume overload, and acidemia that are refractory to medical therapy. The initiation of dialysis helps in attenuating the symptoms of uremia, but only renal transplantation ameliorates the "residual syndrome" and is the renal replacement therapy of choice. Lowering the daily protein intake to 0.6–0.8 g/kg body weight/day has been used to slow down the progression of chronic kidney disease in patients with a GFR of less than 45 ml/min and to mitigate uremic symptoms and transition to dialysis in more advanced chronic kidney disease [38, 39]. The need for renoprotection should be balanced with the risk of protein energy malnutrition which is a predictor of poor prognosis in these patients. Hence, it is best not to lower protein intake to less than 0.8 g/kg body weight/day and to consider a temporary increase in protein intake to 1 g/kg body weight/day in times of acute illness and catabolic states or when the patient has protein energy malnutrition.

Conclusion

CKD is a global health problem and is associated with significant morbidity and mortality, especially cardiovascular consequences. Early detection and altering the modifiable factors and aiming at the underlying cause is the key in assessing, monitoring, and preventing the CKD progression.

Acknowledgements Not applicable.

Competing Interests The authors declare that they have no competing interests.

Availability of Data and Materials Data sharing is not applicable to this article as no datasets were generated or analyzed during this study.

Consent for Publication This is not applicable for this review.

Ethics Approval and Consent to Participate Not applicable.

Funding Funding information is not applicable.

References

1. Kidney Disease: Improving Global Outcomes (KDIGO) CKD Work Group. KDIGO 2012 Clinical practice guideline for the evaluation and management of chronic kidney disease. Kidney Int Suppl. 2013;3:1–150.
2. Chapter 2: definition, identification, and prediction of CKD progression. Kidney Int Suppl (2011). 2013;3(1):63–72.
3. Sharaf El Din UA, Salem MM, Abdulazim DO. Stop chronic kidney disease progression: time is approaching. World J Nephrol. 2016;5(3):258–73.
4. Kuro OM. A phosphate-centric paradigm for pathophysiology and therapy of chronic kidney disease. Kidney Int Suppl (2011). 2013;3(5):420–6.
5. Eftimovska N, Stojceva-Taneva O, Polenakovic M. Slow progression of chronic kidney disease and what it is associated with. Prilozi. 2008;29(1):153–65.
6. Stevens RJ, Evans J, Oke J, Smart B, Hobbs FDR, Holloway E, et al. Kidney age, not kidney disease. CMAJ. 2018;190(13):E389–E93.
7. Li L, Astor BC, Lewis J, Hu B, Appel LJ, Lipkowitz MS, et al. Longitudinal progression trajectory of GFR among patients with CKD. Am J Kidney Dis. 2012;59(4):504–12.
8. Yang L. How acute kidney injury contributes to renal fibrosis. Adv Exp Med Biol. 2019;1165:117–42.
9. Thakar CV, Christianson A, Himmelfarb J, Leonard AC. Acute kidney injury episodes and chronic kidney disease risk in diabetes mellitus. Clin J Am Soc Nephrol. 2011;6(11):2567–72.

10. Sibony M, Gasc J-M, Soubrier F, Alhenc-Gelas F, Corvol P. Gene expression and tissue localization of the two isoforms of angiotensin I converting enzyme. Hypertension. 1993;21(6_pt_1):827–35.
11. Brewster UC, Perazella MA. The renin-angiotensin-aldosterone system and the kidney: effects on kidney disease. Am J Med. 2004;116(4):263–72.
12. Cortes P, Riser BL, Yee J, Narins RG. Mechanical strain of glomerular mesangial cells in the pathogenesis of glomerulosclerosis: clinical implications. Nephrol Dial Transplant. 1999;14(6):1351–4.
13. Culleton BF, Larson MG, Parfrey PS, Kannel WB, Levy D. Proteinuria as a risk factor for cardiovascular disease and mortality in older people: a prospective study. Am J Med. 2000;109(1):1–8.
14. Ruggenenti P, Perna A, Mosconi L, Pisoni R, Remuzzi G. Urinary protein excretion rate is the best independent predictor of ESRF in non-diabetic proteinuric chronic nephropathies. "Gruppo Italiano di Studi Epidemiologici in Nefrologia" (GISEN). Kidney Int. 1998;53(5):1209–16.
15. Koye DN, Magliano DJ, Reid CM, Jepson C, Feldman HI, Herman WH, et al. Risk of progression of nonalbuminuric CKD to end-stage kidney disease in people with diabetes: the CRIC (Chronic Renal Insufficiency Cohort) Study. Am J Kidney Dis. 2018;72(5):653–61.
16. Hemmelgarn B, Zhang J, Manns B, Tonelli M, Larsen E, Ghali W, et al. Progression of kidney dysfunction in the community-dwelling elderly. Kidney Int. 2006;69(12):2155–61.
17. Srivastava A, Kaze AD, McMullan CJ, Isakova T, Waikar SS. Uric acid and the risks of kidney failure and death in individuals with CKD. Am J Kidney Dis. 2018;71(3):362–70.
18. Bundy JD, Bazzano LA, Xie D, Cohan J, Dolata J, Fink JC, et al. Self-reported tobacco, alcohol, and illicit drug use and progression of chronic kidney disease. Clin J Am Soc Nephrol. 2018;13(7):993–1001.
19. Cedillo-Couvert EA, Hsu JY, Ricardo AC, Fischer MJ, Gerber BS, Horwitz EJ, et al. Patient experience with primary care physician and risk for hospitalization in Hispanics with CKD. Clin J Am Soc Nephrol. 2018;13(11):1659–67.
20. Schrauben SJ, Hsu JY, Rosas SE, Jaar BG, Zhang X, Deo R, et al. CKD Self-management: phenotypes and associations with clinical outcomes. Am J Kidney Dis. 2018;72(3):360–70.
21. Cedillo-Couvert EA, Ricardo AC, Chen J, Cohan J, Fischer MJ, Krousel-Wood M, et al. Self-reported medication adherence and CKD progression. Kidney Int Rep. 2018;3(3):645–51.
22. Choi AI, Weekley CC, Chen SC, Li S, Kurella Tamura M, Norris KC, et al. Association of educational attainment with chronic disease and mortality: the Kidney Early Evaluation Program (KEEP). Am J Kidney Dis. 2011;58(2):228–34.
23. Volkova N, McClellan W, Klein M, Flanders D, Kleinbaum D, Soucie JM, et al. Neighborhood poverty and racial differences in ESRD incidence. J Am Soc Nephrol. 2008;19(2):356–64.
24. Siemens TA, Riella MC, Moraes TP, Riella CV. APOL1 risk variants and kidney disease: what we know so far. J Bras Nefrol. 2018;40(4):388–402.
25. Wasser WG, Tzur S, Wolday D, Adu D, Baumstein D, Rosset S, et al. Population genetics of chronic kidney disease: the evolving story of APOL1. J Nephrol. 2012;25(5):603–18.
26. Genovese G, Friedman DJ, Ross MD, Lecordier L, Uzureau P, Freedman BI, et al. Association of trypanolytic ApoL1 variants with kidney disease in African Americans. Science. 2010;329(5993):841–5.
27. Foster MC, Coresh J, Fornage M, Astor BC, Grams M, Franceschini N, et al. APOL1 variants associate with increased risk of CKD among African Americans. J Am Soc Nephrol. 2013;24(9):1484–91.
28. Freedman BI, Julian BA, Pastan SO, Israni AK, Schladt D, Gautreaux MD, et al. Apolipoprotein L1 gene variants in deceased organ donors are associated with renal allograft failure. Am J Transplant. 2015;15(6):1615–22.
29. Kopp JB, Nelson GW, Sampath K, Johnson RC, Genovese G, An P, et al. APOL1 genetic variants in focal segmental glomerulosclerosis and HIV-associated nephropathy. J Am Soc Nephrol. 2011;22(11):2129–37.

30. Divers J, Núñez M, High KP, Murea M, Rocco MV, Ma L, et al. JC polyoma virus interacts with APOL1 in African Americans with nondiabetic nephropathy. Kidney Int. 2013;84(6):1207–13.
31. Meyer TW, Hostetter TH. The pathophysiology of uremia. Brenner & Rector's the kidney. Philadelphia: Elsevier, Inc; 2016. p. 1807–21.
32. Vanholder R, Gryp T, Glorieus G. Urea and chornic kidney disease: the comeback of the century? (in uraemia research). Nephrol Dial Transplant. 2017;12:4–12.
33. Meyer TW, Hostetter TH. Uremia. N Engl J Med. 2007;27:1316–25.
34. Duranton F, Cohen G, De Smet R, Rodriguez M, Jankowski J, Vanholder R, et al; European Uremic Toxin Work Group. Normal and pathologic concentrations of uremic toxins. J Am Soc Nephrol. 2012;23:1258–70.
35. Meyer TW, Hostetter TH. Approaches to uremia. J Am Soc Nephrol. 2014;25:2151–8.
36. Depner TA. Uremic toxicity: urea and beyond. Semin Dial. 2001;14:246–51.
37. Rogan A, McCarthy K, McGregor G, Hamborg T, Evans G, Hewins S. Quality of life measures predict cardiovascular health and physical performance in chronic renal failure patients. PLoS One. 2017;12(9):e0183926.
38. Kalantar-Zadeh K, Fouque D. Nutritional management of chronic kidney disease. N Engl J Med. 2017;377:1765–76.
39. Kovesdy CP, Kalantar-Zadeh K. Back to the future: restricted protein intake for conservative management of CKD, triple goals of renoprotection, uremia mitigation and nutritional health. Int Urol Nephrol. 2016:725–9.

Chapter 6
Diabetic Kidney Disease

Omar H. Maarouf

Introduction

Diabetic kidney disease (DKD) is a form of chronic kidney disease caused by heterogeneous factors in the setting of diabetes [1, 2]. The term DKD is introduced by the Kidney Disease Outcomes Quality Initiative (KDOQI) committee in their clinical practice guidelines in 2007 [2]. This term is used when diabetes is assumed to be the cause of kidney disease without a tissue diagnosis through a kidney biopsy. This is to make a distinction with diabetic nephropathy whereby a kidney biopsy confirms that diabetes is the culprit behind tissue damage resulting in chronic kidney disease (CKD). DKD is interwoven into cardiovascular disease and its mortality [3] making the study of its pathogenesis and potential therapies quite complicated [4].

Pathogenesis

It is believed that hyperglycemia of diabetes leads to the formation of advanced glycation end-products (AGE) complicated by increased reactive oxygen species. These byproducts will incite in situ inflammation leading to tissue damage and fibrosis at the levels of the glomerulus and its capillaries, tubule, and interstitium which constitutes CKD. Deposits of these glycosylation byproducts in the matrix were thoroughly described back in 1936 by Drs. Kimmelstiel and Wilson [5]

O. H. Maarouf (✉)
Division of Nephrology, Department of Medicine, Thomas Jefferson University, Philadelphia, PA, USA
e-mail: omar.maarouf@jefferson.edu

© Springer Nature Switzerland AG 2022
J. McCauley et al. (eds.), *Approaches to Chronic Kidney Disease*,
https://doi.org/10.1007/978-3-030-83082-3_6

whereby these classic lesions in the glomerular mesangium are now known as Kimmelstiel-Wilson nodules. Advanced glycation end products (AGEs) can lead to the activation of molecular pathways which increases local inflammation in the kidney in DKD leading to tissue fibrosis [6]. This is complicated by mesangial cell activation and expansion through the TGFβ pathway [7]. This upregulation of pro-inflammatory and profibrotic factors help recruit macrophages to the kidney furthering inflammation and worsening kidney tissue damage. Sustained insult to the kidney tissue will lead to the DKD progression to end-stage kidney disease (ESKD) [8].

Many studies showed that controlling the blood sugar is a pillar in preventing further progression of DKD as shown by long-term follow-up results of the Action in Diabetes and Vascular Disease [9]. Not only can hyperglycemia cause inflammation and fibrosis in the kidney, it can also alter the glomerular hemodynamic response. It is believed that uncontrolled serum sugar leads to renin-angiotensin-aldosterone system (RAAS) activation [10]. This RAAS activation is thought to lead to preferential afferent glomerular arteriolar vasodilation and efferent glomerular arteriolar vasoconstriction leading to increased intra-glomerular pressure and glomerular hyper-filtration (See Fig. 6.1).

The tubules affect glomerular filtration through a tubuloglomerular feedback system [11]. During hyperglycemia, the glomerular's hemodynamic response to hyperglycemia is affected by the proximal tubule handling of sugar [1, 12]. Increased delivery of sugar in the proximal tubule amplifies proximal tubule expression of sodium-glucose co-transporter-2 (SGLT2) channels increasing sugar reabsorption which drags sodium chloride (NaCl) with sugar and increases salt reabsorption.

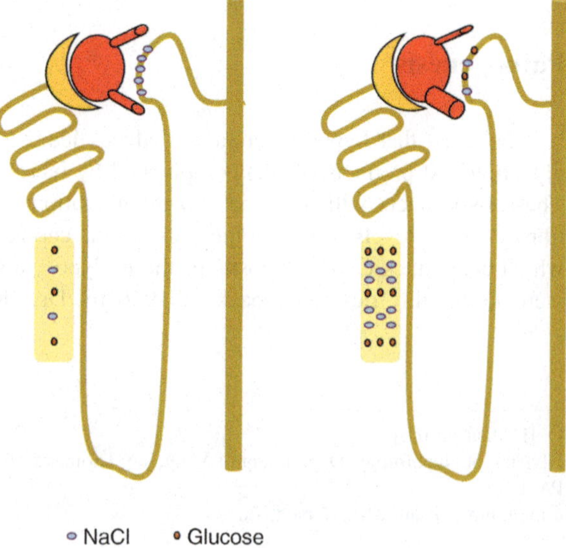

Fig. 6.1 Comparing normal renal physiology to diabetic kidney disease. Increased glucose delivery in the proximal tubule results in an increase in sodium glucose cotranspoter 2 inhibitor (SGLT2i) channels reabsorbing more glucose resulting in NaCl drag. Decreased NaCl delivery in maculae densa leads to tubuloglomerular feedback with afferent arteriole dilation and efferent arteriole constriction resulting in hyperfiltration basic pathophysiology of DKD

This results in decreased sodium chloride delivery to the macula densa. Thus, the macula densa will erroneously sense a decrease in glomerular filtration due to decreased NaCl delivery. Consequently, the afferent arteriole dilates through the tubuloglomerular feedback (TGF) leading to glomerular *hyperfiltration*. There is a differential increased response of the afferent arteriole to vasodilators like nitric oxide and prostanoids in contrast to increased vasoconstriction in the efferent arteriole to ligands like angiotensin II and endothelin 1 [13]. Both afferent vasodilation and efferent vasoconstriction lead to increased intraglomerular pressure causing hyperfiltration in DKD (see Fig. 6.1).

In DKD, hyperfiltration in the glomeruli is further complicated by decreased compliance of the arteriole [14]. The decrease in compliance decreases the autoregulatory potential of the kidneys. All of these factors lead to increased intraglomerular pressure. This tonic increase in pressure in the glomerulus will injure the glomerular structures in the nephron including podocytes, mesangial cells, and endothelial cells of the arterioles and capillaries feeding into the various nephrons. This structural injury will result in DKD progression to ESKD [15].

In DKD patients with hypertension, high blood pressure will further exacerbate hyperfiltration in the glomeruli of DKD patients. This results in further increasing the intraglomerular pressure which will perpetuate the kidney tissue injury in DKD [16].

Existing conventional therapies to slow DKD progression through RAAS blockade [17, 18] are only partially effective, and a significant remaining risk threatens DKD patients to progress to ESKD. Both studies RENAAL and IDNT show a risk reduction of only ~20% against DKD progression [19].

Incidence and Prevalence

Close to 30% of diabetics develop DKD which is the leading cause of end-stage kidney disease (ESKD) worldwide [19]. Approximately, half of the DKD patients have increased albuminuria (i.e., a urine albumin-to-creatinine ratio $\geq$ 30 mg/g) [20]. Despite this high prevalence of DKD, kidney disease awareness is surprisingly poor in the United States where only 10% of diabetics with stage 3 CKD (eGFR 30–59 mL/min/1.73 m^2) are aware of their kidney disease [21].

In type 2 diabetes, it is harder to define DKD. Type 2 diabetes can go undiagnosed for years resulting in a delay in the diagnosis and treatment of diabetes. Unlike type 1 diabetes, the disease onset of DKD in type 2 diabetes is usually beyond 40 years of age [22].

The incidence of albuminuria in type 2 diabetes is three times as much as type 1 diabetes [22]. DKD can present in a similar fashion to other CKD diseases like membranous nephropathy or paraproteinemia. DKD patients present with varying ranges of proteinuria. They also show signs of hypervolemia including lower extremity edema. Therefore, improved recognition of diabetic and nondiabetic kidney disease (NDKD) is crucial in the search of potential therapeutics [23].

Risk Factors

Age

According the CDC report in 2018, the risk DKD increases with age reaching a third of the population in the seventh decade of life. Diabetic kidney disease is an indolent disease that increases with age as longer exposure to diabetes predisposes to progressive kidney disease.

Race/Ethnicity

DKD is more prevalent in the African American and Latino communities [24]. Given that race is a social construct and not a biologic one [25], there is an increased prevalence of DKD among the population with low socioeconomic status given the lack of access to health care and healthy food and lifestyle, including exercise [26].

Obesity

Diabetic kidney disease often coexists with obesity leading to pathogenic features such as glomerular hyperfiltration, progressive albuminuria, podocyte injury, and FSGS [27]. The pathologic feature of obesity-related kidney injury is glomerular hypertrophy and adaptive focal segmental glomerulosclerosis [28]. Obesity can lead to type II diabetes and worsen the clinical course of type I [29]. Obesity and diabetes are quite interrelated risk factors for cardiovascular disease and CKD progression in DKD.

Uncontrolled Blood Sugar

There is overwhelming evidence that controlling blood sugar hinders DKD progression in both types 1 and 2 diabetes [30, 31]. Lower HbA1c results in the reversal of hyperfiltration which defines DKD [32]. Good control of blood sugar has been shown to improve albuminuria [33] and halt the rapid decline in kidney function [31].

Hypertension

Uncontrolled blood pressure leads to worsening albuminuria and DKD progression [34].

As the onset of diabetes is well-defined in type 1 diabetes, the incidence of hypertension in DKD rises significantly with age. In type 2 diabetes, half of these patients are hypertensive at the time of diagnosis. Most studies have shown that good control of blood pressure delays DKD progression independent of the class of the antihypertensive drug. In the ALLHAT trial, diabetic patients had a better outcome using low dose chlorthalidone compared to amlodipine and lisinopril as these patients achieved a lower blood pressure [35].

Multiple studies showed the benefit of using ACE inhibitors and angiotensin II receptor blockers (ARBs) to protect against the progression of DKD in types 1 and 2 diabetes especially in patients with microalbuminuria [36, 37].

When blood pressure is slightly above goal, monotherapy can be sufficient to attain blood pressure goals in diabetics with hypertension. Combination therapy is eventually required in most patients where the ACCOMPLISH trial showed the benefit of adding a long-acting dihydropyridine to the ACE inhibitor or ARB. If the patient has signs of hypervolemia like lower extremity edema or congestive heart failure, adding a loop diuretic (not a thiazide) will be helpful in controlling both the blood pressure and hypervolemia.

If we need to add more antihypertensive drugs, a beta-blocker like carvedilol may be the drug of choice with its superior benefit on sugar and microalbuminuria control.

Upon the results of the SPRINT study, we suggest a goal blood pressure of 125–130/80 mmHg which is similar to the current American Diabetes Association (ADA) guidelines [38].

Albuminuria

It has long been described in diabetic patients that microalbuminuria (30 to 300 mg/g or mg/day) is predictive of diabetic kidney disease and its progression. Later studies showed that worsening macroalbuminuria in non-insulin-dependent diabetics is predictive of DKD progression [39–41].

Recent evidence showed that significant proteinuria is not necessary for DKD progression [42]. With good diabetes control, proteinuria can regress [43, 44] even in those with nephrotic range proteinuria [45]. An interesting report from Italy involving protocol kidney biopsy in patients with diabetes and albuminuria showed only a third with typical diabetic changes while another third showed normal tissue [46]. The most important predictor of DKD progression is not the degree of proteinuria but the eGFR change with rapid decline leading to CKD progression [47].

DKD progression is variable and dependent on a myriad of factors including the patients' characteristics complicated by diabetes and other cardiovascular disease risk control. The average annual rate of GFR decline in DKD is 3 ml/min/1.73 m^2 [43, 48].

Analyzing data from the Third National Health and Nutrition Examination Survey, the researchers found out that a third of patients with the DKD do not have significant albuminuria [49]. The degree of microalbuminuria contributed to developing microvascular disease, particularly in type I diabetes [50]. By contrast, the prevalence of macrovascular disease is similar between nonalbuminuric and albuminuric DKD [51, 52]. In the third NHANES study, only a third of patients had retinopathy where proliferative retinopathy in the presence of DKD correlates with severity of tissue injury.

Role of Kidney Biopsy

The role of kidney biopsy in DKD is important when the change in urine albumin or decrease in GFR is unexpected. In the United States, most biopsies are performed when patients with DKD have CKD stage 4 or when the albuminuria has progressed to nephrotic range [53]. Data from a single-center cohort of over 600 patients with diabetes that had a kidney biopsy showed that only a third had DKD alone. Another third showed additional pathology and the last third showed nondiabetes kidney disease [54]. In this study, multivariate analysis showed that each added year of DM reduced the odds of NDRD by 5% where diabetes duration more of than 12 years was the best predictor (58% sensitivity, 73% specificity) of DN alone.

Pathology

Unlike type 1 diabetes patients who largely develop classical diabetic glomerulopathy, patients with type 2 diabetes present with various pathologic findings on their kidney biopsy [55–57].

The earliest pathology in DKD is the thickening of the glomerular basement membrane. The most classical pathology in the kidney of diabetics involves mesangial expansion complicated by segmental mesangiolysis, in which nodular is referred to as "Kimmelstiel-Wilson nodules" (See Fig. 6.2). As DKD advances, the tissue will show signs of podocyte injury including foot process effacement, and glomerulosclerosis (see Figs. 6.3 and 6.4).

Vascular injury is also seen in DKD due to subendothelial deposits of plasma proteins. This vascular injury is evident as arteriolar hyalinosis and arteriosclerosis of larger vessels. The final common pathway that mediates the progression of DKD into ESKD is tubulointerstitial fibrosis (see Table 6.1).

Progression

The natural history of DKD remains not well defined, whereby patients with DKD do not conform to a classic pattern of progression. In the United Kingdom Prospective Diabetes Study (UKPDS), less than half of patients with DM2 (40%)

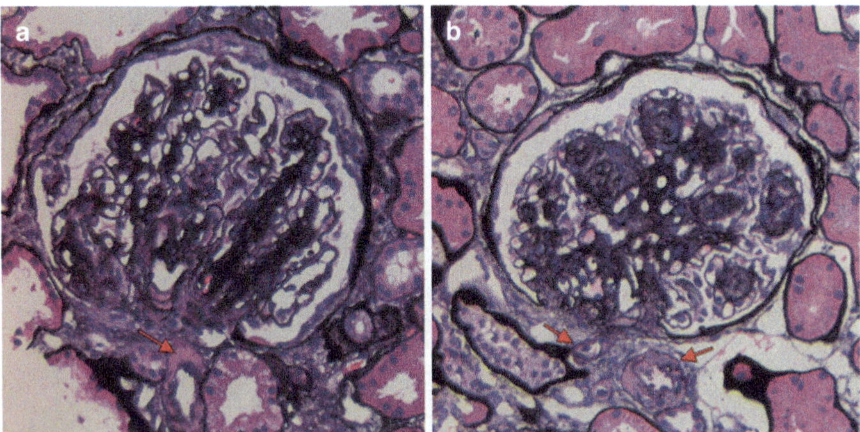

Fig. 6.2 (**a**) Diabetic nephropathy with diffuse mesangial expansion and arteriolar hyalinosis (red arrow). (**b**) Diabetic nephropathy with nodular mesangial expansion (Kimmelstiel-Wilson nodules) and concomitant hyalinosis of afferent and efferent arterioles (red arrows; Jones silver stain). (Adapted from Ref. [55])

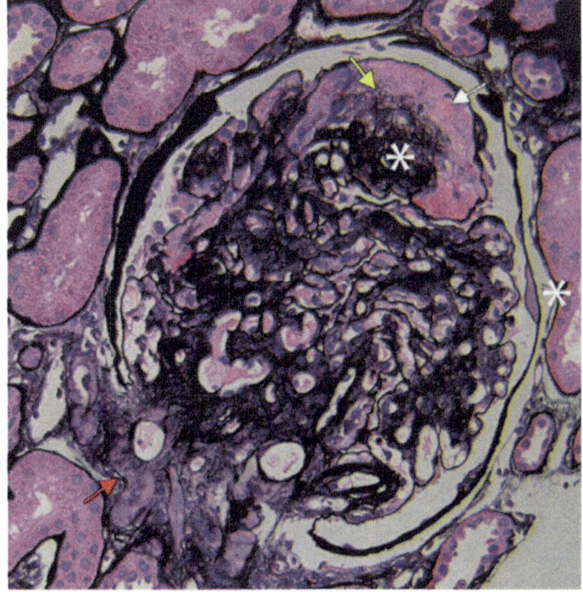

Fig. 6.3 Advanced diabetic nephropathy with Kimmelstiel-Wilson nodule (upper asterisk) with adjacent mesangiolysis (yellow arrow) and a microaneurysm (white arrow) with prominent arteriolar hyalinosis (red arrow). There is a capsular drop (lower asterisk) on the Bowman capsule (Jones silver stain). (Adapted from Ref. [55])

developed albuminuria at a median of 15 years after diagnosis, and close to third developed eGFR<60 ml/min per 1.73 m^2 [41]. The lack of albuminuria or compromised renal function does not exclude DKD structural changes in the kidney. An autopsy study showed a lack of correlation between histopathologic changes and DKD's severity and duration. Remarkably, a fifth of patients with DKD structural tissue changes did not have either albuminuria or decreased eGFR [59].

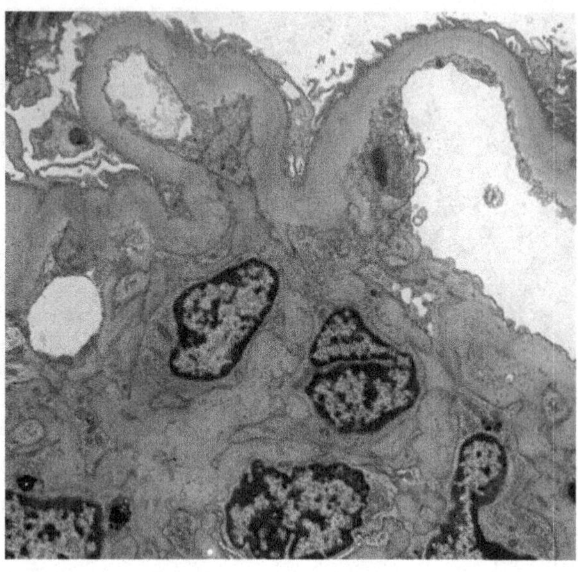

Fig. 6.4 Advanced diabetic nephropathy with prominent thickening of glomerular basement membranes with expanded mesangium, predominantly due to the increased mesangial matrix. There is segmental foot process effacement, indicative of podocyte injury (electron microscopy). (Adapted from Ref. [55])

Table 6.1 International pathologic classification of glomerular changes in diabetic kidney disease [58]

Class	Description	Inclusion criteria
1	Mild or nonspecific light microscopy changes and electron microscopy-proven GBM thickening	GBM > 395 nm in women and > 430 nm in men
2a	Mild mesangial expansion	In >25% of the observed mesangium
2b	Severe mesangial expansion	In >25% of the observed mesangium
3	Nodular sclerosis	Kimmelstiel–Wilson lesion
4	Advanced diabetic glomerulosclerosis	Global glomerular sclerosis in >50% of glomeruli

As for DKD-related complications, some studies showed that predominant tubulointerstitial disease in DKD predisposes these patients to erythropoietin deficiency leading to an increase in anemia prevalence when compared to equivalent eGFR in non-DKD CKD [60]. Remarkably, cardiovascular disease-related deaths in DKD compete with DKD progression to ESKD [61].

Treatment

When there is no direct treatment of diabetic nephropathy, controlling cardiovascular risk factors leads to the delay in the progression of DKD.

Controlling blood sugar is a cornerstone in caring for patients with DKD. In type I DM, the Diabetes Control and Complications Trial (DCCT) involving more than

1300 patients showed that intensive glucose control impairs the development of DKD [62]. ADA recommends an A1C target of <8% for patients with advanced microvascular or macrovascular complications [63].

Blood pressure control is another cornerstone in controlling the incidence of DKD and its progression. This becomes more important in the presence of significant albuminuria (urine albumin excretion >300 mg/day). Evidence of the benefit of RAAS blockade in type I diabetics has been established three decades ago where captopril prevented the cardiovascular outcome of death, ESKD. Captopril delayed progression in DKD in both hypertensive and normotensive patients [64].

As for type 2 diabetes, both the Irbesartan Diabetic Nephropathy Trial (IDNT) [17] and the Reduction of Endpoints in Non-insulin-Dependent Diabetes Mellitus with the Angiotensin II Antagonist Losartan (RENAAL) trial [18] showed delayed DKD progression and reduced ESKD incidence when using ARB to control blood pressure.

Of note, there is no major trial that shows the same benefit in non-albuminuric DKD.

These three trials on the benefit of RAAS blockade through ACEI or ARB prompted the investigation into the benefit of the combination. Two large RCTs (the Veterans Affairs Nephropathy in Diabetes study (VA NEPHRON-D) [65] and Ongoing Telmisartan Alone and in Combination with Ramipril Global Endpoint Trial (ONTARGET) [66]) showed an unexpectedly worse renal outcome from the combination ACEI+ARB therapy. The VA NEPHRON-D trial had to be halted prematurely.

Diabetic patients with kidney disease are at increased CV risk. Dyslipidemia is a known CV risk factor where statin therapy in DKD is recommended [67].

Sodium-glucose co-transporter-2 (SGLT2) inhibitors (SGLT2i) are a new category of drugs recently developed to control blood sugars and have sparked great interest in the renal community given its apparent benefit in cardiovascular disease outcome including decreased overall mortality.

SGLT2i blocks glucose reabsorption in the proximal tubule through SGLT2 channels leading to substantial glycosuria. In diabetes, the increased expression of SGLT2i channels results in increased glucose reabsorption in the proximal tubular (PT). This glucose reabsorption causes a drag of NaCl from the urinary space into the PT leading to salt retention. Thus, the decreased NaCl delivery to macula densa (MD) leads to increased intraglomerular pressure through a tubular-glomerular feedback mechanism with afferent arteriole dilation and increased GFR and subsequent hyperfiltration. Inhibiting these channels leads to increased Na delivery to the MD and subsequently decreased intra-glomerular pressure and restoration of GFR (see Fig. 6.5).

The best evidence on the effect of SGLT2i comes from the Canagliflozin and Renal Events in Diabetes with Established Nephropathy Clinical Evaluation (CREDENCE) trial involving patients with DKD and urine ACR >300 mg/g. The CREDENCE trial showed improved renal and cardiovascular outcome and decreased overall mortality [68]. In a metanalysis of several trials of people with diabetes, SGLT2i reduced ESKD and renal death [69]. They also showed that the benefit of SGLT2i is independent of baseline albuminuria. In these studies, SGLT2i

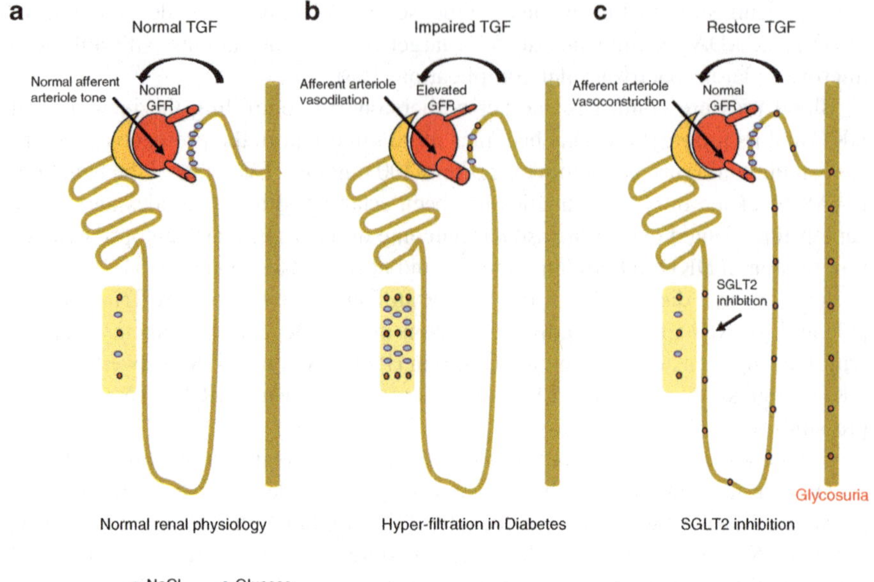

Fig. 6.5 Proposed tubuloglomerular feedback (TGF) mechanisms in normal physiology, diabetic nephropathy, and after sodium-glucose co-transporter (SGLT) 2 inhibition. (**a**) Under physiological conditions, TGF signaling maintains a stable glomerular filtration rate. (**b**) Under chronic hyperglycemic conditions (diabetes mellitus), increased proximal SGLT2-mediated reabsorption of sodium (Na+) and glucose impairs this feedback mechanism and increased renal perfusion. (**c**) SGLT2 inhibition blocks proximal tubule glucose and sodium reabsorption leading to increased sodium delivery to the macula densa and restored arteriolar tone reducing hyperfiltration

drugs reduce major cardiovascular events in patients with cardiovascular disease irrespective of sugar control.

Heart failure is a major cardiovascular complication of diabetes. After several trials showing the impressive effect on cardiovascular outcome, researchers have studied these new classes of drugs in diabetics with heart failure. In the DAPA-HF trial, the investigators studied the drug dapagliflozin in more than 4700 patients with the new New York heart Association classes 2, 3, or 4 and ejection fraction below 40%. These patients were randomized comparing dapagliflozin to placebo. They showed a clear benefit in the group taking the drug with a significant reduction in heart failure outcome and death from cardiovascular causes [70]. Another group of investigators had a similar finding of significant reduction in cardiovascular death or hospitalization in patients with heart failure using the drug empagliflozin [71]. Interestingly, this effect was regardless of the presence or absence of diabetes.

Another class of diabetes drugs with an improved renal outcome is the Glucagon-like peptide-1 receptor agonist (GLP-1-RA). These drugs improve outcome by decreasing albuminuria incidence. These drugs are safer in diabetic patients with advanced DKD [72–74].

There are no published trials evaluating renal outcome in DKD using GLP1-RA. In trials designed to assess cardiovascular outcomes in patients with

Table 6.2 Various newer hypoglycemic drug trials

Study	Drug	Patients	Outcome	Reference
SGLT2i				
CREDENCE	Canaglifozin	4401 patients eGFR: 30–89[a] uACR 0.3–5 g/g + CVD + RAAS blockade	30% RR ↓ MAKE[b]	Perkovic. New England Journal of Medicine. 2019;380:2295–2306
EMPA-REG Outcome	Empaglifozin	7020 patients eGFR ≥ 30[a] + RAAS blockade	10–60% RR ↓ MAKE[b]	Wanner. New England Journal of Medicine. 2016;375:323–334
GLP1 RA				
LEADER	Liraglutide	9340 patients eGFR ≥ 30[a] + CVD + RAAS blockade	20% RR ↓ kidney[c]	Mann, New England Journal of Medicine. 2017;377:839–848
AWARD-7	Dulaglutide	577 patients eGFR: 15–59[a] +RAAS blockade	eGFR higher 5–10% At 52 weeks	Tuttle. Lancet Diabetes Endocrinol. 2018;6:605–617

[a]eGFR: ml/min per 1.73 m^2

[b]MAKE (major adverse kidney event): a composite of ESKD, a doubling of the serum creatinine level, or death from renal or cardiovascular causes

[c]Kidney outcome: new-onset persistent macroalbuminuria, persistent doubling of the Scr level and eGFR of 45 ml or less per min/1.73 m^2, need renal-replacement therapy, or death

diabetes, GLP1-RA agents reduced renal outcome. A prespecified secondary analysis of the LEADER trial of liraglutide led to lower rates of the development and progression of diabetic kidney disease than placebo [72]. In another study designed to assess the efficacy and safety of dulaglutide in patients with type 2 diabetes and moderate-to-severe chronic kidney disease, the AWARD-7 trial showed that once-weekly dulaglutide abridged decline in eGFR. Please see Table 6.2 for a summary of the latest major trials of the newer hypoglycemic agents.

Following DKD Patient During Treatment to Control CV Risk Factors

DKD patients should be followed every 3–6 months, with assessments of blood pressure, volume status, and estimated glomerular filtration rate (eGFR) based on serum creatinine, serum potassium, glycated hemoglobin (A1C), and an evaluation of urine albumin and/or total protein. Whenever RAAS blockade is initiated, renal function should be followed in 1–2 weeks from treatment changes including the potassium level. An elevation in serum creatinine by a third above baseline is expected and is considered acceptable. This might be a sign that RAAS blockade is decreasing intraglomerular pressure and thus not a reason to discontinue therapy with these drugs. Similarly, blood pressure should be closely followed to ensure adequate control.

If hyperkalemia ensues, moderate elevation in potassium should be managed without adjusting the RAAS blockade unless the change is clinically significant.

Like RAAS blockade, clinical parameters including serum creatinine, serum potassium, blood pressure, and volume status should be followed closely in the first few weeks of commencing a sodium-glucose co-transporter 2 (SGLT2) inhibitor.

Referring patients with DKD to a nephrology service is similar to nondiabetic patients with CKD, including CKD (eGFR <30 ml/min/1.73 m^2), rapid decline in eGFR, significant proteinuria, uncontrolled hypertension, and difficult-to-manage complications of CKD (e.g., hyperkalemia, anemia). Many other nephrologists including the author of this chapter would recommend referral to nephrology when eGFR is below 60 ml/min/1.73 m^2 bearing in mind that eGFR might be higher due to hyper-filtration.

Despite good control of these CV risk factors, a considerable proportion of patients with DKD will progress to ESKD. Strong risk factors include a rapid decline in eGFR and increased albuminuria. Using available protective therapies to control CV disease can alleviate the renal decline in DKD. SGLT2 inhibitors are promising drugs that can delay or even reverse kidney disease in DKD. Of note, people with DKD are at particularly high risk of cardiovascular events, including CV death prior to progressing to ESKD. Thus, cardiovascular protective therapies are critical in DKD patients.

References

1. Vallon V, Komers R. Pathophysiology of the diabetic kidney. Compr Physiol. 2011;1(3):1175–232.
2. KDOQI. KDOQI clinical practice guidelines and clinical practice recommendations for diabetes and chronic kidney disease. Am J Kidney Dis. 2007;49(2 Suppl 2):S12–154.
3. Afkarian M, Sachs MC, Kestenbaum B, Hirsch IB, Tuttle KR, Himmelfarb J, et al. Kidney disease and increased mortality risk in type 2 diabetes. J Am Soc Nephrol. 2013;24(2): 302–8.
4. Alicic RZ, Rooney MT, Tuttle KR. Diabetic kidney disease: challenges, progress, and possibilities. Clin J Am Soc Nephrol. 2017;12(12):2032–45.
5. Kimmelstiel P, Wilson C. Intercapillary lesions in the glomeruli of the kidney. Am J Pathol. 1936;12(1):83–98.7.
6. Bierhaus A, Humpert PM, Morcos M, Wendt T, Chavakis T, Arnold B, et al. Understanding RAGE, the receptor for advanced glycation end products. J Mol Med (Berl). 2005;83(11):876–86.
7. Ziyadeh FN, Hoffman BB, Han DC, Iglesias-De La Cruz MC, Hong SW, Isono M, et al. Long-term prevention of renal insufficiency, excess matrix gene expression, and glomerular mesangial matrix expansion by treatment with monoclonal antitransforming growth factor-beta antibody in db/db diabetic mice. Proc Natl Acad Sci U S A. 2000;97(14):8015–20.

8. Tesch GH. Macrophages and diabetic nephropathy. Semin Nephrol. 2010;30(3):290–301.
9. Zoungas S, Chalmers J, Neal B, Billot L, Li Q, Hirakawa Y, et al. Follow-up of blood-pressure lowering and glucose control in type 2 diabetes. N Engl J Med. 2014;371(15): 1392–406.
10. Brenner BM. Hemodynamically mediated glomerular injury and the progressive nature of kidney disease. Kidney Int. 1983;23(4):647–55.
11. Cherney DZ, Perkins BA, Soleymanlou N, Maione M, Lai V, Lee A, et al. Renal hemodynamic effect of sodium-glucose cotransporter 2 inhibition in patients with type 1 diabetes mellitus. Circulation. 2014;129(5):587–97.
12. Fioretto P, Zambon A, Rossato M, Busetto L, Vettor R. SGLT2 Inhibitors and the diabetic kidney. Diabetes Care. 2016;39(Suppl 2):S165–71.
13. Helal I, Fick-Brosnahan GM, Reed-Gitomer B, Schrier RW. Glomerular hyperfiltration: definitions, mechanisms and clinical implications. Nat Rev Nephrol. 2012;8(5):293–300.
14. Hill JV, Findon G, Appelhoff RJ, Endre ZH. Renal autoregulation and passive pressure-flow relationships in diabetes and hypertension. Am J Physiol Renal Physiol. 2010;299(4): F837–44.
15. Hostetter TH. Hyperfiltration and glomerulosclerosis. Semin Nephrol. 2003;23(2):194–9.
16. Tuttle KR, Bakris GL, Bilous RW, Chiang JL, de Boer IH, Goldstein-Fuchs J, et al. Diabetic kidney disease: a report from an ADA Consensus Conference. Diabetes Care. 2014;37(10):2864–83.
17. Lewis EJ, Hunsicker LG, Clarke WR, Berl T, Pohl MA, Lewis JB, et al. Renoprotective effect of the angiotensin-receptor antagonist irbesartan in patients with nephropathy due to type 2 diabetes. N Engl J Med. 2001;345(12):851–60.
18. Brenner BM, Cooper ME, de Zeeuw D, Keane WF, Mitch WE, Parving HH, et al. Effects of losartan on renal and cardiovascular outcomes in patients with type 2 diabetes and nephropathy. N Engl J Med. 2001;345(12):861–9.
19. Fioretto P, Dodson PM, Ziegler D, Rosenson RS. Residual microvascular risk in diabetes: unmet needs and future directions. Nat Rev Endocrinol. 2010;6(1):19–25.
20. Afkarian M, Zelnick LR, Hall YN, Heagerty PJ, Tuttle K, Weiss NS, et al. Clinical manifestations of kidney disease among US adults with diabetes, 1988–2014. JAMA. 2016;316(6): 602–10.
21. Duru OK, Middleton T, Tewari MK, Norris K. The landscape of diabetic kidney disease in the United States. Curr Diab Rep. 2018;18(3):14.
22. Koye DN, Shaw JE, Reid CM, Atkins RC, Reutens AT, Magliano DJ. Incidence of chronic kidney disease among people with diabetes: a systematic review of observational studies. Diabet Med. 2017;34(7):887–901.
23. Anders HJ, Huber TB, Isermann B, Schiffer M. CKD in diabetes: diabetic kidney disease versus nondiabetic kidney disease. Nat Rev Nephrol. 2018;14(6):361–77.
24. Laster M, Shen JI, Norris KC. Kidney disease among African Americans: a population perspective. Am J Kidney Dis. 2018;72(5 Suppl 1):S3–7.
25. Eneanya ND, Yang W, Reese PP. Reconsidering the consequences of using race to estimate kidney function. JAMA. 2019;322(2):113–4.
26. Nicholas SB, Kalantar-Zadeh K, Norris KC. Socioeconomic disparities in chronic kidney disease. Adv Chronic Kidney Dis. 2015;22(1):6–15.
27. Bayliss G, Weinrauch LA, D'Elia JA. Pathophysiology of obesity-related renal dysfunction contributes to diabetic nephropathy. Curr Diab Rep. 2012;12(4):440–6.
28. D'Agati VD, Chagnac A, de Vries AP, Levi M, Porrini E, Herman-Edelstein M, et al. Obesity-related glomerulopathy: clinical and pathologic characteristics and pathogenesis. Nat Rev Nephrol. 2016;12(8):453–71.
29. Corbin KD, Driscoll KA, Pratley RE, Smith SR, Maahs DM, Mayer-Davis EJ, et al. Obesity in type 1 diabetes: pathophysiology, clinical impact, and mechanisms. Endocr Rev. 2018;39(5):629–63.
30. Skupien J, Warram JH, Smiles AM, Niewczas MA, Gohda T, Pezzolesi MG, et al. The early decline in renal function in patients with type 1 diabetes and proteinuria predicts the risk of end-stage renal disease. Kidney Int. 2012;82(5):589–97.

31. Zoppini G, Targher G, Chonchol M, Ortalda V, Negri C, Stoico V, et al. Predictors of estimated GFR decline in patients with type 2 diabetes and preserved kidney function. Clin J Am Soc Nephrol. 2012;7(3):401–8.
32. Tuttle KR, Bruton JL, Perusek MC, Lancaster JL, Kopp DT, DeFronzo RA. Effect of strict glycemic control on renal hemodynamic response to amino acids and renal enlargement in insulin-dependent diabetes mellitus. N Engl J Med. 1991;324(23):1626–32.
33. Perkins BA, Ficociello LH, Silva KH, Finkelstein DM, Warram JH, Krolewski AS. Regression of microalbuminuria in type 1 diabetes. N Engl J Med. 2003;348(23):2285–93.
34. Ku E, McCulloch CE, Mauer M, Gitelman SE, Grimes BA, Hsu CY. Association between blood pressure and adverse renal events in type 1 diabetes. Diabetes Care. 2016;39(12):2218–24.
35. Officers A, Coordinators for the ACRGTA, Lipid-Lowering Treatment to Prevent Heart Attack T. Major outcomes in high-risk hypertensive patients randomized to angiotensin-converting enzyme inhibitor or calcium channel blocker vs diuretic: the Antihypertensive and Lipid-Lowering Treatment to Prevent Heart Attack Trial (ALLHAT). JAMA. 2002;288(23):2981–97.
36. Captopril reduces the risk of nephropathy in IDDM patients with microalbuminuria. The Microalbuminuria Captopril Study Group. Diabetologia. 1996;39(5):587–93.
37. Viberti G, Mogensen CE, Groop LC, Pauls JF. Effect of captopril on progression to clinical proteinuria in patients with insulin-dependent diabetes mellitus and microalbuminuria. European Microalbuminuria Captopril Study Group. JAMA. 1994;271(4):275–9.
38. Group SR, Wright JT Jr, Williamson JD, Whelton PK, Snyder JK, Sink KM, et al. A randomized trial of intensive versus standard blood-pressure control. N Engl J Med. 2015;373(22):2103–16.
39. Mogensen CE, Christensen CK. Predicting diabetic nephropathy in insulin-dependent patients. N Engl J Med. 1984;311(2):89–93.
40. Nelson RG, Bennett PH, Beck GJ, Tan M, Knowler WC, Mitch WE, et al. Development and progression of renal disease in Pima Indians with non-insulin-dependent diabetes mellitus. Diabetic Renal Disease Study Group. N Engl J Med. 1996;335(22):1636–42.
41. Adler AI, Stevens RJ, Manley SE, Bilous RW, Cull CA, Holman RR, et al. Development and progression of nephropathy in type 2 diabetes: the United Kingdom Prospective Diabetes Study (UKPDS 64). Kidney Int. 2003;63(1):225–32.
42. Krolewski AS, Niewczas MA, Skupien J, Gohda T, Smiles A, Eckfeldt JH, et al. Early progressive renal decline precedes the onset of microalbuminuria and its progression to macroalbuminuria. Diabetes Care. 2014;37(1):226–34.
43. de Boer IH, Afkarian M, Rue TC, Cleary PA, Lachin JM, Molitch ME, et al. Renal outcomes in patients with type 1 diabetes and macroalbuminuria. J Am Soc Nephrol. 2014;25(10):2342–50.
44. Yokoyama H, Araki S, Honjo J, Okizaki S, Yamada D, Shudo R, et al. Association between remission of macroalbuminuria and preservation of renal function in patients with type 2 diabetes with overt proteinuria. Diabetes Care. 2013;36(10):3227–33.
45. Rossing K, Christensen PK, Hovind P, Parving HH. Remission of nephrotic-range albuminuria reduces risk of end-stage renal disease and improves survival in type 2 diabetic patients. Diabetologia. 2005;48(11):2241–7.
46. Fioretto P, Mauer M, Brocco E, Velussi M, Frigato F, Muollo B, et al. Patterns of renal injury in NIDDM patients with microalbuminuria. Diabetologia. 1996;39(12):1569–76.
47. Krolewski AS. Progressive renal decline: the new paradigm of diabetic nephropathy in type 1 diabetes. Diabetes Care. 2015;38(6):954–62.
48. Gaspari F, Ruggenenti P, Porrini E, Motterlini N, Cannata A, Carrara F, et al. The GFR and GFR decline cannot be accurately estimated in type 2 diabetics. Kidney Int. 2013;84(1):164–73.
49. Kramer HJ, Nguyen QD, Curhan G, Hsu CY. Renal insufficiency in the absence of albuminuria and retinopathy among adults with type 2 diabetes mellitus. JAMA. 2003;289(24):3273–7.
50. Nelson RG, Knowler WC, Pettitt DJ, Saad MF, Charles MA, Bennett PH. Assessment of risk of overt nephropathy in diabetic patients from albumin excretion in untimed urine specimens. Arch Intern Med. 1991;151(9):1761–5.
51. Thorn LM, Gordin D, Harjutsalo V, Hagg S, Masar R, Saraheimo M, et al. The presence and consequence of nonalbuminuric chronic kidney disease in patients with type 1 diabetes. Diabetes Care. 2015;38(11):2128–33.

52. Ito H, Takeuchi Y, Ishida H, Antoku S, Abe M, Mifune M, et al. High frequencies of diabetic micro- and macroangiopathies in patients with type 2 diabetes mellitus with decreased estimated glomerular filtration rate and normoalbuminuria. Nephrol Dial Transplant. 2010;25(4):1161–7.
53. Mottl AK, Gasim A, Schober FP, Hu Y, Dunnon AK, Hogan SL, et al. Segmental sclerosis and extracapillary hypercellularity predict diabetic ESRD. J Am Soc Nephrol. 2018;29(2):694–703.
54. Sharma SG, Bomback AS, Radhakrishnan J, Herlitz LC, Stokes MB, Markowitz GS, et al. The modern spectrum of renal biopsy findings in patients with diabetes. Clin J Am Soc Nephrol. 2013;8(10):1718–24.
55. Najafian B, Fogo AB, Lusco MA, Alpers CE. AJKD atlas of renal pathology: diabetic nephropathy. Am J Kidney Dis. 2015;66(5):e37–8.
56. Osterby R. Morphometric studies of the peripheral glomerular basement membrane in early juvenile diabetes. I. Development of initial basement membrane thickening. Diabetologia. 1972;8(2):84–92.
57. Adler S. Diabetic nephropathy: linking histology, cell biology, and genetics. Kidney Int. 2004;66(5):2095–106.
58. Tervaert TW, Mooyaart AL, Amann K, Cohen AH, Cook HT, Drachenberg CB, et al. Pathologic classification of diabetic nephropathy. J Am Soc Nephrol. 2010;21(4):556–63.
59. Klessens CQ, Woutman TD, Veraar KA, Zandbergen M, Valk EJ, Rotmans JI, et al. An autopsy study suggests that diabetic nephropathy is underdiagnosed. Kidney Int. 2016;90(1):149–56.
60. Thomas MC, Cooper ME, Rossing K, Parving HH. Anaemia in diabetes: is there a rationale to TREAT? Diabetologia. 2006;49(6):1151–7.
61. Saran R, Robinson B, Abbott KC, Bragg-Gresham J, Chen X, Gipson D, et al. US Renal data system 2019 annual data report: epidemiology of kidney disease in the United States. Am J Kidney Dis. 2020;75(1 Suppl 1):A6–7.
62. Group DER, de Boer IH, Sun W, Cleary PA, Lachin JM, Molitch ME, et al. Intensive diabetes therapy and glomerular filtration rate in type 1 diabetes. N Engl J Med. 2011;365(25):2366–76.
63. American DA. 6. Glycemic targets: standards of medical care in diabetes-2019. Diabetes Care. 2019;42(Suppl 1):S61–70.
64. Lewis EJ, Hunsicker LG, Bain RP, Rohde RD. The effect of angiotensin-converting-enzyme inhibition on diabetic nephropathy. The Collaborative Study Group. N Engl J Med. 1993;329(20):1456–62.
65. Fried LF, Emanuele N, Zhang JH, Brophy M, Conner TA, Duckworth W, et al. Combined angiotensin inhibition for the treatment of diabetic nephropathy. N Engl J Med. 2013;369(20):1892–903.
66. Investigators O, Yusuf S, Teo KK, Pogue J, Dyal L, Copland I, et al. Telmisartan, ramipril, or both in patients at high risk for vascular events. N Engl J Med. 2008;358(15):1547–59.
67. American Diabetes A. 10. Cardiovascular disease and risk management: standards of medical care in diabetes-2020. Diabetes Care. 2020;43(Suppl 1):S111–S34.
68. Perkovic V, Jardine MJ, Neal B, Bompoint S, Heerspink HJL, Charytan DM, et al. Canagliflozin and renal outcomes in type 2 diabetes and nephropathy. N Engl J Med. 2019;380(24): 2295–306.
69. Neuen BL, Young T, Heerspink HJL, Neal B, Perkovic V, Billot L, et al. SGLT2 inhibitors for the prevention of kidney failure in patients with type 2 diabetes: a systematic review and meta-analysis. Lancet Diabetes Endocrinol. 2019;7(11):845–54.
70. McMurray JJV, Solomon SD, Inzucchi SE, Kober L, Kosiborod MN, Martinez FA, et al. Dapagliflozin in patients with heart failure and reduced ejection fraction. N Engl J Med. 2019;381(21):1995–2008.
71. Packer M, Anker SD, Butler J, Filippatos G, Pocock SJ, Carson P, et al. Cardiovascular and renal outcomes with empagliflozin in heart failure. N Engl J Med. 2020;383(15):1413–24.
72. Mann JFE, Orsted DD, Brown-Frandsen K, Marso SP, Poulter NR, Rasmussen S, et al. Liraglutide and renal outcomes in type 2 diabetes. N Engl J Med. 2017;377(9):839–48.
73. Tuttle KR, Lakshmanan MC, Rayner B, Busch RS, Zimmermann AG, Woodward DB, et al. Dulaglutide versus insulin glargine in patients with type 2 diabetes and moderate-to-severe

chronic kidney disease (AWARD-7): a multicentre, open-label, randomised trial. Lancet Diabetes Endocrinol. 2018;6(8):605–17.
74. Gerstein HC, Colhoun HM, Dagenais GR, Diaz R, Lakshmanan M, Pais P, et al. Dulaglutide and renal outcomes in type 2 diabetes: an exploratory analysis of the REWIND randomised, placebo-controlled trial. Lancet. 2019;394(10193):131–8.

Chapter 7
Hypertensive Kidney Disease

Jesse M. Goldman

Introduction and Epidemiology

Definitions

The best definition of hypertensive kidney disease is kidney damage due only to hypertension. Yet, progressive kidney disease of any etiology usually results in the development of hypertension which overlays and contributes to ongoing renal injury. Over time, research has led to a better understanding of how hypertension causes kidney disease and additionally to revision of the target blood pressure to best avoid the contribution of hypertension to progressive kidney disease.

Resistant hypertension: This is defined as blood pressure not at target blood pressure goal while on adequate doses of three (or more) antihypertensive agents of different classes [1]. Classically, one agent must be a diuretic, though it is recognized that some individuals may be unable to tolerate diuretics due to complaints of urinary incontinence, gout episodes, or various side effects of other diuretics. Despite the inability to tolerate a diuretic, many of these individuals should still be classified as resistant hypertension.

Chronic kidney disease (CKD): whether due entirely to hypertension, or to another cause, CKD is defined as kidney damage for ≥ 3 months due to structural or functional abnormalities of the kidney, with or without decreased glomerular filtration rate (GFR). It is usually recognized when kidney function declines to stage 3 CKD. That is, when GFR is <60 ml/min/1.73/^{2} [2]. Within the spectrum of hypertensive kidney disease, it is appropriate to use the classification system devised by the National Kidney Foundation (NKF) of CKD stages 1–5, each higher stage being

J. M. Goldman (✉)
Division of Nephrology, Department of Medicine, Sidney Kimmel School of Medicine, Thomas Jefferson University, Philadelphia, PA, USA
e-mail: Jesse.goldman@jefferson.edu

© Springer Nature Switzerland AG 2022
J. McCauley et al. (eds.), *Approaches to Chronic Kidney Disease*,
https://doi.org/10.1007/978-3-030-83082-3_7

Table 7.1 Stages of chronic kidney disease (CKD)

Stage	Description	GFR (mL/min/1.73 m^2)
1	Kidney damage with normal or ↑ GFR	≥90
2	Kidney damage with mild ↓ GFR	60–89
3	Moderate ↓ GFR	30–59
4	Severe ↓ GFR	15–29
5	Kidney failure	<15 (or dialysis)

From: Nation Kidney Foundation K/DOKI guidelines 2020

associated with increasing cardiovascular and mortality risk. Stage 3 kidney disease has been further divided into stage 3a (GFR 59–45 ml/min) and stage 3b (GFR 44–30 ml/min), since epidemiologic studies have suggested that this transition is a tipping point from patients less likely to progress to renal failure (stage 3a) and those at higher risk more likely to progress to renal failure (stage 3b); Table 7.1.

The optimal levels of systolic and diastolic blood pressure in hypertensive CKD are still under debate since the influential SPRINT trial [3] excluded advanced CKD subjects as well as those subjects with stroke or preexisting orthostatic hypotension. Even with these restrictions, the prospective SPRINT trial showed that cardiovascular outcomes were so superior at a target blood pressure <120/80 mm Hg vs. <140/80 mm Hg that the study was prematurely terminated due to benefit in the lower blood pressure target group. However, it is also true that episodes of AKI were more common. These AKI episodes were reversible and did not transition into worsening of progressive CKD. Of note, the SPRINT trial used a specific automated office blood pressure device (AOBP) to decrease any office white coat hypertension effect. These devices may not currently be available in many offices. For that reason, the AHA guidelines recommend a target office blood pressure of <130/80 mm Hg in all CKD patients, but European guidelines recommend <130/80 in most CKD patients but <140/80 in elderly CKD patients [4]. This later recommendation is based upon concern for increased episodes of AKI.

Epidemiology of Hypertensive Kidney Disease

After diabetes, hypertensive kidney disease is the most common cause of kidney chronic dysfunction in the USA. Additionally, hypertension is the most common comorbidity seen among all patients with CKD. Both the prevalence and severity of hypertension increase with declining renal function so that the vast majority of people with advanced CKD (of any etiology) are suspected of having some component of hypertensive renal disease contributing to any underlying non-hypertensive kidney disease [5]. That is, the prevalence of difficult-to-control and resistant hypertension increases as GFR decreases, with resistant hypertension rates being reported at greater than 20% among all CKD patients [6]. This sustained elevation in BP, in turn, accelerates the progress of kidney function decline

Table 7.2 Combined risk factors for hypertension and chronic kidney disease

Older age
Obesity
Diabetes mellitus
High dietary sodium intake
Tobacco use
Atherosclerosis
Ethnic minority
Heavy ethanol consumption
Resistant hypertension
Heavy NSAID use
Obstructive sleep apnea
Heavy metal exposure

[4]. This has been termed the "vicious cycle" of hypertension and CKD. As will be discussed in the physiology section of this chapter, hypertension causes and accelerates renal injury when impaired hemodynamic auto-regulation allows the transmission of high systemic pressure to small renal arteries and glomerular capillaries, resulting in glomerular injury and subsequent glomerulosclerosis [7]. Once scarred by hypertension, those sclerotic glomeruli are never replaced but instead lost from contributing to daily kidney function forever. Additionally, CKD is clearly recognized as a risk factor for adverse cardiovascular events independent of blood pressure level [8]. Moreover, CKD and hypertension also share similar risk factors including advanced age, obesity, minority ancestry, and cigarette smoking, as well as established comorbidities such as diabetes mellitus and cardiovascular disease (Table 7.2).

The concept that hypertension is responsible for progressive renal dysfunction was first proposed by Richard Bright in 1836 [9]. HTN and CKD are closely associated with an intermingled cause-and-effect relationship. As mentioned above, blood pressure rises with decline in kidney function, and sustained elevations in BP hasten the progression of kidney disease [10]. This deleterious positive feedback relationship between worsening renal function and elevated BP has been observed in early experimental animal models of kidney injury and repeatedly in human clinical trials of hypertensive kidney disease.

The relative risk of serious renal damage in patients with uncomplicated essential hypertension is low as compared with other cardiovascular complications though, owing to the high prevalence of hypertension in the general population, it remains the second leading cause of end-stage renal disease (ESRD), with the risk being substantially higher among blacks and Latinos. Historically, hypertension-induced renal damage in patients with essential hypertension has been separated into the two distinct clinical and histological patterns: "benign" and "malignant" nephrosclerosis [11]. Benign nephrosclerosis is the pattern observed in the majority of patients with uncomplicated hypertension. Pathologists describe nonspecific vascular lesions of hyaline arteriosclerosis developing slowly with minimal or absent proteinuria. Though focal glomerular obsolescence and nephron loss occur over long periods of time, renal function is not seriously compromised except in susceptible individuals such as those with concurrent diabetes in whom the process follows a more severe and accelerated course. In contrast, "malignant" hypertensive nephrosclerosis is seen with very severe hypertension (malignant phase of essential hypertension) and shows a characteristic of acute disruptive vascular and glomerular injury with prominent fibrinoid necrosis and thrombosis. Ischemic glomeruli are frequent because of vascular injury. In general, GFR decreases with age and this development of CKD accelerates vascular aging and atherosclerotic processes. This is manifested as a decreased vascular compliance and increased arterial stiffness, which increase the development of systolic hypertension (and widened pulse pressure) in older individuals with CKD [12].

The first recognized large clinical trial to randomize individuals with advanced nephropathy to two different levels of blood pressure was the Modification of Diet in Renal Disease (MDRD) study. In this study, patients with chronic kidney disease and high rates of protein excretion were randomly assigned to a low BP group with a goal mean arterial pressure (MAP < 92 mm Hg) and a high blood pressure group (MAP < 107 mm Hg) for 4 years. At the end of the study, subjects in the low BP target group had a significantly slower reduction in GFR decline compared to subjects in the high target BP group [13]. In a meta-analysis of studies in non-diabetic kidney disease (AIPRD) study group, a systolic BP range of 110–129 mm Hg was associated with the lowest risk of kidney disease progression in patients with urine protein >1 g/day [14]. In hypertensive CKD patients with less than 1 g/day of urine protein, the data is less strong.

The Chronic Renal Insufficiency Cohort (CRIC) is an ongoing multicenter, prospective, observational cohort study of 3612 adults with established CKD (moderate stage) with a prevalence of reported hypertension equal to 86%. At the time, this compared with only a 29% hypertension rate reported in the general US population when CRIC started [15, 16]. The CRIC study began in the era (1990s) when 140/90 was the prescribed target blood pressures in the USA. Now (2020) that a blood pressure target of <130/80 is recommended, this led to re-classifying millions of people from normal blood pressure to being diagnosed with hypertension. Even with reclassification, the general population still only has a 45% hypertension prevalence: far lower than that in CKD patients. Among isolated hypertensive kidney disease, the prevalence of hypertension is obviously 100%.

Regarding more severe hypertension, 28.1% of adults with hypertension and CKD in the population-based REGARDS (Reasons for Geographic and Racial Differences in Stroke) study have apparent resistant hypertension [17]. This supports the belief that with advancing stages of CKD and the severity of HTN, clinicians must be vigilant in expecting to increase blood pressure medication as CKD worsens [18]. There is clinical evidence that resistant hypertension in CKD patients is marked by vascular inflammation [19]. Conversely, deteriorating renal function from elevated BP is clearly established by the finding of a direct relationship between the relative risk of developing end-stage kidney disease (ESKD) and BP severity [20]. In a large Japanese health registry, of nearly 100,000 individuals, people with a baseline BP near 180/100 mm Hg were 15 times more likely to develop ESKD than people with a baseline BP of 110/70 mm Hg.

Causes of Hypertensive Kidney Disease

Before describing the pathologic features specific to hypertensive kidney disease, it is helpful to describe the factors contributing to all hypertension in CKD patients.

CKD increases blood pressure through at least four distinct physiologic mechanisms. These include impaired sodium regulation [21], increased sympathetic nervous system (SNS) activity [22], increased renin-angiotensin-aldosterone system (RAAS) [23], and abnormalities in the auto-regulatory system [24]. Though clinical volume overload in CKD may be the most clinically obvious contributor to hypertension via impaired renal sodium excretion, several additional factors add to increased vascular tone in the CKD milieu. These include early vascular senescence which in turn reduced baroreceptor sensitivity, decreased vasodilation resulting from decreased nitric oxide, elevated autonomic sympathetic tone, and increased activity of the renin-angiotensin-aldosterone system and activation of the vasoconstricting endothelin system.

Impaired Sodium Excretion

The result of impaired sodium excretion in hypertensive kidney disease is often clinically obvious especially in advanced hypertensive kidney disease with the manifestation of progressive wight gain, lower extremity edema, jugular venous distension, and pulmonary crackles. However, impaired sodium excretion is present in hypertensive kidney disease well before it is clinically obvious [25]. The INTERSALT study tested both within- and between-population relationships between salt and blood pressure in approximately 10,000 freely living community individuals in several countries around the world. A 24-h urine sodium collection was obtained and a correlation between daily sodium excretion and blood pressure was examined. The study revealed only a very small direct relationship between increased dietary sodium intake and the development of essential hypertension [26], on the order of 4–6 mm Hg. This strongly supports the notion that high sodium diet itself does not cause hypertension. Yet, most hypertensive patients, especially CKD patients, are salt-sensitive hypertension patients. That is, the decreased ability to excrete a normal daily salt load (impaired sodium regulation) in the setting of a low GFR is strongly associated with an increase in BP. Stated simply, high sodium diet doesn't cause hypertension but the majority of hypertensive patients (and especially those with hypertensive kidney disease) exhibit salt-sensitive hypertension.

Sodium restriction improves blood pressure in stage 3 and 4 hypertensive kidney disease [27]. The direct mechanism for this improvement is complex and still unclear [28]. Additionally, chronically high sodium intake contributes to increased arterial stiffness, decreased nitric oxide activity, and the production of vascular inflammatory mediators (such as TGF-β), all favoring an increase in BP [29].

Elevated dietary sodium intake also impairs the BP lowering effect of most antihypertensive agents, but especially diuretics [30].

Therapeutically, it is important for the clinician to reinforce sodium restriction not just to decrease blood pressure directly but also to increase the effectiveness of the pharmacologic regimen. Ninety percent of Americans exceed the recommended daily dietary sodium intake [31]. Though very difficult to achieve chronically, the American Heart Association recommends a daily sodium intake of 1500 mg in patients with hypertensive kidney disease as well as in those with diabetes [32]. A systematic review of 16 studies addressing salt intake and kidney disease set out to establish whether variations in dietary sodium consumption influence renal outcomes in people with CKD [33]. Despite heterogeneity among studies, the result suggested that increased sodium intake is associated with an increased likelihood of reduction of GFR and worsening of albuminuria.

In hypertensive kidney disease, albuminuria is associated with both the duration and severity of the hypertension [34]. The presence of higher levels of proteinuria increases the risk of mortality and myocardial infarction independent of the level of eGFR. Studies have demonstrated that even low levels of urinary albumin are associated with increased risk of CVD in hypertensive nephropathy patients with diabetes. This is independent of the level of kidney dysfunction. In the Third Copenhagen study, hypertensive subjects with microalbuminuria had risk of coronary heart disease. Risk was increased independent of age, sex, renal function, diabetes, hypertension, and plasma lipids [35]. The Chronic Kidney Disease Prognosis Consortium demonstrated that in general practice cohorts, there was an increase in cardiovascular mortality when albumin creatinine ration (ACR) is higher than 30 mg/g (3 mg/mmol). Analysis of data from the Heart Outcomes Prevention Evaluation (HOPE) study demonstrated that any degree of albuminuria is a risk factor for cardiovascular events in individuals with or without diabetes [36].

Several medications impair normal renal sodium excretion. Non-steroidal anti-inflammatory drugs (NSAIDs) inhibit vasodilating renal prostaglandin production, especially prostaglandin E2 and prostaglandin I2. This causes sodium retention and acute kidney injury via compromised blood flow to renal cortical glomeruli [37]. These adverse effects are especially prominent in diabetics, elderly, and hypertensive kidney disease patients. Administration of certain immunosuppressants in CKD patients is commonly associated with hypertension and worsening of hypertensive kidney disease. Glucocorticoids with greater mineralocorticoid effect (e.g., cortisol) clearly increase BP by inducing sodium and water retention. In such cases, use of diuretics is necessary to counteract the sodium-retaining effects and lower BP. Similarly, calcineurin inhibitors (tacrolimus, cyclosporin) induce a salt-sensitive hypertension as a result of increased renal expression of the phosphorylated (active) form of the thiazide-sensitive NaCl co-transporter (NCC) as well as direct afferent arteriolar vasoconstriction [38]. Other agents, though not impairing sodium handling but may adversely affect BP control, include decongestant and diet pills that contain sympathomimetic, amphetamine-like stimulants, oral contraceptives, the antidepressant venlafaxine, and herbal preparations containing ephedra (or ma huang) [39] (Table 7.3).

Table 7.3 Medications causing or worsening hypertension

Alcohol, amphetamines, ecstasy (MDMA and derivatives), and cocaine
Angiogenesis inhibitors (including tyrosine kinase inhibitors and monoclonal antibodies)
Antidepressants (including venlafaxine, bupropion, and desipramine)
ADHD meds: methylphenidate, dexmethylphenidate, and dextroamphetamine
Caffeine (including the caffeine in coffee and energy drinks)
Immunosuppressant: corticosteroids, cyclosporine, tacrolimus
Ephedra and many other herbal products
Erythropoietin
Estrogens (including birth control pills)
Migraine medicines (Ergot alkaloids)
Many over-the-counter medicines such as cough/cold and asthma medicines, particularly when the cough/cold medicine is combined with tranylcypromine or tricyclics
Nasal decongestants
Nicotine
Nonsteroidal anti-inflammatory drugs (NSAIDs): ibuprofen, Naprosyn, feldene, piroxicam, Cox-1 and Cox-2 inhibitors, Volteran gel
Testosterone and other anabolic steroids and performance-enhancing drugs
Herbal supplements such as ephedra, St John's wort, and yohimbine

Specifically, in case of hypertensive kidney disease patients, impaired urinary sodium excretion most commonly contributes to hypertension. Therefore, dietary sodium evaluation is crucial in the evaluation and management of hypertensive kidney disease. The Kidney Disease Improving Global Outcomes (K/DOQI) guidelines recommend limiting sodium intake to 2400 mg/day for CKD patients with hypertension [40]. Randomized trials demonstrate significant BP reduction (as much as −23/9 mm Hg) with sodium restriction in hypertensive kidney disease [41, 42]. A 24-h urine sodium collection, to estimate daily sodium intake, may identify inadequately sodium restricted patients and assist in guiding dietary counseling. Also, importantly, the urinary protein-lowering effects of RAAS inhibitors are dependent upon the concurrence of adequate sodium restriction [43]. That is, urine protein excretion may fail to improve, despite adequate RAAS inhibitor dosing if sodium restriction is inadequate.

Additionally, salt-sensitive hypertensive kidney disease is common in patients with obesity and metabolic syndrome. There are similar mechanisms of hypertension in CKD and obesity-associated hypertension including impaired sodium excretion, increased SNS activity, and activation of the RAAS. Both populations have a high incidence of obstructive sleep apnea (OSA) [44].

When resistant hypertension is present in advanced hypertensive kidney disease, it is often accompanied by diuretic-resistant fluid overload. In this situation, instituting dialysis and removal of volume in dialysis will almost always improve blood pressure.

Renin-Angiotensin-Aldosterone System

The renin-angiotensin-aldosterone system is also inappropriately activated in hypertensive kidney disease. Renin is secreted, in less quantities, mainly from the juxtaglomerular apparatus, the nephron site where the afferent arteriole contacts the distal convoluted tubule. Renin secretion is mainly dependent on the effective delivery of circulating blood volume to the kidney, though SNS stimulation also may induce renin secretion via stimulation of the efferent renal nerves [45]. To clarify, normally volume depletion leads to increased renin secretion while clinical volume overload normally decreases renin secretion. In response to an increase in renin secretion, circulating angiotensin II is increased and subsequent vasoconstriction, salt retention, and aldosterone synthesis increase. RAAS activation increases sodium reabsorption by several mechanisms such as due to the effect of angiotensin II on the proximal convoluted tubule and effect of aldosterone on the distal nephron segments. In addition to mineralocorticoid receptor stimulation, aldosterone has a direct effect on increasing vascular tone [46]. Other mediators such as endothelin, oxidative stress, and inflammation mediators also contribute to hypertensive kidney disease. Endothelins, mainly ET-1A, are potent direct vasoconstrictors. Oxidative stressors such as reactive oxygen species also promote vasoconstriction and the release of renin and increase urinary protein excretion [47]. As will be discussed in the section on the treatment of hypertensive kidney disease, inhibitors of the RAAS system are essential in lowering pressure, proteinuria, and the progression of CKD [48].

Sympathetic Nervous System

SNS activity has been demonstrated to be clearly elevated in hypertensive kidney disease patients [22]. However, due to the complexity of the multiple components of the SNS (norepinephrine, central CNS, adrenal, peripheral nerves, cardiac contractility), measurement of any individual patient's SNS activity and its contribution to BP regulation is not practical. The renal arteries are highly innervated, with many afferent and efferent nerve fibers contributing to elevated blood pressure. Stimulation of efferent renal nerves via β-1 adrenoreceptors stimulates renin secretion and activates RAAS. This results in decreased urinary sodium excretion and an increase in renal vascular resistance [49]. Blocking these renal sympathetic fibers through catheter ablation and thereby decreasing sympathetic nerve activity and sodium retention may prove to be a successful component in treating hypertensive kidney patients [50].

Impaired Renal Autoregulation in CKD

Arteries from vascular beds share functional characteristics. However, prominent differences exist in the myogenic responses to changes in transmural pressure in renal arteries. These responses are greater in renal vessels than in other mesenteric or peripheral arteries. Renal blood flow autoregulation is a vital homeostatic mechanism that protects the kidney from abnormal elevations in arterial pressure [51]. Pressure elevations would ordinarily cause glomerular injury if transmitted unadjusted to the glomerular capillaries. Autoregulation also allows the kidney to maintain a relatively constant blood flow to renal parenchymal tissue and glomerular filtration rate necessary for the clearance of metabolic wastes [52]. Impaired autoregulation in chronic kidney disease can result in elevation of glomerular capillary pressure and progressive glomerular damage (Fig. 7.1). Several factors linking chronic glomerular disorders to impaired autoregulation have been identified, including TGF-β [53] and high sodium diet [54].

Both vascular and tubular mechanisms, unique to the kidney, provides high autoregulatory efficiency that maintains renal blood flow and GFR, stabilizes sodium excretion, and buffers transmission of pressure to the fragile glomerular capillaries, thereby protecting against hypertensive barotrauma. One novel aspect of this myogenic response in the renal vasculature is modulation of its strength and speed by the TGF-β and by a connecting tubule glomerular feedback mechanism. Reactive oxygen species and nitric oxide appear to be modulators of these responses.

Inflammation

The CRIC study (Chronic Renal Insufficiency Cohort) found that among subjects with hypertensive kidney disease, the inflammatory cytokines IL-6 and TFN-α were higher, and among CKD patients with apparent treatment resistant hypertension,

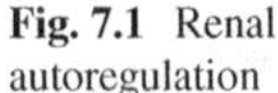

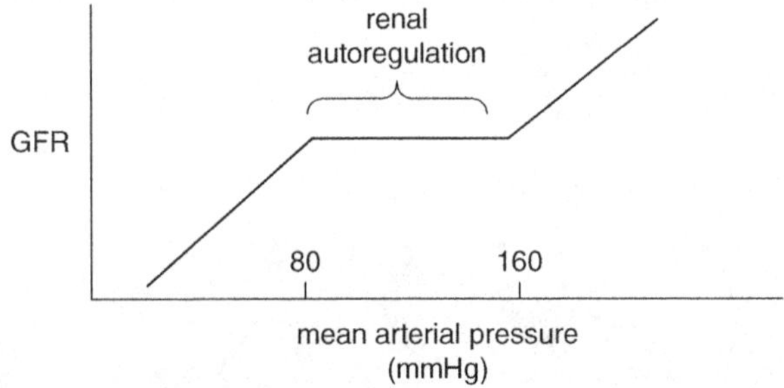

Fig. 7.1 Renal autoregulation

TGF-β levels were lower, compared with CKD patients without resistant hypertension [55]. However, it should be noted that these changes were also associated with lower GFR.

BP Target in Hypertensive Kidney Disease

For patients with an established diagnosis of hypertension in general, the 2017 American Heart association (AHA) guidelines, in collaboration with several other medical societies, issued recommendations that normal blood pressure is a systolic blood pressure <120 mm Hg and diastolic blood pressure <80 mm Hg [56]. Although hypertension is obviously a continuous variable the categories of; elevated blood pressure, stage 1, stage 2 and hypertensive crisis were described (Table 7.4). Each higher category is associated with higher renal and cardiovascular risk.

In the past, several clinical trials, conducted among non-diabetic patients with CKD, failed to demonstrate a benefit from the lower BP target of <130/80 mmHg compared to <140/90 mmHg in slowing the progression of CKD to ESRD [56–58]. Although both the ACCORD [59] and SPRINT trials showed an increase in the risk of serious adverse events with more intensive BP-lowering strategy, the benefit of a BP target of less than 130/80 mm Hg in patients with CKD and proteinuria is supported based on post hoc analyses [60]. Based on the limited clinical trial evidence, almost all of the clinical practice guidelines for the management of BP in hypertensive kidney disease without albuminuria or proteinuria recommend a goal BP of <130/90 mm Hg. The recommendation is for a lower BP target of <130/80 mm Hg for CKD patients with albuminuria or proteinuria as well.

Table 7.4 Blood pressure categories

Blood pressure category	Systolic mm Hg (upper number)		Diastolic mm Hg (lower number)
Normal	Less than 120	and	Less than 80
Elevated	120 – 129	and	Less than 80
High blood pressure (Hypertension) stage 1	130 – 139	or	80 – 89
High blood pressure (Hypertension) stage 2	140 or higher	or	90 or higher
Hypertension crisis (consult your doctor immediately)	Higher than 180	and/or	Higher than 120

From: American Heart Association 2020

Blood Pressure Monitoring and Blood Pressure Patterns in Hypertensive Kidney Disease

In individuals with hypertensive kidney disease, abnormal ambulatory blood pressure monitoring (ABPM) is more strongly associated with worsening of kidney function, higher degree of proteinuria, and greater prevalence of left ventricular hypertrophy (LVH) compared with office blood pressure monitoring [61, 62]. However, since ABPM is not widely reimbursed or available in the USA, it is reserved for individuals with suspected white-coat effect, unexplained adverse symptoms associated with blood pressure medication, or suspected non-dipping hypertensive phenotype when renal function is worsening, despite apparent good control as seen on office or home BP measurements.

ABPM has good ability to predict adverse cardiovascular events among individuals with hypertensive kidney disease as well as in those requiring renal-replacement therapy. For example, among 600 subjects in the AASK Cohort Study, Ku et al. showed a direct association between the difference in office systolic BP and systolic ABPM regarding mortality risk. Those with significantly different in-office readings compared with ABPM readings had a greater cardiovascular risk than individuals with concordant office and ABPM readings [63].

The precise predictive value of home blood pressure monitoring among patients with hypertensive kidney disease is not well understood. Agarwal et al. found in a cohort of 217 military veterans receiving both home BP monitoring and 24-h ABPM that higher home BP was associated with an increased risk of ESRD but not with a composite endpoint of stroke, myocardial infarction, and death. However, higher blood pressures obtained by 24-h ABPM were associated with this composite endpoint [64].

In a cross-sectional study of 5693 hypertensive kidney disease patients, Gorostidi et al. found that a white-coat hypertension effect was present in 36.8% of patients with an office BP ≥140/90 mm Hg. Additionally, masked hypertension was found in 32.1% of patients with an office BP <140/90 mm Hg [65]. Patients with CKD and white-coat effect seem to have a much lower cumulative risk of progressing to end-stage renal disease (ESRD), highlighting the importance of ABPM in hypertensive kidney disease patients [66].

Circadian rhythms of blood pressure are often disturbed in hypertensive kidney disease. A fall in nocturnal BP by approximately 10–20% is normal and confirmed with ambulatory blood pressure monitoring, which characterizes a normal circadian pattern of BP. All individuals regardless of hypertension or CKD status should have normal nocturnal dipping patterns. Hypertensive individuals whose BP consistently fails to dip are at increased risk of kidney disease progression [67] and death. These individuals are labeled non-dippers [68, 69]. A portion of patients with advanced hypertensive kidney disease exhibit a rise in nocturnal BP, termed reverse dipping. This finding is strongly associated with increased cardiovascular events [70]. Due to the adverse events associated with non-dipping and reverse dipping, it has been suggested that hypertensive kidney disease patients take at least part of their blood pressure medication at bedtime in an effort to restore a normal nocturnal dipping pattern [71].

Additionally, a positive association between BP variability and progression of CKD and cardiovascular events has been reported [72]. When ABPM is not available, home BP measurement can provide some information on possible presence of white-coat, masked, or resistant hypertension. Population studies both in general and in CKD demonstrate that home-measured BP is prognostically superior to office BP readings, correlates more closely with ABPM than with office BP measurements, and is more predictive of adverse cardiovascular outcomes [73, 74]. Therefore, out-of-office BP readings, ABPM, or home BP measurement should be used in management.

Masked Hypertension in CKD

Masked hypertension is the converse of white-coat hypertension. It is defined as a normal blood pressure in the clinic but an elevated BP out of the clinic. Patients with CKD have been found to be at higher risk of masked hypertension as compared to the general population [75]. An increased risk of masked hypertension may be due to a greater prevalence of nocturnal non-dipping in the CKD population. Non-dipping blood pressure has been observed to be a strong predictor of CVD, kidney failure, and death. Ambulatory blood pressure monitoring is required to detect non-dipping of blood pressure and is preferred over home blood pressure monitoring to diagnose masked hypertension [76]. If white-coat effect or MH is established, HBPM or ABPM should be used to guide further management decisions.

Resistant Hypertension in Hypertensive Kidney Disease

Resistant hypertension (RH) is common among people with CKD and the prevalence increases as renal function declines [17]. In a study of 10,700 individuals, Tanner found that the prevalence of apparent treatment-resistant hypertension was 15.8%, 24.9%, and 33.4% for those participants with estimated GFR $\geq$ 60, 45–59, and <45 ml/min per 1.73 m [2], respectively. Additionally, after multivariable adjustment, factors such as men, black race, larger waist circumference, diabetes, history of myocardial infarction or stroke, statin use, and lower estimated GFR and higher albumin-to-creatinine ratio levels were associated with apparent treatment-resistant hypertension among individuals with CKD.

In a cross-sectional study of 4265 elderly, hypertensive people with CKD, Kaboré [77] found that a rapid decline in kidney function is more strongly predicted by the presence of resistant hypertension than by the CKD stage itself. Medication non-adherence is a common cause of pseudo-resistant hypertension among CKD patients. This may be due to medication complexity [78].

Role of Hypertension in the Progression of CKD

There is substantial evidence that hypertension is a major factor in the progression of CKD [79]. As previously mentioned, concurrent hypertension and CKD create a "vicious circle" with each condition, if inadequately addressed, contributing to the progression of the other. The dominant "hyper-perfusion theory" holds that systemic hypertension transmits elevated pressure to glomerular capillaries, via hydraulic stress, inducing progressive injury to already damaged glomeruli [80, 81]. Data from the PREVEND study, a prospective, population-based cohort study, provide important information on decline in kidney function in a population [82]. The PREVEND study evaluated 6894 people over a 4-year period and reported loss in eGFR of 2.3 ml/min/4 years in the entire population, 7.2 ml/min/4 years in participants with macroalbuminuria (4300 mg/24 h), and 0.2 ml/min/4 year in participants with impaired renal function. The yearly decline in eGFR among a Japanese general population over 10 years was slightly lower at 0.36 ml/min/year. The rate of eGFR decline was approximately two times higher in those with proteinuria and 1.5 times higher among those with hypertension [83]. Another study of kidney function decline in 74 treated, hypertensive men found that the average rate of renal decline equaled 0.92 ml/min/year [84]. Wright found that among African-Americans with hypertension and a GFR of 20–65 ml/min, the annual decline in GFR equaled approximately 2 ml/year regardless of target pressure achieved [47].

Treatment of Hypertensive Kidney Disease

Use of RAAS Inhibition in CKD

Renin-angiotensin-aldosterone system inhibitors (RAASi) have been repeatedly demonstrated to significantly slow the progression of CKD in randomized controlled trials conducted in adults [85]. The mechanisms by which RAASi slow the progression of CKD include the reduction of proteinuria and optimized BP control [86]. While the benefits of RAASi are certain in hypertensive CKD stages 2–3, there is controversy regarding the role of these agents in stage 4–5 hypertensive CKD. A randomized trial of 224 adults aged 18–70 years with hypertensive CKD stage 4 showed a significantly slower decline in GFR among those treated with an angiotensin-converting enzyme inhibitor (ACEi) compared with placebo [57]. However, there is evidence that fear among clinicians exists that ongoing use of RAASi in advanced stages of CKD will paradoxically result in either life-threatening hyperkalemia or a premature dialysis requirement. In a study by Ku examining patterns of antihypertensive medication use in relation to CKD stage, it was found that during a median follow-up of 7.5 years, the use of RAAS inhibitors decreased from 75% in CKD stage 3 to 37% by stage 5, while the use of calcium channel blockers, diuretics, and β-blockers all increased steadily with advancing CKD. Of note, RAAS inhibition was associated with a 20% lower risk of heart failure and death, regardless of the CKD stage [87].

Prescribing RAASi in hypertensive kidney disease patients has the additional benefit of decreasing cardiovascular risk. Left ventricular hypertrophy is present in 40% of people with hypertensive kidney disease and progressively increases as kidney function declines [88] [89]. In the evaluation of LVH in CKD, several studies suggest that BNP level rises as GFR declines; however, Tagore et al. studied BNP levels in a cohort of 143 clinically euvolemic subjects with hypertensive kidney disease patients without heart disease and found that plasma BNP levels were independent of GFR [90].

A very frequently asked question is as follows: At what level of renal dysfunction should the RAAS inhibitor be stopped in hypertensive chronic kidney disease patients? Since there is good clinical evidence that RAAS blockers are beneficial in slowing the progression of hypertensive kidney disease even at stage 5 CKD (GFR < 15 ml/min), most nephrologists discontinue RAAS inhibitors only when patients are felt to be unreliable in potassium restriction, having blood draws for potassium checks, or in dietary potassium restriction (Table 7.5).

While dual blockade with a combination of an ACEi and an angiotensin receptor blocker (ARB) lowers blood pressure and proteinuria to a greater degree than monotherapy, dual blockade has been associated with significantly higher rates of complications, including hyperkalemia, syncope, and acute kidney injury [91]. It is the recommendation of the author, as well as renal guidelines, to avoid combining ACE-I and ARB therapy in hypertensive kidney disease patients.

Table 7.5 High potassium foods to avoid in CKD stage 4 and 5

Lima beans
Tomato products (whole, juice, sauce)
Salmon
Potatoes and sweet potatoes
Banana
Mushrooms
Melons (cantaloupe, honeydew)
Avocado, beets, Asparagus
Dried fruit (prunes, raisins, apricots, dates)
Citrus fruit (orange, grapefruit, pineapple): whole or juice
Spinach, broccoli, and kale
Peas, cucumber, and zucchini

Diuretics

Several questions immediately arise when a clinician is clear that diuretics are required in a hypertensive kidney disease patient. Which class of diuretic or combination of diuretics should be prescribed? What dose of diuretic should I choose? What should be my goal in prescribing diuretics for this patient? How should I monitor an individual receiving diuretics?

When patients exhibit clear signs of volume overload, sodium excretion must be augmented by titrating diuretics. Many patients may initially receive benefit from a thiazide diuretic for hypertension treatment when normal or only mild (stage 1, 2, or early 3a) kidney disease is present. For most individuals with hypertensive kidney disease, once GFR has declined near 45 ml/min or less, a loop diuretic will be essential to successfully attain and achieve acceptable blood pressure and an edema free state. In fact, the most common reason that blood pressure targets are not achieved in hypertensive kidney disease patients is due to inadequate diuretic administration. Since sodium intake is closely linked to diuretic requirement, a small percent of hypertensive kidney disease patients, who are extremely vigilant in dietary intake, can successfully restrict sodium to 2000 mg daily (or less) and require little if any loop diuretic. However, most individuals are less successful in dietary sodium restriction and may need considerably higher daily dosages. We recommend that hypertensive kidney disease patients weigh themselves daily, at roughly the same time of day while wearing minimal clothing, and to monitor blood pressure at home. This information should be recorded by the patient, and the medical provider should set parameters in advance with triggers to either increase or decrease diuretics. For example, a 70 kg man with stage 4 hypertensive kidney disease (stable GFR = 20 ml/min and creatinine = 4 mg/dl) and blood pressure of 150/90 with signs of volume overload (peripheral edema) may be instructed to increase his furosemide from 20 mg twice daily up to 40 mg po twice daily. Obviously, the result of this change in therapy must be monitored. Patients are advised to seek a weight loss of 0.5–1 lb. per day over the next week with a target weight of perhaps 67–68 kg (loss of 5–7 lbs.). Patients are instructed that if either the weight falls too rapidly (1 kg/day) or blood pressure falls below a desirable levels (systolic <120 mm Hg or diastolic BP <65 mm Hg), then diuretics are held until improvement. Similarly, if weight and BP fail to improve over the next week, then patients are instructed to take an additional 40 mg of furosemide daily in addition to reassessing for hidden sources of dietary sodium. Of note, a repeat serum creatinine test will help guide whether this new lower weight target and blood pressure have compromised renal function.

To inhibit renal sodium reabsorption, loop diuretics (like all diuretics) must first be filtered at the glomerulus. Since stage 4–5 hypertensive kidney disease patients, by definition, have fewer functioning nephrons, these patients require higher dosages of loop diuretics than CKD stage 2 or 3 patients in order to excrete the same daily sodium intake. Furosemide is the most prescribed loop diuretic with a normal half-life (oral dosing) of approximately 2–3 h, which is prolonged in CKD [92] to approximately 6 h. Though K/DOQI guidelines recommend that CKD stages 4–5 patients start furosemide at a dose of 40–80 mg once daily with weekly titration upward by 25–50% [93], it is often desirable to dose furosemide twice or thrice daily [94]. If pill burden or nocturia limits more frequent dosing, then a trial of a different loop diuretic possessing superior pharmacokinetics (bumetanide) or a longer half-life (torsemide) may increase efficacy.

It had been believed that thiazide diuretics were essentially ineffective at GFR < 30 ml/min. However, chlorthalidone, indapamide, and metolazone have longer half-lives than hydrochlorothiazide and, therefore, provide greater net urinary sodium excretion [95]. Clinical trials suggest that long-acting thiazides can successfully reduce BP even in advanced CKD and when combined with loop diuretics [96]. An ongoing study using chlorthalidone in patients with advanced hypertensive kidney disease is being conducted to evaluate the effects on BP and albuminuria (NCT02841280).

One problems is that, among antihypertensive agents, diuretics have the highest rate of non-adherence [97]. Patients with hypertensive kidney disease often report nocturia [98]. Thankfully, hypertensive kidney disease patients seem to be about as adherent to medication as are most other patients [99]. While salt restriction is beneficial in most all diuretic requiring hypertensive kidney disease patients, providers must monitor patients for salt wasting tubular disorders; or volume contraction.

Aldosterone Antagonists in Hypertensive Kidney Disease

Animal studies have shown that aldosterone has an independent role in the development and progression of hypertensive nephropathy and renal fibrosis due to vascular injury. Conversely, aldosterone blockade reduces proteinuria [100]. In humans, RAASi blockade with ACEi or ARB results in only partial suppression of serum aldosterone levels. This phenomenon is termed "aldosterone escape." When hypertensive nephropathy patients are treated with ACEi or ARBs, aldosterone levels decrease in the initial period but subsequently increase within a few months, despite ongoing treatment with ACEi or ARB therapy [101]. This aldosterone escape is associated with an increased excretion of urinary albumin and a decline in GFR. Commercially available aldosterone antagonists include selective (eplerenone) and nonselective antagonists (spironolactone). Both selective and nonselective aldosterone antagonists reduce the risk of cardiovascular mortality and hospitalization in patients with congestive heart failure. In a meta-analysis of 11 trials using ACE or ARB with aldosterone antagonist, proteinuria decreased but additional preservation of renal function could not be convincingly demonstrated. These agents must be used with caution in patients receiving potassium supplementation and in patients with advanced CKD due to the risk of hyperkalemia [102]. Bakris [103] recently found that the selective aldosterone antagonist finerenone slowed progressive renal decline among type 2 diabetics with CKD. It remains to be determined if this also holds true for non-diabetic hypertensive kidney disease.

Since hyperkalemia is often limiting in the ability of clinicians to continue aldosterone antagonists, clinical trials are currently in process to determine whether addition of potassium-binding resins (Kayexalate™, Veltassa™ or Lokalma™) through permitting the continuation of aldosterone antagonism is clinically beneficial.

Dietary Potassium Supplementation

Diets rich in potassium (e.g., DASH) clearly lower blood pressure independent of the amount of sodium ingested. However, given the risk of hyperkalemia, and the absence of clinical studies, a potassium-rich diet cannot be recommended in moderate-to-severe CKD [104].

SGLT-2 Inhibitors

Sodium-glucose co-transporter-2 (SGLT2) inhibitors are glucose-lowering drugs that also lower blood pressure, body weight, and albuminuria and may have direct beneficial effect upon the kidney. Recent randomized, placebo-controlled outcome trials showed that SGLT-2 inhibitors and GLP-1 receptor agonists can reduce the progression of hypertensive kidney disease in addition to reducing cardiovascular events and all-cause mortality in patients with type 2 DM [105].

Post hoc analyses of the EMPA-REG OUTCOME trial found that participants with a history of coronary artery bypass surgery, treated with empagliflozin, had profound reductions in heart failure hospitalizations, nephropathy and cardiovascular and all-cause mortality [106]. Importantly, in the DAPA-CKD trial, 4304 diabetic and non-diabetic participants with GFR 25–75 ml/min and albuminuria received dapagliflozin 10 mg daily or placebo. The study was prematurely terminated for benefit. Among patients with chronic kidney disease, regardless of the presence or absence of diabetes, the risk of a composite of a sustained decline in the GFR of at least 50%, end-stage kidney disease, or death from renal or cardiovascular causes was significantly lower with dapagliflozin than with placebo [107].

Allopurinol

In patients with hypertensive renal disease, there is decreased urinary uric acid excretion, and depending upon gastrointestinal excretion, it may lead to hyperuricemia. So, the prevalence of elevated serum uric acid in patients with hypertensive kidney disease is higher than normal. Elevated serum uric acid has been related to increased risk for the development of hypertension and cardiovascular disease [108]. Chronic hyperuricemia stimulates the renin-angiotensin system and inhibits release of nitric oxide, contributing to renal vasoconstriction and increasing BP. High levels of uric acid may additionally have a pathogenetic role in interstitial inflammation and progression of renal disease. Allopurinol decreases serum uric acid level by inhibiting the enzyme xanthine oxidase. For animal models of established renal diseases, correction of the hyperuricemic state significantly improves BP control, decreases proteinuria, and slows the progression of renal disease [109]. In a prospective, randomized trial [110] of 113 patients with GFR <60 ml/min, patients were randomly assigned to treatment with allopurinol 100 mg/d or usual therapy. Clinical, biochemical, and inflammatory parameters were measured at baseline and at 6, 12, and 24 months of treatment. In the control group, GFR decreased to 3.3 ± 1.2 ml/min, and in the allopurinol group, eGFR increased to 1.3 ± 1.3 ml/min after 24 months. Allopurinol treatment slowed down renal disease progression independently of age, gender, diabetes, C-reactive protein, albuminuria, and use of renin-angiotensin system blockers. Long-term follow-up of this group continued to show benefit [111]. Also, in the Gonryo study [112], among 178 hypertensive kidney disease patients with GFR <45 mL/min, oral allopurinol was prescribed for 67 patients. During follow-up, over a mean of 18.4 months, 28 primary cardiovascular events occurred. Use of allopurinol was a significant beneficial factor (hazard ratio = 0.342) $p = 0.0434$.

Aspirin and Clopidogrel

The benefits of aspirin in people with hypertensive kidney disease was demonstrated by a *post hoc* analysis of the Hypertension Optimal Treatment (HOT) trial [113]. This study reported that among every 1000 persons with eGFR <45 ml/min treated for 3.8 years, 76 major cardiovascular events and 54 all-cause deaths were prevented, though 27 excess major bleeds occurred. The Clopidogrel for Reduction of Events During Observation (CREDO) trial concluded that clopidogrel in mild or moderate CKD may not have the same beneficial effect as it has in people without CKD. Subjects with normal renal function who received 1 year of clopidogrel had a marked reduction in death, MI, or stroke compared with those who received placebo (10.4% versus 4.4%, $P < 0.001$), whereas those with mild and moderate CKD did not have a significant difference in outcomes with clopidogrel therapy versus placebo [114].

Weight Loss for Treatment of Hypertensive Kidney Disease

When lifestyle modification is unsuccessful in achieving weight loss goals, pharmacologic intervention may be recommended. Yet, additional considerations are necessary in patients with CKD. In particularly, orlistat is associated with precipitation of calcium oxalate nephrolithiasis and lorcaserin is contraindicated when eGFR < 30 ml/min due to increased cardiovascular risk [115].

Evaluation for Renal Artery Stenosis in Hypertensive Kidney Disease

Recent trials in hypertensive CKD patients have found that vascular stenting of atherosclerotic renal artery narrowing provides no benefit beyond optimized medical management [116, 117]. Optimal medical management includes use of RAASi medication, additional medication to achieve target blood pressures, smoking cessation, and lipid lowering treatment. Routine screening for RAS in the setting of CKD is therefore discouraged and should only be pursued in patients who have a high likelihood of benefitting from intervention, since these patients were excluded from these trials. Such patients include those with a solitary kidney, severe resistant hypertension, recurrent episodes of "flash pulmonary edema," refractory heart failure, recurrent acute kidney injury (AKI) following introduction of ACEi or ARB, or otherwise unexplained progressive renal insufficiency.

Hypertensive Emergency in Hypertensive Kidney Disease

Hypertensive renal emergency is defined as acute kidney injury due to marked elevation in blood pressure. Though approximately 1% of patients with hypertension are reported to experience an episode of hypertensive emergency, only a small fraction of these events are pure AKI with the majority of patients presenting with concurrent CVA, encephalopathy or acute heart failure [118]. As has been discussed above, most CKD is worsened in a hypertensive environment. However, when the upper limit of renal auto-regulatory is greatly exceeded, then rapid renal injury may develop as seen in malignant hypertension (Fig. 7.2). It may be initially difficult to determine whether a patient has acute kidney injury due to malignant hypertension. For example, a 50-year-old woman with a history of hypertension and CKD (creatinine 1.7 mm/dl from 6 months ago) presents to an emergency department after motor vehicle accident (MVA) with markedly elevated blood pressures (systolic BP 200 mm Hg, diastolic BP 130 mm Hg) and plasma creatinine of 4.2 mg/dl. There are at least two distinct possibilities. One possibility is that, yes, the patient has AKI due to hypertensive renal crisis. Alternatively, there is accelerated hypertension due to

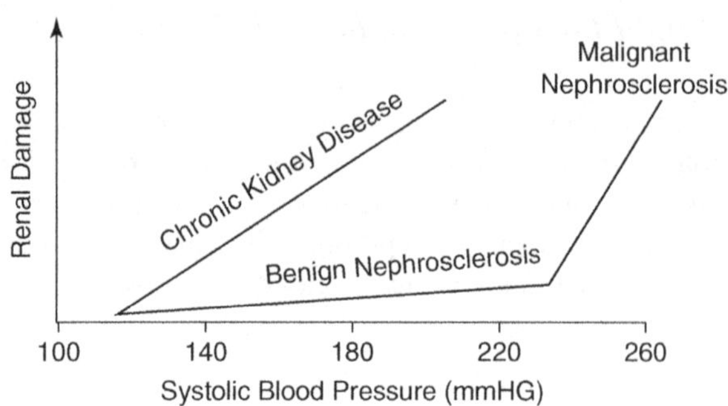

Fig. 7.2 Patterns of kidney injury in hypertension

the MVA and gradual worsening of renal insufficiency from another cause such as NSAID or cocaine use. Discriminating between these two possibilities may be difficult. Examination of a peripheral blood smear demonstrating schistocytes favors hypertensive renal emergency. Having another associated manifestation of hypertensive emergency such as subarachnoid hemorrhage makes hypertensive renal crisis more likely. Excluding other causes of AKI such as hypovolemia, a history of NSAID, or recent radiocontrast exposure use may provide alternative explanations for the rise in creatinine.

The factors leading to the rapid and severe BP elevations in patients with hypertensive emergency are poorly understood. The rapidity of onset suggests a triggering factor superimposed on preexisting hypertensive nephropathy. The release of vasoconstricting substances from the injured vessel wall is believed to be responsible for both the initiation and continuation of renal hypertensive crisis. Mild to moderate increases in BP do not affect renal perfusion because of autoregulatory mechanisms. Instead, severe BP elevations above the autoregulatory limits lead to transmission of pressure to small distal vessels and glomerular capillaries. This elevated pressure in small renal arterioles causes endothelial cell injury and dysfunction. Endothelial cell dysfunction leads to increased vascular wall permeability, cell proliferation, and activation of the coagulation cascade and platelet deposition. In turn, this leads ultimately to fibrinoid necrosis of small renal blood vessels, release of vasoconstrictor substances, and direct renal parenchymal ischemia. The initial vascular damage leads to a cycle of further vascular injury, tissue ischemia, and release of more vasoconstrictor substances. Renal ischemia activates the renin-angiotensin-aldosterone system, vasopressin, and endothelin, and catecholamines play important roles in the pathogenesis of renal injury in hypertensive emergency [119]. Clinically, this may be indistinguishable from thrombocytopenia purpura (TTP) with hemolysis, thrombocytopenia, AKI, and CNS abnormalities.

Prognosis

Individuals with inadequately treated hypertension are more likely to develop end-organ damage, including carotid intima-media thickening, LVH, worsening of renal function, and microalbuminuria [120]. These subgroups all have an unfavorable prognosis and are significantly more likely to suffer the outcomes of death, myocardial infarction, congestive heart failure, stroke, or CKD over time compared to those who have achieved target blood pressure levels [121]. It should not be surprising to learn that this risk increases further if patients have CKD [122].

References

1. Daugherty SL, Powers JD, Magid DJ, Tavel HM, Masoudi FA, Margolis KL, O'Connor PJ, Selby JV, Ho PM. Incidence and prognosis of resistant hypertension in hypertensive patients. Circulation. 2012;125(13):1635–42. Pubmed.
2. Webster AC, Nagler EV, Morton RL, Masson P. Chronic kidney disease. Lancet. 2017;389(10075):1238–52. Pubmed.
3. SPRINT Research Group, Wright JT Jr, Williamson JD, Whelton PK, Snyder JK, Sink KM, Rocco MV, Reboussin DM, Rahman M, Oparil S, Lewis CE, Kimmel PL, Johnson KC, Goff DC Jr, Fine LJ, Cutler JA, Cushman WC, Cheung AK, Ambrosius WT. A randomized trial of intensive versus standard blood-pressure control. N Engl J Med. 2015;373(22):2103–16. Pubmed.
4. Unger T, Borghi C, Charchar F, Khan NA, Poulter NR, Prabhakaran D, Ramirez A, Schlaich M, Stergiou GS, Tomaszewski M, Wainford RD, Williams B, Schutte AE. 2020 International Society of Hypertension Global Hypertension Practice Guidelines. Hypertension. 2020;75(6):1334–57. Pubmed.
5. Muntner P, Anderson A, Charleston J, Chen Z, Ford V, Makos G, et al. Hypertension awareness, treatment, and control in adults with CKD: results from the Chronic Renal Insufficiency Cohort (CRIC) Study. Am J Kidney Dis. 2010;55:441–51. Pubmed.
6. Sakhuja A, Textor SC, Taler SJ. Uncontrolled hypertension by the evidence-based guideline: results from NHANES 2011–2012. J Hypertens. 2015;33:644–51. Pubmed.
7. Bidani AK, Polichnowski AJ, Loutzenhiser R, Griffin KA. Renal microvascular dysfunction, hypertension and CKD progression. Curr Opin Nephrol Hypertens. 2013;22:1–9. Pubmed.
8. Mahmoodi BK, et al. Associations of kidney disease measures with mortality and end-stage renal disease in individuals with and without hypertension: a meta-analysis. Lancet. 2012;380(9854):1649–61. Pubmed.
9. Bright R. Tabular view of the morbid appearances in 100 cases connected with albuminous urine. Guys Hosp Rep. 1836;1(2):380–400.
10. Bakris GL, Williams M, Dworkin L, et al. Preserving renal function in adults with hypertension and diabetes: a consensus approach. National Kidney Foundation Hypertension and Diabetes Executive Committees Working Group. Am J Kidney Dis. 2000;36(3):646–61. Pubmed.
11. Olson JL. Hypertension: essential and secondary forms. In: Jennette JC, Olson JL, Schwartz MM, Silva FG, editors. Heptinstall's pathology of the kidney, vol. 2. 5th ed. Philadelphia: Lippincott-Raven; 1998. p. 943–1002.
12. Briet M, Boutouyrie P, Laurent S, London GM. Arterial stiffness and pulse pressure in CKD and ESRD. Kidney Int. 2012;82:388–400. Pubmed.
13. Klahr S, Levey AS, Beck GJ, Caggiula AW, Hunsicker L, Kusek JW, Striker G. The effects of dietary protein restriction and blood-pressure control on the progression of chronic renal disease. Modification of Diet in Renal Disease Study Group. N Engl J Med. 1994;330(13):877–84. Pubmed.
14. Jafar TH, Stark PC, Schmid CH, Landa M, Maschio G, de Jong PE, de Zeeuw D, Shahinfar S, Toto R, Levey AS, AIPRD Study Group. Progression of chronic kidney disease: the role of blood pressure control, proteinuria, and angiotensin-converting enzyme inhibition: a patient-level meta-analysis. Ann Intern Med. 2003;139(4):244–52. Pubmed.
15. Lash JP, Go AS, Appel LJ, et al. Chronic Renal Insufficiency Cohort (CRIC) Study: baseline characteristics and associations with kidney function. Clin J Am Soc Nephrol. 2009;4(8):1302–11. Pubmed.

16. Egan BM, Zhao Y, Axon RN. US trends in prevalence, awareness, treatment, and control of hypertension, 1988–2008. JAMA. 2010;303(20):2043–50. Pubmed.
17. Tanner RM, Calhoun DA, Bell EK, et al. Prevalence of apparent treatment-resistant hypertension among individuals with CKD. Clin J Am Soc Nephrol. 2013;8:1583–90. Pubmed.
18. Cai G, Zheng Y, Sun X, Chen X. Prevalence, awareness, treatment, and control of hypertension in elderly adults with chronic kidney disease: results from the survey of prevalence, awareness, and treatment rates in chronic kidney disease patients with hypertension in China. J Am Geriatr Soc. 2013;61(12):2160–7. Pubmed.
19. Chen J, Bundy JD, Hamm LL, et al. Inflammation and apparent treatment-resistant hypertension in patients with chronic kidney disease. Hypertension. 2019;73(4):785–93. Pubmed.
20. Tozawa M, Iseki K, Iseki C, Kinjo K, Ikemiya Y, Takishita S. Blood pressure predicts risk of developing end-stage renal disease in men and women. Hypertension. 2003;41(6):1341–5. Pubmed.
21. Pimenta E, Gaddam KK, Oparil S, Aban I, Husain S, Dell'Italia LJ, et al. Effects of dietary sodium reduction on blood pressure in subjects with resistant hypertension: results from a randomized trial. Hypertension. 2009;54:475–81. Pubmed.
22. Kaur J, Young BE, Fadel PJ. Sympathetic overactivity in chronic kidney disease: consequences and mechanisms. Int J Mol Sci. 2017;18(8):1682. Published 2017 Aug 2. Pubmed. https://doi.org/10.3390/ijms18081682.
23. Remuzzi G, Perico N, Macia M, Ruggenenti P. The role of renin-angiotensin-aldosterone system in the progression of chronic kidney disease. Kidney Int Suppl. 2005;99:S57–65. Pubmed.
24. Kaur M, Chandran DS, Jaryal AK, Bhowmik D, Agarwal SK, Deepak KK. Baroreflex dysfunction in chronic kidney disease. World J Nephrol. 2016;5(1):53–65. Pubmed.
25. Welsh CE, Welsh P, Jhund P, Delles C, Celis-Morales C, Lewsey JD, Gray S, Lyall D, Iliodromiti S, Gill JMR, Sattar N, Mark PB. Urinary sodium excretion, blood pressure, and risk of future cardiovascular disease and mortality in subjects without prior cardiovascular disease. Hypertension. 2019;73(6):1202–9. Pubmed.
26. Stamler J. The INTERSALT study: background, methods, findings, and implications. Am J Clin Nutr. 1997;65(2 Suppl):626S–42S. Pubmed.
27. Saran R, Padilla RL, Gillespie BW, Heung M, Hummel SL, Derebail VK, Pitt B, Levin NW, Zhu F, Abbas SR, Liu L, Kotanko P, Klemmer P. A randomized crossover trial of dietary sodium restriction in stage 3-4 CKD. Clin J Am Soc Nephrol. 2017;12(3):399–407. Pubmed.
28. Chamarthi B, Williams JS, Williams GH. A mechanism for salt-sensitive hypertension: abnormal dietary sodium-mediated vascular response to angiotensin-II. J Hypertens. 2010;28(5):1020–6. Pubmed.
29. Hovater MB, Sanders PW. Effect of dietary salt on regulation of TGF-beta in the kidney. Semin Nephrol. 2012;32:269–76. Pubmed.
30. Luft FC, Weinberger MH. Review of salt restriction and the response to antihypertensive drugs: satellite symposium on calcium antagonists. Hypertension. 1988;11:I-229–32. Pubmed.
31. Jackson SL, King SM, Zhao L, Cogswell ME. Prevalence of excess sodium intake in the United States - NHANES, 2009-2012. MMWR Morb Mortal Wkly Rep. 2016;64(52):1393–7. Pubmed.
32. Cook NR, Appel LJ, Whelton PK. Lower levels of sodium intake and reduced cardiovascular risk. Circulation. 2014;129(9):981–9. Pubmed.
33. Jones-Burton C, Mishra SI, Fink JC, et al. An in-depth review of the evidence linking dietary salt intake and progression of chronic kidney disease. Am J Nephrol. 2006;26:268–75. Pubmed.
34. Sarnak MJ. Cardiovascular complications in chronic kidney disease. Am J Kidney Dis. 2003;41:11–7. Pubmed.
35. Klausen K, Borch-Johnsen K, Feldt-Rasmussen B, et al. Very low levels of microalbuminuria are associated with increased risk of coronary heart disease and death independently of renal function, hypertension, and diabetes. Circulation. 2004;110:32–5. Pubmed.
36. Mann JF, Gerstein HC, Yi QL, Lonn EM, Hoogwerf BJ, Rashkow A, Yusuf S. Development of renal disease in people at high cardiovascular risk: results of the HOPE randomized study. J Am Soc Nephrol. 2003;14(3):641–7. Pubmed.

37. Johnson AG, Nguyen TV, Day RO. Do nonsteroidal anti-inflammatory drugs affect blood pressure? Ann Intern Med. 1994;121:289–300. Pubmed.
38. Hoorn EJ, Walsh SB, McCormick JA, Fürstenberg A, Yang CL, Roeschel T, et al. The calcineurin inhibitor tacrolimus activates the renal sodium chloride cotransporter to cause hypertension. Nat Med. 2011;17:1304–9. Pubmed.
39. Mansoor GA. Herbs and alternative therapies in the hypertension clinic. Am J Hypertens. 2001;14:971–5. Pubmed.
40. Kidney Disease Outcomes Quality Initiative, (K/DOQI). K/DOQI clinical practice guidelines on hypertension and antihypertensive agents in chronic kidney disease. Am J Kidney Dis. 2004;43(5 Suppl 1):1. Pubmed.
41. McMahon EJ, Bauer JD, Hawley CM, et al. A randomized trial of dietary sodium restriction in CKD. J Am Soc Nephrol. 2013;24(12):2096–103. Pubmed.
42. Pimenta E, Gaddam KK, Oparil S, et al. Effects of dietary sodium reduction on blood pressure in subjects with resistant hypertension: results from a randomized trial. Hypertension. 2009;54(3):475–81. Pubmed.
43. Lambers Heerspink HJ, Holtkamp FA, Parving HH, Navis GJ, Lewis JB, Ritz E, de Graeff PA, de Zeeuw D. Moderation of dietary sodium potentiates the renal and cardiovascular protective effects of angiotensin receptor blockers. Kidney Int. 2012;82(3):330–7. Pubmed.
44. Nicholl DD, Ahmed SB, Loewen AH, Hemmelgarn BR, Sola DY, Beecroft JM, et al. Declining kidney function increases the prevalence of sleep apnea and nocturnal hypoxia. Chest. 2012;141:1422–30. Pubmed
45. Davis JO, Freeman RH. Mechanisms regulating renin release. Physiol Rev. 1976;56(1):1–56. Pubmed.
46. Briet M, Schiffrin EL. Vascular actions of aldosterone. J Vasc Res. 2013;50:89–99. Pubmed.
47. Araujo M, Wilcox CS. Oxidative stress in hypertension: role of the kidney. Antioxid Redox Signal. 2014;20:74–101. Pubmed.
48. Gaudreault-Tremblay MM, Foster BJ. Benefits of continuing RAAS inhibitors in advanced CKD. Clin J Am Soc Nephrol. 2020;15(5):592–3. Pubmed.
49. DiBona GF, Kopp UC. Neural control of renal function. Physiol Rev. 1997;77:75–197. Pubmed.
50. Sanders MF, Blankestijn PJ. Chronic kidney disease as a potential indication for renal denervation. Front Physiol. 2016;7:220. Pubmed.
51. Carlström M, Wilcox CS, Arendshorst WJ. Renal autoregulation in health and disease. Physiol Rev. 2015;95(2):405–511. Pubmed.
52. Navar LG, Inscho EW, Majid SA, Imig JD, Harrison-Bernard LM, Mitchell KD. Paracrine regulation of the renal microcirculation. Physiol Rev. 1996;76:425–536. Pubmed.
53. Sharma K, Cook A, Smith M, Valancius C, Inscho EW. TGF-beta impairs renal autoregulation via generation of ROS. Am J Physiol Renal Physiol. 2005;288(5):F1069–77. Pubmed.
54. Fellner RC, Cook AK, O'Connor PM, Zhang S, Pollock DM, Inscho EW. High-salt diet blunts renal autoregulation by a reactive oxygen species-dependent mechanism. Am J Physiol Renal Physiol. 2014;307(1):F33–40. Pubmed.
55. Ishigami J, Taliercio J, I Feldman H, Srivastava A, Townsend R, L Cohen D, et al. CRIC Study Investigators. Inflammatory Markers and Incidence of Hospitalization With Infection in Chronic Kidney Disease. Am J Epidemiol. 2020;189(5):433–44. https://doi.org/10.1093/aje/kwz246. PMID: 31673705; PMCID: PMC7306687.
56. Carey RM, Whelton PK. 2017 ACC/AHA Hypertension Guideline Writing Committee. Prevention, detection, evaluation, and management of high blood pressure in adults: synopsis of the 2017 American College of Cardiology/American Heart Association Hypertension Guideline. Ann Intern Med. 2018;168(5):351–8. Pubmed.
57. Wright JT Jr, Bakris G, Greene T, Agodoa LY, Appel LJ, Charleston J, et al. Effect of blood pressure lowering and antihypertensive drug class on progression of hypertensive kidney disease: results from the AASK trial. JAMA. 2002;288:2421–31. Pubmed.

58. Ruggenenti P, Perna A, Loriga G, Ganeva M, Ene-Iordache B, Turturro M, et al. Bloodpressure control for renoprotection in patients with non-diabetic chronic renal disease (REIN-2): multicentre, randomised controlled trial. Lancet. 2005;365:939–46. Pubmed.
59. Action to Control Cardiovascular Risk in Diabetes Study Group, Gerstein HC, Miller ME, Byington RP, Goff DC Jr, Bigger JT, Buse JB, Cushman WC, Genuth S, Ismail-Beigi F, Grimm RH Jr, Probstfield JL, Simons-Morton DG, Friedewald WT. Effects of intensive glucose lowering in type 2 diabetes. N Engl J Med. 2008;358(24):2545–59. Pubmed.
60. Upadhyay A, Earley A, Haynes SM, Uhlig K. Systematic review: blood pressure target in chronic kidney disease and proteinuria as an effect modifier. Ann Intern Med. 2011;154:541–8. Pubmed.
61. Drawz PE, Alper AB, Anderson AH, Brecklin CS, Charleston J, Chen J, et al. Chronic renal insufficiency cohort study investigators: masked hypertension and elevated nighttime blood pressure in CKD: prevalence and association with target organ damage. Clin J Am Soc Nephrol. 2016;11:642–52. Pubmed.
62. Scheppach JB, Raff U, Toncar S, Ritter C, Klink T, Störk S, et al. Blood pressure pattern and target organ damage in patients with chronic kidney disease. Hypertension. 2018;72:929–36. Pubmed.
63. Ku E, Hsu RK, Tuot DS, Bae SR, Lipkowitz MS, Smogorzewski MJ, et al. Magnitude of the difference between clinic and ambulatory blood pressures and risk of adverse outcomes in patients with chronic kidney disease. J Am Heart Assoc. 2019;8:e011013. Pubmed.
64. Agarwal R, Andersen MJ. Blood pressure recordings within and outside the clinic and cardiovascular events in chronic kidney disease. Am J Nephrol. 2006;26:503–10. Pubmed.
65. Gorostidi M, Sarafidis PA, Sierra A, Banegas JR, Ruilope LM, et al. Differences between office and 24-hour blood pressure control in hypertensive patients with CKD: a 5,693-patient cross-sectional analysis from Spain. AmJ Kidney Dis. 2013;62(2):P285–94. Pubmed.
66. Agarwal R, Andersen MJ. Prognostic importance of ambulatory blood pressure recordings in patients with chronic kidney disease. Kidney Int. 2006;69:1175–80. Pubmed.
67. Davidson MB, Hix JK, Vidt DG, Brotman DJ. Association of impaired diurnal blood pressure variation with a subsequent decline in glomerular filtration rate. Arch Intern Med. 2006;166(8):846–52. Pubmed.
68. Boggia J, Li Y, Thijs L, et al. Prognostic accuracy of day versus night ambulatory blood pressure: a cohort study. Lancet. 2007;370(9594):1219–29. Pubmed.
69. Liu M, Takahashi H, Morita Y, et al. Non-dipping is a potent predictor of cardiovascular mortality and is associated with autonomic dysfunction in haemodialysis patients. Nephrol Dial Transplant. 2003;18(3):563–9. Pubmed.
70. Wang C, Ye Z, Li Y, et al. Prognostic value of reverse dipper blood pressure pattern in chronic kidney disease patients not undergoing dialysis: prospective cohort study. Sci Rep. 2016;6:34932. Pubmed.
71. Hermida RC, Smolensky MH, Ayala DE, Fernández JR, Moyá A, Crespo JJ, Mojón A, Ríos MT, Fabbian F, Portaluppi F. Abnormalities in chronic kidney disease of ambulatory blood pressure 24 h patterning and normalization by bedtime hypertension chronotherapy. Nephrol Dial Transplant. 2014;29(6):1160–7. Pubmed.
72. Ciobanu AO, Gherghinescu CL, Dulgheru R, Magda S, Dragoi Galrinho R, Florescu M, et al. The impact of blood pressure variability on subclinical ventricular, renal and vascular dysfunction, in patients with hypertension and diabetes. Maedica. 2013;8:129–36. Pubmed.
73. Cohen DL, Huan Y, Townsend RR. Home blood pressure monitoring in CKD. Am J Kidney Dis. 2014;63:835–42. Pubmed.
74. Niiranen TJ, Ha¨nninen MR, Johansson J, Reunanen A, Jula AM. Home measured blood pressure is a stronger predictor of cardiovascular risk than office blood pressure: the Finn-Home study. Hypertension. 2010;55:1346–135. Pubmed.
75. Agarwal R, Pappas MK, Sinha AD. Masked uncontrolled hypertension in CKD. J Am Soc Nephrol. 2016;27:924–32. Pubmed.
76. Drawz PE, Beddhu S, Kramer HJ, Rakotz M, Rocco MV, Whelton PK. Blood pressure measurement: a KDOQI perspective. Am J Kidney Dis. 2020;75(3):426–34. Pubmed.

77. Kaboré J, Metzger M, Helmer C, Berr C, Tzourio C, Massy ZA, et al. Kidney function decline and apparent treatment-resistant hypertension in the elderly. PLoS One. 2016;11(1):e0146056. Pubmed.
78. Schmitt KE, Edie CF, Laflam P, Simbartl LA, Thakar CV. Adherence to antihypertensive agents and blood pressure control in chronic kidney disease. Am J Nephrol. 2010;32(6):541–8. Pubmed.
79. Dworkin LD. Impact of antihypertensive therapy on progression of experimental renal disease. J Hum Hypertens. 1996;10(10):663–8. Pubmed.
80. Hostetter TH, Olson JL, Rennke HG, Venkatachalam MA, Brenner BM. Hyperfiltration in remnant nephrons: a potentially adverse response to renal ablation. Am J Phys. 1981;241(1):F85–93. https://doi.org/10.1152/ajprenal.1981.241.1.F85. Pubmed.
81. Brenner BM, Meyer TW, Hostetter TH. Dietary protein intake and the progressive nature of kidney disease: the role of hemodynamically mediated glomerular injury in the pathogenesis of progressive glomerular sclerosis in aging, renal ablation, and intrinsic renal disease. N Engl J Med. 1982;307(11):652–9. https://doi.org/10.1056/NEJM198209093071104. Pubmed.
82. Halbesma N, Kuiken DS, Brantsma AH, et al. Macroalbuminuria is a better risk marker than low estimated GFR to identify individuals at risk for accelerated GFR loss in population screening. J Am Soc Nephrol. 2006;17:2582–90. Pubmed.
83. Imai E, Horio M, Yamagata K, et al. Slower decline of glomerular filtration rate in the Japanese general population: a longitudinal 10-year follow-up study. Hypertens Res. 2008;31:433–41. Pubmed.
84. Lindeman RD, Tobin JD, Shock NW. Association between blood pressure and the rate of decline in renal function with age. Kidney Int. 1984;26:861–8. Pubmed.
85. Hou FF, Zhang X, Zhang GH, Xie D, Chen PY, Zhang WR, Jiang JP, Liang M, Wang GB, Liu ZR, Geng RW. Efficacy and safety of benazepril for advanced chronic renal insufficiency. N Engl J Med. 2006;354:131–40. Pubmed.
86. Strippoli GF, Bonifati C, Craig M, Navaneethan SD, Craig JC. Angiotensin converting enzyme inhibitors and angiotensin IIreceptor antagonists for preventing the progression of diabetic kidney disease. Cochrane Database Syst Rev. 2006;CD006257. Pubmed.
87. Ku E, McCulloch CE, Vittinghoff E, Lin F. Use of antihypertensive agents and association with risk of adverse outcomes in chronic kidney disease: focus on angiotensin-converting enzyme inhibitors and angiotensin receptor blockers. J Am Heart Assoc. 2018;7(19). Pubmed.
88. Middleton RJ, Parfrey PS, Foley RN. Left ventricular hypertrophy in the renal patient. J Am Soc Nephrol. 2001;12(5):1079–84. Pubmed.
89. Levin A, Singer J, Thompson CR, et al. Prevalent left ventricular hypertrophy in the predialysis population: identifying opportunities for intervention. Am J Kidney Dis. 1996;27:347–54. Pubmed.
90. Tagore R, Ling LH, Yang H, et al. Natriuretic peptides in chronic kidney disease. Clin J Am Soc Nephrol. 2008;3:1644–51. Pubmed.
91. ONTARGET Investigators, Yusuf S, Teo KK, Pogue J, et al. Telmisartan, ramipril, or both in patients at high risk for vascular events. N Engl J Med. 2008;358(15):1547–59. Pubmed.
92. Brater DC. Clinical pharmacology of loop diuretics. Drugs. 1991;41(Supplement 3):14–22. ISSN *0012-6667*. Pubmed.
93. Levey AS, Rocco MV, Anderson S, Andreoli SP, Bailie GR, Bakris GL, Callahan MB, Greene JH, Johnson CA, Lash JP, McCullough PA, Miller ER, Nally JV, Pirsch JD, Portman RJ, Sevick MA, Sica D, Wesson DE, Agodoa L, et al. K/DOQI clinical practice guidelines on hypertension and antihypertensive agents in chronic kidney disease. Am J Kidney Dis. 2004;43(5 SUPPL. 1):i–S290. Pubmed.
94. Brater DC. Diuretic therapy. N Engl J Med. 1998;339:387–95. Pubmed.
95. Agarwal R, Sinha AD, Pappas MK, Ammous F. Chlorthalidone for poorly controlled hypertension in chronic kidney disease: an interventional pilot study. Am J Nephrol. 2014;39(2):171–82. Pubmed.

 96. Cirillo M, Marcarelli F, Mele AA, Romano M, Lombardi C, Bilancio G. Parallel-group 8-week study on chlorthalidone effects in hypertensives with low kidney function. Hypertension. 2014;63(4):692–7. Pubmed.
 97. Gupta P, Patel P, Štrauch B, et al. Risk factors for nonadherence to antihypertensive treatment. Hypertension. 2017;69(6):1113–20. Pubmed.
 98. Plantinga L, Lee K, Inker LA, Saran R, Yee J, Gillespie B, Rolka D, Saydah S, Powe NR, CDC CKD Surveillance Team. Association of sleep-related problems with CKD in the United States, 2005-2008. Am J Kidney Dis. 2011;58(4):554–64. Pubmed.
 99. Muntner P, Judd SE, Krousel-Wood M, McClellan WM, Safford MM. Low medication adherence and hypertension control among adults with CKD: data from the REGARDS (Reasons for Geographic and Racial Differences in Stroke) study. Am J Kidney Dis. 2010;56(3):447–57. Pubmed.
100. Aldigier JC, Kanjanbuch T, Ma LJ, Brown NJ, Fogo AB. Regression of existing glomerulosclerosis by inhibition of aldosterone. J Am Soc Nephrol. 2005;16(11):3306–14. Pubmed.
101. Staessen J, Lijnen P, Fagard R, Verschueren LJ, Amery A. Rise in plasma concentration of aldosterone during long-term angiotensin II suppression. J Endocrinol. 1981;91(3):457–65. Pubmed.
102. Navaneethan SD, Nigwekar SU, Sehgal AR, Strippoli GF. Aldosterone antagonists for preventing the progression of chronic kidney disease: a systematic review and meta-analysis. Clin J Am Soc Nephrol. 2009;4(3):542–51. Pubmed.
103. Bakris GL, Agarwal R, Ankar SD, et al. Effect of finerenone on chronic kidney disease outcomes in type 2 diabetes. N Engl J Med. 2020; https://doi.org/10.1056/NEJMoa2025845. Pubmed.
104. Tyson CC, Davenport CA, Lin PH, et al. DASH diet and blood pressure among black Americans with and without CKD: the Jackson Heart Study. Am J Hypertens. 2019;32(10):975–82. Pubmed.
105. Kelly MS, Lewis J, Huntsberry AM, Dea L, Portillo I. Efficacy and renal outcomes of SGLT2 inhibitors in patients with type 2 diabetes and chronic kidney disease. Postgrad Med. 2019;131(1):31–42. Pubmed.
106. Verma S, Mazer CD, Fitchett D, et al. Empagliflozin reduces cardiovascular events, mortality and renal events in participants with type 2 diabetes after coronary artery bypass graft surgery: subanalysis of the EMPA-REG OUTCOME® randomised trial. Diabetologia. 2018;61(8):1712–23. Pubmed.
107. Heerspink HJL, Stefánsson BV, Correa-Rotter R, Chertow GM, Greene T, Hou FF, Mann JFE, McMurray JJV, Lindberg M, Rossing P, Sjöström CD, Toto RD, Langkilde AM, Wheeler DC, DAPA-CKD Trial Committees and Investigators. Dapagliflozin in patients with chronic kidney disease. N Engl J Med. 2020;383(15):1436–46. Pubmed.
108. Gagliardi AC, Miname MH, Santos RD. Uric acid: a marker of increased cardiovascular risk. Atherosclerosis. 2009;202(1):11–7. https://doi.org/10.1016/j.atherosclerosis.2008.05.022. Pubmed.
109. Johnson RJ, Kang DH, Feig D, Kivlighn S, Kanellis J, Watanabe S, Tuttle KR, Rodriguez-Iturbe B, Herrera-Acosta J, Mazzali M. Is there a pathogenetic role for uric acid in hypertension and cardiovascular and renal disease? Hypertension. 2003;41(6):1183–90. Pubmed.
110. Goicoechea M, de Vinuesa SG, Verdalles U, Ruiz-Caro C, Ampuero J, Rincón A, Arroyo D, Luño J. Effect of allopurinol in chronic kidney disease progression and cardiovascular risk. Clin J Am Soc Nephrol. 2010;5(8):1388–93. Pubmed.
111. Goicoechea M, Garcia de Vinuesa S, Verdalles U, Verde E, Macias N, Santos A, Pérez de Jose A, Cedeño S, Linares T, Luño J. Allopurinol and progression of CKD and cardiovascular events: long-term follow-up of a randomized clinical trial. Am J Kidney Dis. 2015;65(4):543–9. Pubmed.
112. Terawaki H, Nakayama M, Miyazawa E, et al. Effect of allopurinol on cardiovascular incidence among hypertensive nephropathy patients: the Gonryo study. Clin Exp Nephrol. 2013;17:549–53. Pubmed.

113. Jardine MJ, Ninomiya T, Perkovic V, et al. Aspirin is beneficial in hypertensive patients with chronic kidney disease: a post-hoc subgroup analysis of a randomized controlled trial. J Am Coll Cardiol. 2010;56:956–65. Pubmed.
114. Best PJ, Steinhubl SR, Berger PB, et al. The efficacy and safety of shortand long-term dual antiplatelet therapy in patients with mild or moderate chronic kidney disease: results from the Clopidogrel for the Reduction of Events During Observation (CREDO) trial. Am Heart J. 2008;155:687–93. Pubmed.
115. Scirica BM, Bohula EA, Dwyer JP, Qamar A, Inzucchi SE, McGuire DK, Keech AC, Smith SR, Murphy SA, Im K, Leiter LA, Gupta M, Patel T, Miao W, Perdomo C, Bonaca MP, Ruff CT, Sabatine MS, Wiviott SD, CAMELLIA-TIMI 61 Steering Committee and Investigators. Lorcaserin and renal outcomes in obese and overweight patients in the CAMELLIA-TIMI 61 trial. Circulation. 2019;139(3):366–75. Pubmed.
116. Cooper CJ, Murphy TP, Cutlip DE, et al. Stenting and medical therapy for atherosclerotic renal-artery stenosis. N Engl J Med. 2014;370(1):13–22. Pubmed.
117. Bax L, Woittiez AJ, Kouwenberg HJ, et al. Stent placement in patients with atherosclerotic renal artery stenosis and impaired renal function: a randomized trial. Ann Intern Med. 2009;150(12):840–1. Pubmed.
118. Varon J, Marik PE. Clinical review: the management of hypertensive crises. Crit Care. 2003;7(5):374–84. Pubmed.
119. Patel HP, Mitsnefes M. Advances in the pathogenesis and management of hypertensive crisis. Curr Opin Pediatr. 2005;17(2):210–4. Pubmed.
120. Cuspidi C, Macca G, Sampieri L, Michev I, Salerno M, Fusi V, et al. High prevalence of cardiac and extracardiac target organ damage in refractory hypertension. J Hypertens. 2001;19:2063–70. Pubmed.
121. Daugherty SL, Powers JD, Magid DJ, Tavel HM, Masoudi FA, Margolis KL, et al. Incidence and prognosis of resistant hypertension in hypertensive patients. Circulation. 2012;125:1635–42. Pubmed.
122. De Nicola L, Gabbai FB, Agarwal R, Chiodini P, Borrelli S, Bellizzi V, et al. Prevalence and prognostic role of resistant hypertension in chronic kidney disease patients. J Am Coll Cardiol. 2013;61:2461–7. Pubmed.

Chapter 8
Infection-Related Kidney Disease

Goni Katz-Greenberg and Yasmin Brahmbhatt

Introduction

Infections are a leading cause of increased morbidity and mortality in patients with chronic kidney disease (CKD) [1]. Patients with CKD experience immune dysfunction which is independent of the etiology of their CKD, and this may increase their risk of acquiring infections.

All types of organisms, including bacteria, viruses, fungi, and parasites, have been identified as triggers for the development of kidney injury, either acute or chronic [2]. The clinical manifestations can vary from acute kidney injury (AKI) to acute or chronic glomerulonephritis (GN), nephrotic syndrome, and rapidly progressive GN. Infections can cause kidney injury by either direct invasion of the kidney or indirectly by immune-mediated mechanisms [3].

This chapter provides an overview of how viruses, bacteria, fungi, and parasites cause kidney injury and how some treatments for these infections can affect kidney function. Due to the HIV epidemic and the high prevalence of hepatitis B and C in the USA, this chapter begins with a discussion on the pathophysiology of kidney disease with HIV, hepatitis B, and hepatitis C and how highly active anti-retroviral therapy (HAART) affects kidney function. The chapter then moves on to how other viruses such as hantavirus and dengue virus can cause kidney disease, followed by how bacterial infections cause kidney-related issues such as post-streptococcal glomerulonephritis and infection-related glomerulonephritis. The chapter concludes with kidney involvement with mycobacterial and parasitic infections.

G. Katz-Greenberg
Division of Nephrology, Department of Medicine, Duke University School of Medicine, Durham, NC, USA
e-mail: goni.katzgreenberg@duke.edu

Y. Brahmbhatt (✉)
AstraZeneca, Philadelphia, PA, USA
e-mail: Yasmin.Brahmbhatt@astrazeneca.com

© Springer Nature Switzerland AG 2022
J. McCauley et al. (eds.), *Approaches to Chronic Kidney Disease*,
https://doi.org/10.1007/978-3-030-83082-3_8

Virus-Induced Kidney Disease

Virus-induced kidney injury can occur as a result of direct damage to the cells or as a consequence of systemic and local responses of the host immune systems (innate and adaptive) [4].

Human Immunodeficiency Virus (HIV)

Worldwide, an estimated 37 million people are living with HIV infection, and 1.7 million new infections are diagnosed annually. In the USA and dependent areas in 2018, 37,832 new patients were diagnosed with HIV. Of these cases, 69% were gay, bisexual, and other men who have sex with men, 24% were heterosexuals, and 7% people who inject drugs [5].

Studies on the optimal CKD screening and monitoring strategies among HIV-positive individuals are lacking. Until such studies exist, current CKD guidelines should be followed. CKD screening is recommended at the time of HIV diagnosis and HAART initiation or modification [6].

HIV infection is a known risk factor for kidney disease and can cause both acute kidney injury and chronic kidney disease through an array of different mechanisms. The approach to evaluating kidney disease in a patient with HIV infection involves differentiating acute kidney injury from chronic kidney disease and is shown in Fig. 8.1. An association between HIV and kidney disease was recognized in the 1980s after cases of acquired immunodeficiency syndrome (AIDS) were identified [8, 9]. Between 2 and 17% of HIV-infected patients will develop some form of kidney disease [10]. The spectrum of HIV-associated renal diseases includes diseases that are directly associated with infection, HIV-associated nephropathy (HIVAN), those that are linked to the infection of systemic immune response; HIV-associated immune-complex kidney disease (HIVICK), those that develop as a consequence of superinfections, and those that are associated with the treatment of HIV infection. Given the different manifestations of kidney disease which can accompany HIV infection, a renal biopsy may be necessary to determine the diagnosis for all patients with HIV who present with kidney disease.

With the introduction of HAART, the life expectancy of people living with HIV resembles that of the general population. With the HIV population aging, there has been an increase in age-related co-morbidities such as cardiovascular disease and CKD. Additionally, these patients' burden of comorbidities is increased due to an aging phenomenon thought to be driven by a pro-inflammatory state in patients with HIV [11].

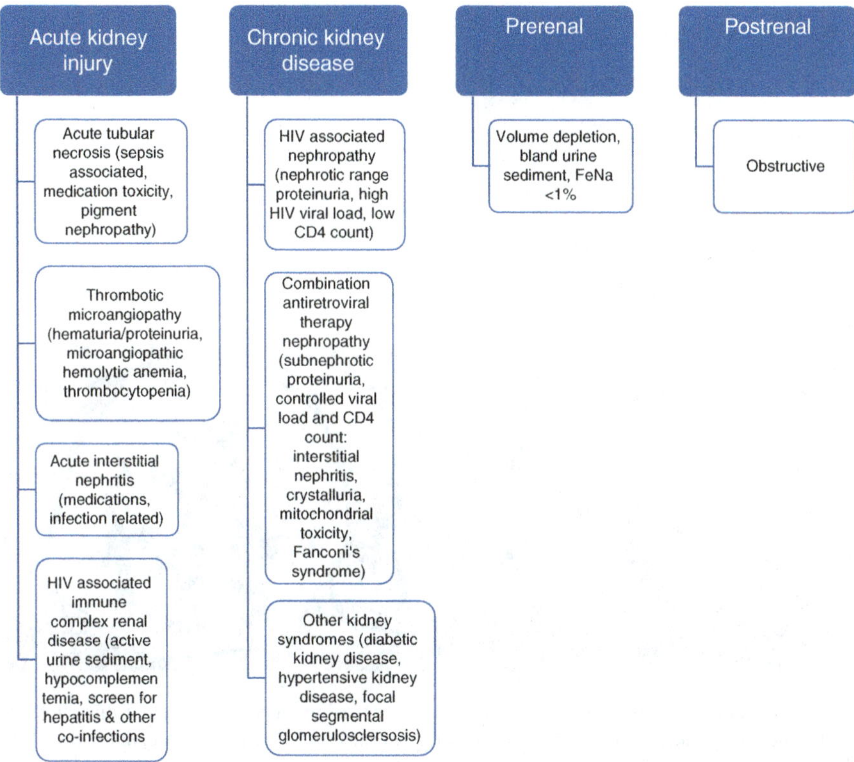

Fig. 8.1 Mechanisms of kidney injury with HIV. (Adapted from Cohen et al. [7])

Human Immunodeficiency Virus–Associated Nephropathy (HIVAN)

Prior to HAART, HIVAN was the most common cause of kidney disease and the prevalence ranged between 3.5 and 10%. Patients with HIVAN would rapidly progress to end-stage kidney disease (ESKD). The typical presentation of patients with HIVAN consisted of nephrotic-range proteinuria and decreased renal function [12]. Since the introduction of HAART, the prevalence of HIVAN has decreased dramatically. The highest rates are reported in Sub-Saharan Africa. In the USA, HIVAN occurs primarily in patients of African-American descent, particularly in those with markedly reduced CD4 counts and high viral loads. HIVAN probably arises because of complex interactions among host factors (especially genetics), pathogen expression (renal viral protein expression), and environmental and socioeconomic factors (the most important of which may be access to care and ART with effective viral suppression).

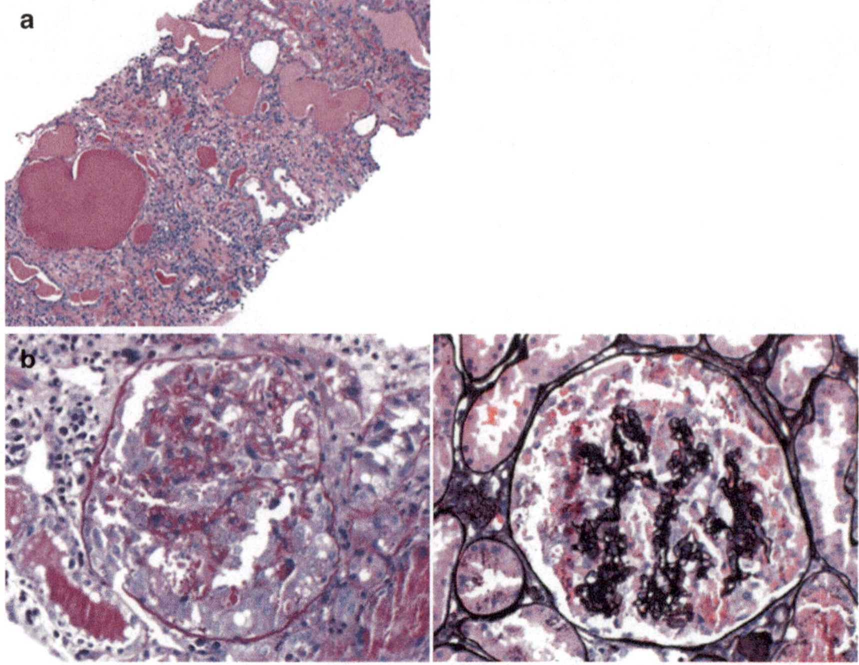

Fig. 8.2 Histology of HIVAN. (**a**) Light microscopy revealing microcystic tubular dilatation. (**b**) Light microscopy and silver stain showing collapsing lesion. (Courtesy of Alejandro Best MD, Arkana Laboratories)

The typical histologic lesion on a renal biopsy in HIVAN is collapsing focal segmental glomerulosclerosis (FSGS). Other histologic findings include tubular microcystic dilatation, interstitial inflammation and fibrosis, and tubuloreticular inclusion bodies [13] (Fig. 8.2).

APOL1 Gene

Given that HIV-positive African Americans have a higher risk of developing CKD, focal segmental glomerulosclerosis (FSGS), and HIVAN, it has long been postulated that genetics may play a role [14]. APOL1 gene variants help in killing *Trypanosoma brucei*, the cause of African sleeping sickness, and the increased genetic predisposition to kidney disease development is due to variants in APOL1 gene, which encodes the apolipoprotein L1. The most common allele of the APOL1 gene is G0; however, the variants G1 and G2 are considered renal risk variants and are associated with increased risk of developing HIVAN. They are also associated with non-HIV CKD such as FSGS, not otherwise specified (NOS), and hypertension-associated nephrosclerosis. The frequency of these risk alleles is approximately 50% in West African blacks and 35% in African Americans [13]. Recent research shows that among patients with biopsy-proven HIVAN, 79% carried two copies of APOL1 risk alleles (G1/G2, G1/G1, or G2/G2) as compared to 2% in the general population [15].

Treatment of HIVAN involves combined anti-retroviral therapy (cHAART), while adjunctive therapies include RAAS blockade and prednisone. In those who progress to ESKD, dialysis remains the mainstay of management, and there is now good evidence that kidney transplantation can be very effective in those with controlled HIV disease.

HIV-Associated Immune Complex Kidney Disease (HIVICK)

HIVICK is defined as glomerular immune complex deposition in the setting of HIV infection. In recent years, the incidence of HIVICK has increased and it is now the most common diagnosis of kidney biopsy of HIV-positive patients. The exact reason for the increased incidence is unknown. It has been postulated that the modulation of the immune system following treatment with ART may cause immune reconstitution and immune complex deposition. It also could be due to the incidence of HIVAN decreasing [16]. HIVICK includes a wide variety of renal lesions including membranous nephropathy, MPGN, lupus nephritis, and IgA nephropathy among others. In contrast to HIVAN, HIVICK is typically diagnosed several years following the patients testing positive for HIV [17].

Similar to HIVAN, there are four main ways to treat HIVICK: (1) combined HAART, (2) immunosuppressants (steroids have been used in certain cases), (3) renin-angiotensin aldosterone blockade, and (4) treatment of underlying co-morbidities [16].

Treatment of HIV with HIV-Associated Anti-Retro-Viral Therapy (HAART)

The most significant development in HIV in the past 40 years since it was first identified was the advent of HAARTs which have significantly improved the prognosis and delayed the progression of HIV. Their effectiveness and widened use have brought new challenges to light including HAART-induced nephrotoxicity, immune-mediated kidney injury, and risk factors for CKD. There are five classes of HAARTs with each one targeting a different step of the virus's replication and infection. Treatment is usually initiated by a combination of drugs from different classes. Many of these medications are partly eliminated in the kidney and require dose adjustment when prescribed to patients with CKD. Serum creatinine is not always a reliable measurement, especially when HIV patients have muscle wasting, but remains the standard of care when estimating GFR.

Protease Inhibitors (PI)

Indinavir (10–20%), lopinavir, and atazanavir are all associated with nephrolithiasis [18].

Indinavir precipitates in the lumen of the distal tubules, due to its insolubility at urine pH of >3.5, and forms clear crystalline casts within the tubular lumens, which are surrounded by a lymphoplasmacytic infiltrate. On urinalysis, the crystals can appear rectangular, starburst shaped, or fan shaped. It has also been associated with acute and chronic tubulointerstitial nephritis and rarely with papillary necrosis. Given its many toxicities, and with emergence of newer PIs, indinavir has fallen out of favor. Atazanavir is a widely used PI due to its high antiviral activity, tolerability, and once-daily dosing. Atazanavir has recently been reported to cause crystalline nephropathy, crystalluria-related interstitial nephritis, and urolithiasis [19]. Nelfinavir and saquinavir have been associated with urolithiasis as well.

Nucleotide Reverse Transcriptase Inhibitors (NRTI)

Most NRTIs are excreted 30–70% via the urinary tract and thus require dose adjustment for abnormal renal function. Abacavir is metabolized in the liver and only 1% of the parent drug is excreted in the urine and, therefore, does not require dose adjustment with kidney disease [20].

Tenofovir disoproxil fumarate (TDF) has been used for almost 20 years and remains a first-line option for treatment of patients with HIV. TDF is the pro-drug of the active agent tenofovir. Tenofovir undergoes renal elimination by a combination of filtration and tubular secretion. About 1% of the drug is protein bound and it requires dose adjustment for eGFR < 50 ml/min [21]. TDF has been linked to a wide range of renal complications from mild proximal tubulopathy to fulminant Fanconi's syndrome. Studies reveal that TDF is associated with a 14% increased risk of CKD [22]. Interestingly several studies have shown that 12 months following the discontinuation of TDF, the risk for CKD is similar to that of HIV-positive patients who were never exposed to TDF [23].

Following two randomized non-inferiority trials in 2015 [24], tenofovir alafenamide fumarate (TAF) was introduced. TAF is a more efficient prodrug than TDF and requires a 90% lower effective dose; therefore, it is less toxic to the kidneys and the bones, making it an attractive alternative to TDF [11].

Non-nucleotide Reverse Transcriptase Inhibitors (NNRTI)

This class of HAART primarily undergo hepatic metabolism by the CYP450 system with little to no urinary excretion. There have been case reports that have linked efavirenz to both interstitial nephritis and nephrolithiasis [25].

Hepatitis C Virus (HCV)

There are between 64 and 103 million people worldwide who are estimated to have chronic HCV infection [26]. HCV infection remains the most frequent chronic viral infection in the USA and is a common comorbidity in patients with CKD [27]. While the main cause of morbidity and mortality in people infected with HCV is associated with liver disease (i.e., cirrhosis, decompensated cirrhosis, hepatocellular carcinoma), extra-hepatic manifestations are common and include mixed cryoglobulinemia, CKD, cardiovascular disease, type 2 diabetes mellitus, lymphoproliferative disorders, porphyria cutanea tarda, lichen planus, and depression. Infection with the HCV virus is often diagnosed in the chronic stage of the disease which could occur decades following the initial infection. HCV is a blood-borne virus, and while the acute infection is often asymptomatic, 60–80% of people will develop chronic HCV infection.

The pathogenesis of kidney injury in HCV is multifactorial and includes the host's immune response and involves the deposition of circulating immune complexes which are composed of HCV antigens, anti-HCV antibodies, and complement factors in the kidney.

While the most recognized renal manifestation of HCV infection is glomerulonephritis, which is caused by an immune complex-mediated response, other forms of kidney injury by the virus include direct cytopathic effect, atherosclerosis, insulin resistance, and chronic inflammation (Fig. 8.3) [28]. Additionally, previous studies have shown that patients with chronic HCV infection have a more rapid progression of CKD and an almost twofold increased risk of developing ESKD compared to HCV-negative controls [29].

Cryoglobulins are immunoglobulins which precipitate in cooled serum and dissolve on rewarming. About 50% of patients with chronic HCV have circulating cryoglobulins, but fewer than 5% will develop mixed cryoglobulinemia syndrome which manifests as a small vessel vasculitis where renal involvement is seen in about 30% of cases. Patients with cryoglobulinemic GN typically present with hypertension, proteinuria, and microscopic hematuria, as well as some degree of renal insufficiency. It can also present as an acute nephritic or, less likely, acute nephrotic syndrome [28]. The pathological pattern of injury in cryoglobulinemia is usually membranoproliferative glomerulonephritis (MPGN), with eosinophilic intraluminal thrombi, a double-contoured basement membrane, and mesangial proliferation visible on light microscopy; subendothelial deposits are typically seen on electron microscopy and immunofluorescence confirms that the deposits consist of IgM, IgG, and C3 (Fig. 8.4).

GN associated with mixed cryoglobulinemic vasculitis and immune complex GN of the membranoproliferative GN type are considered to be the most severe renal manifestation of HCV infection [30].

Other GNs which have been associated with HCV infections and involve the deposition of circulating immune complexes in the kidney include membranous nephropathy, secondary IgA nephropathy, MPGN (without cryoglobulinemia), and two less common GNs – fibrillary and immunotactoid glomerulopathy.

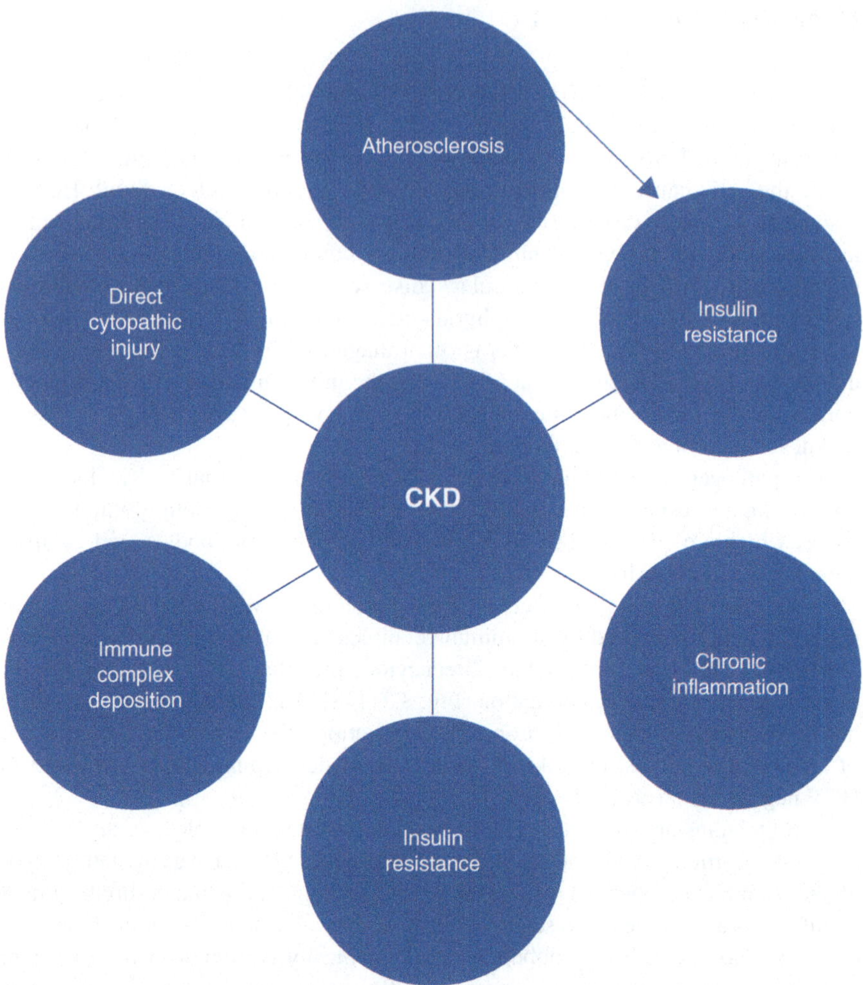

Fig. 8.3 Potential mechanisms of chronic kidney disease in patients with HCV. (Adapted from Fig. 1 in Henson and Sise [28])

HCV Treatment

There is no vaccine for HCV. Until recently, the recommended regimen for chronic HCV-positive patients with CKD included interferon (IFN) with or without ribavirin [27]. However, given the side effect profile and drug-to-drug interactions, only a small subset of patients tolerated this treatment long term.

Direct-acting antiviral agents (DAAs) emerged less than a decade ago. The DAAs have shown to cure more than 95% of patients with chronic HCV infection safely and effectively and have revolutionized the management of HCV infection.

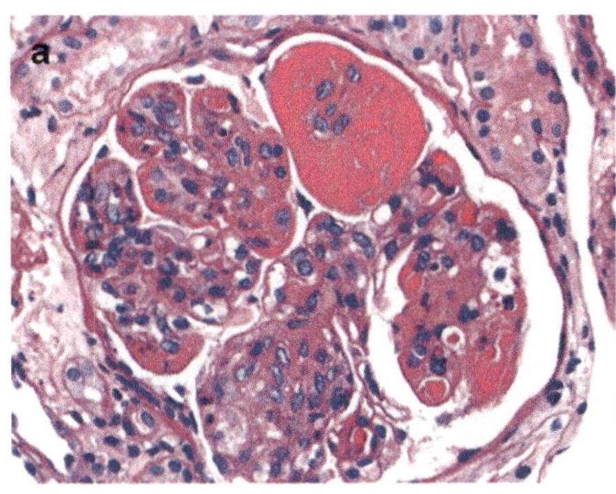
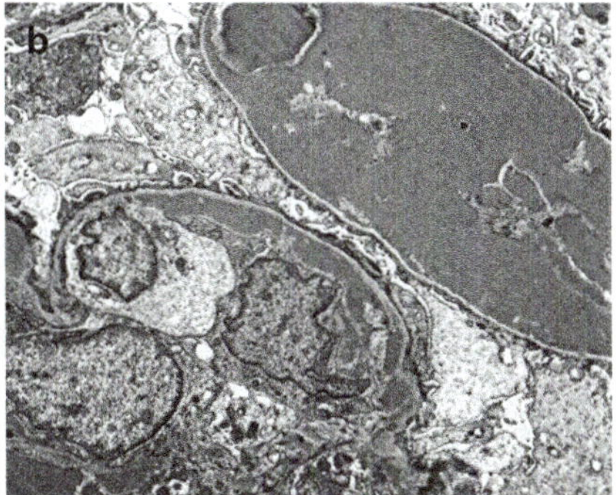

Fig. 8.4 Histology revealing type II cryoglobulinemic membranoproliferative glomerular disease. (**a**) Light microscopy showing endocapillary hypercellularity and large thrombi. (**b**) Electron microscopy revealing subendothelial deposits. (Courtesy of Alejandro Best MD, Arkana Laboratories)

The first DAA, sofosbuvir, was approved by the FDA in 2014 and a sofosbuvir-based IFN-free regimen was introduced. Sofosbuvir is renally eliminated and is not approved for patients with an eGFR < 30 ml/min.

As additional DAAs were introduced to the market and patients with renal impairment were included in clinical trials, studies revealed that patients with HCV-associated GN or mixed cryoglobulinemia were prescribed DAAs with a good response rate. DAAs are now considered the first-line management for cryoglobulinemia as per Kidney Disease Improving Global Outcomes (KDIGO) 2018 guidelines [31].

Hepatitis B Virus

Hepatitis B virus (HBV) is a DNA virus and a member of the Hepadnaviridae family.

Chronic infection (defined as positive serology for HBsAg and anti-HBc antibodies but negative for IgM anti-HBc and anti-HBs antibodies) affects more than 400 million people worldwide, making it the most common chronic viral infection. Of these, 10–20% are co-infected with HCV and 5–10% have co-infection with HIV [32].

Renal disease occurs in 3–5% of patient with chronic HBV and can manifest as immune-complex glomerulonephritis or immune complex-related vasculitis (i.e., polyarteritis nodosa).

The two most common histological patterns associated with HBV are membranous nephropathy (MN) and membranoproliferative GN (MPGN).

Membranous nephropathy (MN) in adults with chronic HBV can manifest as asymptomatic proteinuria but usually presents with nephrotic syndrome and kidney injury with subsequent increased risk of developing renal failure. The liver disease

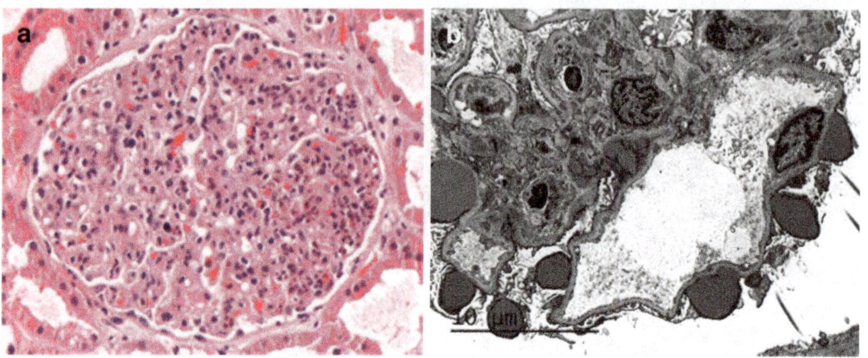

Fig. 8.5 Secondary IgA nephropathy induced by hepatitis B virus. (**a**) Light microscopy revealing endocapillary hypercellularity with neutrophils. (**b**) Electron microscopy revealing subepithelial-like deposits. (Courtesy of Alejandro Best MD, Arkana Laboratories)

is usually apparent at time of diagnosis. On electron microscopy, the appearance of subepithelial immune complex deposits is identical to that of idiopathic MN. In HBV, the antigen present in the immune-complex can be HBsAg, HBcAg, or HBeAg. HBeAg is the smallest of the three antigens and can be isolated from the glomerulus in about 90% of patients with biopsy-proven MN and HBV. Interestingly there has been conflicting data whether anti-PLA2R Ab positivity confirms the diagnosis of idiopathic MN versus HBV-associated MN [33, 34].

Membranoproliferative glomerulonephritis (MPGN) is the second most common GN in patients with chronic HBV. Liver disease is often present, although it can be asymptomatic at time of diagnosis. MPGN usually presents as nephritic syndrome, with or without nephrotic-range proteinuria. The appearance on biopsy is usually of MPGN type 1, with a lobular appearance of the glomerulus, and mesangial, subendothelial, and subepithelial immune deposits. The typical antigen seen in HBV-associated MPGN is HBsAg given its size (40-50kD). A subset of patients will present with cryoglobulinemia, especially if there is a concurrent infection with HCV.

IgA nephropathy has been reported with HBV viral transcripts seen in the mesangium. This is thought to be a result of chronic liver disease, which causes impaired clearance of circulating IgA immune complexes (Fig. 8.5).

HBV Treatment

Hepatitis B virus can survive outside the body for over a week. During that time, the virus can still cause infection if it enters the body of someone who is not infected. The HBV vaccination series is recommended in high-risk populations which include people whose sex partners have hepatitis B, sexually active persons who are not in a long-term monogamous relationship, persons seeking evaluation or treatment for a sexually transmitted disease, men who have sex with other men, people who share needles, syringes, or other drug injection, health care and public safety workers at risk for exposure through bodily fluids, travelers to regions with increased rates of hepatitis B, people with chronic liver disease, kidney disease, HIV infection, and diabetes.

Universal HBV vaccination has been shown to successfully reduce childhood cases of HBV membranous nephropathy related to horizontal transmission of the virus, but it will have no effect on HBV MN due to vertical acquisition of HBV which still represents an important transmission vector in developing countries.

Kidney Disease Improving Global Outcomes (KDIGO) recommends the use of interferon or oral antiviral agents that consist of either nucleotide (adefovir dipivoxil, TDF, TAF) or nucleoside (lamivudine, entecavir, and telbivudine) reverse transcription inhibitors for treatment of HBV-related GN and vasculitis [35]. In the treatment of HBV MN, lamivudine has been the most commonly used agent associated with an initial remission of viremia and complete resolution of the MN lesion in 75–80% of patients. However, lamivudine is associated with a 20% per year resistance rate. For this reason, either entecavir or tenofovir has now been recommended as first-line therapy. A more detailed description of TDF and TAF is under the HCV section of this chapter.

Hepatitis E Virus

Hepatitis E virus (HEV) infection is now increasingly recognized in many countries of the developed world. HEV can cause GN in both immunocompetent and immunosuppressed patients. Many cases of GN which include MPGN with and without mixed cryoglobulinemia, MGN, and IgAN have been described [36]. Decline in estimated glomerular filtration rate with HEV infection has been shown in kidney transplant recipients.

Other Virus-Associated Renal Disease

Flaviviruses

The global incidence of flavivirus infection has increased in recent decades and now expands from endemic tropical and subtropical areas to non-endemic areas. Most disease-causing flavivirus are mosquito borne (arbovirus) and include dengue, yellow fever, Japanese encephalitis, Zika, and West Nile fever. The disease caused by flavivirus is usually asymptomatic or self-limited, mild, and febrile illness. In other cases, the infection can cause a multisystem disease, with high morbidity and mortality.

Dengue Virus

Dengue is a worldwide infection with 40% of the global population living in endemic areas, especially Southeast Asia and Pacific Islands. Infections occur through the bite of the female mosquito *Aedes aegyptii*. Dengue is classified into specific syndromes: dengue fever, dengue hemorrhagic fever, and dengue shock syndrome. AKI occurs in 10–33% of patients and is usually associated with dengue hemorrhagic fever and dengue shock syndrome [3]. AKI results from ATN as a consequence of hypovolemia and capillary leak and/or rhabdomyolysis. GN is also well described which may result from immune-complex deposition or because of direct viral entry into renal tissue. The presence of hematuria and proteinuria (both sub-nephrotic and nephrotic) helps distinguish these cases from typical ATN. Treatment strategies remain limited to supportive management in all categories of dengue.

Hantavirus

Hantaviruses are RNA viruses that belong to the Bunyaviridae family with wild rodent as reservoir. Renal involvement may occur in up to 30–40% of cases. Two syndromes can develop: hemorrhagic fever with renal syndrome (HFRD) and hantavirus pulmonary syndrome (HPS). HFRS manifests clinically with sudden onset of flu-like syndrome with fever, myalgia, and headache followed by gastrointestinal symptoms and AKI with oliguria. HFRS leads to renal edema and retroperitoneal leakage of fluid. Acute tubulointerstitial nephritis with mononuclear cells and CD8+ cell infiltration is the most prominent finding in the renal histopathology. HFRS occurs primarily in Europe and Asia. HPS is observed in North America, Mexico, and Panama with very high mortality rate of up to 30–40% within 24–48 hours of admission. Hantavirus and other rodent-borne disease like leptospirosis have been implicated as one of the potential explanations for Mesoamerican nephropathy. Management for hantavirus infection remains conservative, and preventive strategies with vaccination are limited as an approved vaccine for hantavirus infection is still underway.

Coronavirus-19

At the time of this writing, the coronavirus-19 pandemic has affected millions of people across the world. Acute kidney injury is frequently observed in patients who develop ARDS with this virus. ARDS-associated AKI may be due to several causes including an inflammatory/immune reaction characterized by an enhanced release of circulating mediators able to interact and damage kidney cells [37]. Kidney

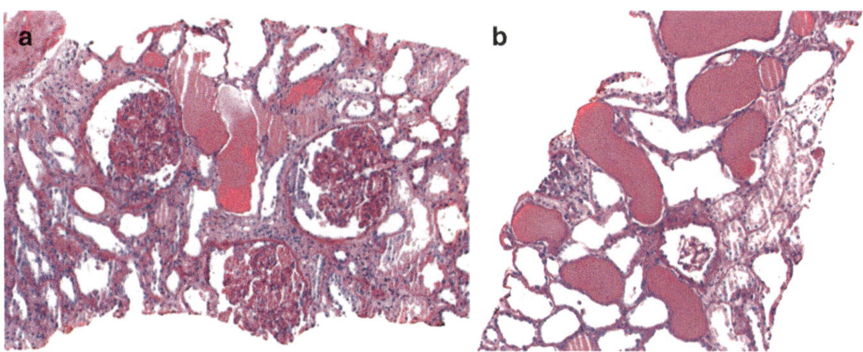

Fig. 8.6 Histopathology revealing Coronavirus-associated FSGS. (**a**) Light microscopy showing collapsing lesion. (**b**) Light microscopy revealing microcystic tubular dilatation. (Courtesy of Alejandro Best MD, Arkana Laboratories)

epithelial cell viral infection may worsen the local inflammatory response and consequently the incidence and the duration of AKI episodes. Few kidney biopsies have been done, which have revealed acute tubular necrosis, FSGS, a microvascular injury syndrome mediated by activation of complement pathways, and an associated procoagulant state. Recent research also points to the presence of viral particles in the epithelial cells (Fig. 8.6).

Bacterial Infections

The most common renal manifestation of bacterial infection is acute kidney injury, usually due to hypotension-related sepsis or acute tubular necrosis (ATN) and is not part of the scope of this chapter. It is important to note, however, that as many as 20% of critically ill patient may have irreversible kidney damage following ATN, and another 40% have incomplete renal recovery which may subsequently lead to CKD [38].

Post-streptococcal Glomerulonephritis

Infections (bacterial, viral, or parasitic) are an important trigger for the development of acute GN [3]. The term post-streptococcal glomerulonephritis (PSGN) historically referred to glomerulonephritis following a streptococcal upper respiratory tract or skin infection mostly in childhood. Patients are classically children and young adults who had a recent streptococcal infection, with a 2–3:1 male predominance. The latency period is 10–21 days from the onset of bacterial infection to presentation, with some of the infections not clinically apparent. Clinical presentation ranges from asymptomatic hematuria, with or without proteinuria, to acute nephritic syndrome (including AKI, hematuria, proteinuria, edema, and new-onset or worsening hypertension).

In the past several decades, there had been a shift in the epidemiology and course of this entity, and it is now referred to as infection-associated glomerulonephritis or infection-related glomerulonephritis (IRGN) [39].

Infection-Related Glomerulonephritis

The incidence of IRGN has decreased in recent decades in developed countries due to improved hygiene and more access to antibiotic treatment. Studies from the last 2 decades show a male: female predominance of 1.5–3:1 and an increase in the incidence in the elderly [40]. About half of the adults in developed countries with IRGN are immunocompromised. Diabetes and alcoholism are two major risk factors in the USA and in Europe, respectively [41]. The two most common pathogens in IRGN are streptococcus and staphylococcus. The latter is as common as the former in developed countries, especially in diabetic patients and the elderly. Most of the staphylococcus-related GN are caused by *S. aureus*, with greater incidence of methicillin-resistant staphlococcus aureus (MRSA) than methicillin-sensitive staphlococcus aureus (MSSA). Gram-negative bacteria are detected in about 10% of cases of IRGN, with *Escherichia coli* being the most common. The most common sites of infection are skin and upper respiratory tract, but other sites, such as the lungs, heart, bone, or urinary tract, are also common.

Diagnosis is made by renal biopsy which demonstrates mesangial and endothelial cell swelling or proliferation, with an influx of neutrophils. Immunofluorescence reveals granular mesangial and capillary wall deposits of IgG and/or C3. The electron microscopy reveals subepithelial immune deposits, also known as "humps."

The disease is usually followed by a clinical recovery over days to weeks. Previously, long-term prognosis was considered excellent; however, we now know that there is an increased risk for lifetime development of CKD [42].

Mycobacterial Infections

Tuberculosis (TB) remains a major cause of morbidity in Southeast Asia and Western Pacific Regions, and with the emergence of multi-drug resistance and co-infection with HIV, it is expected to pose greater challenges. The most common cause of tuberculosis (TB) is *Mycobacterium tuberculosis*. However, some cases can be caused by other *Mycobacterium* species in the *M. tuberculosis* complex (MAC) TB can manifest with pulmonary and extra-pulmonary symptoms. Involvement of the genitourinary tract is seen in 6–8% of all cases of extra-pulmonary TB [39]. Hematogenous spread of the *Mycobacterium* to the kidney with gradual, asymptomatic progression of the disease leads to a delay in diagnosis. Involvement of urinary bladder and ureters leads to obstructive nephropathy. Extensive destructive caseous lesions, ulceration, and dystrophic calcification involving renal parenchyma lead to CKD. Renal involvement can also present as granulomatous interstitial nephritis [40]. TB is the most common cause of secondary amyloidosis in the Indian subcontinent [43, 44]. Diagnosis of renal involvement in TB is usually difficult due to poor culture techniques and poor sensitivity of nucleic acid-based tests. Treatment with anti-tubercular agents usually will not reverse the progression to CKD.

Fungal Infections

Major risks for fungal infections are older age, female gender, prolonged antibiotic use, indwelling catheter, prior surgical procedures, mechanical ventilation, parenteral nutrition, diabetes mellitus, and an immunocompromised state. Most common organisms are *Candida albicans* species as well as non-albicans; less common fungi are filamentous fungi (*Mucor, Aspergillus, Penicillium*); and rare endemic fungi (Blastomyces, Mucormycetes, Histoplasma, Coccidioides). Spread may be ascending (candida) or hematogenous (aspergillus or endemic fungi). Diagnostic tests to evaluate colonization from infection have not been standardized. However, presence of filamentous fungi like *Aspergillus* sp. and endemic fungus, e.g., Blastomyces, almost always reflects infection. Symptomatic patients usually present with urinary tract obstruction from masses of fungal elements (fungus balls). Angio-invasion by fungi may lead to numerous renal micro abscesses and extensive renal infarcts leading to renal dysfunction. Systemic treatment and surgical removal of the obstructing mass are usually required. The prognosis of angio-invasive fungal infection with mucormycosis and aspergillus is poor with high mortality [3].

Protozoan and Parasitic Infections

Out of 342 parasites that infect humans, about 20 of them are associated with kidney disease, which varies from AKI to GN, amyloidosis, urological disorders, and malignancy.

Malaria

Malaria may cause AKI in 2–39% of cases. *Plasmodium falciparum* infection has been reported to cause kidney disease in up to 60% cases [45]. Kidney involvement can also occur with *P. malariae, P. vivax, P. knowlesi,* and *P. ovale*. Renal injury can occur due to renal ischemia because of hemorrhagic changes produced by malarial parasites, intravascular hemolysis, volume depletion, rhabdomyolysis, or systemic inflammatory response syndrome (SIRS). Artesunate is the antimalarial of choice for malaria with kidney involvement. A small number of patients present with glomerular involvement without systemic signs. Acute GN caused by *P. falciparum* usually manifests with microhematuria and mild proteinuria and uncommonly with nephritic syndrome, but renal dysfunction is rare in this situation. Renal histology shows mesangial hypercellularity with infiltration of pigment-laden macrophages and parasitized red cells as well as endocapillary proliferation. Treatment with antimalarials usually normalizes urinary abnormalities. *Plasmodium malariae* may be associated with steroid-resistant nephrotic syndrome, known as tropical nephrotic syndrome. Kidney biopsy shows proliferative pattern with granular deposits of IgG, IgM, and C3 indicating an immune-complex medicated injury. Prognosis is poor as it usually progresses to ESRD despite anti-malarial treatment.

Leptospirosis

Leptospirosis is caused by a spirochete of genus *Leptospira* and is a zoonosis that is endemic in tropical regions. Infection is transmitted to humans through animal urine. Due to high sero-prevalence in endemic areas, it has been implicated in the development of Mesoamerican nephropathy [46]. Renal injury can vary from mild proteinuria, abnormal urinary sediment, tubular dysfunction, and AKI usually due to interstitial nephritis. Renal involvement is usually non-oliguric AKI as a part of multi-organ involvement, along with pulmonary hemorrhage and acute respiratory distress syndrome.

Leishmaniasis

Leishmaniasis is caused by genus Leishmania with humans as reservoir and sand fly as vector. It primarily affects the reticuloendothelial system, and renal involvement is associated with visceral leishmaniasis. It presents with fever, malaise, weight loss, hepatosplenomegaly, and lymphadenopathy. Renal histology can vary from chronic interstitial nephritis, MPGN, and amyloid deposits [47].

Schistosomiasis

Schistosomiasis is endemic in South America, the Far East, and Africa. It primarily affects the lower urinary tract producing a granulomatous response around its ova that produces pseudotubercles in the bladder mucosa which consolidate to form sessile masses and ulcers. Presentation is usually with microscopic to macroscopic hematuria. Progressive disease leads to fibrosis and bladder calcifications, resulting in outflow obstruction or vesicoureteral reflux and, finally, chronic pyelonephritis. Secondary bacterial infection with pseudomonas or proteus is commonly associated with disease. Immune-complex-mediated renal disease occurs in patients with *S. mansoni and S. japonicum* but not with *S. haematobium*. Severe disease is usually symptomatic and progressive even after eradication of infection [48]. Immune-mediated tubulointerstitial nephritis has also been described with *S. mansoni*. Antiparasitic treatment is very effective in early bladder disease but not in advanced and chronic disease involving kidneys. Urological surgery including urinary stenting may be required for the relief of obstructive nephropathy.

Filariasis

Wuchereria bancrofti and Onchocerca volvulus are the two filarial parasites associated with kidney disease. They are transmitted via infected mosquitoes. *W. bancroftis* is endemic in sub-Saharan Africa and Southeast Asia. The disease usually presents with tropical eosinophilic pneumonia, chyluria with hematuria, and elephantiasis [49]. Few patients may present with nephritic syndrome and immune-complex-mediated proliferative GN [50]. *O. volvulus* is rarely associated with minimal change disease or chronic sclerosing GN with progressive renal impairment. Once established, anti-filarial treatment is ineffective in reversing renal disease.

Conclusion

In summary, patients with certain infectious diseases should be screened for kidney involvement via thorough history, physical examination, and basic laboratory tests. Inter-disciplinary collaboration with infectious disease specialists and nephrologists is very important and a carefully drafted treatment plan with ongoing monitoring is required in most cases for optimal outcomes.

References

1. Wang HE, Gamboa C, Warnock DG, Muntner P. Chronic kidney disease and risk of death from infection. Am J Nephrol. 2011;34(4):330–3361. https://www.karger.com/Article/Abstract/330673. https://doi.org/10.1159/000330673.
2. Satoskar AA, Parikh SV, Nadasdy T. Epidemiology, pathogenesis, treatment and outcomes of infection-associated glomerulonephritis. Nat Rev Nephrol. 2019. https://www.ncbi.nlm.nih.gov/pubmed/31399725.; https://doi.org/10.1038/s41581-019-0178-8.

3. Prasad N, Patel MR. Infection-induced kidney diseases. Front Med. 2018;5:327. https://www.ncbi.nlm.nih.gov/pubmed/30555828. https://doi.org/10.3389/fmed.2018.00327.

4. Bruggeman LA. Common mechanisms of viral injury to the kidney. Adv Chronic Kidney Dis. 2019;26(3):164–70.

5. https://www.cdc.gov/hiv/statistics/overview/ataglance.html. Last Accessed 22 Apr 2020.

6. Swanepoel CR, Atta MG, D'Agati VD, et al. Kidney disease in the setting of HIV infection: conclusions from a kidney disease: improving global outcomes (kdigo) controversiesconference.Nephrology.2018;22(6):84–100.https://doi.org/10.24884/1561-6274-2018-22-6-84-100.

7. Cohen SD, Kopp JB, Kimmel PL. Kidney disease associated with human immunodeficiency virus infection. N Engl J Med. 377:2363–74. https://doi.org/10.1056/NEJMra150846.

8. Rao TK, Filippone EJ. Associated focal and segmental glomerulosclerosis in the acquired immunodeficiency syndrome. N Engl J Med. 1984;310:669–73.

9. D'Agati V, Suh J, Carbone L, Cheng J, Appel G. Pathology of HIV-associated nephropathy: a detailed morphologic and comparative study. Kidney Int. 1989;35(6):1358–70. https://www.sciencedirect.com/science/article/pii/S0085253815345762. https://doi.org/10.1038/ki.1989.135.

10. Hou J, Nast C. Changing concepts of HIV infection and renal disease. Curr Opin Nephrol Hypertens. 2018;27:144–52. https://doi.org/10.1097/MNH.0000000000000400.

11. Milburn J, Jones R, Levy JB. Renal effects of novel antiretroviral drugs. Nephrol Dial Transpl. 2017;32(3):434–9. https://www.ncbi.nlm.nih.gov/pubmed/27190354. https://doi.org/10.1093/ndt/gfw064.

12. Cohen SD, Kopp JB, Kimmel PL. Kidney diseases associated with human immunodeficiency virus infection. N Engl J Med. 2017;377(24):2363–74. https://doi.org/10.1056/NEJMra1508467.

13. Rosenberg AZ, Naicker S, Winkler CA, Kopp JB. HIV-associated nephropathies: epidemiology, pathology, mechanisms and treatment. Nat Rev Nephrol. 2015;11(3):150–60. https://www.ncbi.nlm.nih.gov/pubmed/25686569. https://doi.org/10.1038/nrneph.2015.9.

14. Atta MG, Estrella MM, Skorecki KL, et al. Association of APOL1 genotype with renal histology among black HIV-positive patients undergoing kidney biopsy. Clin J Am Soc Nephrol. 2016;11(2):262–70. https://www.ncbi.nlm.nih.gov/pubmed/26668025. https://doi.org/10.2215/CJN.07490715.

15. Kasembeli AN, Duarte R, Ramsay M, et al. APOL1 risk variants are strongly associated with HIV-associated nephropathy in black South Africans. J Am Soc Nephrol. 2015;26(11):2882–90. https://www.ncbi.nlm.nih.gov/pubmed/25788523. https://doi.org/10.1681/ASN.2014050469.

16. Nobakht E, Cohen SD, Rosenberg AZ, Kimmel PL. HIV-associated immune complex kidney disease. Nat Rev Nephrol. 2016;12(5):291–300. https://www.ncbi.nlm.nih.gov/pubmed/26782145. https://doi.org/10.1038/nrneph.2015.216.

17. Booth JW, Hamzah L, Jose S, et al. Clinical characteristics and outcomes of HIV-associated immune complex kidney disease. Nephrol Dial Transpl. 2016;31(12):2099–107. https://www.ncbi.nlm.nih.gov/pubmed/26786550. https://doi.org/10.1093/ndt/gfv436.

18. Wang LC, Osterberg EC, David SG, Rosoff JS. Recurrent nephrolithiasis associated with atazanavir use. BMJ Case Rep. 2014;2014(jan08 1):bcr2013201565. https://doi.org/10.1136/bcr-2013-201565.

19. Daudon M, Frochot V, Bazin D, Jungers P. Drug-induced kidney stones and crystalline nephropathy: pathophysiology, prevention and treatment. Drugs. 2018;78(2):163–201. https://www.ncbi.nlm.nih.gov/pubmed/29264783. https://doi.org/10.1007/s40265-017-0853-7.

20. Berns JS, Kasbekar N. Highly active antiretroviral therapy and the kidney: an update on antiretroviral medications for nephrologists. Clin J Am Soc Nephrol. 2006;1(1):117–29. http://cjasn.asnjournals.org/content/1/1/117.abstract. https://doi.org/10.2215/CJN.00370705.

21. Kearney BP, Flaherty JF, Shah J. Tenofovir disoproxil fumarate: clinical pharmacology and pharmacokinetics. Clin Pharmacokinet. 2004;43(9):595–612. https://search.proquest.com/docview/66648977.

22. Achhra AC, Nugent M, Mocroft A, Ryom L, Wyatt CM. Chronic kidney disease and anti-retroviral therapy in HIV-positive individuals: recent developments. Curr HIV/AIDS Rep. 2016;13(3):149–57. https://www.ncbi.nlm.nih.gov/pubmed/27130284. https://doi.org/10.1007/s11904-016-0315-y.
23. Ryom L, Mocroft A, Kirk O, et al. Association between antiretroviral exposure and renal impairment among HIV-positive persons with normal baseline renal function: the D:A:D study. Int J Infect Dis. 2013;207:1359–69. https://hal.archives-ouvertes.fr/hal-01101122.
24. Sax PE, Wohl D, Yin MT, et al. Tenofovir alafenamide versus tenofovir disoproxil fumarate, coformulated with elvitegravir, cobicistat, and emtricitabine, for initial treatment of HIV-1 infection: two randomized, double-blind, phase 3, non-inferiority trials. Lancet. 2015;385(9987):2606–15. https://www.clinicalkey.es/playcontent/1-s2.0-S014067361560616X. https://doi.org/10.1016/S0140-6736(15)60616-X.
25. McLaughlin M, Guerrero A, Merker A. Renal effects of non-tenofovir antiretroviral therapy in patients living with HIV. Drugs Context. 2018; https://doi.org/10.7573/dic.212519.
26. Fabrizi F, Messa P. The epidemiology of HCV infection in patients with advanced CKD/ESRD: a global perspective. Semin Dial. 2019;32(2):93–8. https://onlinelibrary.wiley.com/doi/abs/10.1111/sdi.12757. https://doi.org/10.1111/sdi.12757.
27. Bruchfeld A, Lindahl K. Direct acting anti-viral medications for hepatitis C: clinical trials in patients with advanced chronic kidney disease. Semin Dial. 2019;32(2):135–40. https://onlinelibrary.wiley.com/doi/abs/10.1111/sdi.12762. https://doi.org/10.1111/sdi.12762.
28. Henson JB, Sise ME. The association of hepatitis C infection with the onset of CKD and progression into ESRD. Semin Dial. 2019;32(2):108–18. https://onlinelibrary.wiley.com/doi/abs/10.1111/sdi.12759. https://doi.org/10.1111/sdi.12759.
29. Molnar MZ, Alhourani HM, Wall BM, et al. Association of hepatitis C viral infection with incidence and progression of chronic kidney disease in a large cohort of US veterans. Hepatology. 2015;61(5):1495–502. https://onlinelibrary.wiley.com/doi/abs/10.1002/hep.27664. https://doi.org/10.1002/hep.27664.
30. Cacoub P, Comarmond C. Considering hepatitis C virus infection as a systemic disease. Semin Dial. 2019;32(2):99–107. https://onlinelibrary.wiley.com/doi/abs/10.1111/sdi.12758. https://doi.org/10.1111/sdi.12758.
31. Gordon CE, Berenguer MC, Doss W, et al. Prevention, diagnosis, evaluation, and treatment of hepatitis C virus infection in chronic kidney disease: synopsis of the kidney disease: improving global outcomes 2018 clinical practice guideline. Ann Intern Med. 2019;171(7):496. https://search.proquest.com/docview/2308474090. https://doi.org/10.7326/M19-1539.
32. Kupin WL. Viral-associated GN: hepatitis B and other viral infections. Clin J Am Soc Nephrol. 2017;12(9):1529–33. https://www.ncbi.nlm.nih.gov/pubmed/27797900. https://doi.org/10.2215/CJN.09180816.
33. Xie Q, Li Y, Xue J, et al. Renal phospholipase A2 receptor in hepatitis B virus-associated membranous nephropathy. Am J Nephrol. 2015;41(4–5):345–53. https://www.karger.com/Article/Abstract/431331. https://doi.org/10.1159/000431331.
34. Berchtold L, Zanetta G, Dahan K, et al. Efficacy and safety of rituximab in hepatitis B virus–associated PLA2R-positive membranous nephropathy. Kidney Int Rep. 2018;3(2):486–91. https://www.sciencedirect.com/science/article/pii/S2468024917303959. https://doi.org/10.1016/j.ekir.2017.09.009.
35. KDIGO clinical practice guideline for glomerulonephritis; chapter 9: infection-related glomerulonephritis. Kidney Int Suppl. 2012;2(2):200–8.
36. Bazerbachi F, Haffar S, Garg SK, Lake JR. Extra-hepatic manifestations associated with hepatitis E virus infection: a comprehensive review of the literature. Gastroenterol Rep. 2016;4(1):1–15. https://www.ncbi.nlm.nih.gov/pubmed/26358655. https://doi.org/10.1093/gastro/gov042.
37. Fanelli V, Fiorentino M, Cantaluppi V, et al. Acute kidney injury in SARS-CoV-2 infected patients. Crit Care. 2020;24(1):1–155. https://search.proquest.com/docview/2391273673. https://doi.org/10.1186/s13054-020-02872-z.

38. Schiffl H. Renal recovery from acute tubular necrosis requiring renal replacement therapy: a prospective study in critically ill patients. Nephrol Dial Transplant. 2006;21(5):1248–52. https://www.ncbi.nlm.nih.gov/pubmed/16449291. https://doi.org/10.1093/ndt/gfk069.
39. Nasr SH, Radhakrishnan J, D'Agati VD. Bacterial infection–related glomerulonephritis in adults. Kidney Int. 2013;83(5):792–803. https://doi.org/10.1038/ki.2012.407.
40. Nasr SH, Fidler ME, Valeri AM, et al. Postinfectious glomerulonephritis in the elderly. J Am Soc Nephrol. 2011;22(1):187–95. https://www.ncbi.nlm.nih.gov/pubmed/21051737. https://doi.org/10.1681/ASN.2010060611.
41. Moroni G, Pozzi C, Quaglini S, et al. Long-term prognosis of diffuse proliferative glomerulonephritis associated with infection in adults. Nephrol Dial Transplant. 2002;17(7):1204–11. https://www.ncbi.nlm.nih.gov/pubmed/12105242. https://doi.org/10.1093/ndt/17.7.1204.
42. Hoy WE, White AV, Dowling A, et al. Post-streptococcal glomerulonephritis is a strong risk factor for chronic kidney disease in later life. Kidney Int. 2012;81(10):1026–32. https://www.sciencedirect.com/science/article/pii/S0085253815551983. https://doi.org/10.1038/ki.2011.478.
43. Daher EDF, da Silva GB Jr, Barros EJG. Renal tuberculosis in the modern era. Am J Trop Med Hyg. 2013;88(1):54–64. https://www.ncbi.nlm.nih.gov/pubmed/23303798. https://doi.org/10.4269/ajtmh.2013.12-0413.
44. Oliveira B, Jayawardene S, Shah S. Single-center experience of granulomatous interstitial nephritis—time for a new approach? Clin Kidney J. 2017;10(2):249–54. https://www.ncbi.nlm.nih.gov/pubmed/28396742. https://doi.org/10.1093/ckj/sfw119.
45. Barsoum RS. Malarial acute renal failure. J Am Soc Nephrol. 2000;11:2147–54.
46. Riefkohl A, Ramirez-Rubio O, Laws RL, et al. Leptospira seropositivity as a risk factor for Mesoamerican nephropathy. Int J Occup Environ Health. 2017;23:1–10. https://doi.org/10.1080/10773525.2016.1275462.
47. Dutra M, Martinelli R, de Carvalho EM, Rodrigues LE, Brito E, Rocha H. Renal involvement in visceral leishmaniasis. Am J Kidney Dis. 1985;6:22–7. https://doi.org/10.1016/S0272-6386(85)80034-2.
48. Barsoum RS. Schistosomiasis and the kidney. Semin Nephrol. 2003;23:34–41. https://doi.org/10.1053/snep.2003.50003a.
49. Nag VL, Sen M, Dash NR, Bansal R, Kumar M, Maurya AK. Hematuria without chyluria: it could still be due to filarial etiology. Trop Parasitol. 2016;6:151. https://doi.org/10.4103/2229-5070.190834.
50. Van Velthuysen ML, Florquin S. Glomerulopathy associated with parasitic infections. Clin Microbiol Rev. 2000;13:55–66. https://doi.org/10.1128/CMR.13.1.55.

Chapter 9
Hepatorenal Syndrome

Maitreyee M. Gupta and Xiaoying Deng

Renal dysfunction is common in patients with advanced liver disease and acute liver injury. The renal dysfunction in liver diseases is manifested as a pre-renal or parenchymal disease. The pre-renal causes include pre-renal acute kidney injury secondary to diuretics therapy, NSAIDs use, GI fluid loss, or any condition that leads to hypovolemia; acute tubular necrosis (ATN) with granular (muddy brown) casts in urine sediment analysis in the setting of sepsis, radiocontrast exposure, and aminoglycoside therapy; or hepatorenal syndrome (HRS). The parenchymal diseases in the setting of advanced liver disease include acute glomerulonephritis from cryoglobulinemia, postinfectious glomerulonephritis, or membranous glomerulonephritis. Hepatorenal syndrome is a severe renal dysfunction and represents the end stage of the decreased renal blood flow (RBF) and decreased glomerular filtration rate (GFR) in the setting of acute liver injury or advanced liver disease with portal hypertension (pHTN). The incidence is about 8% annually in those patients who have ascites. The diagnosis of HRS is by exclusion. The diagnosis criteria of HRS include as follows: (1) presence of cirrhosis and ascites; (2) serum creatinine >1.5 mg/dl or 133 mmol/L; (3) no improvement of serum creatinine after at least 48 h of diuretic withdrawal and volume expansion with albumin (1 g/kg/day, up to maximum 100 g of albumin/day); (4) absence of shock; (5) no current or recent nephrotoxic agent exposure; and (6) absence of renal parenchymal disease as indicated by proteinuria >500 mg/day, microhematuria with >50 red blood cells (RBC) per high-power field, or abnormal renal ultrasound [1, 2]. These criteria were proposed by the International Club of Ascites (ICA) in 2007. It is further classified

M. M. Gupta (✉)
Department of Medicine, Division of Nephrology, Thomas Jefferson University, Philadelphia, PA, USA
e-mail: Maitreyee.gupta@jefferson.edu

X. Deng
Department of Medicine, Division of Nephrology, Sanford Clinic North, North Fargo, ND, USA
e-mail: Xiaoying.deng@sanfordhealth.org

© Springer Nature Switzerland AG 2022
J. McCauley et al. (eds.), *Approaches to Chronic Kidney Disease*,
https://doi.org/10.1007/978-3-030-83082-3_9

Table 9.1 Comparison of hepatorenal syndrome subtype 1 and subtype 2

HRS	Type 1	Type 2
Clinical	More severe	Less severe
Serum creatinine	2× increase of the initial, to a level >2.5 mg/dl in 2 weeks	Ascites resistant to diuretics
eGFR	Reduction > 50%	
24 h urine output	<400–500 ml/24 h	
Median survival	1 month	6.7 months

Table 9.2 Classification of HRS proposed in 2015 by ICA in alignment with KDIGO AKI guideline in 2012

HRS-AKI		Diagnosis of cirrhosis and ascites	
		Diagnosis of AKI according to ICA-AKI criteria	
		No response after 2 consecutive days of diuretics withdrawal and plasma volume expansion with albumin 1 g/kg body weight	
		Absence of shock	
		No current or recent use of nephrotoxic agents (NSAIDs, aminoglycosides, iodinated contrast media, etc.)	
		No microscopic signs of structural kidney injury	Absence of proteinuria (>500 mg/dl)
			Absence of microscopic hematuria (>50 RBC/high-power field)
			Normal finding on renal ultrasound
AKI stages	Stage 1	Increase in sCr ≥ 0.3 mg/dl or increase in sCr ≥ 1.5–2-fold from baseline	
	Stage 2	Increase in sCr ≥ 2–3-fold from baseline	
	Stage 3	Increase in sCr > 3-fold from baseline or ≥4.0 mg/dl with acute increase ≥0.3 mg/dl or initiation of renal replacement therapy	

Modified from references [2, 8–10]

as rapidly developing acute kidney injury (AKI), HRS type 1, or slowly progressive chronic kidney disease (CKD), HRS type 2 (Table 9.1). HRS type 1 is a more serious condition than HRS type 2. HRS type 1 is defined as a doubling of the initial serum creatinine to a level >2.5 mg/dl (220 micromol/L) or a 50% decrease of the initial 24 h creatinine clearance in less than 2 weeks, often with oliguria with 24-h urine output less than 400–500 ml/24 h. HRS type 2 is defined as less renal impairment as those observed in type 1, characterized by a slower course of moderate renal failure and serum creatinine between 1.5 and 2.5 mg/dl, mainly the patients with ascites that are resistant to diuretic treatment [3–7]. Patients with HRS type 2 can develop into type 1 after exposure to infection or other predisposed conditions. This classification was then modified to adapt to the new AKI diagnosis criteria proposed in 2012 by KDIGO (Kidney Disease: Improving Global Outcomes) in 2015 (Table 9.2) [11]. AKI is then defined as any increase of creatinine from baseline by as 0.3 mg/dl or any increase of creatinine by 50% above baseline within a 48-hour period (Table 9.2). The above two classifications are mainly focused on serum creatinine, which is a poor serum marker of renal function impairment in

Table 9.3 New classification of HRS proposed by ICA in 2019

Old classification	New classification	Subtype	Criteria
HRS-1	HRS-AKI		1. Absolute Cr increase ≥0.3 mg/dl within 48 h and/or 2. Urine output <0.5 ml/kg 6 h or 3. Percentage increase in sCr ≥ 50% from most recent outpatient sCr within 3 months as baseline
	HRS-NAKI	HRS-AKD	1. eGFR < 60 ml/min/1.73 m² for <3 months in the absence of other structural causes 2. Percentage increase in sCr < 50% using the most recent outpatient sCr within 3 months as baseline
		HRS-CKD	1. eGFR < 60 ml/min/1.73 m² for ≥3 months in the absence of other structural causes

Modified from reference [1]

cirrhotic patients. Creatinine can be affected by several factors including assay interference with bilirubin, reduced hepatic creatinine synthesis, muscle wasting, and malnutrition from chronic liver diseases [12]. Since these classifications do not accurately reflect the clinical scenario, a newer classification based on pathophysiological characterization of HRS has been proposed by ICA lately. Patients with cirrhosis and AKI can be divided into distinct subgroups according to the underlying pathology [2, 13]. Causes of AKI in cirrhotic patients other than HRS AKI (acute) are identified in the new classification, and it includes pre-renal hypovolemia caused by bleeding, excessive diuretic use, or any excessive fluid loss; bile acid nephropathy; acute tubular injury; acute tubular necrosis; and AKI caused by intrinsic renal causes including acute interstitial nephritis (AIN). This type of AKI is collectively referred as non-HRS AKI (HRS-NAKI), which is very different from HRS type 1 (HRS-1), a functional disorder of the kidney without structural abnormality. HRS-NAKI is further divided into HRS-AKD (subacute) and HRS-CKD (chronic) (Table 9.3). CKD represents a collective disease carrying renal parenchyma structural changes resulted from any cause, including glomerulonephropathy, interstitial renal disease, and causes associated with comorbid disease such as diabetes mellitus (DM) and hypertension (HTN) [1]. The newer classification removed the time limit of 2 weeks and serum creatinine of 2.5 mg/dl, a cornerstone for the diagnosis of HRS in the past.

Epidemiology

The lack of accurate renal function assessment in cirrhotic patients and evolving diagnosis criteria and complexity of cirrhosis limit the accurate diagnosis of HRS; the incidence of HRS is largely unknown. It is likely that HRS occurs more commonly than we expected. A few reports are available in hospitalized patients. AKI is found in 25–50% of cirrhotic patients who were admitted to hospitals [14, 15]. AKI is caused by etiologies in three different categories, including pre-renal, renal parenchymal, and post-renal. The common causes of pre-renal disease in cirrhotic patients are hypovolemia and HRS-AKI. This accounts for 60–70% causes of HRS-AKI and 11–20% of all causes of AKI [16, 17]. Intrinsic renal causes account for 30% of all causes in cirrhotic patients and include ischemic injury and acute tubular necrosis (ATN), acute glomerulonephritis (GN), and acute interstitial nephritis (AIN). The post-renal causes are less than 1% [16, 18]. Based on new criteria, more than half of the cirrhotic patients who were admitted to hospitals had AKI. HRS and ATN are more common in stage 2 and 3 AKI [19]. In outpatient setting, the incidence is varying, ranging from 8% to 54% for HRS and 11–21% for ATN, based on KDIGO and ICA criteria (Table 9.2) [16, 20, 21]. The incidence and prevalence of HRS vary dramatically based on which criteria were used and how rigorously the criteria were followed. A large cohort study is needed to determine the precise incidence and prevalence of HRS based on new criteria, especially in outpatient setting.

Pathophysiology of HRS

HRS-AKI

HRS-AKI develops with progressive reduction in renal blood flow as a result of splanchnic vasodilation and renovascular constriction in the setting of portal hypertension. Cardiac dysfunction, adrenal insufficiency, and ongoing inflammation in those cirrhotic patients also contribute significantly. As revealed in Fig. 9.1, the classic theory regarding development of AKI in cirrhotic patients is severe reduction in kidney function caused by severe systemic vasodilation and subsequent renal vasoconstriction. Increased portal hypertension and shear stress on the portal blood vessels cause endothelial cells to produce vasodilators such as nitric oxide (NO) and prostanoids [3, 22, 23]. These vasodilators work locally to cause severe splanchnic vasculature dilation leading to decreased renal blood perfusion. The effective mean arterial blood pressure is thus decreased, which then activates renin-angiotensin-aldosterone axis and visceral sympathetic system to increase cardiac output and heart rates to compensate for the decreased effective mean arterial blood pressure. The locally increased vasopressin and endothelin secretion also contribute to reduced intra-glomerular blood flow. As liver disease worsens, the splanchnic vasodilation and renal vasoconstriction get worse, leading to functional renal impairment without structural abnormality. Aldosterone and vasopressin can also cause water and sodium retention and further worsen ascites [24, 25].

About 50% cirrhotic patients have cirrhotic cardiomyopathy with abnormal response to both physiological and pathological stresses [26]. The cardiac output is low due to persistent systemic vasodilation, which predisposes these patients to HRS-AKI and is associated with poor prognosis. Any condition that worsens hypotension such as beta-blocker use leading to inadequate renal blood perfusion can further jeopardize renal impairment.

Adrenal insufficiency is seen in about 25% of decompensated cirrhotic patients [27]. Adrenal insufficiency can downregulate beta-adrenergic receptors and modulate

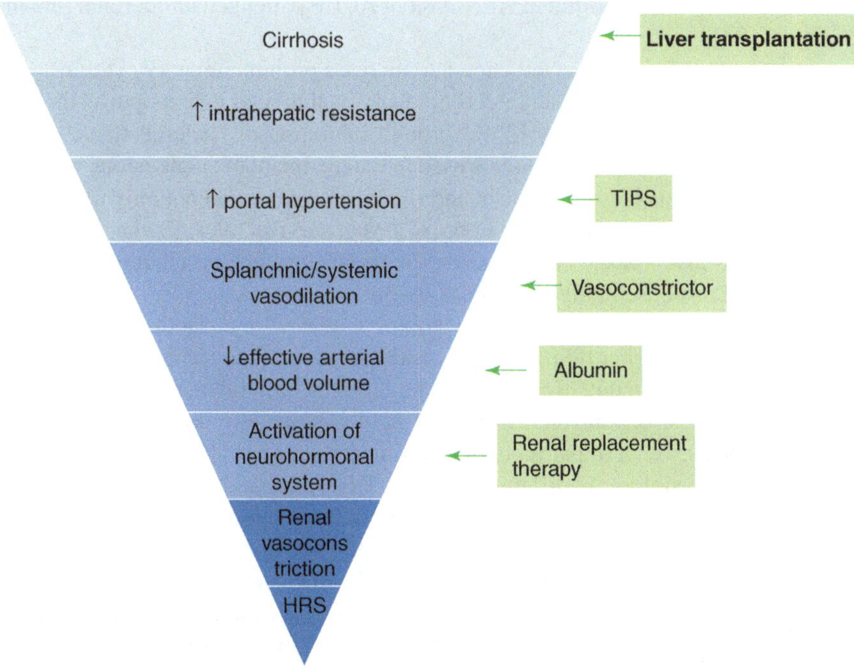

Fig. 9.1 Pathophysiology of HRS and treatment strategy based on pathophysiology

the effects of catecholamines on myocardial contraction and vascular responsiveness, worsen stroke volume and heart rates, and further decrease cardiac output.

Systemic inflammation is another key factor that predisposes to AKI in advanced liver disease patients. The mechanism is not very clear, but observational studies noticed an increase in mortality of those patients with systemic inflammation and increased proinflammatory cytokine levels than those without. The inflammatory cascade is likely triggered by bacterial translocation and endotoxemia in the setting of portal hypertension [28–31].

HRS-NAKI

Unlike the significant hemodynamic dysfunction occurring in HRS-AKI, systemic inflammation and bacterial translocation play critical role in the pathophysiology of HRS-NAKI. Several recent studies demonstrated that 29 serum cytokines and nonmercaptalbumin were markedly elevated in acute-on-chronic liver failure (ACLF), which is characterized with multi-organ failure and unfavorable responses to albumin and terlipressin treatment [32]. The severity of renal failure was closely related to cytokines, not renin or copeptin levels. The kidney biopsy also revealed structural abnormalities including chronic tubulointerstitial injury, glomerular and vascular injury, and increased Toll-like receptor 4 and caspase-3, which have not been reported in HRS-AKI or ACLF patients without renal impairment [33, 34].

Bacterial translocation is well known to increase proinflammatory cytokines and lipopolysaccharides, which can directly induce renal tubular cell apoptosis through the caspase-mediated pathway [35]. Through inhibition of bacterial translocation and endotoxin production, antibiotics used in the treatment of spontaneous bacterial peritonitis (SBP) such as norfloxacin and rifaximin were found not only to delay or decrease incidence of AKI but also improve 1-year survival rates. Further, the extent of ACLF was also associated with response to terlipressin and albumin treatment with reduced response in higher grades [36–38].

Bile acid also contributes to the development of AKI in cirrhotic patients given worse outcome in higher bilirubin levels and less response to terlipressin treatment [39, 40]. Bile acid can directly injure renal tubules or form tubular bile acid casts to cause tubular obstruction. Increasing bile acid clearance by norursodeoxycholic acid can decrease renal impairment in experimental animals [41].

The pathophysiology is different between HRS-AKI and HRS-NAKI; there is also overlap as HRS-AKI persists. Research found that about 60% of HRS-AKI did not respond to albumin and terlipressin treatment; the unresponsiveness increases with time. The persistent renal parenchymal ischemia could promote inflammatory changes within the renal interstitium and tubular cell death and evolve into HRS-NAKI over time [42]. Patient's residual renal function is hardly recovered once HRS-AKI persists for more than 6 weeks even with liver transplantation.

Clinical Manifestations

HRS is functional impairment of the kidneys. Most patients will present with a progressive increase in serum creatinine with bland or normal urine sediment and no or minimal proteinuria with urinary protein less than 500 mg daily. Since HRS is pre-renal, urine sodiun is typically less than 10 MEQ/L. Some patients may have oliguria with less than 400 ml in 24-hour urine output. Some patients may not have any oliguria especially in the early stage of the diseases.

The onset of renal failure is insidious. The HRS can be triggered by precipitating factors, such as spontaneous bacterial peritonitis (SBP), acute GI blood loss, or hypovolemia from over diuresis. Diuretics alone would not cause any HRS but can cause azotemia, especially in the setting of rapid fluid removal without apparent edema patients. The azotemia induced by diuretics improves once diuretics are discontinued.

Diagnosis

Serum creatinine is not very accurate in the setting of chronic advanced liver disease. Creatinine levels in cirrhotic patients can overestimate the impaired renal function as most cirrhotic patients produce less creatinine and BUN from their failing livers; they are malnourished with less muscle mass and increased muscle wasting, and they have increased renal tubule creatinine secretion. The increased volume distribution could further dilute creatinine levels; the serum hyperbilirubinemia can interfere with the creatinine assay in the lab. All of these can lead to overestimation of the impaired renal function. The new criteria proposed by ICA (Table 9.3) allow the trend of creatinine to be used instead of actual creatinine levels. If creatinine increases more than 0.3 mg/dl and/or more than or equal to 50% from baseline, AKI can be diagnosed. The diagnostic criteria of HRS according to ICA-AKI criteria are listed in Tables 9.2 and 9.3.

Since the above criteria are unable to provide any information on HRS-AKI and HRS-NAKI, extensive research efforts have been offered to look for a better biomarker. Several biomarkers including neutrophil gelatinase-associated lipocalin (NGAL), interleukin-18, liver-type fatty acid binding protein (L-FABP), kidney injury molecule-1, Toll-like receptor 4, π-glutathione S-transferase, and α-glutathione S-transferase have been assessed in great details in the setting of AKI and liver cirrhosis [43]. HRS is very difficult to differentiate from ATN clinically. Urinary NGAL can help in diagnosis of ATN as the level increased to 417 µg/L in ATN versus only 30 µg/L in pre-renal azotemia, 82 µg/L in CKD, and 76 µg/L in HRS. Urinary NGAL level is unable to differentiate pre-renal azotemia and HRS. There is also an overlap between these conditions.

Differential Diagnosis

Distinguishing HRS from other renal impairment is very important clinically as HRS is irreversible, while ATN and most causes of pre-renal diseases are generally reversible. HRS is diagnosed based on clinical criteria and is a diagnosis of exclusion. All other conditions must be ruled out before the diagnosis of HRS.

First, the secondary renal impairment from glomerulonephritis and vasculitis in chronic liver disease needs to be ruled out. Mixed cryoglobulinemia syndrome, membranoproliferative glomerulonephritis (MPGN) type I, membranous nephropathy, and polyarteritis nodosa (PAN) should be evaluated for possible underlying HCV and HBV infection. The urine sediments usually contain red blood cells, red cell casts, or other casts and also have significant proteinuria, which is an important feature of renal parenchymal damage.

Secondly, cirrhosis may be secondary to underlying hepatic steatosis or nonalcoholic fatty liver disease; diabetic nephropathy needs to be ruled out. A previous prospective study indicated that pre-renal or infection-associated kidney injury was more common than HRS after analyzing 562 patients with cirrhosis and renal impairment in one single center [44]. Some cirrhotic patients may have chronic kidney disease before the HRS; on the other hand, patients with ongoing infection especially SBP in the absence of septic shock can have HRS, as up to 18% of cirrhotic patients have persistent abnormal renal impairment despite successful antibiotics treatment for peritonitis [5]. Postinfectious IgA nephropathy can be ruled out by active urinary sediment.

Thirdly, acute tubular necrosis (ATN) needs to be ruled out. Patients with cirrhosis can develop ATN after GI bleeding, SBP, exposure to radiocontrast, sepsis, hypotension, a course of NSAIDs use, or aminoglycoside therapy. The history, rapid increase in serum creatinine, oliguria, and positive urinary sediment analysis showing muddy brown casts/granular/epithelial casts all help in the diagnosis of ATN. The fractional excretion of sodium is usually more than 2% versus less than 1% in HRS patients [45]. Of note, some cirrhotic patients with ATN may have lower fractional excretion of sodium in the setting of persistent renal ischemia induced by liver disease. In addition, marked hyperbilirubinemia can cause granular and epithelial cell casts without ATN. Some biomarkers might be helpful such as NGAL once it is officially available and verified by a large clinical trial.

Pre-renal disease is difficult to distinguish from HRS. Pre-renal disease can be induced in cirrhotic patients by GI fluid/blood losses, over diuresis, and NSAIDs use to block renal vasodilation from prostaglandins, a key factor to maintain renal perfusion in the setting of portal hypertension. HRS only can be clinched as diagnosis, after no improvement in renal function with discontinuation of diuresis, discontinuation of any potential nephrotoxins, and a trial of fluid repletion.

Kidney biopsy is not needed when diagnosing HRS as HRS does not cause any renal parenchymal changes, only functional abnormality. A specific, subtle, and reversible renal lesion, called the reflux of proximal convoluted tubular epithelium into Bowman's space, can be seen in about 71.4% autopsied HRS kidneys as reported before [46]. Transjugular kidney biopsy can be performed if the biopsy results will impact on treatment and if such treatment could outweigh the potential harms associated with the invasive procedure.

Treatment

The ideal treatment for HRS is a recovery of liver function by treating underlying acute or chronic liver diseases. Once liver function is recovered, the renal impairment will improve. It has been confirmed in many liver transplantation recipients. If liver function recovery is impossible, the treatment of HRS is supportive. The treatment approaches are largely decided by the following factors: the care levels that will be offered to the patient, whether inpatient admission or in outpatient setting; ICU, monitored or floor level of care; the availability of certain medications, for which there is national and regional variability; and whether patient is a candidate for liver transplantation (Fig. 9.1).

Management of HRS remains a clinical challenge. The early initiation of treatment may increase the likelihood of the resolution of HRS as it bears extremely high mortality. Several approaches are available now as we have better understanding of pathophysiology of HRS. Some agents may not be available in certain countries in the world, but mounting evidence may promote an early approval of their use in those countries.

Medical Management

As previously stated, once HRS is diagnosed, all diuretics should be discontinued, as well as all other offensive agents. Diagnostic and therapeutic paracentesis in couple with albumin administration should be carried as needed to rule out SBP and compartment syndrome, as well as to decrease intra-abdominal pressure to improve renal perfusion. Intravenous albumin administration is a part of standard care in HRS-NAKI patients secondary to pre-renal causes from hypovolemia, GIB. It is also very important in the diagnosis of HRS-AKI based on ICA diagnosis criteria [47]. Albumin is believed to work on HRS through the following effects/actions. Albumin could increase oncotic pressure, improve capillary permeability, solubilization, transport and metabolism via its negative electric charges; it also can serve as antioxidant via its N-terminal metal binding (Cys-34) and improve hemostatic effect by a higher concentration of Cys-34 N-terminal; albumin can stabilize endothelium and modulate immunization by increasing intracellular glutathione and decreasing tumor necrosis factor (TNF)-induced nuclear factor (NF)-kappa B activation, an endotoxin-binding inactivation [48–50]. However, due to decreased sodium and water excretion in the kidneys of cirrhotic patients, caution should be exercised when albumin is administered to these patients who are susceptible to significant fluid retention and pulmonary edema.

As demonstrated in Fig. 9.1, treatment tailored to vasoconstriction is the main stream of therapy and also first line in the treatment of HRS. The vasoconstrictive agents need to be used with intravenous albumin. Terlipressin is the most commonly used vasopressin analog outside of the United States. Terlipressin has not been approved by FDA to be used in the United States yet. Terlipressin is synthesized peptide and contains 12 amino acids, an analogue of vasopressin. It acts at V1 receptors located in splanchnic circulation, causes vasoconstriction to decrease portal circulation blood flow, decreases portal pressure, and shifts blood to systemic circulation. Terlipressin not only can increase systemic blood volume by constricting splanchnic circulation as above but it also can decrease renin and angiotensin release and dilate renal blood vessels to improve renal function. Terlipressin with albumin could reverse 23.7% HRS patients with creatinine decreased to less than 1.5 mg/dl, whereas albumin alone only can achieve similar reversal in 15.2% patients [51, 52]. Other researchers reported higher response rates, ranging between 25% and 75% [53–57]. The terlipressin can be given as an intravenous bolus at starting dose of 0.5–1 mg every 4–6 h, with a progressive up-titrating to a maximum dose of 2 mg every 4 h. The dose titration is based on responses of serum creatinine. No response is defined as a decrement of creatinine is less than 25% of baseline. The response is also associated with initial serum creatinine levels and grade of acute on chronic liver failure [38, 55]. Patients with creatinine at 3–5 mg/dl responded well to terlipressin and no response if baseline creatinine was greater than 5.6 mg/dl [55]. To achieve HRS reversal, a sustained rise in mean arterial pressure is required. Therefore, terlipressin should be maintained until complete response or at least 14 days. Other clinicians proposed continuous infusion at 2–12 mg/day of

Table 9.4 Comparison of vasoconstrictors in HRS

	Midodrine	Terlipressin	Norepinephrine
Route	Oral		
Response rate	Limited, similar to albumin alone	40–50%	40–50%
Monitoring levels	None	Monitored bed	ICU bed
Safety	Safe	GI, ischemia	Ischemia, GI, ARDS
Cost	$	Not available in USA	$$
Rationale	*	***	**

$ indicates cost
* indicates strength of studied benefits in improving renal function in HRS

terlipressin, which is as effective as bolus [58]. The most severe side effects are possible myocardial ischemia and intestinal ischemia from the vasoconstriction. The patient should be placed in monitored bed when terlipressin is administered.

The alternative vasoconstrictor is norepinephrine. Norepinephrine is nonselective alpha- and beta-adrenergic agonist and frequently used as a pressor support in hypotension/shock patients. Its use has to be in the ICU setting with central line to avoid peripheral ischemia. It has been shown in small studies to be effective in reserving HRS by increasing arterial blood pressures [59–61]. Norepinephrine can be given at 0.05–0.1 µg/kg/min up to 2 µg/kg/min intravenously. The side effects are arrhythmia, myocardial infarction, and peripheral ischemia. Several studies have been conducted to compare its use in HRS with terlipressin head to head; norepinephrine is inferior to terlipressin in reversal of HRS and overall survival [59–62].

The use of midodrine and octreotide was started in 1999 when a small study revealed that five patients benefited from its use [63]. Midodrine is a prodrug that converts to desglymidodrine, an alpha 1 agonist, which acts at systemic alpha1 receptors to increase blood pressure. It can be given at the doses of 5–15 mg three times daily by mouth. Octreotide can reduce blood flow in splanchnic circulation by inhibiting release of several hormones including glucagon, vasoactive peptide, secretin, motilin, serotonin, and pancreatic polypeptide. The doses are 100–300 µg three times daily by subcutaneously injection. The combination use of midodrine and octreotide can decrease more serum creatinine as compared to albumin alone (40% versus 10%) and improve mortality (43% versus 71%) [6]. However, recent small study revealed that the combination use is inferior to terlipressin in terms of HRS reversal [53] (Table 9.4).

TIPS

Transjugular intrahepatic portosystemic shunt (TIPS) could decrease portal hypertension and reverse the circulatory changes and associated inflammation, in turn to improve renal function. A small study did reveal improved serum creatinine and possible survival benefits [64]. In type 1 HRS, 50% of patients achieved HRS reversal and survived more than 3 months [65]. In type 2 HRS, most patients achieved HRS reversal and ascites control, and 70% of patients survived more than 1 year. However, more than 50% patients developed hepatoencephalopathy and responded to medical treatment of hepatoencephalopathy [66]. Therefore, increased incidence of hepatoencephalopathy and worsening liver disease limit its use.

Renal Replacement Therapy

Hemodialysis AKI requiring renal replacement therapy is increasing over years in the United States [67]. Initiation of renal replacement therapy in HRS is controversial given its high mortality. The current census is to use renal replacement therapy as a bridge for those patients who are listed for liver transplantation as study revealed that the mortality is similar between HRS and ATN who received hemodialysis [68]. Other studies demonstrated that the severity of illness and the number of organ failure in ACLF are more predictive of 28-day survival than the causes of AKI; some clinicians believe that it is reasonable to initiate renal replacement treatment regardless of the liver transplantation candidacy [68, 69]. The ideal initiation time of renal replacement therapy in this patient population is not studied yet. The initiation of renal replacement therapy should be individualized based on patient's volume status, abnormal electrolytes, acid and base, and diuretic tolerances, as well as responses to medical management.

MARS Liver support system, also called albumin dialysis with molecular absorbent recirculating system (MARS), is being used to bridge HRS patients to eventual liver transplantation (Fig. 9.2). The study on its use is very limited; a large clinical trial is needed before any conclusion can be drawn. A very limited study revealed no significant difference on 28-day survival between the patients who underwent MARS therapy and those who did not receive MARS but standard medical treatments [70, 71].

Liver Transplantation

The only definitive treatment for HRS is liver transplantation. The renal recovery and patient survival after liver transplantation are significantly higher than those with acute tubular necrosis and comparable with those with no or stage 1 AKI [72]. In a large study using the Scientific Registry of Transplant Recipients, a cohort of 2112 patients who received acute renal replacement therapy before liver transplantation, only 91% patients had complete renal recovery, about 9% still need chronic renal replacement therapy 6 months out of their liver transplantation [73, 74]. The reasons for those 9% patients or others who did not have renal recovery after the

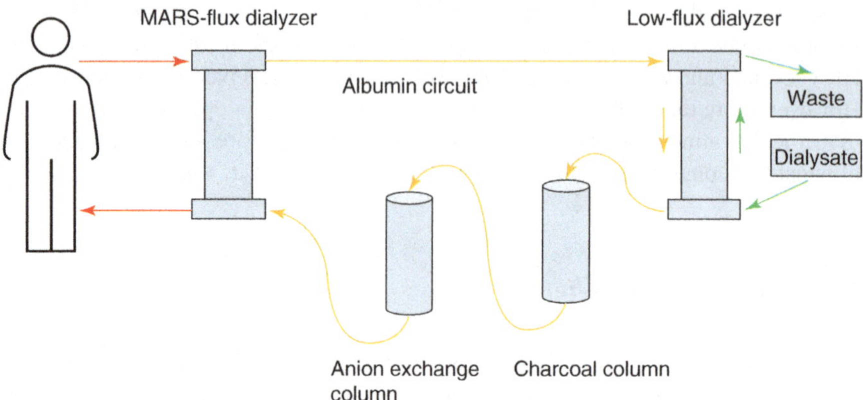

Fig. 9.2 Diagram of molecular absorbent and recirculating system (MARS)

liver transplantation are unclear. Whether the delayed recovery is secondary to pre-existing comorbidities, unknown or undiagnosed intrinsic renal parenchymal disease prior to the transplantation, perioperative events, or immunosuppression posttransplantation remains further investigation.

Simultaneous liver and kidney transplantation are increasing over past several years after the introduction of organ allocation based on MELD scores [75, 76]. It accounts for 10% of liver transplantation in the United States at present [77]. The driving force for the increased dual transplantation is largely secondary to predicted lack of renal recovery and increased mortality post liver transplantation [78]. In liver transplantation alone patients, about up to 20% will develop some degree renal impairment, and about 2% will benefit from dual liver and kidney transplantation [79, 80]. The indication for simultaneous liver-kidney transplantation is included in Table 9.5.

Inflammation plays an important role in the development of HRS. Controlling ongoing inflammation may help prevent or reverse hepatorenal syndrome in theory. There is no related study yet; it might open another door to effectively treat and reverse HRS.

Prevention

HRS is better to be prevented than treated. The strategy to prevent HRS is to prevent the progression of chronic liver diseases in the well-compensated patients; reverse decompensated cirrhosis; avoid any agents or condition that could impair renal blood perfusion including NSAIDs. Intravenous albumin repletion in therapeutic paracentesis and in combination with prophylactic and therapeutic antibiotics use for spontaneous bacterial peritonitis has been shown to decrease the incidence of AKI in cirrhotic patients [36]. The albumin should be given at 1.5 g/kg on day 1 followed by 1 g/kg on day 3 for SBP and 8 g/L of removed ascites in large volume

Table 9.5 Indication for simultaneous liver-kidney transplantation, cited and adapted from OPTN Simultaneous Liver Kidney (SLK) Allocation Policy [81]

Transplant nephrology decides the following	The following should be documented in the chart, at least one of the following in each category
CKD with eGFR≤ 60 ml/min for 90 consecutive days	Patients need regular HD treatment Patients calculated/measured creatinine clearance or eGFR ≤ 35 ml/min at the time of registration on the kidney transplant waiting list
Sustained AKI	On HD for at least 6 consecutive weeks Calculated/measured creatinine clearance or eGFR ≤ 25% for at least 6 consecutive weeks and documented every 7 days Patients have combination of the above two for 6 consecutive weeks
Metabolic diseases	Hyperoxaluria Atypical HUS from mutations in factor H and possibly factor I Familial non-neuropathic systemic amyloid Methylmalonic aciduria

Adapted from reference [81]

paracentesis. If cost is not a concern; one clinical trial revealed that a long-term administration of albumin in decompensated cirrhotic patients could decrease rates of SBP and HRS and improve survival [82]. There is no demonstrated benefit if albumin is administered in non-SBP infection in cirrhotic patients. Many cirrhotic patients with ascites are on diuretics. The diuretics should be discontinued without hesitation, when serum creatinine starts to increase. Beta-blockers are very effective and widely used in cirrhosis to prevent variceal bleeding. However, the decreased cardiac output may predispose those patients to AKI as reported [83]. Therefore, clinician should consult hepatology and carefully weigh the benefits and risks of continuation of nonselective beta-blocker use in this patient population.

Prognosis

HRS is frequently a fatal complication of cirrhosis; the median survival is about 1 and 6.7 months, respectively [84]. This prognosis is much worse than those cirrhotic patients with ascites without renal impairment. The mortality rates of the type 1 HRS exceed more than 50% after 1 month without liver transplantation [44]. Current available treatment of terlipressin and norepinephrine only can reverse 40–50% of cases; the only definitive treatment is liver transplantation. The early diagnosis thus appears important. The current diagnosis of HRS is based on clinical grounds, and introduction of urinary NGAL to differentiate ATN might offer a practical means for early diagnosis. Data on predictors of response to treatment suggest that treatment should be started as early as possible [44]. Early diagnosis and early treatments will be optimal goal to interrupt the pathophysiology and eventually reverse the HRS. Research to identify biomarkers and treatment options is largely needed to improve the outcomes of HRS patients.

References

1. Angeli P, Garcia-Tsao G, Nadim MK, Parikh CR. News in pathophysiology, definition and classification of hepatorenal syndrome: a step beyond the International Club of Ascites (ICA) consensus document. J Hepatol. 2019;71(4):811–22.
2. Angeli P, Gines P, Wong F, Bernardi M, Boyer TD, Gerbes A, et al. Diagnosis and management of acute kidney injury in patients with cirrhosis: revised consensus recommendations of the International Club of Ascites. J Hepatol. 2015;62(4):968–74.
3. Gines P, Schrier RW. Renal failure in cirrhosis. N Engl J Med. 2009;361(13):1279–90.
4. Arroyo V, Gines P, Gerbes AL, Dudley FJ, Gentilini P, Laffi G, et al. Definition and diagnostic criteria of refractory ascites and hepatorenal syndrome in cirrhosis. International Ascites Club. Hepatology. 1996;23(1):164–76.
5. Salerno F, Gerbes A, Gines P, Wong F, Arroyo V. Diagnosis, prevention and treatment of hepatorenal syndrome in cirrhosis. Gut. 2007;56(9):1310–8.
6. Esrailian E, Pantangco ER, Kyulo NL, Hu KQ, Runyon BA. Octreotide/Midodrine therapy significantly improves renal function and 30-day survival in patients with type 1 hepatorenal syndrome. Dig Dis Sci. 2007;52(3):742–8.
7. International club of ascites. Guidelines: criteria for the diagnosis of hepatorenal syndrome: 2019. Available from: http://www.icascites.org/about/guidelines/.
8. Kellum JA, Lameire N. Diagnosis, evaluation, and management of acute kidney injury: a KDIGO summary (part 1). Crit Care. 2013;17(1):204.
9. Nadim MK, Durand F, Kellum JA, Levitsky J, O'Leary JG, Karvellas CJ, et al. Management of the critically ill patient with cirrhosis: a multidisciplinary perspective. J Hepatol. 2016;64(3):717–35.
10. Palevsky PM, Liu KD, Brophy PD, Chawla LS, Parikh CR, Thakar CV, et al. KDOQI US commentary on the 2012 KDIGO clinical practice guideline for acute kidney injury. Am J Kidney Dis. 2013;61(5):649–72.
11. Andrassy KM. Comments on 'KDIGO 2012 clinical practice guideline for the evaluation and management of chronic kidney disease'. Kidney Int. 2013;84(3):622–3.
12. Francoz C, Glotz D, Moreau R, Durand F. The evaluation of renal function and disease in patients with cirrhosis. J Hepatol. 2010;52(4):605–13.
13. Wong F, Nadim MK, Kellum JA, Salerno F, Bellomo R, Gerbes A, et al. Working party proposal for a revised classification system of renal dysfunction in patients with cirrhosis. Gut. 2011;60(5):702–9.
14. Piano S, Rosi S, Maresio G, Fasolato S, Cavallin M, Romano A, et al. Evaluation of the acute kidney injury network criteria in hospitalized patients with cirrhosis and ascites. J Hepatol. 2013;59(3):482–9.
15. Piano S, Fasolato S, Salinas F, Romano A, Tonon M, Morando F, et al. The empirical antibiotic treatment of nosocomial spontaneous bacterial peritonitis: results of a randomized, controlled clinical trial. Hepatology. 2016;63(4):1299–309.
16. Garcia-Tsao G, Parikh CR, Viola A. Acute kidney injury in cirrhosis. Hepatology. 2008;48(6):2064–77.
17. Fang JT, Tsai MH, Tian YC, Jenq CC, Lin CY, Chen YC, et al. Outcome predictors and new score of critically ill cirrhotic patients with acute renal failure. Nephrol Dial Transplant. 2008;23(6):1961–9.
18. Hartleb M, Gutkowski K. Kidneys in chronic liver diseases. World J Gastroenterol. 2012;18(24):3035–49.
19. Huelin P, Piano S, Sola E, Stanco M, Sole C, Moreira R, et al. Validation of a staging system for acute kidney injury in patients with cirrhosis and association with acute-on-chronic liver failure. Clin Gastroenterol Hepatol. 2017;15(3):438–45.e5.
20. Salerno F, Cazzaniga M, Merli M, Spinzi G, Saibeni S, Salmi A, et al. Diagnosis, treatment and survival of patients with hepatorenal syndrome: a survey on daily medical practice. J Hepatol. 2011;55(6):1241–8.

21. Planas R, Montoliu S, Balleste B, Rivera M, Miquel M, Masnou H, et al. Natural history of patients hospitalized for management of cirrhotic ascites. Clin Gastroenterol Hepatol. 2006;4(11):1385–94.
22. Martin PY, Gines P, Schrier RW. Nitric oxide as a mediator of hemodynamic abnormalities and sodium and water retention in cirrhosis. N Engl J Med. 1998;339(8):533–41.
23. Martin PY, Ohara M, Gines P, Xu DL, St John J, Niederberger M, et al. Nitric oxide synthase (NOS) inhibition for one week improves renal sodium and water excretion in cirrhotic rats with ascites. J Clin Invest. 1998;101(1):235–42.
24. Sola E, Gines P. Renal and circulatory dysfunction in cirrhosis: current management and future perspectives. J Hepatol. 2010;53(6):1135–45.
25. Kastelan S, Ljubicic N, Kastelan Z, Ostojic R, Uravic M. The role of duplex-doppler ultrasonography in the diagnosis of renal dysfunction and hepatorenal syndrome in patients with liver cirrhosis. Hepato-Gastroenterology. 2004;51(59):1408–12.
26. Krag A, Bendtsen F, Henriksen JH, Moller S. Low cardiac output predicts development of hepatorenal syndrome and survival in patients with cirrhosis and ascites. Gut. 2010;59(1): 105–10.
27. Acevedo J, Fernandez J, Prado V, Silva A, Castro M, Pavesi M, et al. Relative adrenal insufficiency in decompensated cirrhosis: relationship to short-term risk of severe sepsis, hepatorenal syndrome, and death. Hepatology. 2013;58(5):1757–65.
28. Wiest R, Lawson M, Geuking M. Pathological bacterial translocation in liver cirrhosis. J Hepatol. 2014;60(1):197–209.
29. Navasa M, Follo A, Filella X, Jimenez W, Francitorra A, Planas R, et al. Tumor necrosis factor and interleukin-6 in spontaneous bacterial peritonitis in cirrhosis: relationship with the development of renal impairment and mortality. Hepatology. 1998;27(5):1227–32.
30. Maiwall R, Chandel SS, Wani Z, Kumar S, Sarin SK. SIRS at admission is a predictor of AKI development and mortality in hospitalized patients with severe alcoholic hepatitis. Dig Dis Sci. 2016;61(3):920–9.
31. Shah N, Mohamed FE, Jover-Cobos M, Macnaughtan J, Davies N, Moreau R, et al. Increased renal expression and urinary excretion of TLR4 in acute kidney injury associated with cirrhosis. Liver Int. 2013;33(3):398–409.
32. Claria J, Arroyo V, Moreau R. The acute-on-chronic liver failure syndrome, or when the innate immune system Goes astray. J Immunol. 2016;197(10):3755–61.
33. Trawale JM, Paradis V, Rautou PE, Francoz C, Escolano S, Sallee M, et al. The spectrum of renal lesions in patients with cirrhosis: a clinicopathological study. Liver Int. 2010;30(5): 725–32.
34. Shah N, Dhar D, El Zahraa Mohammed F, Habtesion A, Davies NA, Jover-Cobos M, et al. Prevention of acute kidney injury in a rodent model of cirrhosis following selective gut decontamination is associated with reduced renal TLR4 expression. J Hepatol. 2012;56(5):1047–53.
35. Jo SK, Cha DR, Cho WY, Kim HK, Chang KH, Yun SY, et al. Inflammatory cytokines and lipopolysaccharide induce Fas-mediated apoptosis in renal tubular cells. Nephron. 2002;91(3):406–15.
36. Fernandez J, Navasa M, Planas R, Montoliu S, Monfort D, Soriano G, et al. Primary prophylaxis of spontaneous bacterial peritonitis delays hepatorenal syndrome and improves survival in cirrhosis. Gastroenterology. 2007;133(3):818–24.
37. Dong T, Aronsohn A, Gautham Reddy K, Te HS. Rifaximin decreases the incidence and severity of acute kidney injury and hepatorenal syndrome in cirrhosis. Dig Dis Sci. 2016;61(12):3621–6.
38. Piano S, Schmidt HH, Ariza X, Amoros A, Romano A, Husing-Kabar A, et al. Association between grade of acute on chronic liver failure and response to terlipressin and albumin in patients with hepatorenal syndrome. Clin Gastroenterol Hepatol. 2018;16(11):1792–800.e3.
39. van Slambrouck CM, Salem F, Meehan SM, Chang A. Bile cast nephropathy is a common pathologic finding for kidney injury associated with severe liver dysfunction. Kidney Int. 2013;84(1):192–7.

40. Barreto R, Fagundes C, Guevara M, Sola E, Pereira G, Rodriguez E, et al. Type-1 hepatorenal syndrome associated with infections in cirrhosis: natural history, outcome of kidney function, and survival. Hepatology. 2014;59(4):1505–13.
41. Krones E, Eller K, Pollheimer MJ, Racedo S, Kirsch AH, Frauscher B, et al. NorUrsodeoxycholic acid ameliorates cholemic nephropathy in bile duct ligated mice. J Hepatol. 2017;67(1): 110–9.
42. Davenport A, Sheikh MF, Lamb E, Agarwal B, Jalan R. Acute kidney injury in acute-on-chronic liver failure: where does hepatorenal syndrome fit? Kidney Int. 2017;92(5):1058–70.
43. Belcher JM. Acute kidney injury in liver disease: role of biomarkers. Adv Chronic Kidney Dis. 2015;22(5):368–75.
44. Martin-Llahi M, Guevara M, Torre A, Fagundes C, Restuccia T, Gilabert R, et al. Prognostic importance of the cause of renal failure in patients with cirrhosis. Gastroenterology. 2011;140(2):488–96.e4.
45. Diamond JR, Yoburn DC. Nonoliguric acute renal failure associated with a low fractional excretion of sodium. Ann Intern Med. 1982;96(5):597–600.
46. Kanel GC, Peters RL. Glomerular tubular reflux--a morphologic renal lesion associated with the hepatorenal syndrome. Hepatology. 1984;4(2):242–6.
47. Arroyo V, Fernandez J. Pathophysiological basis of albumin use in cirrhosis. Ann Hepatol. 2011;10(Suppl 1):S6–14.
48. Garcia-Martinez R, Caraceni P, Bernardi M, Gines P, Arroyo V, Jalan R. Albumin: pathophysiologic basis of its role in the treatment of cirrhosis and its complications. Hepatology. 2013;58(5):1836–46.
49. Caraceni P, Domenicali M, Tovoli A, Napoli L, Ricci CS, Tufoni M, et al. Clinical indications for the albumin use: still a controversial issue. Eur J Intern Med. 2013;24(8):721–8.
50. Arroyo V, Garcia-Martinez R, Salvatella X. Human serum albumin, systemic inflammation, and cirrhosis. J Hepatol. 2014;61(2):396–407.
51. Boyer TD, Sanyal AJ, Wong F, Frederick RT, Lake JR, O'Leary JG, et al. Terlipressin plus albumin is more effective than albumin alone in improving renal function in patients with cirrhosis and hepatorenal syndrome type 1. Gastroenterology. 2016;150(7):1579–89.e2.
52. Wong F, Pappas SC, Boyer TD, Sanyal AJ, Bajaj JS, Escalante S, et al. Terlipressin improves renal function and reverses hepatorenal syndrome in patients with systemic inflammatory response syndrome. Clin Gastroenterol Hepatol. 2017;15(2):266–72.e1.
53. Cavallin M, Kamath PS, Merli M, Fasolato S, Toniutto P, Salerno F, et al. Terlipressin plus albumin versus midodrine and octreotide plus albumin in the treatment of hepatorenal syndrome: a randomized trial. Hepatology. 2015;62(2):567–74.
54. Martin-Llahi M, Pepin MN, Guevara M, Diaz F, Torre A, Monescillo A, et al. Terlipressin and albumin vs albumin in patients with cirrhosis and hepatorenal syndrome: a randomized study. Gastroenterology. 2008;134(5):1352–9.
55. Boyer TD, Sanyal AJ, Garcia-Tsao G, Blei A, Carl D, Bexon AS, et al. Predictors of response to terlipressin plus albumin in hepatorenal syndrome (HRS) type 1: relationship of serum creatinine to hemodynamics. J Hepatol. 2011;55(2):315–21.
56. Sanyal AJ, Boyer T, Garcia-Tsao G, Regenstein F, Rossaro L, Appenrodt B, et al. A randomized, prospective, double-blind, placebo-controlled trial of terlipressin for type 1 hepatorenal syndrome. Gastroenterology. 2008;134(5):1360–8.
57. Arora V, Maiwall R, Rajan V, Jindal A, Muralikrishna Shasthry S, Kumar G, et al. Terlipressin is superior to noradrenaline in the management of acute kidney injury in acute on chronic liver failure. Hepatology. 2020;71(2):600–10.
58. Cavallin M, Piano S, Romano A, Fasolato S, Frigo AC, Benetti G, et al. Terlipressin given by continuous intravenous infusion versus intravenous boluses in the treatment of hepatorenal syndrome: a randomized controlled study. Hepatology. 2016;63(3):983–92.
59. Alessandria C, Ottobrelli A, Debernardi-Venon W, Todros L, Cerenzia MT, Martini S, et al. Noradrenalin vs terlipressin in patients with hepatorenal syndrome: a prospective, randomized, unblinded, pilot study. J Hepatol. 2007;47(4):499–505.

60. Sharma P, Kumar A, Shrama BC, Sarin SK. An open label, pilot, randomized controlled trial of noradrenaline versus terlipressin in the treatment of type 1 hepatorenal syndrome and predictors of response. Am J Gastroenterol. 2008;103(7):1689–97.
61. Singh V, Ghosh S, Singh B, Kumar P, Sharma N, Bhalla A, et al. Noradrenaline vs. terlipressin in the treatment of hepatorenal syndrome: a randomized study. J Hepatol. 2012;56(6):1293–8.
62. Nassar Junior AP, Farias AQ, LA DA, Carrilho FJ, Malbouisson LM. Terlipressin versus norepinephrine in the treatment of hepatorenal syndrome: a systematic review and meta-analysis. PLoS One. 2014;9(9):e107466.
63. Angeli P, Volpin R, Gerunda G, Craighero R, Roner P, Merenda R, et al. Reversal of type 1 hepatorenal syndrome with the administration of midodrine and octreotide. Hepatology. 1999;29(6):1690–7.
64. Song T, Rossle M, He F, Liu F, Guo X, Qi X. Transjugular intrahepatic portosystemic shunt for hepatorenal syndrome: a systematic review and meta-analysis. Dig Liver Dis. 2018;50(4):323–30.
65. Wadei HM, Mai ML, Ahsan N, Gonwa TA. Hepatorenal syndrome: pathophysiology and management. Clin J Am Soc Nephrol. 2006;1(5):1066–79.
66. Arroyo V, Fernandez J. Management of hepatorenal syndrome in patients with cirrhosis. Nat Rev Nephrol. 2011;7(9):517–26.
67. Nadkarni GN, Simoes PK, Patel A, Patel S, Yacoub R, Konstantinidis I, et al. National trends of acute kidney injury requiring dialysis in decompensated cirrhosis hospitalizations in the United States. Hepatol Int. 2016;10(3):525–31.
68. Allegretti AS, Parada XV, Eneanya ND, Gilligan H, Xu D, Zhao S, et al. Prognosis of patients with cirrhosis and AKI who initiate RRT. Clin J Am Soc Nephrol. 2018;13(1):16–25.
69. Angeli P, Rodriguez E, Piano S, Ariza X, Morando F, Sola E, et al. Acute kidney injury and acute-on-chronic liver failure classifications in prognosis assessment of patients with acute decompensation of cirrhosis. Gut. 2015;64(10):1616–22.
70. Banares R, Catalina MV, Vaquero J. Liver support systems: will they ever reach prime time? Curr Gastroenterol Rep. 2013;15(3):312.
71. Banares R, Nevens F, Larsen FS, Jalan R, Albillos A, Dollinger M, et al. Extracorporeal albumin dialysis with the molecular adsorbent recirculating system in acute-on-chronic liver failure: the RELIEF trial. Hepatology. 2013;57(3):1153–62.
72. Nadim MK, Genyk YS, Tokin C, Fieber J, Ananthapanyasut W, Ye W, et al. Impact of the etiology of acute kidney injury on outcomes following liver transplantation: acute tubular necrosis versus hepatorenal syndrome. Liver Transpl. 2012;18(5):539–48.
73. Sharma P, Goodrich NP, Schaubel DE, Guidinger MK, Merion RM. Patient-specific prediction of ESRD after liver transplantation. J Am Soc Nephrol. 2013;24(12):2045–52.
74. Sharma P, Goodrich NP, Zhang M, Guidinger MK, Schaubel DE, Merion RM. Short-term pretransplant renal replacement therapy and renal nonrecovery after liver transplantation alone. Clin J Am Soc Nephrol. 2013;8(7):1135–42.
75. Nadim MK, Davis CL, Sung R, Kellum JA, Genyk YS. Simultaneous liver-kidney transplantation: a survey of US transplant centers. Am J Transplant. 2012;12(11):3119–27.
76. Nadim MK, Sung RS, Davis CL, Andreoni KA, Biggins SW, Danovitch GM, et al. Simultaneous liver-kidney transplantation summit: current state and future directions. Am J Transplant. 2012;12(11):2901–8.
77. Asch WS, Bia MJ. New organ allocation system for combined liver-kidney transplants and the availability of kidneys for transplant to patients with stage 4-5 CKD. Clin J Am Soc Nephrol. 2017;12(5):848–52.
78. Srinivas TR, Stephany BR, Budev M, Mason DP, Starling RC, Miller C, et al. An emerging population: kidney transplant candidates who are placed on the waiting list after liver, heart, and lung transplantation. Clin J Am Soc Nephrol. 2010;5(10):1881–6.
79. Chopra A, Cantarovich M, Bain VG. Simultaneous liver and kidney transplants: optimizing use of this double resource. Transplantation. 2011;91(12):1305–9.

80. Puri V, Eason J. Simultaneous liver-kidney transplantation. Curr Transpl Rep. 2015;2(4):297–302.
81. OPTN/UNOS Kidney Transplantation Committee. Simultaneous Liver Kidney (SLK) Allocation Policy 2015 [cited 26 Nov 2019]. Available from: https://optn.transplant.hrsa.gov/media/1192/0815-12_SLK_Allocation.pdf.
82. Caraceni P, Riggio O, Angeli P, Alessandria C, Neri S, Foschi FG, et al. Long-term albumin administration in decompensated cirrhosis (ANSWER): an open-label randomised trial. Lancet. 2018;391(10138):2417–29.
83. Serste T, Melot C, Francoz C, Durand F, Rautou PE, Valla D, et al. Deleterious effects of beta-blockers on survival in patients with cirrhosis and refractory ascites. Hepatology. 2010;52(3):1017–22.
84. Alessandria C, Ozdogan O, Guevara M, Restuccia T, Jimenez W, Arroyo V, et al. MELD score and clinical type predict prognosis in hepatorenal syndrome: relevance to liver transplantation. Hepatology. 2005;41(6):1282–9.

Chapter 10
Lupus Nephritis

Omar H. Maarouf

Introduction

Systemic lupus erythematosus (SLE) is a chronic multisystem autoimmune disease that predominantly affects women of childbearing age where it can often involve the kidneys.

Lupus nephritis (LN) is common in patients with SLE. LN is the most common cause of kidney injury in SLE. Noteworthy, men with SLE have likely more aggressive disease with increased rates of renal and cardiovascular involvement and are more likely to progress to end-stage renal disease (ESRD) than women [1].

Patients that show manifestation of SLE at a younger age are more likely to develop LN. SLE without nephritis presents later in life. LN classically develops early in the disease course within the first 3 years of SLE diagnosis. It can also be contemporaneous with SLE diagnosis. LN likely develops at a younger age and involve the female sex, with a predilection for non-European ancestry. Of note, Black and Hispanic patients have a worse disease course with increased predilection to progress to ESRD than white patients [2].

In proliferative LN, a third can progress to end-stage kidney disease (ESKD). Early clinical response to induction immunosuppressive therapy protects against progression to ESKD whereby 10-year kidney survival in clinical responders can be as high as 90%. In contrast, partial response to immunotherapy decreases kidney survival down to 50%. Unfortunately, the renal survival drops significantly in non-responders to ~10%. Mortality in LN is quite variable among different series ranging in between 15% and 25% [3].

O. H. Maarouf (✉)
Division of Nephrology, Department of Medicine, Thomas Jefferson University, Philadelphia, PA, USA
e-mail: omar.maarouf@jefferson.edu

© Springer Nature Switzerland AG 2022
J. McCauley et al. (eds.), *Approaches to Chronic Kidney Disease*,
https://doi.org/10.1007/978-3-030-83082-3_10

Being an autoimmune disease, the effect of genetics on the disease course is quite evident. As in most autoimmune diseases, gene modifications in HLA molecules capture auto-antigens activating our immune response in lupus nephritis [4]. Interestingly, gene modifications in HLA-DR4 and HLA-DR11 might protect against LN, while HLA-DR3 and HLA-DR15 modifications can increase the risk of LN. The occurrence of these risk alleles alone does not necessarily lead to LN as many patients with LN do not have these high-risk variants. More gene modifications in HLA molecules are likely to be discovered as we look for more gene variants in LN. These genetic variations likely have a role in the racial and ethnic disparities of lupus and LN [5].

Pathophysiology

Formation of autoantibodies directed against auto-antigens is key in the disease process of LN, leading to immune complex (IC) formation and accumulation of circulating immune complexes (IC) in glomeruli. This IC can form in situ when autoantibodies target intrinsic glomerular antigens leading to the activation of our complement system to clear local injury. The sustained stimulus in autoimmune diseases leads to a dysregulated immune response enhancing local inflammation which leads to propagating the local kidney injury. The autoimmune response is further stimulated by apoptotic debris (including chromatin) that might be incompletely cleared by our complement system response. These apoptotic debris activate intrarenal dendritic cells (DCs) forming plasmacytoid DCs (pDCs) which activate T cells. When these T cells activate B cells, they enhance the production of anti-chromatin antibodies. The inflammatory response to intraglomerular injury leads to sustained complement system activation in an attempt to clear the local injury. This tonic response of the complement system activation results in tissue injury and further inflammation, through both classic and alternate pathways [6].

T- and B-cell interactions stimulate interstitial plasma cell generation in the kidney interstitium leading to clonally restricted autoantibody-producing plasma cells. This cascade of inflammatory response is facilitated by intrarenal DC producing interferon-α (IFN-α) which augments autoreactive B-cell activation and its reciprocal interaction in T-cell activation. These interactions further activate the immune response leading to an amplified plasma cell response producing autoantibodies in the kidney interstitium. C1q component of the complement system is vital for IC clearance whereby antibodies to C1q impair IC clearance [7]. This prolonged local injury and inflammation attract neutrophils to try and clear this inflammation, but the sustained local injury leads to neutrophil apoptosis. These apoptotic bodies release neutrophil extracellular traps (NETs) which trap more neutrophils. This propagates the local injury further whereby local immune cell responders like pDCs release IFN-α further augmenting the inflammatory response by enhancing the intrarenal autoimmunity and inflammation leading to kidney tissue injury which can

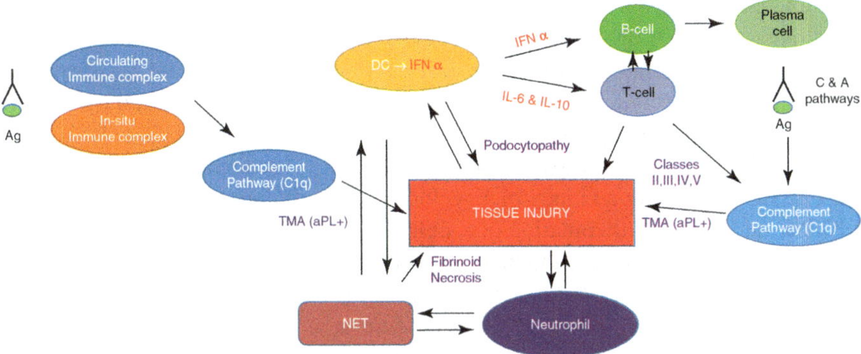

Fig. 10.1 These schemata summarize the principal components of the immune system that contribute to LN pathogenesis and elucidate current understanding on the autoimmune response in LN. Circulating plasmacytoid dendritic cells are recruited into the kidney and release IFN-α which stimulates antigen-presenting cells and promotes B-cell differentiation into plasma cells. B cells present autoantigens to T cells which leads to T-cell activation and release of proinflammatory cytokines such as IL-6. Neutrophils are attracted to clear inflammation. Sustained autoimmune response can lead to NET formation and further the local inflammation leading to increased inflammatory injury and tissue fibrosis if not treated

cause tissue fibrosis if this dysregulated auto-immune response is not abrogated (see Fig. 10.1) [8].

Diagnosis

Lupus nephritis is usually asymptomatic, and thus screening in high-risk individuals can help in earlier diagnosis of LN in SLE patients. Serum creatinine, urine protein, and urine sediment are the main labs that can be used to screen for LN. An active urine sediment manifested in the presence of blood and/or protein on urine dipstick in a patient with SLE is suggestive of LN. However, UA as a screening tool can be inaccurate depending on the urine concentration and adequacy of collection. Red blood cells found in UA can be from a non-glomerular source like menstruation or a kidney stone. The urine should be analyzed using microscopy looking for signs of glomerular bleeding like dysmorphic RBCs, or the gold standard of diagnosis is an RBC cast. The findings in a UA are affected by the varying urine concentrations. We can control for varying urine concentrations by measuring urine creatinine and determine the urine protein to creatinine ratio. It is also important to measure urine albumin concurrently to confirm that the proteinuria is mainly albuminuria. When deciding on starting or changing the immunosuppression regimen, it is advised to confirm the level of proteinuria using 24-hour urine collection. We can also measure the urine protein to creatinine ratio in the 24-hour urine collection to control for errors of collection.

Clinicians caring for patient with SLE have to be wary of discrepancies between the clinical presentation of patients with lupus nephritis and kidney pathologic findings [9]. Class IV lupus nephritis can present with minimal signs of lupus nephritis [10, 11]. SLE patients with nonsignificant proteinuria (<1 g/24 h) can have significant kidney involvement with proliferative LN (classes III or IV) [12, 13].

Changes in clinical findings of LN may not be reflected in the renal pathology of the disease compelling a kidney biopsy. Increase in proteinuria might either reflect LN flare and kidney inflammation or a sign of progression of LN to kidney fibrosis [14]. Of note, a sharp increase in proteinuria can reflect a new class V LN (membranous nephropathy) or advanced proliferative lesion. Most nephrologists would order a kidney biopsy in SLE patients when proteinuria is greater than 0.5 g especially when associated with rising serum creatinine. This becomes more essential in the early phases of LN.

A rise in creatinine and blood pressure with a non-active UA in addition to a subnephrotic proteinuria likely points toward endothelial injury resulting in thrombotic microangiopathy (TMA). In this scenario, we also have to look for the presence of concurrent antiphospholipid syndrome (APLAS) when the blood pressure control is worsening. Those patients with APLAS and LN dictate anticoagulation in addition to immunotherapy to prevent propagation of the vascular injury. The concurrent presence of proteinuria and hematuria in the urine sediment suggests active inflammation [15].

Given these inconsistencies between the clinical presentation and the renal pathology in LN, many nephrologists have a low threshold to pursue the gold standard for diagnosis and classification of LN through percutaneous kidney biopsy [16]. When the screening tests for LN are positive, we usually pursue a kidney biopsy. The threshold of proteinuria to pursue a kidney biopsy is not well defined. Nevertheless, proteinuria greater than 500–1000 mg per day is an equitable mark to obtain a kidney biopsy. Early in the disease course, proteinuria usually reflects kidney glomerular inflammation as the kidney will likely not show any scarring or fibrosis.

Another form of renal injury not related to glomerular inflammation is TMA/ antiphospholipid nephropathy involving direct endothelial injury independent of inflammation. This injury can represent 25% of kidney involvement in LN and can be associated with proliferative lesions. Another form of a nonimmune complex related injury is lupus podocytopathy which is present in 1–2% of SLE patients. Those patients with lupus podocytopathy present with nephrotic syndrome like class V LN making it clinically challenging to differentiate their diagnosis. Electron microscopy (EM) will thus be crucial to distinguish these two entities. In lupus podocytopathy, EM will show diffuse foot process effacement as in class V LN but subendothelial or subepithelial deposits will be absent. Lupus podocytopathy often behaves like minimal change disease whereby their response to corticosteroid treatment alone is quite rapid. A few other lesions that are less common include acute tubular necrosis, tubulointerstitial nephritis, renovascular disease, or nephrotoxicity from medications.

As stated above, clinical findings might not correlate with the activity in kidney tissues. Some nephrologists prefer to do protocol repeat biopsies to better follow on their LN patients. Repeated renal biopsies have risks of bleeding and infection and are controversial whereby most nephrologists do not pursue protocol biopsies. This procedure is invasive in patients that can be high risk with elevated blood pressure or low platelets. Nevertheless, literature involving observational studies on protocol kidney biopsies shows remarkable finding whereby patients with a complete clinical response showed significant persistent histologic activity in 20–50% of cases. On the other hand, half of patients thought to have achieved partial remission with persistent proteinuria (with urine protein excretion >500 mg per day) showed no histologic activity on repeat biopsy but tissue fibrosis – explaining the ongoing proteinuria [17].

Guidelines about LN diagnosis have been put forward by the LN working group in 2016. These guidelines will aid in defining LN pathology and aid nephrologist to better select immunosuppressive treatments for LN. The early pathologic change in LN is mesangial hypercellularity where the new consensus raises the cutoff from three to four cells in the mesangial area. Thus, the presence of greater than four cells in the mesangial area defines class II LN. Once inflammatory cells are spotted in the kidney tissue whether in the mesangial or endothelial area, it represents a higher grade of inflammation defined as classes III and IV. When the inflammatory response is not cleared, persistent sub-endothelial deposits are seen as wire loops on light microscopy, while hyaline thrombi reflect hyaline masses within the capillary lumen. Endothelial injury in LN is common and manifested as endothelial cell swelling of inflammation. The other cause of endothelial cell swelling is thrombotic microangiopathy when there are no signs of inflammation. Crescents represent sheets of cells in the outer glomerulus composed of parietal epithelial cells and inflammatory cells specially monocytes and/or macrophages. Thus, crescents clearly denote proliferative lesions.

Another critical lesion in lupus nephritis is fibrinoid necrosis which reflects a break in the glomerular basement membrane or mesangial matrix. This pathology is similar to ANCA-associated vasculitis. Pathologists have increased their focus on chronic lesions which is usually a sign of fibrosis – irreversible tissue damage which cannot be treated. When these chronic lesions are present in the glomerulus, it signifies glomerular sclerosis or in the interstitium forming interstitial fibrosis leading to tubular atrophy and renal failure. Please see Figs. 10.2 and 10.3 which, respectively, illustrate the tissue pathology in various classes of LN whereby Fig. 10.2 is a cartoon schema of localized pathologies, while Fig. 10.3 depicts representations of light microscopy findings.

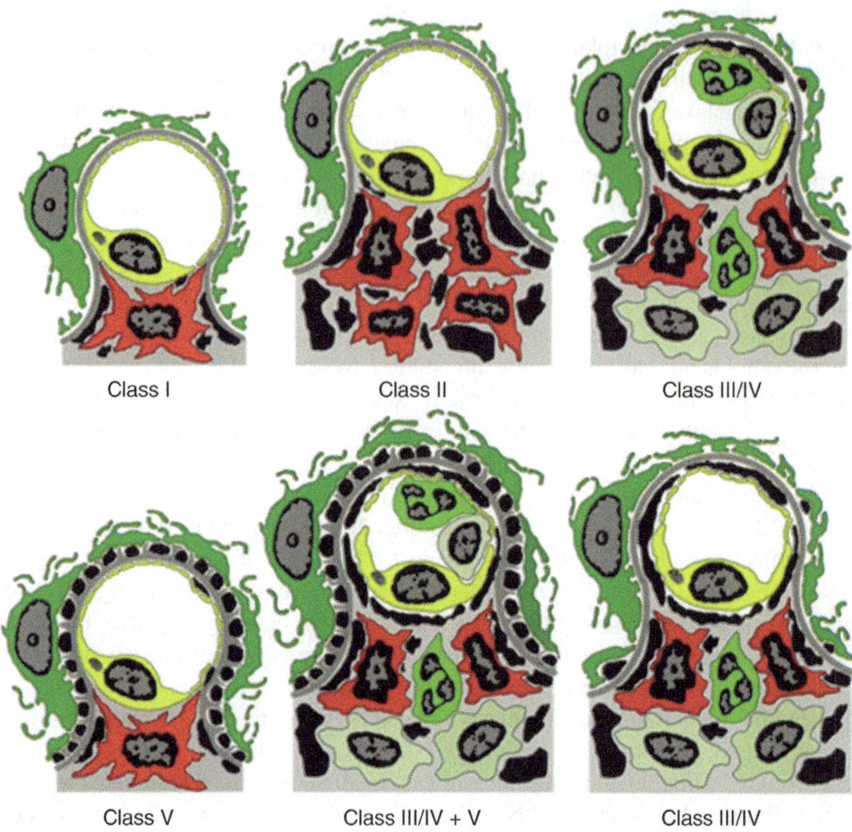

Fig. 10.2 Cartoon depicting the ultrastructural changes of a single glomerular capillary affected by lupus glomerulonephritis: Class I with mesangial immune deposits (*black*) but no mesangial cell (*red*) hypercellularity or influx of leukocytes. Class II with mesangial immune deposits and mesangial cell hypercellularity but no influx of leukocytes; class III/IV (*upper right*) with mesangial and capillary influx of leukocytes; class III/IV (*lower right*) with subendothelial capillary wall immune deposits that can be seen by LM and mesangial but no capillary influx of leukocytes (*dark green* neutrophils and *light green* monocytes/macrophages); class III/IV + V with an influx of leukocytes and numerous subepithelial immune deposits in addition to subendothelial deposits; and class V with numerous subepithelial immune deposits but no influx of leukocytes (podocyte = *outer green* cell, endothelial cell = *yellow* cell, mesangial cell = *red* cell, neutrophil = *green* cell with segmented nucleus, monocyte/macrophage = *light green*). *LM* light microscopy (Adapted from reference [17])

Treatment

Clinical Response Definitions

Achieving complete remission (CR) is the primary target in treating LN [18]. CR is usually defined as a reduction in protein excretion to less than 0.5 g per day with

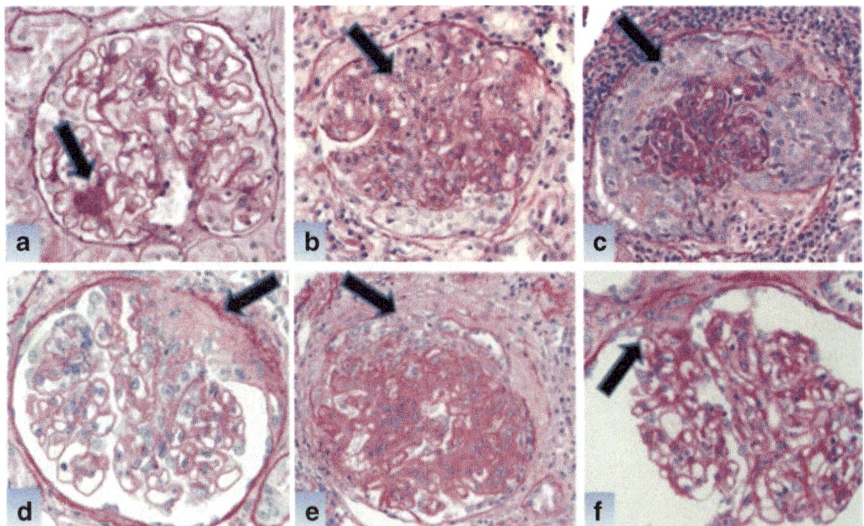

Fig. 10.3 Examples of glomerular lesions in LN. *Arrows* point to typical examples. (**a**) Mesangial hypercellularity, (**b**) endocapillary hypercellularity, (**c**) cellular crescent, (**d**) fibrous crescent, (**e**) fibrocellular crescent, (**f**) adhesion. PAS (periodic acid-Schiff) stain (Adapted from reference [17])

serum creatinine level within 15% of previous baseline. Partial remission (PR) is defined as achieving greater than 50% reduction in proteinuria to non-nephrotic levels, with serum creatinine level within 25% of previous baseline. Patients who do not meet criteria for CR or PR are considered nonresponders. Of note, the level of hematuria is not used as a criterion of remission given that urine sediment microscopy can be variable depending on adequacy of collection and handling of urine. However, the finding of an RBC cast is used as a sign of active LN. Urine protein is the only screening parameter that predicted long-term renal response [19]. The Euro-Lupus Nephritis Trial revealed that a urine protein excretion of less than 0.8 g per day at 1 year was the best predictor of renal response in LN [20]. The other two screening tools, serum creatinine and microscopic hematuria, did not predict the clinical course of LN.

Treatment Protocols (Please See Table 10.1 for a Summary)

The histologic findings of the kidney biopsy and the clinical presentation determine the appropriate treatment regimen for patients with LN [22].

The treatment protocol should also be based on the probable pathophysiology of LN whether during presentation or a flare.

Plasmacytoid dendritic cells (pDCs) release interferon-α (IFN-α) promoting the production of antigen-presenting cells, stimulating autoreactive B-cell

Table 10.1 Induction and maintenance treatments for LN [21]

Medication	Regimen	Dose
LN induction first-line therapies		
CYC	IV CYC (NIH)	0.75–1 g/m^2 monthly ×6; reduce dose by ¼ for eGFR <20 ml/min
	IV CYC (low dose)	0.5 g q2weeks × 6 months
	Oral CYC	1.5 mg/kg/day × 3–6 months; reduce doss by ¼ for eGFR < 20 ml/min
MMF	Oral	1–1.5 g BID (Myfortic 770 mg BID) × 6 months
LN induction emerging therapies		
Rituximab	IV	1 g × 2 on days 1 and 14
Multi-target	CNI and MMF	Tacrolimus 0.05 mg/kg/day (trough: 4–6 ng/ml) *or* CYC 3–5 mg/kg/day (trough: *unclear*) MMF 0.5–1 BID × 6 months
LN maintenance		
MMF	Oral	0.5–1 g BID
Azathioprine	Oral	1.5–2 mg/kg/day

differentiation into plasma cells, and increasing the production of CD4 helper T cells and CD8 memory T cells. This tonic immune response increases local inflammation and feeds autoantibody production by activated B cells leading to immune complex formation [7, 23].

When these circulating immune complexes deposit in the kidney tissue, pDCs are again activated which can further complement pathway activation. pDC activation leads to augmented B- and T-cell responses. B- and T-cell responses are reciprocally activated resulting in sustained stimulation of the autoimmune response encompassing interleukins like IL-2 and IL-17 [24, 25].

In selecting the treatment regimen of LN, a nephrologist should address the dysregulated response of both the inflammatory and autoimmune component of immune activation in the acute and chronic phases of LN.

The complement pathway has two main arms to clear circulating immune complexes and apoptotic debris. The classic pathway impedes the formation of large immune complexes, while the alternative pathway solubilizes immune complexes [26]. During a dysregulated response as in autoimmune activation, the tonic activation of both complement pathways leads to tissue damage during lupus nephritis [27].

The histopathologic lesions in LN are separated into two broad categories: non-proliferative versus proliferative. Non-proliferative lesions usually lack inflammatory cell infiltration of the local tissue and include mesangial hypercellularity as seen in class II LN and class V without nephrotic syndrome. On the other hand, proliferative lesions involve infiltration of inflammatory cells that necessitate immunosuppression such as those that belong to classes III, IV, and V with nephrotic syndrome.

This initial phase of treatment is the induction phase and classically lasts 3–6 months.

Once the induction phase ends, a prolonged maintenance phase of treatment follows. During the maintenance phase, nephrologists would slowly taper drugs that suppress both the immune anti-inflammatory responses. The maintenance medications are slowly tapered to limit the risk of a LN flare. Therefore, the maintenance phase of treatment can last several years. We do not have good evidence on the appropriate duration of the maintenance component of LN treatment.

Induction Therapy

Prior to the introduction of corticosteroids to treat LN, the patient survival rate in LN was alarmingly low at around 17% at 5 years [28]. Corticosteroids have dramatically improved patient survival rates for proliferative disease to 55% at 5 years. In the early 1980s, cyclophosphamide was introduced as an induction treatment which drastically improved survival up to 80% [29].

Nowadays, the proliferative phase of LN is treated with a combination of an immunosuppressive agent with oral steroids. These induction protocols commonly include cyclophosphamide (CYC) or mycophenolate mofetil (MMF). Despite years of use of these induction therapies and their supporting evidence, none of these anti-proliferative drugs are approved by the US Food and Drug Administration (FDA) to treat LN. The use of these anti-proliferative drugs in treating LN remains off-label. Presently, corticosteroids are the only FDA-approved drug to treat LN.

CYC proved to be an effective immunomodulatory agent in LN induction therapy. However, it is associated with serious side effects like premature ovarian failure whereby the majority of patients with LN flares are women of childbearing age. It also carries a higher risk of future malignancies. This prompted a group of researchers in Europe to test the potency of a lower CYC dose to alleviate its unwelcomed side effects. Euro-Lupus Nephritis Trial (ELNT) compared the standard dose (NIH) regimen CYC ($0.5–1$ g/m^2 monthly pulses for 6 months, total dose exposure of $9–12$ g) with a low-dose IV CYC regimen of 500 mg every 2 weeks for 6 doses (total dose exposure of 3 g) [30].

The 10-year outcome of this study is very promising [31]. The lower dose was equally effective for short-term remission induction (54% remission for low-dose vs 46% in high-dose cyclophosphamide at 1 year) and long-term kidney function conservation. As anticipated, fewer adverse events were documented in patients treated with low-dose cyclophosphamide. One limitation of this European study is that most participants were predominantly white.

To further mitigate the side effect profile of CYC, the researchers of the Aspreva Lupus Management Study (ALMS) replaced it with another agent, MMF [32]. Their study was a prospective multiethnic cohort of 370 patients that compared MMF (3 g per day) with CYC (NIH regimen dosing) as induction treatment for LN. At both time points of 6 months and 3.5 years, those researchers showed similar efficacy when it comes to both total (CR plus PR) response and CR at 56% in the MMF group (8.6% CR) and 53% in the cyclophosphamide group (8.1% CR) at 6 months. After 3.5 years of follow-up, CR rates increased and continued to be similar between both cohorts (62% for the MMF cohort and 59% for the CYC cohort) [33]. Of note, the MMF cohort did have a higher gastrointestinal toxicity profile and a higher total dropout rate. Other adverse event rates were similar between both cohorts. Unlike CYC, MMF did not increase the risk for either infertility or malignancy. Given the childbearing female dominant population with LN, MMF has generally replaced CYC as the first-line induction treatment for proliferative LN.

Maintenance Therapy

There are two major objectives of maintenance therapy. One is to maintain the therapeutic effect of induction treatment over a long period of time without its toxicity. The other objective is to maintain suppression of the autoimmune response to thwart LN flares.

In mostly white participants (the MAINTAIN nephritis trial, $n = 105$), the MAINTAIN researchers revealed similar time to first LN flare when comparing maintenance dosing of both MMF and azathioprine [34]. However, in multiethnic participants (ALMS maintenance trial, $n = 227$), the ALMS researchers revealed that MMF (2 g per day) is superior to azathioprine (2 mg/kg per day) in preventing treatment failure (16.4% vs 32.4%, respectively, $P = 0.003$) [33]. Treatment failure was defined as a composite end point of death, acute kidney injury requiring renal replacement therapy, doubling of serum creatinine level, LN flare, or need for rescue therapy. Thus, the treatment of choice for LN maintenance has become MMF in most instances. The optimal maintenance treatment duration is not well defined due to lack of good evidence. Many experts recommend that maintenance treatment duration be at least 3 years.

Emerging Therapies and Protocols

As the earliest treatment of LN, corticosteroids (CS) remain the corner stone of induction and maintenance therapy of LN. CS are effective in rapidly inhibiting the inflammatory response of a lupus flare. However, their toxic side effect profile is well known to be unfavorable. A group of investigators wanted to study the effect of a lower total dose of CS during LN induction treatment. They launched a prospective pilot study (rituxilup study) of 50 participants with proliferative LN including classes III, IV, or V. Oral CS was not used during induction phase, but patients were administered 2 boluses of IV methylprednisolone (500 mg each) 2 weeks apart in addition to 2 concurrent doses of rituximab and were then maintained on MMF [35]. At 1-year follow-up, 52% of patients achieved CR which is analogous to response rates in the literature for LN induction using standard high-dose CS treatment. The rituxilup study is quite intriguing in that the classic approach to treat LN with high-dose CS during the induction phase exposes patients to unwarranted risk of CS with no clear benefit. Additional evidence from large prospective trials is needed to better assess the dose and duration of CS in LN induction treatment.

Antimalarials in LN

Antimalarial drugs are immunomodulatory agents that block toll-like receptor signaling on pDC, reducing production of IFN-α and downstream pro-inflammatory cytokines suppressing the innate immune component of the LN autoimmune response. This characteristic property of antimalarials makes them key components in both the induction and maintenance phase of LN treatment. Additionally, antimalarials are thought to have antithrombotic effects. These drugs are safe in pregnancy making them more attractive in childbearing age females. The recommended dose of hydroxychloroquine is 5 mg per kg per day (maximum dose of 400 mg per day) in SLE patients [36]. Patients started on antimalarials should have a baseline eye examination and be yearly evaluated afterward by an ophthalmologist to screen for retinal toxicity from these drugs.

B-cell Depletion

The dysregulated autoimmune B-cell response is at the corner stone of the LN flare pathophysiology. There are a few observational studies aiming at B cells showing improved clinical response after B-cell depletion with rituximab, a monoclonal antibody against CD20. Nonetheless, a well-conducted prospective phase III Lupus Nephritis Assessment with Rituximab (LUNAR) Study did not show that rituximab improved the clinical response during induction treatment of LN [37]. However, this effect was seen at a longer follow-up. The LUNAR investigators showed significant discrepancy in peripheral blood B-cell depletion in patients with lupus nephritis treated with rituximab from the LUNAR trial. The LUNAR study showed that achievement of complete peripheral depletion of B cells is crucial for disease response in the kidney. The investigators also demonstrate the benefit of the duration and briskness of complete peripheral depletion at their longer follow-up study [38].

Various clinical trials are ongoing to inhibit the autoreactive B-cell response by rituximab especially in situations of disease resistance or improving maintenance therapy to prevent relapse. This becomes critical in patients that are intolerant or refractory to MMF or azathioprine.

A new and more potent anti-CD20 ligand obinutuzumab is being evaluated in a couple prospective RCTs. Another target of the B-cell response that can be inhibited is the circulating B-cell activating factor (BAFF) which is upregulated during the LN flare. Suppression of BAFF with belimumab, a humanized monoclonal antibody against BAFF, is FDA approved for non-renal SLE. Trials testing belimumab are in the pipeline to improve LN induction and maintenance treatment plans by blocking the autoreactive B-cell response.

Calcineurin inhibitors (CNIs) can suppress the autoimmune B-cell response in LN. A Chinese prospective study of 302 patients compared 6 months of a combination of tacrolimus (4 mg per day) and MMF (1 g per day) with NIH regimen IV CYC. At the 6-month follow-up, the combination or multitarget group is significantly superior to IV CYC in achieving CR (46% vs 26%, respectively, $P < 0.001$). However, this advantage of the multitarget approach is peculiarly lost at longer follow-up of just 18 months. This is a good illustration that we should be cautious of studies in LN of short-term outcome. LN is a protracted disease that we better perform clinical studies of long follow-up duration. CNIs affect the hemodynamics of the kidney glomeruli and can also stabilize the cytoskeleton. These features can mask its ability to suppress the autoimmune response. Currently, Phase III Aurinia Lupus Nephritis (AURA-LV) trial is ongoing to study the effect of adding a novel calcineurin inhibitor voclosporin to the standard of care using MMF in a multiethnic population [39].

Management of Class V LN

Class V lupus nephritis, also known as membranous LN, is different from primary membranous nephropathy that it does not usually remit spontaneously. We limit treatment using immunosuppression to patients presenting with nephrotic-range proteinuria. Class V LN is not common; thus, recruiting those patients to clinical trials is quite challenging. There is scarcity of literature on the optimum treatment regimen for these patients. We also have limited data from subgroup analysis in several trials showing that the efficacy of MMF is similar to that of the NIH regimen cyclophosphamide in this patient population [40].

Pregnancy and LN

As this disease is prevalent in women of childbearing age, patients with LN who want to become pregnant should be encouraged to delay their family planning till LN is thought to be inactive for at least 6 months. Immunosuppressive treatment should never be stopped as these women attempt to conceive. Pregnancy during active disease will likely lead to harmful consequences. Most pregnancies in SLE patients that occur without active LN or extrarenal lupus activity have an uncomplicated course. In a prospective cohort study of 71 pregnancies in patients with mostly quiescent LN, researchers show that preterm birth occurred in about a third of these pregnancies at 30.8%, while LN flares ensued in 20% of those patients; preeclampsia or HELLP (hemolysis, elevated liver enzyme levels, and a low platelet count) syndrome, in 11%; and fetal loss, in 8.4% [41, 42]. Treating a renal flare in pregnant patients can be challenging.

A few of the available immunosuppressive medications are considered safe in pregnancy. CNIs are among the likely safe IS drugs that can be continued throughout pregnancy. Azathioprine, corticosteroids, and hydroxychloroquine are among other immunosuppression medications that can be considered safe during pregnancy. Thus, CNI alone or in combinations with azathioprine is a good regimen to prescribe in a LN flare during pregnancy. Nephrologists are quite careful when prescribing CS in pregnancy for its increased risk for gestational diabetes. So, we reserve CS in pregnancy as an add-on IS medication if further immunosuppression is warranted. If a kidney biopsy is required to establish the diagnosis or check for relapse during pregnancy, it can be performed safely up to 20 weeks of gestation.

Dialysis and Transplantation in LN

ESKD patients with LN have a comparable 5-year survival rates as other ESKD patients without LN. As many other conditions, kidney transplantation in LN offers better overall survival and fewer cardiovascular and infectious complications than patients with LN receiving dialysis.

Many nephrologists keep their ESKD patients with LN on dialysis for several [1–4] months before they start the kidney transplantation process to ensure disease latency. Remarkably, a study of more than 4700 patients with LN showed that a wait time on dialysis of more than 3 months can be harmful with twofold increased risk for graft failure compared with those with fewer than 3 months receiving dialysis [43]. Along the same line, preemptive transplantation in individuals with LN and advanced chronic kidney disease had better allograft and overall survival without an increased risk of LN recurrence posttransplantation.

The recurrence of LN in kidney allografts varies in the range of 2–11% over a period of 4–5 years. The paradigm in preemptive kidney transplantation in LN has shifted whereby KT is not reserved for those receiving dialysis for more than 6 months [44].

Conclusion

Our knowledge of clinical mechanisms behind LN pathogenesis has substantially progressed over the last two decades. However, the progress in improving outcome has been modest. Despite these advances in knowledge and subsequent therapeutics, advanced chronic kidney disease and kidney failure rates remain markedly elevated and unchanged for two decades. We believe that the future of LN therapy should utilize a multi-targeted goals to better control the inflammatory and autoimmune responses of the kidney during a LN flare. This might also decrease disease recurrence and reduce the side effect profile of each of these drugs when used alone at higher doses.

References

1. Chen YE, Korbet SM, Katz RS, Schwartz MM, Lewis EJ, Collaborative Study Group. Value of a complete or partial remission in severe lupus nephritis. Clin J Am Soc Nephrol. 2008;3(1):46–53.
2. Danchenko N, Satia JA, Anthony MS. Epidemiology of systemic lupus erythematosus: a comparison of worldwide disease burden. Lupus. 2006;15(5):308–18.
3. Tektonidou MG, Dasgupta A, Ward MM. Risk of end-stage renal disease in patients with lupus nephritis, 1971-2015: a systematic review and Bayesian meta-analysis. Arthritis Rheumatol. 2016;68(6):1432–41.
4. Iwamoto T, Niewold TB. Genetics of human lupus nephritis. Clin Immunol. 2017;185:32–9.
5. Munroe ME, James JA. Genetics of lupus nephritis: clinical implications. Semin Nephrol. 2015;35(5):396–409.
6. Birmingham DJ, Hebert LA. The complement system in lupus nephritis. Semin Nephrol. 2015;35(5):444–54.
7. Gallagher KM, Lauder S, Rees IW, Gallimore AM, Godkin AJ. Type I interferon (IFN alpha) acts directly on human memory CD4+ T cells altering their response to antigen. J Immunol. 2009;183(5):2915–20.
8. Lech M, Anders HJ. The pathogenesis of lupus nephritis. J Am Soc Nephrol. 2013;24(9):1357–66.
9. Giannico G, Fogo AB. Lupus nephritis: is the kidney biopsy currently necessary in the management of lupus nephritis? Clin J Am Soc Nephrol. 2013;8(1):138–45.
10. Gonzalez-Crespo MR, Lopez-Fernandez JI, Usera G, Poveda MJ, Gomez-Reino JJ. Outcome of silent lupus nephritis. Semin Arthritis Rheum. 1996;26(1):468–76.
11. Zabaleta-Lanz M, Vargas-Arenas RE, Tapanes F, Daboin I, Atahualpa Pinto J, Bianco NE. Silent nephritis in systemic lupus erythematosus. Lupus. 2003;12(1):26–30.
12. Christopher-Stine L, Siedner M, Lin J, Haas M, Parekh H, Petri M, et al. Renal biopsy in lupus patients with low levels of proteinuria. J Rheumatol. 2007;34(2):332–5.
13. Hsieh YP, Wen YK, Chen ML. The value of early renal biopsy in systemic lupus erythematosus patients presenting with renal involvement. Clin Nephrol. 2012;77(1):18–24.
14. De Rosa M, Azzato F, Toblli JE, De Rosa G, Fuentes F, Nagaraja HN, et al. A prospective observational cohort study highlights kidney biopsy findings of lupus nephritis patients in remission who flare following withdrawal of maintenance therapy. Kidney Int. 2018;94(4):788–94.
15. Malvar A, Pirruccio P, Alberton V, Lococo B, Recalde C, Fazini B, et al. Histologic versus clinical remission in proliferative lupus nephritis. Nephrol Dial Transplant. 2017;32(8):1338–44.
16. Parikh SV, Alvarado A, Malvar A, Rovin BH. The kidney biopsy in lupus nephritis: past, present, and future. Semin Nephrol. 2015;35(5):465–77.
17. Bajema IM, Wilhelmus S, Alpers CE, Bruijn JA, Colvin RB, Cook HT, et al. Revision of the International Society of Nephrology/Renal Pathology Society classification for lupus nephritis: clarification of definitions, and modified National Institutes of Health activity and chronicity indices. Kidney Int. 2018;93(4):789–96.
18. Kidney Disease: Improving Global Outcomes (KDIGO). Chapter 12: lupus nephritis. Kidney Int Suppl (2011). 2012;2(2):221–32.
19. Dall'Era M, Cisternas MG, Smilek DE, Straub L, Houssiau FA, Cervera R, et al. Predictors of long-term renal outcome in lupus nephritis trials: lessons learned from the Euro-Lupus Nephritis cohort. Arthritis Rheumatol. 2015;67(5):1305–13.

20. Tamirou F, Lauwerys BR, Dall'Era M, Mackay M, Rovin B, Cervera R, et al. A proteinuria cut-off level of 0.7 g/day after 12 months of treatment best predicts long-term renal outcome in lupus nephritis: data from the MAINTAIN Nephritis Trial. Lupus Sci Med. 2015;2(1):e000123.
21. Parikh SV, Almaani S, Brodsky S, Rovin BH. Update on lupus nephritis: core curriculum 2020. Am J Kidney Dis. 2020;76(2):265–81.
22. Parikh SV, Rovin BH. Current and emerging therapies for lupus nephritis. J Am Soc Nephrol. 2016;27(10):2929–39.
23. Ramos HJ, Davis AM, Cole AG, Schatzle JD, Forman J, Farrar JD. Reciprocal responsiveness to interleukin-12 and interferon-alpha specifies human CD8+ effector versus central memory T-cell fates. Blood. 2009;113(22):5516–25.
24. Foster MH. T cells and B cells in lupus nephritis. Semin Nephrol. 2007;27(1):47–58.
25. Crispin JC, Oukka M, Bayliss G, Cohen RA, Van Beek CA, Stillman IE, et al. Expanded double negative T cells in patients with systemic lupus erythematosus produce IL-17 and infiltrate the kidneys. J Immunol. 2008;181(12):8761–6.
26. Schifferli JA, Steiger G, Hauptmann G, Spaeth PJ, Sjoholm AG. Formation of soluble immune complexes by complement in sera of patients with various hypocomplementemic states. Difference between inhibition of immune precipitation and solubilization. J Clin Invest. 1985;76(6):2127–33.
27. Birmingham DJ, Irshaid F, Nagaraja HN, Zou X, Tsao BP, Wu H, et al. The complex nature of serum C3 and C4 as biomarkers of lupus renal flare. Lupus. 2010;19(11):1272–80.
28. Cameron JS. Lupus nephritis. J Am Soc Nephrol. 1999;10(2):413–24.
29. Austin HA 3rd, Klippel JH, Balow JE, le Riche NG, Steinberg AD, Plotz PH, et al. Therapy of lupus nephritis. Controlled trial of prednisone and cytotoxic drugs. N Engl J Med. 1986;314(10):614–9.
30. Houssiau FA, Vasconcelos C, D'Cruz D, Sebastiani GD, Garrido Ed Ede R, Danieli MG, et al. Immunosuppressive therapy in lupus nephritis: the Euro-Lupus Nephritis Trial, a randomized trial of low-dose versus high-dose intravenous cyclophosphamide. Arthritis Rheum. 2002;46(8):2121–31.
31. Houssiau FA, Vasconcelos C, D'Cruz D, Sebastiani GD, de Ramon Garrido E, Danieli MG, et al. The 10-year follow-up data of the Euro-Lupus Nephritis Trial comparing low-dose and high-dose intravenous cyclophosphamide. Ann Rheum Dis. 2010;69(1):61–4.
32. Appel GB, Contreras G, Dooley MA, Ginzler EM, Isenberg D, Jayne D, et al. Mycophenolate mofetil versus cyclophosphamide for induction treatment of lupus nephritis. J Am Soc Nephrol. 2009;20(5):1103–12.
33. Dooley MA, Jayne D, Ginzler EM, Isenberg D, Olsen NJ, Wofsy D, et al. Mycophenolate versus azathioprine as maintenance therapy for lupus nephritis. N Engl J Med. 2011;365(20):1886–95.
34. Houssiau FA, D'Cruz D, Sangle S, Remy P, Vasconcelos C, Petrovic R, et al. Azathioprine versus mycophenolate mofetil for long-term immunosuppression in lupus nephritis: results from the MAINTAIN Nephritis Trial. Ann Rheum Dis. 2010;69(12):2083–9.
35. Condon MB, Ashby D, Pepper RJ, Cook HT, Levy JB, Griffith M, et al. Prospective observational single-centre cohort study to evaluate the effectiveness of treating lupus nephritis with rituximab and mycophenolate mofetil but no oral steroids. Ann Rheum Dis. 2013;72(8):1280–6.
36. Pons-Estel GJ, Alarcon GS, McGwin G Jr, Danila MI, Zhang J, Bastian HM, et al. Protective effect of hydroxychloroquine on renal damage in patients with lupus nephritis: LXV, data from a multiethnic US cohort. Arthritis Rheum. 2009;61(6):830–9.
37. Rovin BH, Furie R, Latinis K, Looney RJ, Fervenza FC, Sanchez-Guerrero J, et al. Efficacy and safety of rituximab in patients with active proliferative lupus nephritis: the Lupus Nephritis Assessment with Rituximab study. Arthritis Rheum. 2012;64(4):1215–26.
38. Diedrichs DR, Gomez JA, Huang CS, Rutkowski DT, Curtu R. A data-entrained computational model for testing the regulatory logic of the vertebrate unfolded protein response. Mol Biol Cell. 2018;29(12):1502–17.
39. Rovin BH, Solomons N, Pendergraft WF 3rd, Dooley MA, Tumlin J, Romero-Diaz J, et al. A randomized, controlled double-blind study comparing the efficacy and safety of dose-ranging

voclosporin with placebo in achieving remission in patients with active lupus nephritis. Kidney Int. 2019;95(1):219–31.
40. Radhakrishnan J, Moutzouris DA, Ginzler EM, Solomons N, Siempos II, Appel GB. Mycophenolate mofetil and intravenous cyclophosphamide are similar as induction therapy for class V lupus nephritis. Kidney Int. 2010;77(2):152–60.
41. Buyon JP, Kim MY, Guerra MM, Laskin CA, Petri M, Lockshin MD, et al. Predictors of pregnancy outcomes in patients with lupus: a cohort study. Ann Intern Med. 2015;163(3):153–63.
42. Moroni G, Doria A, Giglio E, Imbasciati E, Tani C, Zen M, et al. Maternal outcome in pregnant women with lupus nephritis. A prospective multicenter study. J Autoimmun. 2016;74:194–200.
43. Jorge A, Wallace ZS, Lu N, Zhang Y, Choi HK. Renal transplantation and survival among patients with lupus nephritis: a cohort study. Ann Intern Med. 2019;170(4):240–7.
44. Sabucedo AJ, Contreras G. ESKD, transplantation, and dialysis in lupus nephritis. Semin Nephrol. 2015;35(5):500–8.

Chapter 11
Onconephrology

Maria P. Martinez Cantarin and Christina Mejia

Introduction

The National Cancer Institute Surveillance, Epidemiology, and End Results (SEER) program reported that approximately 15.3 million people in the United States had cancer of any site in 2016 [1]. Also, approximately 1.7 million new cases of cancer were diagnosed in 2019. The number of people living with cancer has been increasing during the past few years in part due to improved patient survival with more modern approaches to cancer therapy. The 5-year survival of cancer patients was around 69% in 2011 compared to 49–55% in the 1970s–1980s with traditional chemotherapy [1]. The unintended consequence of improved cancer survival is that more patients will likely experience the short- and long-term side effects of cancer treatment. More patients with cancer will also develop chronic conditions like chronic kidney disease (CKD) which carry their own impact on morbidity and mortality.

Caring for patients with both cancer and kidney disease poses a significant challenge to the medical team. Cancer populations are often vulnerable and have a multitude of risk factors for acute kidney injury including treatment-related nephrotoxicity. CKD, on other hand, may be a consequence of a specific cancer itself or due to comorbidities like hypertension and diabetes similar to the general population. As cancer survival improves, more patients with cancer will live long enough to reach end-stage renal disease (ESRD) requiring renal replacement therapy. Although the approach to the diagnosis and treatment of most kidney diseases

M. P. Martinez Cantarin (✉)
Medicine-Nephrology, Sidney Kimmel Medical College at Thomas Jefferson University, Philadelphia, PA, USA
e-mail: maria.p.martinezcantarin@jefferson.edu

C. Mejia
Medicine-Nephrology, Johns Hopkins University, Baltimore, MD, USA
e-mail: cmejia5@jh.edu

© Springer Nature Switzerland AG 2022
J. McCauley et al. (eds.), *Approaches to Chronic Kidney Disease*,
https://doi.org/10.1007/978-3-030-83082-3_11

is similar among cancer patients and the general population, we will discuss below conditions and issues unique to cancer patients which highlights the growing need for onconephrology training.

Assessment of Kidney Function in Cancer Patients

Kidney function is commonly expressed in terms of creatinine clearance or glomerular filtration rate (GFR). Accurate measurement of kidney function among cancer patients is important as it is considered in the choice and dosing of chemotherapeutic drugs and because kidney injury can complicate the clinical course of cancer patients. However, reliable measurement of kidney function in this population is often challenging due to the limitations in the tools available to the clinician. Serum creatinine-based formulas like the Cockroft and Gault (CG), the Modification of Diet in Renal Disease (MDRD), and the CKD Epidemiology Collaboration (CKD-EPI) are easy to use and estimate the glomerular filtration rate (eGFR). The Kidney Disease: Improving Global Outcomes (KDIGO) recommends the use of CKD-EPI in the general population [2]. Cancer patients, however, often suffer from sarcopenia resulting in decreased creatinine generation. Serum creatinine-based formulas tend to overestimate kidney function in this setting and may lead to unwanted drug toxicity. The underestimation of kidney function is equally worrisome as it may lead to sub-therapeutic dosing and treatment failure. Despite losing favor in clinical practice, the CG formula developed back in 1976 is still the basis of most drug-dosing recommendations for adjustment for kidney function. The CG formula predates the standardization of Cr assays, is seldomly reported by standard laboratories, and is less accurate in the elderly, the age group in which the majority of cancer patients fall into [3, 4]. The largest study that validated eGFR formulas among cancer patients was by Janowitz and colleagues in 2017 [5]. Among 2582 cancer patients, the CKD-EPI formula when adjusted to body surface area was the most accurate published formula compared against chromium-51 (51Cr) EDTA excretion as the gold standard. More accurate measures of kidney function include inulin and iothalamate clearance, but they are expensive and mostly used in research settings. 24-hour urine creatinine clearance measurement can be utilized but may be cumbersome particularly in non-hospitalized patients. Cystatin C is not affected by differences in muscle mass or diet and is relatively inexpensive. This can be used to estimate GFR either alone or in conjunction with serum creatinine using CKD-EPI cystatin C equations. However, cystatin C can increase in states of high cell turnover and non-Hodgkin's B-cell lymphoma limiting its use in certain cancers [6]. There are no clear recommendations on the best method to determine kidney function among cancer patients.

Tubular function is an important aspect of kidney function that is often neglected. Among cancer patients, attention to tubular function is necessary as many chemotherapeutic drugs cause tubular toxicity that may lead to acid-base and electrolyte abnormalities. Measuring urinary beta-2 microglobulin, a marker of proximal tubular injury, and calculating for the fractional excretion of urinary ions may be valuable tests as serum creatinine and blood urea nitrogen (BUN) may remain normal with tubular dysfunction [5, 7].

Acute Kidney Injury in Cancer Patients

Acute kidney injury (AKI) often complicates the clinical course of cancer patients. In a Danish study of 37,267 cancer patients, the 1-year risk of AKI after cancer diagnosis was 17%, and the 5-year risk was around 27% [8]. In a US cancer center, among 3558 patients admitted over 3 months, 12% had AKI based on the RIFLE (Risk, Injury, Failure, Loss, ESRD) criteria [9]. The risk of AKI may depend on the underlying malignancy with renal cancer, multiple myeloma, and liver cancer being associated with the highest risk [8]. Other risk factors include underlying diabetes, iodinated contrast exposure, chemotherapy, and antibiotic use [9]. Similar to the general population, AKI in cancer patients results in higher costs of hospitalization, longer hospital stay, and increased morbidity and mortality [10]. In a Brazilian cohort of 288 cancer patients in an intensive care unit, mortality rates were 49%, 62%, and 87% for patients with RIFLE criteria R, I, and F, respectively, compared to 13.6% in those without AKI [11].

Based on pathophysiology, the causes of AKI among cancer patients can be divided into prerenal, intrinsic, and postrenal similar to how we approach AKI in the general population (Table 11.1). AKI in cancer patients can also be classified as being cancer-related (caused by the cancer itself), therapy-related, or cancer-nonspecific. Cancer-nonspecific causes include volume depletion, iodinated contrast exposure, medications (e.g., non-steroidal anti-inflammatory drugs [NSAIDs], angiotensin-converting enzyme inhibitors [ACEIs], antibiotics, diuretics), ischemic acute tubular necrosis (ATN), sepsis, and renal vein or artery occlusion. In a cohort of 975 patients admitted in a medical-surgical intensive care unit, 32% had AKI with shock/ischemia and sepsis accounting for the majority of cases [12]. The management of cancer-nonspecific causes of AKI follow recommendations for the general population. Hypovolemia, shock, and sepsis should be approached aggressively as cancer patients can be frail and immunocompromised. Nephrotoxic medications and iodinated contrast should be avoided if possible, but their use should be weighed against their benefits if it can alter the course of treatment (e.g., cancer staging) and the goals of care (e.g., palliative vs curative). Despite the inaccuracy of estimates of GFR in AKI, appropriate dose adjustment of medications should still be attempted. Consultation with pharmacy should be considered to avoid over- or under-dosing chemotherapeutic drugs and life-saving antibiotics. Medical teams should also pay attention to medications commonly prescribed to cancer patients, like renally excreted analgesic medications. Morphine and other opioids have metabolites that may accumulate with reduced kidney function and can result in life-threatening neurologic and respiratory depression. Gabapentin and baclofen are also commonly

Table 11.1 Causes of acute kidney injury in cancer patients

Mechanism of AKI	Causes
Prerenal	Volume depletion Cardiorenal syndrome/heart failure Hepatorenal syndrome Drugs
Intrinsic	
Glomerular	Paraprotein-related diseases, thrombotic microangiopathy, atheroembolism, paraneoplastic glomerulonephritis
Vasculature	Renal vein/artery thrombosis
Interstitium	Medications, paraprotein-related disease, infections/sepsis
Tubular	Cast nephropathy Tumor lysis syndrome Ischemic acute tubular necrosis Nephrotoxins, iodinated contrast Rhabdomyolysis
Postrenal	Renal calculi Papillary necrosis Tumor invasion of the ureter/bladder Bladder or prostate malignancy Retroperitoneal fibrosis post-surgery/radiation

used analgesic medications that require dose adjustment for eGFR and can lead to neurotoxicity at high doses.

The incidence of AKI requiring dialysis among critically ill cancer patients ranges from 2% to 5% [8–10]. The indications for initiating dialysis among cancer patients are similar to those without cancer. These include acid-base and electrolyte abnormalities that are refractory to medical management, volume overload with oliguria, and uremia. Active cancer should not be a hindrance to offering dialysis to patients especially in the setting of a reversible process. However, it is important to recognize that dialysis is an invasive procedure and also carries its own risks (e.g., bleeding from dialysis access insertion, infection, arrhythmias, hemodynamic changes). Factors like cancer prognosis, previously set goals of care, advanced directives, and baseline physical function/frailty prior to the acute illness should all be part of the discussion before initiating dialysis. The cost of hospitalization increases by around 21% for patients with AKI who require dialysis [10]. Furthermore, 10–15% of those who required dialysis for AKI will progress to ESRD [8].

Tumor Lysis Syndrome

Tumor lysis syndrome (TLS) results from the rapid release of intracellular substances into the extracellular compartment due to destruction of cancer cells. It often occurs in response to therapy but can rarely occur spontaneously in certain cancers. TLS is characterized by hyperuricemia, hyperkalemia, and hyperphosphatemia with secondary hypocalcemia due to calcium binding to phosphate. AKI results for uric acid and calcium phosphate precipitation in the tubule. Since the development of effective hypouricemic agents, calcium phosphate precipitation is now a more dominant process in AKI from TLS. The Cairo-Bishop definition is used for the laboratory and clinical diagnosis of TLS (Table 11.2) [13].

Acute lymphoblastic leukemia (ALL), non-Hodgkin's lymphoma, and acute myeloid leukemia (AML) are the most common malignancies associated with TLS [13, 14]. With the emergence of more effective anticancer drugs, TLS is being increasingly seen in cancers not historically associated with it like chronic lymphocytic leukemia. Tumor-related risk factors for developing TLS include high cell proliferation rate, increased chemosensitivity of the cancer, and a large tumor burden (organ infiltration, bone marrow involvement, elevated lactate dehydrogenase [LDH]) [15]. Certain parameters for different hematologic malignancies are used to identify which patients are at high, moderate, or low risk of developing TLS (e.g., AML with WBC count $\geq 100 \times 10^9$/L or lymphoblastic lymphoma with LDH $\geq 2 \times$ upper limit of normal are considered high risk) [16]. Other risk factors for TLS include pre-treatment hyperuricemia (>7.5 mg/dl), prior kidney disease/AKI, exposure to other nephrotoxins, acidic urine, oliguria, volume depletion, and a higher calcium phosphate product ($>60mg^2/dl^2$) [13, 17]. TLS with AKI is associated with a fivefold increased risk of death within 6 months compared to the absence of AKI [14].

Preventive strategies for TLS include aggressive intravenous or oral hydration with at least 3 L/m^2 per day to achieve a urine output of 80–100 ml/m^2/hour [13]. Loop diuretics should be used when oliguria with volume overload occurs. Allopurinol and/or rasburicase can be given prophylactically to patients who have an intermediate or high risk for developing TLS. Febuxostat can also be used instead of allopurinol but is more expensive. Urine alkalinization is no longer recommended as it can promote calcium phosphate deposition and may worsen AKI [13]. Close monitoring of electrolytes and LDH should be done during chemotherapy for early detection. When TLS occurs, aggressive medical management of electrolyte derangements should be done to avoid organ damage and life-threatening events like cardiac dysrhythmias. Hypouricemic medications should be administered

Table 11.2 The Cairo-Bishop definition of tumor lysis syndrome in adults

Laboratory[a]	Clinical[b]
Uric acid ≥ 8 mg/dL[c]	Increase in creatinine ≥ 1.5 ULN
Potassium ≥ 6 mEq/L[c]	Cardiac arrhythmia
Phosphorus > 4.5 mg/dL[c]	Seizure
Calcium ≤ 7 mg/dl[c]	

Abbreviations: *ULN* upper limit of normal
[a]≥2 of the laboratory changes within 3 days before or 7 days after chemotherapy
[b]Clinical tumor lysis syndrome refers to laboratory tumor lysis syndrome and at least one clinical complication and can be graded based on severity of clinical complication
[c]or a 25% increase from baseline

promptly. With severe hyperkalemia, medications that shift potassium intracellularly should be given as a temporizing measure, but eventual excretion from the body should be the goal. Exogenous sources of potassium and phosphate (intravenous or dietary) should be limited, and binders can be administered. Calcium replacement is only indicated for severe or symptomatic hypocalcemia (electrocardiogram changes, dysrhythmias, tetany) as excessive repletion will promote calcium phosphate binding and precipitation. Indications for renal replacement include oliguria or anuria, volume overload not responding to diuretics, refractory hyperkalemia, symptomatic hypocalcemia, and a calcium phosphate product $>70mg^2/dl^2$ [13, 17, 18]. The efficiency of intermittent hemodialysis varies depending on the size of dialyzer used and the duration of treatment. Uric acid and potassium are rapidly lowered by intermittent hemodialysis treatments lasting 4–6 hours. In severe hyperkalemia, intermittent hemodialysis may be done first to rapidly lower potassium levels followed by continuous renal replacement therapy (CRRT) to avoid a rebound effect [14]. Phosphate clearance is slower and time dependent due to its large volume of distribution. It may require more frequent treatments if intermittent hemodialysis is planned, and continuous renal replacement therapy is a better option in cases of severe hyperphosphatemia. Peritoneal dialysis is less efficient and is not commonly done for TLS. TLS complicated by AKI is associated with higher in-hospital and 6-month mortality, even after adjusting for severity of illness [19].

Therapy-Related Acute Kidney Injury

Cancer therapy has greatly evolved in the past century. In the first half of the twentieth century, therapy options for cancer were limited to radiotherapy and traditional chemotherapeutic drugs. As the effects of these treatments were not specific to cancer cells, patients suffered from numerous side effects. The 1980s harbored in the era of targeted therapy. Tyrosine kinase inhibitors and monoclonal antibodies were developed to act against specific molecular targets like altered oncogenes or tumor suppressor genes that were responsible for tumor growth and progression. Targeted therapy is efficacious against cancer cells and has limited effects on normal cells improving the tolerability of chemotherapy. In 2010, immunotherapy started taking center stage by targeting immune tolerance that allows certain cancers to proliferate.

The kidneys are particularly susceptible to drug toxicity due to its role in drug metabolism and excretion. Certain anticancer drugs are toxic to certain segments of the nephron or the interstitium resulting in varied renal manifestations depending on which segment is affected. Electrolyte abnormalities are common in proximal tubulopathies, proteinuria occurs in glomerular involvement or podocytopathies, and thrombotic microangiopathy (TMA) can develop with insult to the vasculature and causes hypertension and proteinuria. As newer anticancer drugs come into play, it is important for the clinician to be familiar with their associated toxicities. As the indications for immunotherapy grow, clinicians may start encountering immune-mediated nephrotoxicity more frequently than the typical tubular toxicities that are observed with traditional chemotherapeutic drugs.

Traditional Chemotherapeutic Agents

Platinum Salts

Cisplatin and its analogues carboplatin and oxaliplatin exert their anticancer effect by cross-linking with purine bases resulting in interference with DNA replication and repair. These agents are commonly used in head and neck, gynecologic, testicular, and lung cancer. Several mechanisms have been described in the literature including direct proximal and distal tubular epithelial cell toxicity, renal vasoconstriction, and pro-inflammatory effects [20]. Cisplatin-induced nephrotoxicity can therefore present with a Fanconi-like syndrome (phosphate and potassium wasting, glucosuria in the setting of normoglycemia, hypouricemia, aminoaciduria, and tubular acidosis), TMA, and AKI. In a recent study of 821 adults treated with cisplatin for various cancers, AKI occurred in 31.5% with a median decline in eGFR by ~10 ml/min per 1.73 m^2 [21]. Risk factors for developing AKI with platinum salts include older age, higher peak plasma concentrations, previous cisplatin therapy, pre-existing kidney disease, and concomitant use of other nephrotoxic agents like amphotericin or aminoglycoside [22–24]. AKI is usually non-oliguric as urine output is preserved due to the kidney's decreased ability to concentrate urine. Preventive measures include using lower doses or alternative agents, maintaining adequate hydration with normal saline infusion, and correction of hypomagnesemia. Other "nephroprotective" strategies like the use of amifostine, sodium thiosulfate, N-acetylcysteine, or theophylline are more controversial. Cisplatin-induced AKI is generally reversible with dose reduction, but the drug should be discontinued when severe and progressive kidney dysfunction occurs with a ≥50% increase in serum creatinine from baseline or presence of oliguria. When cisplatin therapy is associated with TMA or hemolytic uremic syndrome (HUS), it should also be discontinued. Carboplatin and oxaliplatin are thought to be less nephrotoxic and may be considered as alternatives to cisplatin.

Methotrexate and Pemetrexed

Methotrexate (MTX) inhibits the dihydrofolate reductase enzyme resulting in a shortage of thymidylate and purines required for nucleic acid synthesis. MTX is used in acute lymphoblastic leukemia, lymphomas, osteosarcoma, and gestational trophoblastic disease. Around 90% of MTX is excreted in the urine unchanged. Drugs that inhibit renal excretion of MTX like NSAIDs, phenytoin, proton pump inhibitors (PPIs), and sulfamethoxazole/trimethoprim can lead to toxicity. The incidence of AKI with MTX has historically been reported to be as high as 30–50% [4]. A more recent study reported a much lower incidence of just 1.8% in 3887 patients with osteosarcoma [25]. Lower doses of MTX do not commonly result in nephrotoxicity. At doses ≥ 500 mg/m^2, MTX can precipitate in the tubules causing obstruction and direct tubular injury. Acidic urine, volume depletion, elevated plasma concentration, and mutations in the multidrug resistance protein 2 (MRP2) transporter in the proximal tubule all promote MTX precipitation [4, 26]. MTX has also been associated with a transient decline in eGFR occurring within a week of initiation and is thought to be due to arteriolar and mesangial constriction [27].

Intravenous hydration and urine alkalinization (targeting a urine pH of 7.0–8.0) can be used to decrease tubular precipitation of MTX. Leucovorin and thymidine can restore DNA synthesis in normal hematopoietic and enteric cells and are used as rescue therapy. Urgent hemodialysis has been used to decrease MTX levels when it is markedly elevated in the serum with signs of organ damage such as elevated hepatic enzymes, AKI, myelosuppression, or neurologic dysfunction. Depending on the modality and duration of treatment, around 50–80% of MTX can be removed with hemodialysis. The use of high-flux hemodialysis appears to result in the greatest decrease in MTX levels with a single treatment [25]. After discontinuation of hemodialysis, a rebound increase in serum MTX levels is expected and may necessitate additional treatment sessions. Peritoneal dialysis is generally ineffective in reducing MTX levels. The recombinant enzyme carboxypeptidase G2 (glucarpidase) cleaves MTX into inactive metabolites. It can rapidly decrease MTX levels by 97–99% within 30 minutes of administration and can be used instead of hemodialysis when available [28, 29].

Pemetrexed is a derivative of MTX and is used in the treatment of advanced non-small cell lung cancer (NSCLC) and pleural mesotheliomas. Similar to MTX, 70–90% of the drug is excreted in the urine unchanged. It has been associated with acute tubular necrosis (ATN), acute tubulointerstitial nephritis (ATIN), renal tubular acidosis (RTA), and diabetes insipidus based on case reports [30–32].

Ifosfamide and Cyclophosphamide

Ifosfamide and cyclophosphamide are alkylating agents that inhibit DNA synthesis by causing DNA strand breaking. Ifosfamide is used in the treatment of patients with lymphomas, sarcomas, and testicular and ovarian cancers. Cyclophosphamide is commonly used in lymphomas, leukemias, and breast cancer. Nephrotoxicity can present as AKI from ATN, proximal tubular dysfunction with Fanconi syndrome, RTA types 1 and 2, and nephrogenic diabetes insipidus (DI). Risk factors for nephrotoxicity include the concomitant use of platinum salts, pre-existing kidney disease, nephrectomy, and renal irradiation. Nephrotoxicity is commonly dose dependent, but there have been reports of it being sporadic [4, 33]. Both syndrome of inappropriate antidiuretic hormone (SIADH) and nephrogenic DI have been reported with cyclophosphamide. Nephrotoxicity resulting from these alkylating agents can be managed with drug discontinuation, adequate hydration, and electrolyte repletion. Lastly, ifosfamide and cyclophosphamide can cause hemorrhagic cystitis from accumulation of the toxic metabolite acrolein that triggers an intense inflammatory reaction. Mesna inactivates acrolein and has been used in the prevention of hemorrhagic cystitis in conjunction with aggressive hydration and forced diuresis in patients receiving high-dose cyclophosphamide or ifosfamide.

Nitrosoureas

Nitrosoureas are alkylating agents that deactivate a variety of reductases leading to inhibition of DNA synthesis [34]. Carmustine (BiCNU), streptozotocin, and lomustine (CCNU) belong to this group and are used for treatment of gliomas, central nervous system tumors, lymphomas, and melanoma. It is also administered prior to bone marrow stem cell transplant. These agents result in nephrotoxicity by causing direct proximal tubular cell injury, chronic interstitial nephritis, and AKI. Hypotension also occurs during carmustine infusion and can lead to renal hypoperfusion. Nephrotoxicity usually manifests 2–3 weeks after drug administration but can also be delayed presenting months to years after the drug has been discontinued. Forced diuresis during infusion can prevent nephrotoxicity [35]. Infusion-related hypotension can be addressed with slower infusion rates, administration of vasopressors, and holding antihypertensive medications prior to infusion [4].

Gemcitabine and Mitomycin C

Gemcitabine is a pyrimidine antimetabolite that inhibits the ribonucleotide reductase and DNA polymerase. It is used for pancreatic cancer, bladder cancer, and NSCLC. Mitomycin C (MMC) is an antibiotic that acts as an alkylating agent and is used in some gastrointestinal cancers. Nephrotoxicity for these agents is in the form of TMA with hemolytic anemia, thrombocytopenia, and AKI. Gemcitabine-induced TMA is rare, with a reported incidence of 0.015–0.4% [36–38]. Immune and non-immune mechanisms are proposed but are not well understood. The development of TMA seems to be dependent on the cumulative dose received. It can have a delayed presentation occurring 3–18 months after drug discontinuation [37]. Clinical presentation can be similar to HUS or thrombotic thrombocytopenic purpura (TTP) with more prominent neurologic symptoms. New-onset or worsening hypertension was found to precede the diagnosis of TMA [36]. Discontinuation of the medication is recommended when TMA develops. Plasmapheresis has been used in some case reports [39].

Targeted Therapy

Vascular Endothelial Growth Factor (VEGF) Inhibitors

VEGF functions as the main growth factor that controls angiogenesis by binding to VEGF receptors with tyrosine kinase activity on the vascular endothelium. The US Food and Drug Association (FDA) has approved several VEGF inhibitors including monoclonal antibodies against VEGF (bevacizumab) or its receptor (ramucirumab). Tyrosine kinase inhibitors (TKI) are small molecules that block the intracellular domain of the VEGF receptor. Compared to the monoclonal antibodies, TKIs (sunitinib, sorafenib, pazopanib) have the advantage of oral bioavailability but are less specific and may inhibit other tyrosine kinase receptors. Aflibercept is another VEGF inhibitor that works by acting as a decoy receptor trapping VEGF before it binds to its endothelial receptor. VEGF inhibitors are used in renal cell cancer and a variety of other solid tumors. The monoclonal antibodies are used in cervical, ovarian, breast, and colorectal cancer. TKIs have been used in hepatocellular, thyroid, and small cell lung cancer (SCLC).

In the kidney, VEGF is important to maintain podocyte and endothelial function which explain the nephrotoxicity associated with VEGF inhibitors. Proteinuria has been reported in 21–64% of patients receiving VEGF inhibitors, and nephrotic syndrome can occur in 1–2% of patients [4, 40]. Minimal change disease (MCD), focal segmental sclerosis (FSGS), and even proliferative glomerulonephritis have been reported in kidney biopsies of patients treated with VEGF inhibitors [40–44]. TMA is a feared complication of VEGF inhibitors and results from endothelial injury. The incidence of TMA with VEGF inhibitor therapy is unknown, and the development of TMA warrants drug discontinuation. TKIs have also been associated with acute and chronic interstitial nephritis, hypophosphatemia, and nephrogenic DI [20, 45]. Renal effects of VEGF inhibitors manifest around 6 months after initiating therapy [44]. AKI is often reversible with drug discontinuation, while proteinuria often decreases but may be persistent [45].

Hypertension (HTN) develops in around 13–40% of patients treated with VEGF inhibitors and is dose dependent [41, 43]. It is thought to develop due to the downregulation of nitric oxide production and impaired natriuresis. The development of HTN actually correlates with better response to anticancer treatment and does not warrant drug discontinuation [26, 41]. ACEIs or angiotensin receptor blockers (ARBs) are reasonable choices for blood pressure control, especially in the setting of concomitant proteinuria [45]. However, there are no recommendations on the preferred antihypertensive agent for patients with VEGF inhibitor-induced HTN.

BRAF Inhibitors

B-raf proteins are involved in signal transmission for cell growth via the MAPK pathway [20]. BRAF inhibitors like vemurafenib and dabrafenib have been approved for the treatment of advanced melanoma with BRAF mutations. Various renal toxicities have been reported in patients treated with BRAF inhibitors, ranging from AKI, metabolic derangements (hypokalemia, hyponatremia, hypophosphatemia) [41], acute tubulointerstitial nephritis (AIN), podocytopaties, and granulomatous formation in the glomeruli. A decline in eGFR can occur within 2 months of initiation of therapy [20].

Anaplastic Lymphoma Kinase (ALK) Inhibitors

Anaplastic lymphoma kinase (ALK) is found in various tumors like Hodgkin's lymphoma, NSCLC, and rhabdomyosarcoma and is the target of ALK inhibitors like crizotinib. In a study of 38 patients with NSCLC treated with crizotinib, Brosnan et al. reported a decline in eGFR by 24% from baseline around 2 weeks after treatment [46]. It is unclear whether the decline in eGFR is due to true AKI or is a result of decreased creatinine secretion by the proximal tubule, as both have been described in the literature. A small decline in eGFR does not usually warrant discontinuation of therapy, but careful monitoring of renal function is recommended when this happens. Renal cyst progression has also been documented with crizotinib therapy, but malignant transformation has not been reported [41].

Proteasome Inhibitors

Proteasome inhibitors exert their antitumor effect by impairing proteasome function leading to accumulation of abnormal proteins within cancer cells. Bortezomib and carfilzomib are used in multiple myeloma and have both been associated rarely with TMA, AIN, and AKI [41]. Carfilzomib has also been associated with podocytopathy and a tumor lysis-like syndrome.

Immunotherapy

Immune Checkpoint Inhibitors (ICPI)

T cells have specific surface receptors that when bound to ligands on antigen-presenting cells result in a downregulation of the immune response [47]. These "checkpoints" promote tolerance and survival of certain cancers. Immune checkpoint inhibitors (ICPI) are monoclonal antibodies that bind to these receptors or their ligands, allowing the immune system to go "unchecked" to start attacking cancer cells. Two receptors have been identified, cytotoxic T-lymphocyte-associated antigen 4 (CTLA4) and programmed cell death protein 1 (PD1). Ipilimumab is a monoclonal antibody against CTLA4 and has been approved for the treatment of metastatic melanoma and renal cell cancer [48]. Nivolumab and pembrolizumab are antibodies against PD1 and have been approved in many types of cancer, although they are mainly used for melanoma, NSCLC, head and neck cancer, colon cancer with microsatellite instability, triple negative breast cancer, and renal cell cancer. Cemiplimab is another PD1 inhibitor that has been approved for cutaneous squamous cell cancer. Atezolizumab, durvalumab, and avelumab inhibit the ligand of PD1 (PD-L1) and are now the first line for urothelial cell cancer due to prolonged overall and progression-free survival [48]. The former two are also approved for

NSCLC. Since ICPIs exert its anticancer effect through a form of "autoimmunity," immune-related adverse events (irAE) have been described with ICPIs involving the skin, gastrointestinal tract, endocrine system, and, less commonly, kidneys.

AKI has been reported to occur in 3–17% of patients treated with an ICPI [48, 49]. ICPI-associated AKI (ICPI-AKI) is not clearly defined in literature. It is suspected in the setting of an increase in serum creatinine (usually ≥50% from baseline) with ICPI therapy and in the absence of an alternative etiology. ICPI-AKI is more probable if it occurs concomitantly or following an irAE, sterile pyuria, and/or eosinophilia. In a study of 138 patients with ICPI-AKI, AKI occurred with an irAE in 43% of cases. Rash was the most common irAE associated with ICPI-AKI [50]. Development of AKI occurs around 3.5 months after initiation of ICPI, but has been reported to occur even after a year of an extrarenal irAE [51].

The pathophysiology of ICPI-AKI is still unknown. One hypothesis is that the tubules act as a target of self-reactive T cells, resulting in AIN which is commonly seen on renal biopsies of patients with ICPI-AKI. Another hypothesis is that exposure to certain drugs (acting as direct triggers or as haptens) result in T-cell priming and subsequent ATIN. Prior or concomitant use of proton pump inhibitors (PPIs) has been documented in the majority of patients with ICPI-AKI [49, 50]. Some hypothesize that PPI exposure results in sensitization, although PPIs by itself are known to cause ATIN in the general population. Other risk factors for developing ICPI-AKI include combination therapy with an anti-CTLA4 and an anti-PD-1/PD-L1 agent and a lower baseline eGFR. There is no defining feature that characterizes ICPI-AKI. As mentioned, it can present with sterile pyuria, eosinophilia, and sub-nephrotic range proteinuria similar to ATIN from other etiologies [50].

The National Comprehensive Cancer Network recommends considering a kidney biopsy only for those with a threefold rise in serum creatinine [51]. Some authors advocate for a more lenient approach to performing biopsies even in milder forms of AKI and prior to empiric treatment with corticosteroids if ATIN is suspected, especially in the absence of contraindications to doing a biopsy [48]. Kidney biopsies should also be performed when alternative diagnoses like glomerulonephritis are being considered. Retrospective studies reported the efficacy of steroids in reversing ICPI-AKI. In a study of 138 patients with ICPI-AKI, 85% achieved either complete or partial renal recovery with corticosteroid therapy [50]. Although there are no controlled trials supporting a particular steroid regimen, a dose of 1 mg/kg of prednisone can be considered as a starting dose. Pulse methylprednisolone can be considered for more severe AKI. The use of other immunosuppressive agents like mycophenolic acid and cyclophosphamide has been reported, but data is too sparse to draw any conclusions on their efficacy [48].

Since ICPIs have resulted in improved overall survival for certain cancers, the decision to re-challenge patients who have developed ICPI-AKI is important. The American Society of Clinical Oncology recommends against restarting ICPI in patients who developed severe AKI described as a serum creatinine >3× or >4.0 mg/dL of baseline or a need for dialysis [52]. However, the risk of kidney injury should be carefully weighed against the benefit of a potentially life-saving therapy, and the decision should be individualized. About a quarter of patients who are re-challenged will have a recurrence of AKI [50].

Another unique issue arising from ICPIs is among solid organ transplant (SOT) recipients, including kidney recipients. SOT recipients have a higher risk of cancer compared to the general population due to immunosuppression. Among recipients who develop cancers sensitive to ICPIs, the use of these agents raises the possibility of triggering an episode of rejection as it boosts the immune response. Case reports of rejection after ICPIs have been published, but due to the absence of larger series, it has been difficult to establish a strong association due to confounding factors [53]. For instance, a diagnosis of cancer in a transplant recipient would likely entail a reduction in immunosuppression, which by itself can account for episodes of rejection.

Chimeric Antigen Receptor T-Cell (CAR-T) Therapy

CAR-T therapy is a form of adoptive cell transfer and has been approved by the US FDA for certain cancers in 2017. It involves harvesting a patient's own T cells and bioengineering them to produce surface receptors (chimeric antigen receptors) which attach to a specific tumor antigen (e.g., CD19 on B cells). These CAR-T cells are expanded ex vivo and then infused back into the patient resulting in antitumor activity. CAR-T therapy is approved for children and adults with relapsed and refractory acute lymphoblastic leukemia (tisagenlecleucel) and more recently for large B-cell lymphoma (axicabtagene ciloleucel and tisagenlecleucel). CAR-T is also being studied for a variety of solid tumors.

Immune-mediated nephrotoxicity has been reported with CAR-T therapy. Cytokine release syndrome results in a systemic inflammatory response from a surge in cytokines produced by the CAR-T cells themselves or activated native immune cells. Cytokine release syndrome was observed in >40% of patients receiving CAR-T therapy and may present with fever, shock, cardiac, neurologic symptoms, and AKI [54]. The mechanism of AKI is prerenal due to systemic vasodilation and/or acute tubular injury from renal hypoperfusion. Cardiorenal syndrome can also occur in the setting of cardiovascular compromise. A rise in serum creatinine can be observed 7–10 days after CAR-T infusion. The management of cytokine release syndrome is mainly supportive, but anti-cytokine therapies such as IL6 receptor antagonist tocilizumab and steroids have also been used [55]. Hemophagocytic lymphohistiocytosis and tumor lysis syndrome have also been documented with CAR-T therapy and are also associated with AKI. CAR-T therapy is also associated with electrolyte abnormalities like hypokalemia, hyponatremia, and hypophosphatemia.

Radiation Nephropathy

Radiation is part of the definitive therapy for certain cancers like testicular cancer, lymphomas, or sarcoma. Total body irradiation (TBI) is also performed as part of conditioning prior to hematopoietic stem cell transplantation (TBI-HSCT). Ionizing radiation results in disruption of chemical bonds and production of oxygen radical species that cause injury to DNA and killing cancer cells. During radiation for abdominal, pelvic, or retroperitoneal tumors or during TBI, the kidneys are commonly exposed to ionizing radiation due to their location. A total dose of 23 Gy of photon irradiation to both kidneys is considered the threshold dose that can result to radiation nephropathy [56]. For patients who undergo radiation prior to HSCT, a single dose of 10 Gy can cause kidney injury. Some proposed mechanisms for radiation nephropathy include oxidative stress, increased production of fibrosis transforming growth factor B, vascular injury, and activation of the renin-angiotensin system (RAS) [57]. "Acute" radiation nephropathy actually presents around 6–12 months after irradiation with various symptoms like headaches, dyspnea, fatigue, edema, and malignant hypertension. It can also present with hemolytic uremic syndrome (HUS) or TMA. Proteinuria may be present but is commonly in the non-nephrotic range. Chronic radiation nephropathy can be primary, with the initial presentation occurring ≥18 months after irradiation, or secondary, resulting from an episode of acute radiation nephropathy progressing to CKD. The management of radiation nephropathy is mostly supportive. RAS blockers are a reasonable option for hypertensive patients with proteinuria, although there are no controlled trials proving their benefit. Prevention of radiation injury includes the use of protective shields to limit the volume of the kidneys exposed and fractionated dosing allowing for recovery between treatments.

Hematopoietic Stem Cell Transplantation (HSCT)

The number of patients who undergo hematopoietic stem cell transplantation (HSCT) has continued to increase, and long-term follow-up is available. Most data on outcomes of HSCT are obtained from pediatric populations. AKI and CKD are common complications of HSCT and affect anywhere from 10% to 70% of recipients [57]. AKI is more common in patients who undergo allogenic HSCT compared to autologous transplant (50% vs 10%) [58]. Mechanisms of kidney injury unique to HSCT include graft-versus-host disease (GVHD), hepatic sinusoidal obstruction from veno-occlusive disease/sinusoidal obstruction syndrome (SOS), and calcineurin inhibitor (CNI)-associated nephrotoxicity. GVHD causes injury to the skin, gastrointestinal tract, liver, and kidneys due to an inflammatory cascade leading to activation of cytotoxic T cells. SOS results from injury to the sinusoidal endothelial cells due to conditioning therapy. This results in acute portal hypertension leading to AKI due to decreased renal perfusion and tubular injury. Meanwhile, CNI nephrotoxicity is caused by renal arteriolar vasoconstriction and ischemic injury. TMA can also occur in the setting of both GVHD and CNI use. The use of TBI as conditioning therapy also contributes to the AKI observed after HSCT. AKI develops in up to 70% of patients who undergo myeloablative therapy prior to allogenic HSCT [57]. GVHD can present with nephrotic-range proteinuria, but other glomerulopathies should still be considered. MCD, membranous nephropathy, membranoproliferative glomerulonephritis (MPGN), FSGS, and IgA nephropathy have all been describe after HSCT and can only be diagnosed by kidney biopsy. Among those who require dialysis for AKI, mortality rates range from 55% to 100% [59, 60].

Around 15% of patients who undergo HSCT will develop CKD [57]. The presence of pre-existing CKD has previously excluded patients from receiving an HSCT. However, this has changed over the years with more patients with CKD undergoing HSCT, especially in the setting of multiple myeloma. It is therefore expected that the prevalence of CKD after HSCT will only increase further in the future. The management of CKD after HSCT should be similar to any patient with CKD and proteinuria. Blood pressure control with a RAS blocker is preferred. Consideration should be given to stopping or switching from CNIs to an alternative immunosuppressive agent to prevent further kidney injury. The true incidence of ESRD after HSCT is unknown but is associated with poor outcomes as compared to ESRD from other causes [61].

Cancer-Related Kidney Disease

Paraprotein-Related Kidney Disease

Classification of Paraprotein-Related Diseases

Monoclonal plasma cell disorders result from an abnormal proliferation of a clone of plasma cells producing excessive amounts of paraproteins which may be immunoglobulins (IgG, IgA, IgD, IgE, and IgM) and/or its components (κ or λ light chains). The range of monoclonal disorders includes premalignant diseases such as monoclonal gammopathy of undetermined significance (MGUS), monoclonal gammopathy of renal significance (MGRS), and smoldering multiple myeloma to defined malignancies such as multiple myeloma (MM), Waldenström macroglobulinemia, or chronic lymphocytic leukemia (CLL). MGUS represents a plasma cell monoclonal gammopathy with a small amount of the paraprotein, specifically a serum monoclonal immunoglobulin <30 g/l and <10% monoclonal bone marrow plasma cells with no end organ damage. Multiple myeloma has a higher burden of either paraprotein or end organ damage, and this damage will prompt treatment. For example, active MM is defined after the paraprotein causes end organ damage mainly represented by hypercalcemia, anemia, renal disease characterized by cast nephropathy, and/or bone disease with lytic lesions. Smoldering MM requires a serum monoclonal immunoglobulin levels >30 g/l or >10% monoclonal bone marrow plasma cells without evidence of end organ damage. In 2012, the International Kidney and Monoclonal Gammopathy Research Group (IKMG) introduced the term MGRS after increased recognition of renal disease in patients with a low burden monoclonal gammopathy. Despite the small amount of circulating protein and the fact that there are no other organs involved, the monoclonal gammopathy is associated with monoclonal renal deposits demonstrated by immunofluorescence, and the presentation is different than myeloma kidney or cast nephropathy. Currently, MGRS is defined by a B-cell or plasma cell lymphoproliferative disease with a kidney lesion related to the monoclonal gammopathy but does not cause any other organ damage and does not otherwise meet hematological criteria for specific therapy [62]. Most of the renal diseases associated with monoclonal immunoglobulins will present as deposits of monoclonal immunoglobulin in a specific part of the glomeruli with the exception of C3 glomerulopathy and TMA that do not present with deposits.

Clinical and Histological Manifestations of Renal Involvement in Plasma Cell Dyscrasias

A wide range of renal manifestations can occur with plasma cell disorders. As previously mentioned, renal manifestations of plasma cell dyscrasias can be classified according to paraprotein-dependent and paraprotein-independent mechanisms. Sepsis, hypercalcemia, volume depletion, contrast-induced nephropathy, tumor lysis, and medication toxicity (e.g., bisphosphonates) can occur, and they are independent of the monoclonal protein burden. The most common paraprotein-related kidney diseases are cast nephropathy, monoclonal immunoglobulin deposition disease (MIDD), and light chain amyloidosis (AL) and account for 75% of paraprotein-related kidney disease [63]. Other renal presentations include different glomerulonephritis (membranoproliferative, diffuse proliferative, crescentic, cryoglobulinemia, IgA, minimal change, or membranous glomerulopathy), tubulointerstitial nephritis, immunotactoid and fibrillary glomerulopathy, and TMA.

Renal injury in MGRS results from deposition of paraproteins in the tubular and glomerular basement membranes. The IKMG group generally divides MGRS into diseases with organized or non-organized deposits on histology. The organized deposits can also be classified as fibrillary (immunoglobulin-related amyloidosis and monoclonal and fibrillary glomerulonephritis), microtubular (immunotactoid and cryoglobulinemic glomerulonephritis), or inclusion or crystalline deposits. The non-organized deposits include MIDD (including light chain deposition disease [LCDD] or heavy chain deposition disease [HCDD] or a combination of both) and proliferative glomerulonephritis with monoclonal immunoglobulin deposits. As mentioned, MGRS can also present without monoclonal immunoglobulin deposits as C3 glomerulopathy with monoclonal gammopathy and thrombotic microangiopathy [62].

Patients with active multiple myeloma and renal involvement frequently have acute kidney injury, but other clinical presentations such as different degrees of proteinuria including nephrotic syndrome, nephritic syndrome, rapidly progressive glomerulonephritis, and progressive CKD can also be seen. In contrast, renal involvement in MGRS tends to be more subtle, presenting as urinary abnormalities and mild CKD [64].

Multiple Myeloma

Of all the monoclonal gammopathies, multiple myeloma (MM) requires a specific mention due to its frequency and its common association with kidney disease. MM accounts for 10% of all hematologic malignancies [65]. It is incurable and is characterized by treatment-responsive disease followed by relapsed and refractory disease in its treatment course. MM accounts for 20% of deaths from hematologic malignancies. Renal dysfunction from cast nephropathy is considered the only renal myeloma-defining event and can be used to make the diagnosis of MM in addition to the hematologic criteria. Around 50% of the patients with MM present with renal dysfunction at time of diagnosis with about 25% presenting with a serum creatinine greater than 2 mg/dl and 2–10% even requiring dialysis at presentation [66, 67]. Renal failure in the context of MM is one of the strongest predictors of poor outcomes [68]. As a myeloma-defining event, renal dysfunction is defined as an eGFR <40 ml/min per 1.73 m^2 and a definitive or presumptive diagnosis of cast nephropathy [69]. Cast nephropathy, historically known as myeloma kidney, results from tubular injury from the excessive amounts of filtered free light chains (FLC). In the distal tubules, FLCs bind with Tamm-Horsfall protein resulting in cast formation and intratubular obstruction. This can occur abruptly with rapid development of oliguria. In the proximal tubule, filtered FLCs are reabsorbed via endocytosis and can cause direct proximal tubular injury from the accumulation and degradation of FLCs. Tubulointerstitial fibrosis can result from distal tubule rupture and the release of pro-inflammatory substances with proximal tubular injury [70]. Different paraproteins have different affinity to Tamm-Horsfall proteins resulting in varying degrees in their ability to cause nephrotoxicity. Light chain myeloma accounts for 40–50% of severe cast nephropathy. Volume depletion and markedly elevated levels of serum and urinary FLC are associated with increased risk of renal dysfunction. The proteinuria in MM is composed of Bence-Jones proteins and is not detected by urine dipstick, which detects urinary albumin. Spot or 24-hour urine protein collection can be sent to measure proteinuria in MM. When significant albuminuria is present, paraprotein-related glomerular involvement from MIDD or AL amyloidosis should be considered.

Evaluation of Suspected Monoclonal Gammopathy

Serum protein electrophoresis (SPEP) and urine protein electrophoresis (UPEP) are used to identify monoclonal proteins. They are inexpensive tests but have poor sensitivity in detecting serum FLC and may not always differentiate between polyclonal from monoclonal proteins. Urine electrophoresis provides differentiation between the urine albumin and urine paraprotein excretion which helps with diagnosing, prognosticating, and monitoring of response to therapy. Immunofixation (IF) is now routinely done and has better sensitivity in identifying the monoclonal protein involved. Since it is a qualitative test, it cannot be used to monitor progression or partial response to treatment. The FLC immunoassay has recently been made available and has better precision in detecting FLC. It is used to determine the amount of serum free or unbound λ and κ chains. It is also used to determine the κ:λ free light chain ratio. In kidney dysfunction from other etiologies or in systemic inflammatory conditions, serum FLCs may be elevated, but the κ:λ is mainly preserved. The reference range of κ:λ is normally 0.2–1.65. The range can increase to 0.34–3.10 in patients with significant renal disease such as CKD stage 5 or in hemodialysis patients. In paraprotein diseases, κ:λ will be abnormal, and the absolute value of the involved light chain will be markedly elevated to around 100–200× of the reference range, usually >1000 mg/l. In the clinics, FLC immunoassays should be used to complement but not replace SPEP with IF. Due to the ease of performing serum assays and the rapid results of the newer FLC immunoassays, it may be reasonable to forgo performing a kidney biopsy to diagnose paraprotein-related kidney disease in certain clinical settings. The risk of under-diagnosis of a condition that can be treated versus the risk of the kidney biopsy procedure should be balanced in every patient. Kidney biopsy should, however, be pursued if an alternative diagnosis is being entertained, especially if it may alter treatment in a patient with preserved eGFR. A kidney biopsy would also be the only way to definitively diagnose or differentiate the different kinds of MGRS. It is important to note that these patients may have relatively large kidneys in the setting of paraprotein deposition, and kidney size on ultrasound may not always be a reliable indicator of the chronicity of renal dysfunction. To determine monoclonality on the kidney deposits, immunofluorescence staining for κ, λ light chains, as well as IgG subclasses should be performed.

Treatment of Monoclonal Gammopathies with Renal Involvement

Treatment of patients with paraprotein-related kidney disease is composed of supportive care and treatment directed against the underlying malignancy or clonal cell involved. For cast nephropathy, volume expansion with intravenous crystalloids will decrease the concentration of FLC in the tubules and result in increased tubular flow to flush them out. Forced diuresis with loop diuretics may increase precipitation and is not recommended. Initiation of dexamethasone with chemotherapy should be done immediately to rapidly reduce the burden of FLC in MM. Plasmapheresis does not provide benefit due to the large volume of distribution of light chains, and hemodialysis using high cutoff dialyzers remains controversial. Definitive treatment of MM includes chemotherapy with regimens that include bortezomib and daratumumab and autologous stem cell transplant for those who are eligible for it. These can be performed even for patients with renal failure. Definitive treatment for MGRS will depend on the type of clonal cell identified producing the immunoglobulin. In general, patients with a lesser degree of renal dysfunction at presentation, lower urinary light chain excretion, and hypercalcemia are more likely to have reversible renal dysfunction. With the discovery of effective chemotherapeutic agents, up to 80% of patients with MM will have renal recovery when early reduction in FLC levels is achieved [70]. Response to treatment and improvement in renal function are associated with better overall clinical outcomes in MM.

Leukemia and Lymphoma

Kidney infiltration by leukemia and lymphoma cells is typically asymptomatic and may be suspected when enlarged kidneys are seen on imagining in conjunction with a diagnosis of leukemia and lymphoma. In a review of autopsy findings of several case series, the incidence of infiltrative renal disease with lymphoma ranged from 18% to 61% [71]. Renal injury results from a variety of mechanisms, including tubular compression from infiltrating cells, lysozyme overproduction, ATN, and intrarenal leukostasis. Treatment is directed against the underlying malignancy.

Paraneoplastic Glomerular Disease

A variety of glomerular diseases have been associated with different cancers and are hypothesized to result from a paraneoplastic process. Substances like growth factors, cytokines, or hormones are secreted by cancer cells resulting in an impaired immune response and glomerulonephritis (GN). Paraneoplastic GN thus occurs in the absence of direct tumor invasion. The diagnosis of paraneoplastic GN is difficult to establish, especially since renal manifestations can predate or present years after the diagnosis of cancer. The diagnosis is only truly established if renal manifestations resolve with control of the cancer and recur with cancer recurrence. Detection of tumor antigens or antitumor antibodies in immune deposits on renal biopsy will also support the diagnosis of paraneoplastic GN. Many patients are asymptomatic from their cancer at the time of renal diagnosis, and this frequently predates their cancer diagnosis, emphasizing the need for a high index of suspicion and a thorough cancer workup in the appropriate context.

Membranous nephropathy (MN) is the most common glomerular pathology associated with cancer. In a series of 240 biopsy-proven MN, the largest to date, around 10% of patients had a diagnosis of cancer [72]. MN has been reported in a wide range of cancers including solid tumors like lung, colon, prostate, gastric, breast, and renal cancer as well as hematologic malignancies like AML and CML. Proteinuria can predate the diagnosis of cancer, commonly by a year, but can be delayed by up to 10 years after renal biopsy. The likelihood of MN being secondary to cancer increases with age >65 years and >20 pack per day smoking history. Unlike primary MN, antibodies against PLA_2R are usually absent in paraneoplastic MN, and IgG1 and IgG2 immune deposits are more prominent. MCD is commonly associated with Hodgkin's lymphoma and has also been described in lung, colon, and renal cancer. VEGF is hypothesized to be one factor that may be contributing to the development of MCD with certain cancers due to its ability to increase renal glomerular permeability [73]. MPGN, IgA nephropathy, FSGS, and rapidly progressive GN have all been described associated with cancer. Treatment of paraneoplastic GN is focused on treating the underlying malignancy. It is important, however, to remember that primary and other secondary GNs may coexist with paraneoplastic GNs which may require separate therapy.

Urinary Tract Obstruction

Urinary obstruction can occur from urologic (bladder or prostate) or non-urologic cancers that cause compression or invasion of the urinary tract. Hydronephrosis is usually seen on renal ultrasound, although patients with retroperitoneal tumors or fibrosis causing ureteral obstruction may need more invasive testing. Malignant dissemination to three or more sites, severe hydronephrosis, and a low serum albumin (<3 mg/dl) were factors associated with lower survival among patients requiring urinary diversion. The predicted 6-month survival of patients with 2–3 of these risk factors was only 2% compared to 70% in patients with none [74]. The reported median survival after urinary diversion was around 3–6 months, and around 40–50% will experience complications related to the diversion [75]. In general, overall survival of patients with malignant ureteral obstruction is poor, without even accounting for the severity of post-renal AKI. Close communication between the medical team and urology is necessary.

Renal Cell Carcinoma

The incidence of renal cell carcinoma (RCC) has been increasing through the years and accounts for around 4% of new cases of cancer and 2% of all cancer deaths [1]. The increase may be due to improved detection as half of the cases are diagnosed as incidental findings on imaging. The majority of patients with RCC are asymptomatic with less than 10% of patients reporting the classic triad of hematuria, flank pain, and a palpable abdominal mass. RCC can be associated with production of erythropoietin and parathyroid-related protein and can result in erythrocytosis and hypercalcemia, respectively. Contrast-enhanced CT scan (CECT) and MRI have better sensitivity to detecting malignant lesions as compared to regular ultrasound. Contrast-enhanced ultrasound (CEUS) has the advantage of not using iodinated contrast, which may benefit patients with moderate to severe CKD. A recent meta-analysis reported that CEUS was at the least equally sensitive to CECT in the diagnosis of renal masses [76]. The Bosniak classification categorizes renal cystic masses according to their likelihood of being malignant. Features suggestive of malignancy include heterogeneity, thick and irregular septations and borders, and contrast-enhancing nodules. Larger tumors have a higher chance of being malignant especially if >7 cm [77]. Those that are indeterminate (Class III) or presumed to be malignant (Class IV) require surgical exploration. Historically, clinicians have shied away from pursuing biopsy of renal masses due to fear of percutaneous seeding and bleeding complications. More recently, biopsy has been increasingly performed especially in cases that with inconclusive imaging findings or in high-risk surgical candidates.

The 5-year survival of patients with localized RCC is around 80–90% [78]. Trends in surgical management have changed through the years. Nephron-sparing surgery or partial nephrectomy is now preferred for masses <7 cm and result in a slower decline in eGFR during long-term monitoring. Radical nephrectomy is reserved for masses >7 cm and/or with signs of local invasion. Radiofrequency ablation and cryosurgery are options for small localized masses less than 4 cm and for those who are high-risk surgical candidates. Around 20% of patients present with metastasis, and the 5-year survival for those with distant metastasis is around 12%. ICPI and VEGF inhibitors are now the preferred agents for adjunctive therapy for those with advanced or metastatic RCC.

CKD, ESRD, and Cancer

The epidemiological interaction of CKD, ESRD, and cancer is complex. CKD and ESRD carry a higher risk of developing cancer [79]. CKD and ESRD on dialysis are associated with a higher incidence of lip, thyroid, renal cell, and urinary tract cancers. ESRD patients who received a transplant are at a higher risk of immune-mediated or infection-associated cancers like lymphomas. Even more interesting, incident dialysis by itself carries a worse 5-year survival than common cancers like breast, prostate, and colorectal cancer. Meanwhile, for patients with existing cancer, cancer-related mortality is higher in patients with ESRD [78]. Despite this, there is a paucity of data on safety and efficacy of anticancer therapy in patients with reduced renal function as up to 75% of ongoing clinical trials in cancer exclude patients with reduced renal function [4]. This conundrum poses a challenge to the clinician in terms of the cost-effectiveness of cancer surveillance, diagnosis, and treatment of cancers in advanced CKD or ESRD.

References

1. Cancer of Any Site — Cancer Stat Facts. https://seer.cancer.gov/statfacts/html/all.html. Accessed 24 Aug 2020.
2. CKD Evaluation and Management – KDIGO. https://kdigo.org/guidelines/ckd-evaluation-and-management/. Accessed 24 Aug 2020.
3. Casal MA, Nolin TD, Beumer JH. Estimation of kidney function in oncology implications for anticancer drug selection and dosing. Clin J Am Soc Nephrol. 2019;14(4):587–95. https://doi.org/10.2215/CJN.11721018.

4. Cohen EP, Krzesinski JM, Launay-Vacher V, Sprangers B. Onco-nephrology: core curriculum 2015. Am J Kidney Dis. 2015;66(5):869–83. https://doi.org/10.1053/j.ajkd.2015.04.042.

5. Janowitz T, Williams EH, Marshall A, et al. New model for estimating glomerular filtration rate in patients with cancer. J Clin Oncol. 2017;35(24):2798–805. https://doi.org/10.1200/JCO.2017.72.7578.

6. Mulaomerović A, Halilbašić A, Čičkušić E, Zavašnik-Bergant T, Begić L, Kos J. Cystatin C as a potential marker for relapse in patients with non-Hodgkin B-cell lymphoma. Cancer Lett. 2007;248(2):192–7. https://doi.org/10.1016/j.canlet.2006.07.004.

7. Schardijn GHC, Statius Van Eps LW. β 2 -microglobulin: its significance in the evaluation of renal function. Kidney Int. 1987;32(5):635–41. https://doi.org/10.1038/ki.1987.255.

8. Christiansen CF, Johansen MB, Langeberg WJ, Fryzek JP, Sørensen HT. Incidence of acute kidney injury in cancer patients: a Danish population-based cohort study. Eur J Intern Med. 2011;22(4):399–406. https://doi.org/10.1016/j.ejim.2011.05.005.

9. Salahudeen AK, Doshi SM, Pawar T, Nowshad G, Lahoti A, Shah P. Incidence rate, clinical correlates, and outcomes of AKI in patients admitted to a comprehensive cancer center. Clin J Am Soc Nephrol. 2013;8(3):347–54. https://doi.org/10.2215/CJN.03530412.

10. Lahoti A, Nates JL, Wakefield CD, Price KJ, Salahudeen AK. Costs and outcomes of acute kidney injury in critically ill patients with cancer. J Support Oncol. 2011;9(4):149–55. https://doi.org/10.1016/j.suponc.2011.03.008.

11. Libório AB, Abreu KLS, Silva GB, et al. Predicting hospital mortality in critically ill cancer patients according to acute kidney injury severity. Oncology. 2011;80(3-4):160–6. https://doi.org/10.1159/000329042.

12. Soares M, Salluh JIF, Carvalho MS, Darmon M, Rocco JR, Spector N. Prognosis of critically ill patients with cancer and acute renal dysfunction. J Clin Oncol. 2006;24(24):4003–10. https://doi.org/10.1200/JCO.2006.05.7869.

13. Coiffier B, Altman A, Pui CH, Younes A, Cairo MS. Guidelines for the management of pediatric and adult tumor lysis syndrome: an evidence-based review. J Clin Oncol. 2008;26(16):2767–78. https://doi.org/10.1200/JCO.2007.15.0177.

14. Perry Wilson F, Berns JS. Onco-nephrology: tumor lysis syndrome. Clin J Am Soc Nephrol. 2012;7(10):1730–9. https://doi.org/10.2215/CJN.03150312.

15. Cairo MS, Coiffier B, Reiter A, Younes A. Recommendations for the evaluation of risk and prophylaxis of tumour lysis syndrome (TLS) in adults and children with malignant diseases: an expert TLS panel consensus. Br J Haematol. 2010;149(4):578–86. https://doi.org/10.1111/j.1365-2141.2010.08143.x.

16. Belay Y, Yirdaw K, Enawgaw B. Tumor lysis syndrome in patients with hematological malignancies. J Oncol. 2017; https://doi.org/10.1155/2017/9684909.

17. Howard SC, Jones DP, Pui CH. The tumor lysis syndrome. N Engl J Med. 2011;364(19):1844–54. https://doi.org/10.1056/NEJMra0904569.

18. Jones GL, Will A, Jackson GH, Webb NJA, Rule S, on Behalf of the British Committee for Standards in Haematology. Guidelines for the management of tumour lysis syndrome in adults and children with haematological malignancies on behalf of the British Committee for Standards in Haematology. Br J Haematol. 2015;169(5):661–71. https://doi.org/10.1111/bjh.13403.

19. Darmon M, Guichard I, Vincent F, Schlemmer B, Azoulay L. Prognostic significance of acute renal injury in acute tumor lysis syndrome. Leuk Lymphoma. 2010;51(2):221–7. https://doi.org/10.3109/10428190903456959.

20. Małyszko J, Kozłowska K, Kozłowski L, Małyszko J. Nephrotoxicity of anticancer treatment. Nephrol Dial Transplant. 2017;32(6):924–36. https://doi.org/10.1093/ndt/gfw338.

21. Latcha S, Jaimes EA, Patil S, Glezerman IG, Mehta S, Flombaum CD. Long-term renal outcomes after cisplatin treatment. Clin J Am Soc Nephrol. 2016;11(7):1173–9. https://doi.org/10.2215/CJN.08070715.

22. Kemp G, Rose P, Lurain J, et al. Amifostine pretreatment for protection against cyclophosphamide-induced and cisplatin-induced toxicities: results of a randomized control trial in patients with advanced ovarian cancer. J Clin Oncol. 1996;14(7):2101–12. https://doi.org/10.1200/JCO.1996.14.7.2101.

23. Siegert W, Beyer J, Strohscheer I, et al. High-dose treatment with carboplatin, etoposide, and ifosfamide followed by autologous stem-cell transplantation in relapsed or refractory germ cell cancer: a phase I/II study. J Clin Oncol. 1994;12(6):1223–31. https://doi.org/10.1200/JCO.1994.12.6.1223.
24. Reece PA, Stafford I, Russell J, Khan M, Gill PG. Creatinine clearance as a predictor of ultrafilterable platinum disposition in cancer patients treated with cisplatin: relationship between peak ultrafilterable platinum plasma levels and nephrotoxicity. J Clin Oncol. 1987;5(2):304–9. https://doi.org/10.1200/JCO.1987.5.2.304.
25. Widemann BC, Balis FM, Kempf-Bielack B, et al. High-dose methotrexate-induced nephrotoxicity in patients with osteosarcoma: incidence, treatment, and outcome. Cancer. 2004;100(10):2222–32. https://doi.org/10.1002/cncr.20255.
26. Perazella MA. Onco-nephrology: renal toxicities of chemotherapeutic agents. Clin J Am Soc Nephrol. 2012;7(10):1713–21. https://doi.org/10.2215/CJN.02780312.
27. Howard SC, McCormick J, Pui C, Buddington RK, Harvey RD. Preventing and managing toxicities of high-dose methotrexate. Oncologist. 2016;21(12):1471–82. https://doi.org/10.1634/theoncologist.2015-0164.
28. Widemann BC, Schwartz S, Jayaprakash N, et al. Efficacy of glucarpidase (carboxypeptidase G2) in patients with acute kidney injury after high-dose methotrexate therapy. Pharmacotherapy. 2014;34(5):427–39. https://doi.org/10.1002/phar.1360.
29. Widemann BC, Balis FM, Murphy RF, et al. Carboxypeptidase-G2, thymidine, and leucovorin rescue in cancer patients with methotrexate-induced renal dysfunction. J Clin Oncol. 1997;15(5):2125–34. https://doi.org/10.1200/JCO.1997.15.5.2125.
30. Stavroulopoulos A, Nakopoulou L, Xydakis AM, Aresti V, Nikolakopoulou A, Klouvas G. Interstitial nephritis and nephrogenic diabetes insipidus in a patient treated with pemetrexed. Ren Fail. 2010;32(8):1000–4. https://doi.org/10.3109/0886022X.2010.501930.
31. Glezerman IG, Pietanza MC, Miller V, Seshan SV. Kidney tubular toxicity of maintenance pemetrexed therapy. Am J Kidney Dis. 2011;58(5):817–20. https://doi.org/10.1053/j.ajkd.2011.04.030.
32. Michels J, Spano JP, Brocheriou I, Deray G, Khayat D, Izzedine H. Acute tubular necrosis and interstitial nephritis during pemetrexed therapy. Case Rep Oncol. 2009;2(1):53–6. https://doi.org/10.1159/000208377.
33. Glezerman IG, Jaimes EA. Chemotherapy and kidney injury. Am Soc Nephrol. 2016:1–10. https://www.asn-online.org/education/distancelearning/curricula/onco/Chapter11.pdf
34. Schallreuter KU, Gleason FK, Wood JM. The mechanism of action of the nitrosourea antitumor drugs on thioredoxin reductase, glutathione reductase and ribonucleotide reductase. Biochim Biophys Acta. 1990;1054(1):14–20. https://doi.org/10.1016/0167-4889(90)90199-N.
35. Morris A, Warenius HM, Tobin M. Forced diuresis to reduce nephrotoxicity of streptozotocin in the treatment of advanced metastatic insulinoma. Br Med J (Clin Res Ed). 1987;294(6580):1128. https://doi.org/10.1136/bmj.294.6580.1128.
36. Blake-Haskins JA, Lechleider RJ, Kreitman RJ. Thrombotic microangiopathy with targeted cancer agents. Clin Cancer Res. 2011;17(18):5858–66. https://doi.org/10.1158/1078-0432.CCR-11-0804.
37. Humphreys BD, Sharman JP, Henderson JM, et al. Gemcitabine-associated thrombotic microangiopathy. Cancer. 2004;100(12):2664–70. https://doi.org/10.1002/cncr.20290.
38. Fung MC, Storniolo AM, Nguyen B, Arning M, Brookfield W, Vigil J. A review of hemolytic uremic syndrome in patients treated with gemcitabine therapy. Cancer. 1999;85(9):2023–32. https://doi.org/10.1002/(SICI)1097-0142(19990501)85:9<2023::AID-CNCR21>3.0.CO;2-2.
39. Izzedine H, Isnard-Bagnis C, Launay-Vacher V, et al. Gemcitabine-induced thrombotic microangiopathy: a systematic review. Nephrol Dial Transplant. 2006;21(11):3038–45. https://doi.org/10.1093/ndt/gfl507.
40. Eremina V, Jefferson JA, Kowalewska J, et al. VEGF inhibition and renal thrombotic microangiopathy. N Engl J Med. 2008;358(11):1129–36. https://doi.org/10.1056/NEJMoa0707330.
41. Nussbaum EZ, Perazella MA. Update on the nephrotoxicity of novel anticancer agents. Clin Nephrol. 2018;89(3):149–65. https://doi.org/10.5414/CN109371.

42. Halimi J-M, Azizi M, Bobrie G, et al. Author's personal copy vascular and renal effects of anti-angiogenic therapy Author's personal copy. https://doi.org/10.1016/j.nephro.2008.10.002.
43. Capasso A, Benigni A, Capitanio U, et al. Summary of the International Conference on Onco-Nephrology: an emerging field in medicine. Kidney Int. 2019;96(3):555–67. https://doi.org/10.1016/j.kint.2019.04.043.
44. Izzedine H, Escudier B, Lhomme C, et al. Kidney diseases associated with anti-vascular endothelial growth factor (VEGF): an 8-year observational study at a single center. Med (United States). 2014;93(24):333–9. https://doi.org/10.1097/MD.0000000000000207.
45. Salahudeen AK, Bonventre JV. Onconephrology: the latest frontier in the war against kidney disease. J Am Soc Nephrol. 2013;24(1):26–30. https://doi.org/10.1681/ASN.2012070690.
46. Brosnan EM, Weickhardt AJ, Lu X, et al. Drug-induced reduction in estimated glomerular filtration rate in patients with ALK-positive non-small cell lung cancer treated with the ALK inhibitor crizotinib. Cancer. 2014;120(5):664–74. https://doi.org/10.1002/cncr.28478.
47. Seidel JA, Otsuka A, Kabashima K. Anti-PD-1 and anti-CTLA-4 therapies in cancer: mechanisms of action, efficacy, and limitations. Front Oncol. 2018;8(MAR) https://doi.org/10.3389/fonc.2018.00086.
48. Gupta S, Cortazar FB, Riella LV, Leaf DE. Immune checkpoint inhibitor nephrotoxicity: update 2020. Kidney360. 2020;1(2):130–40. https://doi.org/10.34067/kid.0000852019.
49. Seethapathy H, Zhao S, Chute DF, et al. The incidence, causes, and risk factors of acute kidney injury in patients receiving immune checkpoint inhibitors. Clin J Am Soc Nephrol. 2019;14(12):1692–700. https://doi.org/10.2215/CJN.00990119.
50. Cortazar FB, Kibbelaar ZA, Glezerman IG, et al. Clinical features and outcomes of immune checkpoint inhibitor-associated AKI: a multicenter study. J Am Soc Nephrol. 2020;31(2):435–46. https://doi.org/10.1681/ASN.2019070676.
51. Thompson JA. New NCCN guidelines: recognition and management of immunotherapy-related toxicity. J Natl Compr Canc Netw. 2018;16:594–6. Harborside Press. https://doi.org/10.6004/jnccn.2018.0047.
52. Brahmer JR, Lacchetti C, Schneider BJ, et al. Management of immune-related adverse events in patients treated with immune checkpoint inhibitor therapy: American society of clinical oncology clinical practice guideline. J Clin Oncol. 2018;36(17):1714–68. https://doi.org/10.1200/JCO.2017.77.6385.
53. Venkatachalam K, Malone AF, Heady B, Santos RD, Alhamad T. Poor outcomes with the use of checkpoint inhibitors in kidney transplant recipients. Transplantation. 2020;104(5):1041–7. https://doi.org/10.1097/TP.0000000000002914.
54. Jhaveri KD, Rosner MH. Chimeric antigen receptor T cell therapy and the kidney: what the nephrologist needs to know. Clin J Am Soc Nephrol. 2018;13(5):796–8. https://doi.org/10.2215/CJN.12871117.
55. Brudno JN, Kochenderfer JN. Toxicities of chimeric antigen receptor T cells: recognition and management. Blood. 2016;127(26):3321–30. https://doi.org/10.1182/blood-2016-04-703751.
56. Cohen EP, Robbins MEC. Radiation nephropathy. Semin Nephrol. 2003;23(5):486–99. https://doi.org/10.1016/S0270-9295(03)00093-7.
57. Cohen EP, Pais P, Moulder JE. Chronic kidney disease after hematopoietic stem cell transplantation. Semin Nephrol. 2010;30(6):627–34. https://doi.org/10.1016/j.semnephrol.2010.09.010.
58. Hingorani S. Renal complications of hematopoietic-cell transplantation. N Engl J Med. 2016;374(23):2256–67. https://doi.org/10.1056/NEJMra1404711.
59. Satwani P, Bavishi S, Jin Z, et al. Risk factors associated with kidney injury and the impact of kidney injury on overall survival in pediatric recipients following allogeneic stem cell transplant. Biol Blood Marrow Transplant. 2011;17(10):1472–80. https://doi.org/10.1016/j.bbmt.2011.02.006.
60. Flores FX, Brophy PD, Symons JM, et al. Continuous renal replacement therapy (CRRT) after stem cell transplantation. A report from the prospective pediatric CRRT Registry Group. Pediatr Nephrol. 2008;23(4):625–30. https://doi.org/10.1007/s00467-007-0672-2.
61. Cohen EP, Piering WF, Kabler-Babbitt C, Moulder JE. End-stage renal disease (ESRD) after bone marrow transplantation: poor survival compared to other causes of ESRD. Nephron. 1998;79(4):408–12. https://doi.org/10.1159/000045085.

62. Leung N, Bridoux F, Batuman V, et al. The evaluation of monoclonal gammopathy of renal significance: a consensus report of the International Kidney and Monoclonal Gammopathy Research Group. Nat Rev Nephrol. 2019;15(1):45–59. https://doi.org/10.1038/s41581-018-0077-4.
63. Nasr SH, Valeri AM, Sethi S, et al. Clinicopathologic correlations in multiple myeloma: a case series of 190 patients with kidney biopsies. Am J Kidney Dis. 2012;59(6):786–94. https://doi.org/10.1053/j.ajkd.2011.12.028.
64. Sethi S, Rajkumar SV, D'Agati VD. The complexity and heterogeneity of monoclonal immunoglobulin–associated renal diseases. J Am Soc Nephrol. 2018;29(7):1810–23. https://doi.org/10.1681/ASN.2017121319.
65. Palumbo A, Anderson K. Multiple myeloma. N Engl J Med. 2011;364(11):1046–60. https://doi.org/10.1056/NEJMra1011442.
66. Kyle RA, Gertz MA, Witzig TE, et al. Review of 1027 patients with newly diagnosed multiple myeloma. Mayo Clin Proc. 2003;78(1):21–33. https://doi.org/10.4065/78.1.21.
67. Winearls CG. Acute myeloma kidney. Kidney Int. 1995;48:1347–61. Nature Publishing Group. https://doi.org/10.1038/ki.1995.421.
68. Sathick IJ, Drosou ME, Leung N. Myeloma light chain cast nephropathy, a review. J Nephrol. 2019;32(2):189–98. https://doi.org/10.1007/s40620-018-0492-4.
69. Rajkumar SV, Dimopoulos MA, Palumbo A, et al. International Myeloma Working Group updated criteria for the diagnosis of multiple myeloma. Lancet Oncol. 2014;15(12):e538–48. https://doi.org/10.1016/S1470-2045(14)70442-5.
70. Hutchison CA, Batuman V, Behrens J, et al. The pathogenesis and diagnosis of acute kidney injury in multiple myeloma. Nat Rev Nephrol. 2012;8(1):43–51. https://doi.org/10.1038/nrneph.2011.168.
71. Richmond J, Sherman RS, Diamond HD, Craver LF. Renal lesions associated with malignant lymphomas. Am J Med. 1962;32(2):184–207. https://doi.org/10.1016/0002-9343(62)90289-9.
72. Lefaucheur C, Stengel B, Nochy D, et al. Membranous nephropathy and cancer: epidemiologic evidence and determinants of high-risk cancer association. Kidney Int. 2006;70(8):1510–7. https://doi.org/10.1038/sj.ki.5001790.
73. Lien YHH, Lai LW. Pathogenesis, diagnosis and management of paraneoplastic glomerulonephritis. Nat Rev Nephrol. 2011;7(2):85–95. https://doi.org/10.1038/nrneph.2010.171.
74. Ishioka J, Kageyama Y, Inoue M, Higashi Y, Kihara K. Prognostic model for predicting survival after palliative urinary diversion for ureteral obstruction: analysis of 140 cases. J Urol. 2008;180(2):618–21. https://doi.org/10.1016/j.juro.2008.04.011.
75. Wong L-M, Cleeve LK, Milner AD, Pitman AG. Malignant ureteral obstruction: outcomes after intervention. Have things changed? J Urol. 2007;178(1):178–83. https://doi.org/10.1016/j.juro.2007.03.026.
76. Furrer MA, Spycher SCJ, Büttiker SM, et al. Comparison of the diagnostic performance of contrast-enhanced ultrasound with that of contrast-enhanced computed tomography and contrast-enhanced magnetic resonance imaging in the evaluation of renal masses: a systematic review and meta-analysis. Eur Urol Oncol. 2019; https://doi.org/10.1016/j.euo.2019.08.013.
77. Frank I, Blute ML, Cheville JC, Lohse CM, Weaver AL, Zincke H. Solid renal tumors: an analysis of pathological features related to tumor size. J Urol. 2003;170(6 I):2217–20. https://doi.org/10.1097/01.ju.0000095475.12515.5e.
78. Yanik EL, Clarke CA, Snyder JJ, Pfeiffer RM, Engels EA. Variation in cancer incidence among patients with esrd during kidney function and nonfunction intervals. J Am Soc Nephrol. 2016;27(5):1495–504. https://doi.org/10.1681/ASN.2015040373.
79. Maisonneuve P, Agodoa L, Gellert R, et al. Cancer in patients on dialysis for end-stage renal disease: an international collaborative study. Lancet. 1999;354(9173):93–9. https://doi.org/10.1016/S0140-6736(99)06154-1.

Chapter 12
Complications of Chronic Kidney Disease: Electrolyte and Acid-Base Disorders

Hasan Arif

Acidemia of Chronic Kidney Disease

Epidemiology

Metabolic acidosis is defined as a persistent serum bicarbonate value of less than 22 mEq per L in patients with chronic kidney disease. The prevalence is approximately 15% [1, 2]. Studies such as the Chronic Renal Insufficiency Cohort study (CRIC) and the NephroTest cohort shed light on different degrees of the prevailing metabolic acidosis in various stages of kidney disease. The prevalence of acidosis was 7%, 13%, 37% in stages 2, 3, and 4, respectively, as studied in the CRIC participants [2]. The NephroTest cohort showed a similar trend [1].

Pathophysiology

On a daily basis, the kidney filters and reabsorbs 4000–4500 mEq of bicarbonate. It also has the ability to synthesize bicarbonate to neutralize endogenous acids. Serum bicarbonate levels are known to drop in patients with CKD. Under normal circumstances, adults generate 1 mEq per kg body weight of acid, while children generally generate approximately 2–3 mEq per kg of body weight. The acid generated in the body is neutralized by our internal buffering system. The net acid load of an

H. Arif (✉)
Medicine-Nephrology, Sidney Kimmel Medical College at Thomas Jefferson University, Philadelphia, PA, USA
e-mail: hasan.arif@jefferson.edu

© Springer Nature Switzerland AG 2022
J. McCauley et al. (eds.), *Approaches to Chronic Kidney Disease*,
https://doi.org/10.1007/978-3-030-83082-3_12

individual can be explained by subtracting the bicarbonate generated by the body and the acid excreted by the kidney from the acid generated [3].

$$\text{Net Acid Load} = \text{Acid generated} - (\text{bicarbonate generated} + \text{acid excreted})$$

The amount of acid or bicarbonate generated by the body is dependent on the amount and quality of food ingested, whereas the acid excreted from the kidney is a function of the eGFR and the tubular handling of organic acids.

Diets that are high in fruit and vegetables are low in acid production, whereas proteins (primarily animal-based) lead to a higher generation of acid [3–6]. If the net acid generation is positive, then the body's buffering system curbs it. The renal tubules then generate bicarbonate to replenish the buffer consumed. This results in an unchanged serum bicarbonate level.

In CKD, acidemia occurs as a function of three issues. In no particular order, these three issues are a reduction in the ability of the kidney to remove titratable acids by generating ammonia, its ability to reabsorb filtered bicarbonate, and its ability to generate bicarbonate that has been utilized for buffering [7–10].

Ammonia generation is considerably reduced in CKD even though per functional nephron generation of ammonia is increased [11]. Increased ammonia production promotes fibrosis and eGFR reduction due to complement activation [12]. Acidosis stimulates the production of aldosterone, angiotensin 2, and endothelin to increase tubular acid excretion. An increase in these three hormones promotes further fibrosis [13–16]. Patients with CKD can acidify their urine; however, the degree of acidification is less than those with normal kidney function [13, 17].

CKD patients can have a normal serum bicarbonate values even though they are considered to be in a positive proton balance. The NephroTest course studied patients with CKD stages 1 through 4 for a little over 4 years showing CKD stage 4 patients were in a positive acid balance with normal serum bicarbonate levels. Patients with similar eGFRs can have a wide range of serum bicarbonate values. Concomitant comorbidities such as smoking, renal tubular acidification defects, and high-protein diet can all lead to lower serum bicarbonate levels [7, 18].

Clinical Findings

In the majority of cases, there are no clinical findings due to metabolic acidosis of chronic kidney disease. It is usually identified via serum chemistries with serum bicarbonate of less than 22 mEq per L; however, this is not an absolute. Some advanced CKD patients have a normal serum bicarbonate value. In very rare cases, serum bicarbonate values can be less than 14 mEq per L but are usually greater than 20 mEq per L [4, 18].

The Modified Diet in Renal Disease (MDRD) and the African American Study of Kidney Disease and Hypertension (AASK) showed a direct relationship between eGFR and serum bicarbonate levels [4, 19]. In the MDRD study, CKD patients, who had an eGFR less than 18 mL/minute per 1.73 m^2, had mean serum bicarbonate values of 21 ± 3.9. Only 20% out of 5000 CKD stage 5 patients followed via the VA hospitals had bicarbonate of less than 22 mEq per L [20].

This is further complicated by what we have been traditionally taught about acidemia in CKD. Widmer et al. studied acidemia of CKD and found that initially, a non-gap metabolic acidosis exists that evolved into a non-gap and a high anion gap and finally into a high anion gap metabolic acidosis [21]. This is likely due to the accumulation of sulfates and phosphates as eGFR falls and the kidneys inability to remove them.

Differentials for CKD acidemia are tubulointerstitial kidney disease (TIKD) and hyporeninemic hypoaldosteronism; the latter is associated with a non-gap metabolic acidosis. Distinguishing them is important as treatment targets are different.

Hyperkalemia and severe acidemia are a feature of both TIKD and hyporeninemic hypoaldosteronism and are out of proportion to the renal function.

In normal kidneys, ammonia production is a result of proximal tubular acidification and a trigger to excrete protons. Hyperkalemia diminishes the production of ammonia by raising intracellular pH and preventing the deamination of glutamine to ammonia in the mitochondria. In type 4 RTA or hyporeninemic hypoaldosteronism, the correction of potassium increases the production of ammonia and improves pH [22, 23].

Adverse Effects

Metabolic acidosis of CKD is associated with a plethora of complications. Acidemia leads to chronic inflammation, dissolution of bone, muscle degradation, growth retardation, and dysregulation of insulin. Metabolic acidosis of CKD accelerates the worsening of chronic kidney disease and increases mortality [24].

Acidemia causes dysregulation of insulin growth factor 1. This increases proteolytic enzymes resulting in muscle wasting and a negative nitrogen balance [25–27].

In experimental models, metabolic acidosis can compromise albumin synthesis by the liver. The data on this is conflicting [28]. Certain experimental model studies show acidemia worsening albumin levels in CKD patients [29]. The 3rd National Health and Nutrition Examination Survey (NHANES III) data analysis revealed that low bicarbonate levels in serum correlated with low serum albumin levels in patients with CKD [8, 30].

Smaller controlled trials as well as larger observational study show that metabolic acidosis accelerates CKD progression [14–16, 20, 31]. Shah et al., through an observational model, studied 5000 individuals over a median of 3.4 years. Patients were observed to have a greater than 50% decline in their eGFR or reach any GFR of less than 15 mL/minute for 1.73 m^2 if their bicarbonate concentration was persistently less than 22 mEq per L [32]. In the CRIC study, the patients' were followed for at least 6 years [33]. Approximately 3500 participants were in the study. There was almost a twofold increase in the risk of CKD progression in the form of either decline in eGFR to half its original value or end-stage renal disease in patients who had a persistent serum bicarbonate concentration of less than 22 mEq per L.

Two separate observational studies of least a thousand patients each also showed that if patients' bicarbonate was maintained to a serum value of greater than 22 mEq per L, those patients had a preservation of eGFR and lower incidence of end-stage renal disease. The Multi-Ethnic Study of Atherosclerosis (MESA) studied 1000 patients with eGFRs greater than 60 mL/minute per 1.73 m^2 [34]. Patients who had a bicarbonate value of less than 22 also showed an accelerated decline in eGFR as well as a higher incidence of requiring renal replacement therapy. Another study of more than 1000 patients called the NephroTest showed a similar pattern of worsening eGFR for patients who had lower serum bicarbonate [13].

In metabolic acidosis of CKD, it appears that retention of hydrogen ions in the interstitium is partly responsible for the worsening of chronic kidney disease, even when serum bicarbonate levels are normal [14, 35]. Randomized controlled trials to prove a direct correlation between the severity of CKD and metabolic acidosis of CKD have not been conducted.

Upregulation of endothelin, angiotensin 2, and aldosterone has been implicated as potential mechanisms for the worsening of a metabolic acidosis of CKD [14, 36, 37]. In both human-animal models, it has been noted that the correction of acidemia leads to a reduction of these hormones and a reduced decline in eGFR. In CKD, ammonia production is increased which in turn leads to complement activation and results in fibrosis [12]. In CKD, the ammonia production for residual nephrons is increased. Pro-inflammatory cytokine and chemokine production is stimulated in the kidney in an acidic environment adding to the kidney damage [38]. Hence, in theory, these patients would be at higher risk of progression of CKD.

CKD acidemia can be linked directly and indirectly to cardiovascular disease and hypertension, respectively.

From the literature review, mortality increases in acidemia of chronic kidney disease [39]. CKD registry of the Cleveland Clinic, MDRD, and NHANES III all showed that low serum bicarbonate levels led to higher cardiovascular mortality [30, 39, 40]. Of note, these are observational findings and require randomized controlled trials for confirmation as there is a difference between causation and correlation.

Treatment

Treatment guidelines for acidemia of chronic kidney disease are usually based on expert opinion as randomized controlled trials are not available. Notable organizations such as Kidney Disease: Improving Global Outcomes (KDIGO) and National Kidney Foundation-Kidney Disease Outcomes Quality Initiative (NKF-KDOQI) have recommended a target value of >22 mEq per L [41, 42]. The NKF-KDOQI, which is a US-based renal organization, has recommended that a base preparation be used as treatment if serum bicarbonate levels are less than 22 mEq per L for a value equal to or greater than 22 mEq per L [41]. Renal organizations for both Australia (Care of Australians with Renal Impairment) [43] and the Renal Association of Great Britain (RAGB) [44] also recommend targeting a value of equal to or greater than 22 mEq per L [43, 44].

Studies such as the CRIC shed some light on to the upper limit of treatment values. In this particular study, it was found that there was an increased risk of heart failure and death when adjusting all confounding factors for inflammation medication use and kidney function if serum bicarbonate concentrations were maintained to a value of greater than 26 mEq per L [33].

Most practicing physicians target a range of 22–26 mEq per L [33, 45].

Theoretically, complications of an alkaline administration could be a potential for metastatic tissue calcification. To date, there are no studies that have proven that this occurs [46]. Secondly, most base preparations are sodium-based. There have been short- and long-term studies that have not shown to have significant effects on either systolic or diastolic hypertension, weight gain, or congestive heart failure. Sodium when administered with bicarbonate or other anions leads to lower sodium retention as compared to administration with chloride.

Available Therapeutics

Calculation of Bicarbonate Deficit

Before considering therapeutics for the repletion of serum bicarbonate, we have to calculate how much bicarbonate needs to be administered to the patient.

The formula is as follows:

Desired serum bicarbonate (DHCO3) minus actual serum bicarbonate (AHCO3) multiplied by the volume of distribution (Vd) of serum bicarbonate

Vd is 50% of total body weight (TBW) in women and 60% in men. Below is an example and application of the formula in a 50 kg female.

$$Bicarbonate\ Deficit = DHCO3 - AHCO3 \times (0.5 \times TBW)$$

Female patient with a weight of 50 kg and a serum bicarbonate value of 20 mEq per L. (desired bicarbonate value of 24 mEq per L)

The bicarbonate deficit will be:

$$24 - 20 \times (0.5 \times 50) = 4 \times 25 \times 100\ mEq$$

With this information, now we can decide on therapeutics that are available.

Dietary Management of Metabolic Acidosis of Chronic Kidney Disease

Dietary management of metabolic acidosis though possible is a little tricky to achieve. One study was able to achieve a goal of approximately 24.5 mEq per L by the administration of fruits and vegetables. Dietary fruit and vegetables were designed to provide 50% of the acid load only. Fruits and vegetables are a natural source of potassium which can lead to hyperkalemia in our CKD population. This can be further exacerbated if they are on potassium-sparing blood pressure medications such as angiotensin-converting enzyme inhibitors and angiotensin receptor blockers [47]. In this study, most of the patient population were either CKD stage 3 or 4 and were not on renin-angiotensin-aldosterone system blockers and highly motivated. This avoided the development of hyperkalemia.

Replicating this study in the general population would be very difficult as all these patients were very motivated and were followed by a renal dietitian. Nonetheless, this is still an option for a select group of highly motivated patients.

Pharmaceutical Management

Sodium bicarbonate tablets usually come in aliquots of 300–650 mg per tablet. With their use, one is able to administer at least 3.7–8 mEq of sodium bicarbonate per tablet. These tablets are generally inexpensive and easy to administer. Excessive belching is an unwanted side effect of the administration of these medications. Bicarbonate reacts with hydrochloric acid in the stomach to produce carbon dioxide that gives a feeling of satiety as well as fullness.

Enteric-coated version of these tablets have fewer GI side effects. There are also enteric-coated as well as soft coated capsules containing 500 mg and 1000 mg sodium bicarbonate. The enteric-coated capsules allow for a larger content of sodium bicarbonate getting beyond the stomach for absorption.

Shohl's solution and Bicitra are solutions that provide 1 mEq of bicarbonate for every mL of solution ingested. Both the solutions are citrate-based and metabolized in the liver to produce bicarbonate. As a side effect, they can increase the absorption of aluminum.

Phosphate binders such as calcium acetate, calcium citrate, and sevelamer carbonate as a secondary function can help improve acidemia as they have precursors of bicarbonate.

Sodium Disorder and Chronic Kidney Disease

Epidemiology

Approximately 4–8% of ambulatory and 20–35% of hospitalized patients suffer from hyponatremia defined as the serum sodium of less than 135 mEq per L [48–51]. An association exists between hyponatremia and increased morbidity and mortality [50, 52, 53]. Speculation pertaining to this association could be due to hyponatremia itself versus the severity of the diseases causing hyponatremia.

The prevalence of hypernatremia which is defined as sodium of greater than 145 mEq per L is only about 2% [54]. Poor prognosis is associated with admission to the medical intensive care units. There is extensive data pertaining to the prognosis of this patient population [49, 51, 55, 56].

The incidence, prevalence, and significance of both hyper- and hyponatremia have not been studied in the chronic kidney disease population from a population health study prespective. As chronic kidney disease progresses, the ability of the kidney to concentrate or dilute is progressively impaired. Hence, one can speculate that sodium disorders would have a higher prevalence in the chronic kidney disease population. Kovesdy et al. attempted to answer the question on incidence and prevalence of hyper- and hyponatremia in the CKD population [57]. Over 650,000 US veterans who had CKD were studied with a median follow-up of 5.5 years. 13.5% had hyponatremia and 2% had hypernatremia at baseline. The incidence of hyponatremia was 26% and hypernatremia was 7% [58]. This study sheds some light of the incidence and prevalence of hypo- and hypernatremia in the population.

Similar to potassium, sodium has a U-shaped curve as it relates to all-cause mortality. Even after multivariable adjustment, comorbidities such as cancer, liver disease, or congestive heart failure did not alter these findings. This U-shaped associated with sodium disorders has been corroborated by studies performed in medical intensive care units. Even though the prevalence of hyponatremia is higher, hypernatremia has shown to have a strong association with mortality [49, 56].

Sodium disorders are common in end-stage renal disease patients with hyponatremia being more common than hypernatremia. In one study, the prevalence of hyponatremia in oliguric end-stage renal disease patients on hemodialysis was approximately 29% [59]. In comparison, peritoneal dialysis patients only had an incident of 14.5% [60]. The difference is likely because most PD patients have residual renal function. In hemodialysis patients, the presumption is increased intradialytic water intake. Most hemodialysis patients have no residual renal function. Hence, they exclusively rely on the dialysis treatments for sodium and water homeostasis. Patients with hyponatremia on hemodialysis are also found to have high intradialytic weight gains. There is a strong association of hyponatremia and mortality in end-stage renal disease patients [59, 61, 62]. Studies that have been conducted have adjusted for heart failure, volume overload, the volume of ultra-filtration, and modality of renal replacement therapy, and still this association exists. In peritoneal dialysis, hyponatremia is associated with low residual renal function. Unlike hemodialysis, these patients were found to have a reduction in their total body weight, which is inferring that they have a poor nutritional status [60].

Pathophysiology of Concentrating and Diluting Defects in Chronic Kidney Disease

The Counter-Current Mechanism in Chronic Kidney Disease

To adapt to a terrestrial environment, the kidneys can conserve water under arid conditions by concentrating the urine. Healthy individuals can concentrate urine to approximately 1200 milliosmoles per kg of water to allow for a urine volume of only 500 mL given an osmolar intake of at least 600 milliosmoles per day.

As one progresses through the stages of chronic kidney disease, the ability of the kidney to concentrate is diminished. As CKD advances, the number of function nephrons diminishes. For constant solute intake, the number of osmoles handled per nephron increases. This objects each nephron to undergo significant osmotic diuresis. The ability of the kidney to concentrate is dependent on the generation of a hypertonic interstitium [63]. The thick ascending loop of Henle normal function maintains a corticomedullary osmotic gradient. This allows sodium chloride and urea to concentrate in the medulla, thereby allowing water to be reabsorbed.

The papilla in the inner medulla is the main location where urinary concentration occurs. The health of the inner medulla is crucial in the kidneys' ability to reabsorb water. CKD animal experimental models with equal inulin clearance were studied. One group had their papillae removed, and the other group had intact papilla. Animals with papillectomization were unable to concentrate their urine [64].

Patients who suffer from sickle cell disease [65], medullary cystic disease, autosomal dominant polycystic kidney disease, and papillary necrosis secondary to nonsteroidal anti-inflammatory use also have difficulty in concentrating the urine [66–68]. The above studied animal model can be applied to patients with damaged papilla. Most patients who have papillary damage have concentrating defects that are out of proportion to their glomerular filtration rate.

Vasopressin levels are elevated in chronic kidney disease [68]. Due to the inability of the collecting duct to respond to vasopressin, the urine cannot concentrate. Administration of vasopressin does not restore the ability to concentrate further implying resistance at the receptor level.

Uremic milieu also blunts intracellular response to vasopressin by a reduction in cyclic AMP. This is, in part, secondary to a reduction in receptors for vasopressin [69]. The final result in reduced expression of water channels [70]. These channels are called aquaporins. There are three aquaporin channels in the kidney. Aquaporin 1 is located in the descending loop of Henle. Aquaporins 2 and 3 are located at the luminal and basolateral membranes in the collecting tubule, respectively [71]. Aquaporin 2 can be endocytosed and exocytosed as well as be synthesized by the cells in the collecting tubule to allow for less or more water reabsorption, respectively. It is this aquaporin 2 responsible blunting that finds the results in an inability to reabsorb water.

Chronic kidney disease patients also have difficulty in maximally diluting the urine. This is primarily the result of a dysfunctional ascending loop of Henle which is unable to remove solute from the urine. This relative inability to concentrate or dilute urine to either reabsorb or excrete extra water can lead to hyper- or hyponatremia, respectively.

Clinical Implications

Normal kidneys can dilute urine to 50 mL osmoles per kg water and concentrate it to almost 1200 milliosmoles per kg water. As an example, we will be considering an individual with an intake of 600 milliosmoles per day and hence would need to remove 600 milliosmoles from his circulation on a daily basis via his urinary output. Under extreme conditions, this individual can remove all osmoles in as little as 500 mL of urine (600 milliosmoles per day divided by 1200 milliosmoles per kg water) when challenged with a scarcity of water. This will maintain the individuals' serum sodium within a normal range. The same individual can remove at least 12 L of water in the event of excessive consumption (600 milliosmoles per day divided by 50 milliosmoles per kg water = 12 l). This wide range of flexibility allows for maintaining a normal serum sodium regardless of water intake.

In chronic kidney disease, the diluting or concentrating ability of the kidney is hampered. As stated previously, a patient's osmolar load is usually around 600 milliosmoles per day. In the setting of CKD, the concentrating ability can be limited (reduced to 300 milliosmoles from 1200 milliosmoles per kg water). This particular individual is now mandated to make 2 liters of urine to get rid of the 600 milliosmoles (600/300) that he has consumed in 24 hours. If this particular individual consumes less than 2 L of water a day, they will lose more water than they have consumed and will turn hypernatremic. At the other end, due to chronic kidney disease, the diluting ability is reduced from 50 milliosmoles per kg water to 200 milliosmoles per kg water. Hence, the patient can make approximately 3 L of urine (600/200). If this particular individual drinks more than 3 L of water, they will develop hyponatremia.

Treatment

Chronic kidney disease can cause hyponatremia in itself. However, its treatment is no different than that of patients with normal kidney function [72]. Clinical assessment of the patient for volume status, removal of offending agents, and treating the underlying endocrine or hormonal issues are the cornerstone of any hyponatremia treatment. Certain treatment limitations are outlined below.

Hypovolemic Hyponatremia Secondary to Volume Deficits

Patients with chronic kidney disease are prone to develop hypovolemia. At baseline, they have a higher fractional excretion of sodium, plus due to hypertension are usually on concomitant diuretics [73, 74]. If such a patient developed hyponatremia, these diuretics (loop diuretics) should be discontinued, and administration of normal saline is usually the fluid of choice. Close monitoring is required as these patients can conversely hold on to sodium and can very easily tip into hypervolemia.

Euvolemic/Hypervolemic Hyponatremia

ADH Inhibitors

For patients with chronic kidney disease who developed euvolemic hyponatremia, the removal of offending agents is paramount. Antidepressants, anticonvulsants, and anti-psychotics are the most common class of drugs responsible for SIADH. ADH inhibitors can help with free water removal by antagonizing the effect of vasopressin [75]. Demeclocycline is a synthetic tetracycline with a secondary function of ADH inhibition. It has a nephrotoxic profile in the setting of hepatic insufficiency and can hence further worsen chronic kidney disease. V2 receptors have been studied extensively in the treatment of euvolemic hyponatremia but excluded patients with moderate to severe chronic kidney disease [75, 76]. Shoaf et al. studied pharmacodynamics and pharmacokinetics in chronic kidney disease patients showing that vaptans (V2 blockers) are less successful in patients with a creatinine clearance of less than 15 mL/minute [77]. Patients with advanced kidney disease but a creatinine clearance of greater than 15 mL/minute were able to clear free water under the effect of vaptans but had a delayed response.

Water Restriction

Water restriction has limited efficacy in both patients with normal renal function and chronic kidney disease as it is difficult to implement.

Use of Loop Diuretics

Loops are effective in free water clearance in chronic kidney disease populations either alone or in combination with water restriction. Limitations may be due to the resistance of advanced chronic kidney disease patients to diuretics. Those who are responsive should be monitored closely for their volume status and electrolytes.

Hypernatremia and Chronic Kidney Disease

Hypernatremia can develop in chronic kidney disease in the setting of a lack of free water ingestion and the kidneys' inability to concentrate urine. Treatment includes enteral or parenteral free fluid repletion.

Hyponatremia and End-Stage Renal Disease

Hyponatremia in end-stage renal disease patients without residual renal function is due to excessive intake of water. Two modalities have to be employed in the correction of hyponatremia in end-stage renal disease patients. They are the use of appropriate hemodialysis prescription and restriction of free fluid intake. There is no one size fits all for the correction of hyponatremia in end-stage renal disease patients. There are no prospective randomized controlled trials conducted to study the safety and efficacy of correcting hyponatremia and end-stage renal disease patients. Anecdotally large cohort analysis has shown that using a higher dialysate sodium bath to correct hyponatremia in dialysis patients reduced mortality and hospitalization despite high intradialytic weight gain [61, 62]. Central pontine myelinolysis is a complication of rapid sodium correction. The average time for a hemodialysis prescription is 4 hours. If an appropriate sodium concentration is not prescribed in the dialysate, it can lead to rapid sodium correction during the dialysis session. There is very scarce information on hemodialysis-related osmotic demyelination [78]. One speculative rationale could be that three times a week hemodialysis session does not allow for adaptive mechanisms to develop. Another speculation is that high urea levels help protect the brain from the rapid correction of sodium in dialysis patients.

Patients in need of renal replacement therapy for acute kidney injury, patients who are initiating hemodialysis, or established hemodialysis patients who have not been dialyzed for a considerable period of time are most likely to have issues with rapid correction of hyponatremia.

Patients with severe hyponatremia (<120 mEq per L) are at high risk for rapid correction with conventional renal replacement therapy as dialysis machines have a lower limit of 130 mEq per L of sodium in the dialysate bath. In most practices, these patients either are dialyzed via continuous renal replacement therapy or are administered a hypotonic solution infusion concomitant to hemodialysis.

For peritoneal dialysis patients, using hypertonic rapid exchanges can correct hyponatremia. The hypertonic dextrose solution causes total body water removal without concomitant solute removal and hence results in the correction of hyponatremia. Given the nature of peritoneal dialysis, special focus needs to be placed on potassium [79].

Potassium and Chronic Kidney Disease

Epidemiology

Ninety-eight percent of potassium is present intracellularly. Its main function is to adjust the acid-base balance, to augment cellular metabolism, and finally to create a trans-membrane potential for neuromuscular conduction and function [80]. Serum potassium levels are maintained by excretion of approximately 100 mEq of potassium per day, 95% of which is through the kidney with approximately 5–10 mEq via the gastrointestinal tract around 5 mEq per day via sweat through the skin [80, 81].

The proximal and distal convoluted tubules are two major points of renal potassium control with the latter requiring sodium delivery and the presence of aldosterone.

Hyperkalemia and hypokalemia can contribute to the worsening of kidney disease either directly or indirectly. In the case of hyperkalemia, discontinuation of medications (namely, renin-angiotensin-aldosterone system (RAAS) blockers) that are proven to be renal protective results in the progression of chronic kidney disease [82]. In the case of hypokalemia, due to increased renal ammoniagenesis, there is subsequent activation of the complement system and increased fibrosis [12].

Multiple interventions exist to curb hyperkalemia; however, very little data exists to predict which CKD patient will develop it. Hypokalemia in CKD patients could arise as a result of either diuretic use or poor oral intake or both.

Hyperkalemia in Chronic Kidney Disease

Hyperkalemia is a serum potassium value of greater than 5 mEq/L or mmol/L.

Hyperkalemia can result in severe clinical repercussions, namely, cardiac arrhythmias, that can be fatal [83, 84]. A number of factors play a role in the development of hyperkalemia in the setting of CKD, namely, ingestion of high-potassium foods, dysregulated distribution of potassium between extracellular fluid and intracellular compartment, and the inability to excrete potassium from the body.

The most notable predisposing factor for high serum potassium is chronic kidney disease [84, 85]. The incidence of hyperkalemia in the chronic kidney disease population is approximately 2–35%. In the setting of CKD, certain diseases have a higher association with hyperkalemia, namely, diabetes mellitus and heart failure [86]. Predisposition to hyperkalemia could be due to the use of potassium-sparing medications, insulin deficiency, hyperglycemia, and hyporeninemic hypoaldosteronism [87, 88]. With hyperkalemia, increased mortality is noted in both the general population and chronic kidney disease patients highlighting the importance to maintain levels within a normal range.

Mechanism of Hyperkalemia and Chronic Kidney Disease

As renal function worsens, renal clearance of potassium is diminished. This with the concomitant intake of high-potassium foods results in difficulty maintaining a normal serum potassium value. Chronic kidney disease populations suffer from acidemia. In order to curb hydrogen, it is moved intracellularly to be buffered requiring the extrusion of an intracellularly positive ion, namely, potassium.

Chronic kidney disease patients are plagued with multiple comorbidities. They are at the highest risk for acute kidney injuries which can result in an inability to handle a potassium load. Diabetes mellitus causes hypertonicity due to hyperglycemia in the absence of insulin resulting in increasing extracellular potassium values [89]. This phenomenon is called osmotic drag where glucose being a tonically active agent draws intracellular fluid into the extracellular compartment. This intracellular fluid is rich in potassium, hence leading to hyperkalemia. Diabetic patients can also be suffering from hyporeninemic hypoaldosteronism impairing the kidney's ability to excrete potassium. Concomitantly due to proteinuria, these patients are commonly on renin-angiotensin-aldosterone system blockers that can further impair the kidney's ability to remove the potassium from the circulation [84, 89].

Cardiovascular disease which includes hypertension, coronary artery disease, and congestive heart failure requires medications to prevent fibrotic remodeling. Use of renin-angiotensin-aldosterone system blockers including aldosterone blockers can limit the ability of the kidneys to excrete potassium. Other pharmacological interventions employed in the care of these patients can also interfere with potassium values. Heparin acts as an aldosterone synthase inhibitor, hence reducing aldosterone levels and results in hyperkalemia. Beta-blockers compete with catecholamine and hence prevent intracellular movement of potassium. This is usually seen with nonselective beta-blockers. In the case of cardioselective beta-blockers (B1-selective), the beta 2 receptor is still available for activation.

Hyperkalemia in such a population can result in severe consequences including arrhythmias that can lead to death [90–92]. Discontinuation of these medications can curb hyperkalemia but, in the long run, leads to worsening cardiac and renal fibrosis. Horne et al. showed that patients with potassium of greater than 6 meq/L versus those with less than 5 meq/l had a higher rate of hospitalization and death [91].

The RENAAL study showed a higher incidence of hyperkalemia in the losartan-treated group versus placebo. Lewis et al. showed that RAAS inhibitors are renal protective for CKD patients [82]. Patients were on either irbesartan or placebo. The incidence of hyperkalemia in the irbesartan group was approximately 18% versus 6% in the placebo group [93]. The ONTARGET trial used dual RAAS blockers in proteinuric and chronic kidney disease patients [94]. The study showed a higher percentage of hyperkalemia and acute kidney injury in the dual RAAS-treated group.

When chronic kidney disease patients develop hyperkalemia, either RAAS blockers are discontinued, or their doses are reduced. However, this can lead to an accelerated worsening of chronic kidney disease, earlier initiation of hemodialysis, and increased morbidity and mortality [82]. In contrast, CKD patients who were continued on their RAAS inhibitors at maximally tolerated doses had renal preservation, delayed onset on dialysis, and reduced morbidity and mortality [95].

This then begs the question of therapeutics available for the treatment of hyperkalemia while maintaining the use of RAAS blockers.

Clinical Sequel

Hyperkalemia is graded in severity based on the potassium value with mild hyperkalemia (5.5–6.0), moderate hyperkalemia (6.0–6.5), and severe hyperkalemia (>6.5). This is not the sole criterion as the clinical picture of the patient and electrocardiogram findings also factored into the severity. Patients can exhibit symptoms such as nausea, muscular weakness, paresthesia, cardiac arrhythmias, or cardiac arrests. From an electrocardiographic standpoint, we can see peaked T-waves early on with prolonged PR interval, narrow complex QT interval, and QRS widening indicating evolution into a more severe clinical outcome [96]. These EKG findings have seen approximately 50% of patients suffering from hyperkalemia.

Treatment

Management of hyperkalemia requires a twofold intervention. The initial intervention requires temporization and the acute removal of potassium from the patient's body. Temporizing techniques include intracellular shifting of potassium by the use of insulin and/or beta-agonist [96]. Cardiac membrane action potential stabilizers such as calcium gluconate and calcium chloride are utilized when the QTC prolongation is noted on the EKG. Acute removal of potassium from the body requires the use of diuretics, the use of sodium bicarbonate, and/or renal replacement therapy. Diuretics increase urinary potassium losses. Sodium bicarbonate can be used in hyperkalemia to facilitate the movement of potassium from the extravascular space intracellularly by alkalinizing the pH of blood. It also causes kaliuresis since bicarbonate couples with potassium during the process of excretion.

Mild hyperkalemia can be conservatively managed by dietary modifications. Identification and restriction of potassium-rich foods can help in the reduction of serum potassium in chronic kidney disease patients. However, due to dietary limitations of fruits, vegetables and fiber either can lead to worsening or can cause constipation. Constipation can lead to increased potassium absorption due to a delay in colonic transit time [86, 97].

Hyperkalemia is associated with the use of multiple medications. Heparin and low-molecular-weight heparin, calcineurin inhibitors, nonsteroidal anti-inflammatory drugs, trimethoprim, and beta-blockers are just to name a few [89]. These medications should be adjusted in the setting of chronic kidney disease and hyperkalemia. RAAS inhibitors have already been discussed. The pros of continuation of RAAS blockers are cardiac and renal protection, whereas the cons can lead to acute kidney injury and hyperkalemia.

Hyperkalemia can persist after conservative management. Escalation of already prescribed medications for volume management (diuretics) and chronic kidney disease acidemia (bicarbonate) can help reduce serum potassium values. The use of diuretics is reserved for patients who require volume management as well as blood pressure control. Hypovolemia can occur with the use of diuretics that reduces GFR and can exacerbate hyperkalemia [98].

Multiple pharmaceutical treatments have made their way onto the market for the treatment of hyperkalemia. Exchange resins such as sodium polystyrene sulfonate, calcium polystyrene sulfonate, patiromer, and sodium zirconium cyclosilicate are available for the treatment of chronic hyperkalemia.

Sodium Polystyrene Sulfonate

This medication was approved in 1958, 4 years prior to the FDA requiring safety studies. This is a sodium-based exchange resin. It exchanges sodium for potassium, calcium, and ammonia. It is effective in the distal colon. This medication is administered either orally or rectally. The effectiveness of the oral route has a lag of at least 6–8 hours due to its transit to the distal colon.

Doses between 60 and 80 g can reduce potassium levels by 0.9–1.7 millimoles per L. As per the FDA, the administration should be limited to 3 hours before and after oral medications. Studies have shown that certain medications such as amlodipine, metoprolol, amoxicillin, Lasix, phenytoin, and warfarin are more likely to bind. Patients with chronic kidney disease are at a high risk of gastrointestinal bleed secondary to necrosis. Studies to assess efficacy have not been conducted in chronic kidney disease patients [99].

Calcium Polystyrene Sulfonate

As the name suggests, it is a calcium-based exchange resin which can be administered both orally and in certain cases rectally once diluted with sorbitol. Side effects include constipation, hypercalcemia, and hypercalciuria [99].

Dose between 2.5 and 15 g per day was found to decrease potassium values in 70% of patients by 0.3 mmol/L [100].

Patiromer

Patiromer was approved for the treatment of chronic hyperkalemia in October of 2015. It is a calcium-based resin that exchanges divalent ion for potassium. The product is reconstituted in water and administered orally. The site of action is the large bowel. Constipation, hypomagnesemia, and diarrhea are the top three side effects. Severe hypokalemia (<3.5 meq/l) was seen in 4.7% of the patients studied, and severe hypomagnesemia (<1.7 meq/l) was seen at 9%. Starting dose is 4.2 g twice a day with escalation to a maximum of 16.8 g twice a day. Patients in these studies were able to continue on their RAAS blockers. Reduction in potassium was dose-related [101]. This is not an "as-needed" medication. Over-the-counter medication doses should be limited to 3 hours before and 3 hours after the administration. Medications to be taken into consideration include ciprofloxacin, levothyroxine, and metformin.

Dialysis patients prescribed patiromer showed a reduced serum potassium level without any observed side effects [102].

Sodium Zirconium Cyclosilicate

This is a zirconium-based exchange resin which was approved by the FDA in May 2018. The selective exchange is between potassium and sodium for ammonium and hydrogen in the gastrointestinal tract. It helps with potassium removal via the GI tract. Hence, the most common side effect is diarrhea [103]. The recommended dose is 10 g three times a day. Once normal serum potassium levels are achieved, dose reduction is required to once a day (5–15 g). The preparation has 400 mg of sodium for every 5 g dose. Hence, patients should be monitored for volume overload. Over-the-counter medication dosing should be limited to 2 hours before and 2 hours after.

Renal Replacement Therapy

For advanced CKD patients, persistent hyperkalemia, and resistance to pharmacological therapy, initiation of renal replacement therapy is prudent [86, 96]. The use of a dialysate bath of 2 mEq to 3 mEq is the usual standard. The use of very-low-potassium baths (0–1 meq of K) is usually not recommended as it can cause a sudden shift in potassium leading to arrhythmias and sudden death [96, 104]. There are no formal trials, but observation data exists to suggest this correlation. Modification of the dialysis prescription, frequency, or using new dialysis modalities can be utilized for patients who are persistently hyperkalemic. Patients who suffer from end-stage renal disease are on low-potassium dialysate baths which are adjusted based on their monthly blood works. Hence, a potential for prescribing the incorrect potassium bath exists since these values are not being checked on a daily basis [104].

Hypokalemia in Chronic Kidney Disease

Hypokalemia is defined as the potassium value of less than 3.5 millimoles per L in the serum. In the CKD population, the prevalence is about 1–3%. Prevalence is 1–2% in the hemodialysis population with 5–22% in the peritoneal dialysis population [105–108]. These rates may vary from country to country. Diuretic use results in renal potassium losses [109] with thiazides increasing the risk by five-fold.

Clinical Sequel

Symptomatology is similar to that of hyperkalemia but also includes muscular weakness, paralysis, and respiratory failure in very severe cases. Arrhythmias are also very common in patients with severe hypokalemia. Muscular weakness occurs due to delayed conduction. Electrocardiographic findings of mild hypokalemia are inverted T-waves with severe hypokalemia leading to visible U-waves, QT prolongation, and mild ST depression.

Most studies show that the risk of ventricular tachycardia increases with a potassium value of less than 3.5 mEq per L as published by Coca et al. in the *American Journal of Kidney Diseases* 2005.

Goals of Treatment

Identification of the cause is paramount in helping treat hypokalemia in chronic kidney disease. Diuretic use, poor oral intake, diarrhea, vomiting, and certain high aldosterone states can lead to chronic hypokalemia.

Potassium Preparation

These exist in the form of liquid, tablets, and extended-release tablets. They are known for their large size and unpleasant taste.

An oral potassium phosphate is an option in patients with concomitant low phosphorus. Two different strengths exist. The original provides 3.7 mEq of potassium per tablet with the potassium phosphate neutral prep providing 1.1 mEq of potassium per tablet.

Oral potassium bicarbonate and citrate preparations also exist. They can be used in patients with chronic kidney disease who are prone to develop renal stones and have concomitant acidemia.

Intravenous preparations can be utilized when oral access is not possible. Rapid correction with IV potassium is not advisable as it can lead to life-threatening arrhythmias. On average, every 20 mEq of potassium chloride can result in 0.25–0.5 mEq per L of correction of serum potassium.

Kovesdy et al. in 2018 showed a U-shaped mortality curve for potassium in chronic kidney disease patients by conducting a meta-analysis of 27 international cohorts [110]. Data was analyzed for over 1.2 million patients over a 7-year period. Hypokalemia is a risk for mortality in both hemodialysis and peritoneal dialysis patients. Torlen et al. studied 10,000 peritoneal dialysis patients and 111,000 hemodialysis patients via the DaVita cohort [106]. A U-shaped Kaplan-Meier mortality curve is seen in these patients.

Oral potassium supplementation in peritoneal dialysis patients reduces mortality [111]. The use of RAAS blockade along with aldactone has proven to be beneficial in peritoneal dialysis patients likely due to its action on GI receptors as well as the patient's residual renal function [112]. The Dialysis Outcomes and Practice Patterns Study (DOPPS) showed relatively low potassium (<4.0 meq/l) was not related to all-cause mortality [113].

References

1. Moranne O, Froissart M, Rossert J, Gauci C, Boffa JJ, Haymann JP, M'rad MB, Jacquot C, Houillier P, Stengel B, Fouqueray B, NephroTest Study Group. Timing of onset of CKD-related metabolic complications. J Am Soc Nephrol. 2009;20:164–71.
2. Raphael KL, Zhang Y, Ying J, Greene T. Prevalence of and risk factors for reduced serum bicarbonate in chronic kidney disease. Nephrology (Carlton). 2014;19:648–54.
3. Scialla JJ, Anderson CA. Dietary acid load: a novel nutritional target in chronic kidney disease? Adv Chronic Kidney Dis. 2013;20(2):141–9.
4. Gennari FJ, Hood VL, Greene T, Wang X, Levey AS. Effect of dietary protein intake on serum total CO2 concentration in chronic kidney disease: modification of diet in renal disease study findings. Clin J Am Soc Nephrol. 2006;1(1):52–7.
5. Goraya N, Simoni J, Jo C, Wesson DE. A comparison of treating metabolic acidosis in CKD stage 4 hypertensive kidney disease with fruits and vegetables or sodium bicarbonate. Clin J Am Soc Nephrol. 2013;8(3):371–81.
6. Kanda E, Ai M, Kuriyama R, Yoshida M, Shiigai T. Dietary acid intake and kidney disease progression in the elderly. Am J Nephrol. 2014;39(2):145–52.
7. Kraut JA, Madias NE. Metabolic acidosis: pathophysiology, diagnosis and management. Nat Rev Nephrol. 2010;6(5):274–85.
8. Eustace JA, Astor B, Muntner PM, Ikizler TA, Coresh J. Prevalence of acidosis and inflammation and their association with low serum albumin in chronic kidney disease. Kidney Int. 2004;65(3):1031–40.

9. Madias NE, Kraut JA. Uremic acidosis. In: Seldin DW, Giebisch G, editors. The regulation of acid-base balance. New York: Raven Press; 1989. p. 285–317.
10. Karim Z, Attmane-Elakeb A, Bichara M. Renal handling of NH41 in relation to the control of acid-base balance by the kidney. J Nephrol. 2002;15(suppl 5):S128–34.
11. Simpson DP. Control of hydrogen ion homeostasis and renal acidosis. Medicine. 1971;50(6):503–41.
12. Nath KA, Hostetter MK, Hostetter TH. Increased ammoniagenesis as a determinant of progressive renal injury. Am J Kidney Dis. 1991;17(6):654–7.
13. Vallet M, Metzger M, Haymann JP, et al. Urinary ammonia and long-term outcomes in chronic kidney disease. Kidney Int. 2015;88(1):137–45.
14. Wesson DE, Simoni J. Acid retention during kidney failure induces endothelin and aldosterone production which lead to progressive GFR decline, a situation ameliorated by alkali diet. Kidney Int. 2010;78(11):1128–35.
15. Goraya N, Wesson DE. Does correction of metabolic acidosis slow chronic kidney disease progression? Curr Opin Nephrol Hypertens. 2013;22(2):193–7.
16. Kraut JA. Effect of metabolic acidosis on progression of chronic kidney disease. Am J Physiol Renal Physiol. 2011;300(4):F828–9.
17. Schwartz WB, Hall PW, Hays RM, Relman AS. On the mechanism of acidosis in chronic renal disease. J Clin Invest. 1959;38(1):39–52.
18. Raphael KL, Zhang Y, Ying J, Greene T. Prevalence of and risk factors for reduced serum bicarbonate in chronic kidney disease. Nephrology. 2014;19(10):648–54.
19. Scialla JJ, Appel LJ, Astor BC, et al. Net endogenous acid production is associated with a faster decline in GFR in African Americans. Kidney Int. 2012;82(1):106–12.
20. Kovesdy CP. Metabolic acidosis and kidney disease: does bicarbonate therapy slow the progression of CKD? Nephrol Dial Transplant. 2012;27(8):3056–62.
21. Widmer B, Gerhardt RE, Harrington JT, Cohen JJ. Serum electrolytes and acid base composition: the influence of graded degrees of chronic renal failure. Arch Intern Med. 1979;139(10):1099–102.
22. Kraut JA, Madias NE. Differential diagnosis of nongap metabolic acidosis: value of a systematic approach. Clin J Am Soc Nephrol. 2012;7(4):671–9.
23. Szylman P, Better OS, Chaimowitz C, Rosler A. Role of hyperkalemia in the metabolic acidosis of isolated hypoaldosteronism. N Engl J Med. 1976;294(7):361–5.
24. Kraut JA, Madias NE. Consequences and therapy of the metabolic acidosis of chronic kidney disease. Pediatr Nephrol. 2011;26(1):19–28.
25. May RC, Kelly RA, Mitch WE. Mechanisms for defects in muscle protein metabolism in rats with chronic uremia: the influence of metabolic acidosis. J Clin Invest. 1987;79(4):1099–2003.
26. Graham KA, Reaich D, Channon SM, Downie S, Goodship TH. Correction of acidosis in hemodialysis decreases whole body protein degradation. J Am Soc Nephrol. 1997;8(4):632–7.
27. Mak RH, Cheung W. Energy homeostasis and cachexia in chronic kidney disease. Pediatr Nephrol. 2006;21(12):1807–14.
28. Ballmer PE, McNurlan MA, Hulter HN, Anderson SE, Garlick PJ, Krapf R. Chronic metabolic acidosis decreases albumin synthesis and induces negative nitrogen balance in humans. J Clin Invest. 1995;95(1):39–45.
29. Kleger GR, Turgay M, Imoberdorf R, McNurlan MA, Garlick PJ, Ballmer PE. Acute metabolic acidosis decreases muscle protein synthesis but not albumin synthesis in humans. Am J Kidney Dis. 2001;38(6):1199–207.
30. Raphael KL, Zhang Y, Wei G, Greene T, Cheung AK, Beddhu S. Serum bicarbonate and mortality in adults in NHANES III. Nephrol Dial Transplant. 2013;28(5):1207–13.
31. de Brito-Ashurst I, Varagunam M, Raftery MJ, Yaqoob MM. Bicarbonate supplementation slows progression of CKD and improves nutritional status. J Am Soc Nephrol. 2009;20(9):2075–84.
32. Shah SN, Abramowitz M, Hostetter TH, Melamed ML. Serum bicarbonate levels and the progression of kidney disease: a cohort study. Am J Kidney Dis. 2009;54(2):270–7.

33. Dobre M, Yang W, Pan Q, et al. Persistent high serum bicarbonate and the risk of heart failure in patients with chronic kidney disease (CKD): a report from the Chronic Renal Insufficiency Cohort (CRIC) Study. J Am Heart Assoc. 2015;4(4):1–10.

34. Driver TH, Shlipak MG, Katz R, et al. Low serum bicarbonate and kidney function decline: the Multi-Ethnic Study of Atherosclerosis (MESA). Am J Kidney Dis. 2014;64(4):534–41.

35. Wesson DE, Simoni J, Broglio K, Sheather SJ. Acid retention accompanies reduced GFR in humans and increases plasma levels of aldosterone and endothelin. Am J Physiol Renal Physiol. 2011;300(4):F830–7.

36. Wesson DE, Nathan T, Rose T, Simoni J, Tran RM. Dietary protein induces endothelin-mediated kidney injury through enhanced intrinsic acid production. Kidney Int. 2007;71(3):210–7.

37. Goraya N, Simoni J, Jo CH, Wesson DE. Treatment of metabolic acidosis in patients with stage 3 chronic kidney disease with fruits and vegetables or oral bicarbonate reduces urine angiotensinogen and preserves glomerular filtration rate. Kidney Int. 2014;86(5):1031–8.

38. Raj S, Scott DR, Nguyen T, Sachs G, Kraut JA. Acid stress increases gene expression of proinflammatory cytokines in MadinDarby canine kidney cells. Am J Physiol Renal Physiol. 2013;304(1):F41–8.

39. Menon V, Tighiouart H, Vaughn NS, et al. Serum bicarbonate and long-term outcomes in CKD. Am J Kidney Dis. 2010;56(5):907–14.

40. Navaneethan SD, Schold JD, Arrigain S, et al. Serum bicarbonate and mortality in stage 3 and stage 4 chronic kidney disease. Clin J Am Soc Nephrol. 2011;6(10):2395–402.

41. National Kidney Foundation. KDOQI clinical practice guidelines for bone metabolism and disease in chronic kidney disease 2003. Am J Kidney Dis. 2003;42 (4)(suppl 2):S3–S201.

42. Kidney Disease: Improving Global Outcomes (KDIGO) CKD Work Group. KDIGO 2012 clinical practice guideline for the evaluation and management of chronic kidney disease. Kidney Int. 2013;3(suppl 1):1–150.

43. Chan M, Johnson D. Modification of lifestyle and nutrition intervention for management of early chronic kidney disease. 2015. http://www.cari.org.au/CKD/CKD%20early/Modification_of_Llifestyle_Nutrition_ECKD.pdf. Accessed 1 Feb 2015.

44. Wright M, Jones C. Correction of metabolic acidosis and nutrition in CKD. 2015. www.renal.org/guidelines/modules/nutrition-in-ckd. Accessed 1 Feb 2015.

45. Dobre M, Yang W, Chen J, et al. Association of serum bicarbonate with risk of renal and cardiovascular outcomes in CKD: a report from the Chronic Renal Insufficiency Cohort (CRIC) Study. Am J Kidney Dis. 2013;62(4):670–8.

46. de Solis AJ, Gonzalez-Pacheco FR, Deudero JJ, et al. Alkalinization potentiates vascular calcium deposition in an uremic milieu. J Nephrol. 2009;22(5):647–53.

47. Jun M, Jardine MJ, Perkovic V, Pilard Q, Billot L, Rodgers A, et al. Hyperkalemia and renin-angiotensin aldosterone system inhibitor therapy in chronic kidney disease: a general practice-based, observational study. PLoS One. 2019;14(3):e02131192.

48. Schrier RW, Sharma S, Shchekochikhin D. Hyponatraemia: more than just a marker of disease severity? Nat Rev Nephrol. 2013;9(3):124.

49. Funk GC, Lindner G, Druml W, et al. Incidence and prognosis of dysnatremias present on ICU admission. Intensive Care Med. 2010;36(2):304–11. [PubMed: 19847398].

50. Liamis G, Rodenburg EM, Hofman A, Zietse R, Stricker BH, Hoorn EJ. Electrolyte disorders in community subjects: prevalence and risk factors. Am J Med. 2013;126(3):256–63. [PubMed: 23332973].

51. Stelfox HT, Ahmed SB, Khandwala F, Zygun D, Shahpori R, Laupland K. The epidemiology of intensive care unit-acquired hyponatraemia and hypernatraemia in medical-surgical intensive care units. Crit Care. 2008;12(6):R162. [PubMed: 19094227].

52. Gankam-Kengne F, Ayers C, Khera A, de Lemos J, Maalouf NM. Mild hyponatremia is associated with an increased risk of death in an ambulatory setting. Kidney Int. 2013;83(4):700–6. [PubMed: 23325088].

53. Wald R, Jaber BL, Price LL, Upadhyay A, Madias NE. Impact of hospital-associated hyponatremia on selected outcomes. Arch Intern Med. 2010;170(3):294–302. [PubMed: 20142578].

54. Arampatzis S, Frauchiger B, Fiedler GM, et al. Characteristics, symptoms, and outcome of severe dysnatremias present on hospital admission. Am J Med. 2012;125(11):1125 e1–7. [PubMed: 22939097].
55. Darmon M, Timsit JF, Francais A, et al. Association between hypernatraemia acquired in the ICU and mortality: a cohort study. Nephrol Dial Transplant. 2010;25(8):2510–5. [PubMed: 20167570].
56. Stelfox HT, Ahmed SB, Zygun D, Khandwala F, Laupland K. Characterization of intensive care unit acquired hyponatremia and hypernatremia following cardiac surgery. Can J Anaesth. 2010;57(7):650–8. [PubMed: 20405264].
57. Kovesdy CP, Lott EH, Lu JL, et al. Hyponatremia, hypernatremia, and mortality in patients with chronic kidney disease with and without congestive heart failure. Circulation. 2012;125(5):677–84. [PubMed: 22223429].
58. Argent NB, Burrell LM, Goodship TH, Wilkinson R, Baylis PH. Osmoregulation of thirst and vasopressin release in severe chronic renal failure. Kidney Int. 1991;39(2):295–300. [PubMed: 2002642].
59. Waikar SS, Curhan GC, Brunelli SM. Mortality associated with low serum sodium concentration in maintenance hemodialysis. Am J Med. 2011;124(1):77–84. [PubMed: 21187188].
60. Dimitriadis C, Sekercioglu N, Pipili C, Oreopoulos DG, Bargman JM. Hyponatremia in peritoneal dialysis: epidemiology in a single center and correlation with clinical and biochemical parameters. Perit Dial Int. [published online ahead of print 1 May 2013]. https://doi.org/10.3747/pdi.2012.00085.
61. Hecking M, Karaboyas A, Saran R, et al. Predialysis serum sodium level, dialysate sodium, and mortality in maintenance hemodialysis patients: the Dialysis Outcomes and Practice Patterns Study (DOPPS). Am J Kidney Dis. 2012;59(2):238–48. [PubMed: 21944663].
62. Hecking M, Karaboyas A, Saran R, et al. Dialysate sodium concentration and the association with interdialytic weight gain, hospitalization, and mortality. Clin J Am Soc Nephrol. 2012;7(1):92–100. [PubMed: 22052942].
63. Gilbert RM, Weber H, Turchin L, Fine LG, Bourgoignie JJ, Bricker NS. A study of the intrarenal recycling of urea in the rat with chronic experimental pyelonephritis. J Clin Invest. 1976;58(6):1348–57. [PubMed: 993348].
64. Finkelstein FO, Hayslett JP. Role of medullary structures in the functional adaptation of renal insufficiency. Kidney Int. 1974;6(6):419–25. [PubMed: 4280470].
65. Hatch FE, Culbertson JW, Diggs LW. Nature of the renal concentrating defect in sickle cell disease. J Clin Invest. 1967;46(3):336–45. [PubMed: 6023770].
66. Zittema D, Boertien WE, van Beek AP. Vasopressin, copeptin, and renal concentrating capacity in patients with autosomal dominant polycystic kidney disease without renal impairment. Clin J Am Soc Nephrol. 2012;7(6):906–13. [PubMed: 22516290].
67. Guay-Woodford L. Other cystic diseases. In: Floege J, Johnson R, Feehally J, editors. Comprehensive clinical nephrology, vol. 4. St Louis: Saunders/Elsevier; 2010. p. 543–59.
68. Jawadi MH, Ho LS, Dipette D, Ross DL. Regulation of plasma arginine vasopressin in patients with chronic renal failure maintained on hemodialysis. Am J Nephrol. 1986;6(3):175–81. [PubMed: 3740126].
69. Fine LG, Schlondorff D, Trizna W, Gilbert RM, Bricker N. Functional profile of the isolated uremic nephron. Impaired water permeability and adenylate cyclase responsiveness of the cortical collecting tubule to vasopressin. J Clin Invest. 1978;61(6):1519–27. [PubMed: 207738].
70. Teitelbaum I, McGuinness S. Vasopressin resistance in chronic renal failure. Evidence for the role of decreased V2 receptor mRNA. J Clin Invest. 1995;96(1):378–85. [PubMed: 7615808].
71. Nielsen S, Agre P. The aquaporin family of water channels in kidney. Kidney Int. 1995;48(4):1057–68. [PubMed: 8569067].
72. Thurman J, Berl T. Therapy of dysnatremic disorders. In: Wilcox C, editor. Therapy in nephrology and hypertension, vol. 3. Philadelphia: Elsevier; 2008. p. 337–52.
73. Coleman AJ, Arias M, Carter NW, Rector FC, Seldin DW. The mechanism of salt wastage in chronic renal disease. J Clin Invest. 1966;45(7):1116–25. https://doi.org/10.1172/JCI105418. PMID: 16695913; PMCID: PMC292784.

74. Danovitch GM, Bourgoignie J, Bricker NS. Reversibility of the "salt-losing" tendency of chronic renal failure. N Engl J Med. 1977;296(1):14–9. https://doi.org/10.1056/NEJM197701062960104. PMID: 618364.

75. Rozen-Zvi B, Yahav D, Gheorghiade M, Korzets A, Leibovici L, Gafter U. Vasopressin receptor antagonists for the treatment of hyponatremia: systematic review and meta-analysis. Am J Kidney Dis. 2010;56(2):325–37. [PubMed: 20538391].

76. Schrier RW, Gross P, Gheorghiade M, et al. Tolvaptan, a selective oral vasopressin V2-receptor antagonist, for hyponatremia. N Engl J Med. 2006;355(20):2099–112. [PubMed: 17105757].

77. Shoaf S, Bricmont P, Mallikaarjun S. Pharmacokinetics and pharmacodynamics of oral tolvaptan in subjects with varying degrees of renal function. Kidney Int. [published online ahead of print 18 Sept 2013]. https://doi.org/10.1038/ki203.350.

78. Soupart A, Penninckx R, Stenuit A, Decaux G. Azotemia (48 h) decreases the risk of brain damage in rats after correction of chronic hyponatremia. Brain Res. 2000;852(1):167–72. [PubMed: 10661508].

79. Nolph KD, Hano JE, Teschan PE. Peritoneal sodium transport during hypertonic peritoneal dialysis. Physiologic mechanisms and clinical implications. Ann Intern Med. 1969;70(5):931–41. [PubMed: 5783428].

80. Palmer BF, Clegg DJ. Physiology and pathophysiology of potassium homeostasis. Adv Physiol Educ. 2016;40(4):480–90.

81. Santos BF, Boim MA, Santos OF. Distúrbios do metabolismo do potássio. In: Ajzen H, Schor N, editors. Guia de nefrologia. 3ª ed. Barueri: Manole; 2011. p. 93–105.

82. Brenner BM, Cooper ME, de Zeeuw D, Keane WF, Mitch WE, Parving HH, et al., RENAAL Study Investigators. Effects of losartan on renal and cardiovascular outcomes in patients with type 2 diabetes and nephropathy. N Engl J Med 2001;345(12):861–869.

83. Hayes J, Kalantar-Zadeh K, Lu JL, Turban S, Anderson JE, Kovesdy CP. Association of hypo- and hyperkalemia with disease progression and mortality in males with chronic kidney disease: the role of race. Nephron Clin Pract. 2012;120(1):c8–16.

84. Belmar Vega L, Galabia ER, Bada da Silva J, Bentanachs González M, Fernández Fresnedo G, Piñera Haces C, et al. Epidemiology of hyperkalemia in chronic kidney disease. Nefrologia. 2019;39(3):227–86.

85. Cowan AC, Gharib EG, Weir MA. Advances in the management of hyperkalemia in chronic kidney disease. Curr Opin Nephrol Hypertens. 2017;26(3):235–9.

86. Bianchi S, Aucella F, De Nicola L, Genovesi S, Paoletti E, Regolisti G. Management of hyperkalemia in patients with kidney disease: a position paper endorsed by the Italian Society of Nephrology. J Nephrol. 2019;32(4):499–516.

87. Caravaca-Fontán F, Valladares J, Díaz-Campillejo R, Barroso S, Luna E, Caravaca F. Association of hyperkalemia with clinical outcomes in advanced chronic kidney disease. Nefrologia. 2019;39(5):513–22.

88. Thomsen RW, Nicolaisen SK, Hasvold P, Sanchez RG, Pedersen L, Adelborg K, et al. Elevated potassium levels in patients with chronic kidney disease: occurrence, risk factors and clinical outcomes: a Danish population-based cohort study. Nephrol Dial Transplant. 2018;33(9):1610–20.

89. Kovesdy CP. Management of hyperkalaemia in chronic kidney disease. Nat Rev Nephrol. 2014;10(11):653–62.

90. Tromp J, van der Meer P. Hyperkalaemia: aetiology, epidemiology, and clinical significance. Eur Heart J Suppl. 2019;21(Suppl A):A6–A11.

91. Horne L, Ashfaq A, MacLachlan S, Sinsakul M, Qin L, LoCasale R, et al. Epidemiology and health outcomes associated with hyperkalemia in a primary care setting in England. BMC Nephrol. 2019;20(1):85.

92. Mishima E, Haruna Y, Arima H. Renin-angiotensin system inhibitors in hypertensive adults with non-diabetic CKD with or without proteinuria: a systematic review and meta-analysis of randomized trials. Hypertens Res. 2019;42(4):469–82.

93. Lewis EJ, Hunsicker LG, Clarke WR, Berl T, Pohl MA, Lewis JB, et al. Renoprotective effect of the angiotensin-receptor antagonist irbesartan in patients with nephropathy due to type 2 diabetes. N Engl J Med. 2001;345(12):851–60.

94. Mann JF, Schmieder RE, McQueen M, Dyal L, Schumacher H, Pogue J, et al., ONTARGET Investigators. Renal outcomes with telmisartan, ramipril, or both, in people at high vascular risk (the ONTARGET study): a multicenter, randomized, double-blind, controlled trial. Lancet 2008;372(9638):547–553.

95. Epstein M. Hyperkalemia constitutes a constraint for implementing renin-angiotensin-aldosterone inhibition: the widening gap between mandated treatment guidelines and the real-world clinical arena. Kidney Int Suppl (2011). 2016;6(1):20–8.

96. Vijayakumar S, Butler J, Bakris GL. Barriers to guideline mandated renin-angiotensin inhibitor use: focus on hyperkalemia. Eur Heart J Suppl. 2019;21(Suppl A):A20–7.

97. Cupisti A, Brunori G, Di Iorio BR, D'Alessandro C, Pasticci F, Cosola C, et al. Nutritional treatment of advanced CKD: twenty consensus statements. J Nephrol. 2018;31(4):457–73.

98. Khan YH, Sarriff A, Adnan AS, Khan AH, Mallhi TH. Chronic kidney disease, fluid overload and diuretics: a complicated triangle. PLoS One. 2016;11(7):e0159335.

99. Kim GH. Pharmacologic treatment of chronic hyperkalemia in patients with chronic kidney disease. Electrolyte Blood Press. 2018;17(1):1–6.

100. Yu MY, Yeo JH, Park JS, Lee CH, Kim GH. Long-term efficacy of oral calcium polystyrene sulfonate for hyperkalemia in CKD patients. PLoS One. 2017;12(3):e0173542.

101. Weir MR, Bakris GL, Bushinsky DA, Mayo MR, Garza D, Stasiv Y, et al., OPAL-HK Investigators. Patiromer in patients with kidney disease and hyperkalemia receiving RAAS inhibitors. N Engl J Med 2015;372(3):211–221.

102. Bushinsky DA, Rossignol P, Spiegel DM, Benton WW, Yuan J, Block GA, et al. Patiromer decreases serum potassium and phosphate levels in patients on hemodialysis. Am J Nephrol. 2016;44(5):404–10.

103. Packham DK, Rasmussen HS, Lavin PT, El-Shahawy MA, Roger SD, Block G, et al. Sodium zirconium cyclosilicate in hyperkalemia. N Engl J Med. 2015;372(3):222–31.

104. Abuelo JG. Treatment of severe hyperkalemia: confronting 4 fallacies. Kidney Int Rep. 2017;3(1):47–55.

105. Lee S, Kang E, Yoo KD, et al. Lower serum potassium associated with increased mortality in dialysis patients: a nationwide prospective observational cohort study in Korea. PLoS One. 2017;12:e0171842.

106. Torlen K, Kalantar-Zadeh K, Molnar MZ, et al. Serum potassium and cause-specific mortality in a large peritoneal dialysis cohort. Clin J Am Soc Nephrol. 2012;7:1272–84.

107. Jung JY, Chang JH, Lee HH, et al. De novo hypokalemia in incident peritoneal dialysis patients: a 1-year observational study. Electrolyte Blood Press. 2009;7:73–8.

108. Zanger R. Hyponatremia and hypokalemia in patients of peritoneal dialysis. Semin Dial. 2010;23:575–80.

109. Marti G, Schwarz C, Leichtle AB, et al. Etiology and symptoms of severe hypokalemia in emergency department patients. Eur J Emerg Med. 2014;21:46–51.

110. Kovesdy CP, Matsushita K, Sang Y, et al. Serum potassium and adverse outcomes across the range of kidney function: a CKD prognosis consortium meta-analysis. Eur Heart J. 2018;39:1535–42.

111. Zhang Y, Chen P, Chen J, Wang L, Wei Y, Xu D. Association of low serum potassium levels and risk for all-cause mortality in patients with chronic kidney disease: a systematic review and meta-analysis. Ther Apher Dial. 2018; https://doi.org/10.1111/1744-9987.12753.

112. Langote A, Hiremath S, Ruzicka M, et al. Spironolactone is effective in treating hypokalemia among peritoneal dialysis patients. PLoS One. 2017;12:e0187269.

113. Karaboyas A, Zee J, Brunelli SM, et al. Dialysate potassium, serum potassium, mortality, and arrhythmia events in hemodialysis: results from the Dialysis Outcomes and Practice Patterns Study (DOPPS). Am J Kidney Dis. 2017;69:266–77.

Chapter 13
Anemia in Chronic Kidney Disease

Maria P. Martinez Cantarin and Ubaldo E. Martinez Outschoorn

Introduction

Anemia is defined as an absolute reduction of the total number of circulating red blood cells. Clinically, anemia is diagnosed by a decrease in hemoglobin (Hgb) concentration, decrease in hematocrit, or red blood cell count. The diagnosis of anemia by using a hemoglobin threshold was initially proposed by a WHO expert committee in 1968 and has been widely used clinically and in research studies [1]. By WHO standards, the lower limit of normal Hgb in adult non-pregnant females was considered to be 12 g/dL, while in adult males, it was considered to be 13 g/dL. Several other studies that used a more contemporary cohort of participants and also added race and age as potential variables have also been published with slightly higher Hgb thresholds (women of all ages 12.2 g/dL, young white males 13.7 g/dL, older white males 13.2 g/dL, black males of all ages 11.5 g/dL) [2].

Anemia is a common complication that occurs during chronic kidney disease (CKD). It was initially recognized and described in 1839 by Sir Robert Christison as the loss of blood color in patients with advanced kidney disease [3]. The prevalence of anemia in patients with chronic kidney disease varies depending on the reference Hgb used, but unfortunately many different thresholds for the definition of anemia in CKD have been used, making its prevalence highly variable. As an example, data from the 1990s showed that 68% of pre-dialysis patient had hematocrit less than 30% with 51% of those having a hematocrit less than 28% [4].

M. P. Martinez Cantarin (✉)
Medicine-Nephrology, Sidney Kimmel Medical College at Thomas Jefferson University, Philadelphia, PA, USA
e-mail: maria.p.martinezcantarin@jefferson.edu

U. E. Martinez Outschoorn
Medical Oncology, Sidney Kimmel Medical College at Thomas Jefferson University, Philadelphia, PA, USA
e-mail: ubaldo.martinez-outschoorn@jefferson.edu

© Springer Nature Switzerland AG 2022
J. McCauley et al. (eds.), *Approaches to Chronic Kidney Disease*,
https://doi.org/10.1007/978-3-030-83082-3_13

A more recent report by Stauffer et al., using a definition of anemia of hemoglobin levels less than 12 g/dL in women and less than 13 g/dL in men, determined a prevalence of 15.4% of anemia in patients with kidney disease, which is double the prevalence in the general population. As CKD progresses, the prevalence of anemia rises. At stage 5 CKD, the same study reported a prevalence of anemia of 53.4% [5]. Anemia is almost universal during dialysis. Data from USRDS reports that only 14.5% of hemodialysis patients and 21.4% of peritoneal dialysis patients had hemoglobin levels higher than 12 g/dL in 2017 [6].

Having diabetes and chronic kidney disease increases the risk of anemia. A report by the National Kidney Foundation, Kidney Early Evaluation Program (KEEP), and the definition of anemia based on hemoglobin concentrations less than 12 g/dL for men and less than 11 g/dL for women, showed that the prevalence of anemia and stage 3 CKD was as high as 22.2% and more than half of the population had anemia with stage 4 CKD and diabetes. The greatest difference in anemia prevalence between diabetics and non-diabetics with CKD was for stage 3 CKD, with a prevalence of anemia that was 3 times higher in diabetic patients that in nondiabetic CKD patients [7].

Consequences of Anemia of CKD

Anemia, due to reduced oxygen delivery to organs and tissues, is associated with a plethora of symptoms including fatigue, low energy, weakness, shortness of breath, headaches, sleep disturbances, reduced mental acuity, and cognitive impairment. These symptoms are associated with a significant deterioration in the quality of life of patients with CKD [8–11].

Besides its effects on quality of life, anemia in CKD patients has been associated with increased mortality, cardiovascular diseases including left ventricular hypertrophy (LVH), and hospitalizations. Patients on hemodialysis with hematocrit of less than 30% have increased risk for hospitalizations and mortality [12, 13]. Furthermore, in patients with severe anemia, defined as hemoglobin less than 9 g/dL, every 0.1 g/dL decrease in hemoglobin was associated with increased mortality and cardiac complications including LVH and heart failure [14].

Data from the DOPPS study also has shown that patients with hemoglobin less than 10 g/dL had 29% higher risk of hospitalization than patients with hemoglobin between 11 and 12 g/dL. In this study, for every 0.1 g/dL higher hemoglobin concentrations, patients had a 5% decrease in the relative risk of death and 4% decrease in the relative risk of hospitalization [15]. Similar associations have been found using data from Canadian databases [16]. Hence, some authors have proposed a threshold of 11 gram/deciliter to define the higher risk for complications associated with anemia of chronic kidney disease [16].

The observational studies and the availability of recombinant EPO led to numerous clinical trials evaluating the effect of treatment of anemia in chronic kidney disease on mortality, morbidity, and quality of life. The results of these trials on anemia treatment in CKD, including randomized controlled trials, have shown that normalization or near normalization of hemoglobin in patients with chronic kidney disease does not improve outcomes including quality of life. Furthermore, trials that aimed to improve Hgb to close to normal (>13 g/dL) were associated with higher mortality and cardiovascular complications [17–20].

Pathophysiology

Erythropoietin (EPO), a circulating factor that stimulates erythropoiesis, was initially described in the 1950s [21]. EPO was found to be produced mainly by the kidney [22] and thanks to the purification and cloning of the EPO protein, quantification of its circulating levels was possible by the 1970s [23–25].

EPO has 165 amino acids and it is highly glycosylated. It is secreted to the bloodstream with a half-life of 5–12 hours. At baseline, EPO circulation is continuous at a low level, but in the presence of anemia, EPO levels can increase rapidly up to 100 times the baseline levels. EPO binds to its receptor causing a conformational change and activating intracellular signal transduction pathways that increase cell division and prolong the survival of red blood cell precursors, mainly erythroid burst forming and colony forming units [26].

EPO levels are low relative to the degree of anemia in CKD. Patients without chronic kidney disease, with the same degree of anemia than patients with CKD, had EPO levels 10–100 times higher than patient with CKD [27–29]. Due to these observations, EPO deficiency was thought to be the main cause of anemia in CKD. With the introduction of recombinant human EPO, anemia treatment in patients with CKD was widespread. Despite the potential benefits, initial studies showed significant complications and resistance with administration of recombinant EPO with the goal of achieving hemoglobin levels higher than 11 g/dL [17], raising the question of other potential factors that can contribute to the development of anemia in CKD besides relative EPO deficiency.

The production of EPO by the kidney is regulated by hypoxia-inducible factor (HIF), which is a transcription factor that, as it name indicates, accumulates during hypoxia [30, 31]. HIF is a heterodimer with two isoforms HIF-α (encoded by *HIF1A*) and HIF-β (encoded by *ARNT*) [32]. HIF-α is produced continuously by the kidney cells and it is the isoform that responds primarily to hypoxia. It has three different isoforms, HIF-1α, HIF-2α (encoded by *EPAS*), and HIF-3α (encoded by *HIF3A*), and every isoform regulates different genes [33] and has different tissue restrictions. In the kidney, HIF2α is the main isoform expressed in interstitial cells, endothelium, and glomeruli, whereas HIF1α is mainly expressed by the tubular cells. Of the three isoforms, HIF-2α seems to play a more important role in the regulation of EPO and iron metabolism genes [34]. The activity of HIF-3α is less understood.

HIF-β is also constitutively produced but is not regulated by hypoxia. During hypoxic conditions, HIF-α accumulates and translocates to the nucleus where it binds to HIF-β, and the heterodimer will bind to the hypoxic response regions in the DNA. HIF1α, HIF2α, and HIF3α complexes with HIF1β are termed HIF-1, HIF-2, and HIF3. HIF target genes include EPO, glycolytic genes, and genes involved iron metabolism-angiogenesis. HIF-1 and HIF2 both increase the transcription of hypoxia-related genes, but their specific gene targets, kinetics of activation, and oxygen dependence differ.

The oxygen sensitivity of HIF-α proteins is regulated by prolyl hydroxylase domain enzymes (PHD). PHDs act as an oxygen sensor mechanism by hydroxylating target prolyl residues of HIF-α in normoxia and driving its degradation. Oxygen-dependent hydroxylation of HIF-α increases its affinity for the von Hippel-Lindau tumor suppressor protein (pVHL). Therefore, after prolyl hydroxylation, HIF-α will bind pVHL which will promote HIF ubiquitination and its degradation by the proteasome [35, 36]. PHD have three isoforms: PHD1, PHD2, and PHD3, with PHD2 being the main isoform involved in the regulation of HIF content [37]. All the PHD isoforms have low affinity for oxygen, and low oxygen concentrations significantly reduce PHD catalytic activity. HIFα stabilizers are currently in phase III clinical trials in the USA as a potential alternative treatment of anemia in CKD, and they are approved in Asia.

EPO is mainly produced by peritubular interstitial fibroblast in the kidney. During normoxia, fibroblasts around the cortico-medullary region produce most of the EPO, whereas in hypoxia, EPO production is also shared by fibroblast from the cortex and medulla via HIF-2α stabilization [38]. With the progression of interstitial fibrosis, tubular atrophy, and loss of peritubular capillaries associated with CKD, the kidney cells are exposed to increased levels of hypoxia. Despite hypoxic environment, production and function of HIF cannot match the increasing hypoxic conditions. Besides the relative insufficiency of HIF response to hypoxia, there is also a relative decrease in EPO production due to conversion of renal fibroblasts to myofibroblasts during CKD progression, and myofibroblasts lose their capacity to produce EPO after anemic or hypoxic stimuli [39]. Despite this, the production of EPO by the myofibroblasts in CKD kidneys may be increased by inactivating PHD enzymes using PHD inhibitors.

Ongoing research has shown that the lack of erythropoietin is not the sole cause of anemia in chronic kidney disease. Some studies have postulated uremic-induced inhibitors of erythropoiesis as potential contributors to anemia, although no specific factors have been identified. Studies with radioisotope labeling has shown shortened red blood cells survival in patients with CKD. Other mechanical, metabolic, and nutritional deficiencies have also been proposed as contributors to anemia seen in chronic kidney disease [40, 41].

Currently, it is also widely recognized that alterations in the iron metabolism have an important role in the development of anemia of chronic kidney disease. Patients with kidney disease suffer from both decreased iron intake and decreased iron mobilization, which facilitate an overall state of functional iron deficiency.

Production of red blood cells by the bone marrow is regulated by EPO, but differentiation from erythroblast to reticulocyte is a process that requires iron; hence, iron deficiency will limit EPO responsiveness. Iron is absorbed from the gastrointestinal tract and circulates bound to transferrin. Circulating iron will travel to bone marrow to be used in erythropoiesis or will get stored bound to ferritin in the spleen or liver.

The absorption and movement of iron are regulated by hepcidin. Hepcidin is a protein produced in the liver that promotes the internalization of ferroportin, an iron transporter located in the duodenum, hepatocytes, and macrophages. Expression of ferroportin is needed for iron to be absorbed from the gastrointestinal tract and also for movement of iron from the circulation to the reticuloendothelial system and vice versa. Hepcidin levels follow iron stores with high hepcidin levels seen in iron overload and low hepcidin levels reported in iron deficiency. Another potent inducer of hepcidin is inflammation. Hepcidin levels are elevated in patients with CKD most likely as a consequence of lower excretion, increased inflammation, vitamin D deficiency, and iron overload. HIF suppresses hepcidin production most likely via increased erythropoiesis due to increased EPO production, and recent clinical studies have shown that HIF stabilizers can decrease hepcidin levels. This decrease in hepcidin by HIF stabilizers contributes to optimization of iron metabolism and to the improvement of anemia in CKD independently of the changes in EPO production. Besides the effects on hepcidin, HIF-1 promotes iron utilization as it increases the expression of transferrin, transferrin receptor 1, and ceruloplasmin, and HIF2 enhances absorption of iron by the intestine by upregulation of divalent metal transporter 1 and duodenal cytochrome B.

Reduced iron intake in patients with CKD is most likely multifactorial and includes decreased appetite, exacerbated by uremic anorexia, erratic absorption from the gastrointestinal tract due to increased hepcidin activity, and the use of medications that will interfere with iron absorption. Some of the causes that contribute to the increased iron loss in CKD include the loss of iron from trapped blood in dialyzers, gastrointestinal bleeding due to poor platelet function, anticoagulation with dialysis, use of antiplatelet drugs, and frequent laboratory sampling [42, 43].

Treatment of Anemia in Chronic Kidney Disease

The main treatment of anemia of CKD is recombinant human erythropetin (rHuEPO). The term erythropoiesis-stimulating agents (ESA) currently only involves erythropoietin analogs, but other drugs that are not EPO analogs are being developed for use in anemia of CKD.

Treatment goals with rHuEPO included the avoidance of blood transfusions, improvement of anemia symptoms, and improvement of detrimental outcomes. Initial studies were clear in determining that EPO use in patients with Hgb values of <8 g/dL was able to revert the symptoms associated with severe anemia [8, 10, 11].

Despite the initial data, randomized controlled trials that used EPO analogs for the treatment of anemia in kidney disease targeting Hgb levels close to normal were not able to show an improvement in outcomes. Furthermore, some of those studies were associated with increased mortality and cardiovascular events including stroke.

In 1998, Dr. Besarab published the results of normal hematocrit cardiac trial (NHCT), a randomized controlled trial in high-risk hemodialysis patients with ischemic heart disease or congestive heart failure and anemia [17]. The trial used epoetin alpha as a treatment option with a goal Hgb of 13–15 g/dL versus 9–10 g/dL. The study randomized 1233 patients who were followed for a median time of 14 months. The primary end point was length of time to death or no fatal myocardial infarction. The study showed no significant increase in reaching the primary outcome in the high hematocrit group (RR 1.3). Despite a non-significant trend, this study was halted.

The CHOIR study in 2006 used epoetin alpha in CKD patients with a target Hgb level lower than prior studies (13.5 g/dL versus 11.3 g/dL) [18]. The study enrolled 1432 patients with chronic kidney disease with and without diabetes with a median study duration of 16 months. The primary endpoint was a composite of death, myocardial infarction, hospitalization for CHF, and stroke. This study showed a 34% increased risk to reach the primary endpoint in the higher hemoglobin group compared to the lower hemoglobin group. The study also reported similar changes in quality of life between the groups. The study concluded that targeting higher hemoglobin levels of 13.5 g/dL in patients with CKD was associated with increased risk and no real benefit in the quality of life.

The CREATE study also in 2006 used epoetin beta for treatment of anemia in 603 CKD 3 and 4 patients not on hemodialysis [19]. Their goal Hgb treatment during the study was 13–15 g/dL in the near-normal Hgb target group versus 10.5–11.5 g/dL in the low Hgb target group. Mean follow-up was 3 years. Similar to the NHCT trial, this study showed that the high hemoglobin group did not present a higher risk of first cardiovascular event but a significant increase in the risk of needing dialysis. The study concluded that there was no cardiac benefit to aim for higher hemoglobin rates.

The TREAT trial in 2009 included more than 4000 CKD patients with type 2 diabetes and anemia [20]. It used darboepoetin alfa to achieve a goal Hgb of 13 g/dL. The comparison arm used darboepoetin just as rescue therapy once Hgb levels were below 9 g/dL. The primary endpoint was a composite outcome of death or a cardiovascular event and of death or end-stage renal disease. There were no differences in the rates of the primary outcomes in the high versus rescue hemoglobin targets, but the higher hemoglobin levels were associated with higher risk of stroke.

Besides the cardiovascular effects, data on the use of ESA in the treatment of chemotherapy-associated anemia in patients with cancer showed that ESA use may affect survival rates in patient with head and neck cancer, non-small cell lung cancer, lymphoma, cervical cancer, and breast cancer. In 2019, the American Society of Clinical Oncology and the American Society of Hematology updated their guidelines of ESA use in cancer patients. Both societies currently recommend to avoid the use of ESA in patients with cancer whose treatment intent is cure. The recommendations are based on the known risks and not on clinical trials' data of ESA use [44]. Methoxy polyethylene glycol-epoetin beta (Mircera), the most recently approved ESA analog, is not indicated for the treatment of anemia due to chemotherapy as a dose-ranging study of Mircera was terminated early because of more deaths among patients receiving Mircera than another ESA.

Due to the increasing reports of lack of hard outcome improvement and the possibility of increased harm, the FDA mandated a black box warning for all ESAs stating their risks (increased risk of death, cardiovascular events, thromboembolic events, stroke, and cancer) and recommending its use with the lowest dose as possible to avoid transfusions.

Another feared, although very rare, adverse effect associated with the use of ESA was the development of pure red cell aplasia. Red cell aplasia is a type of normocytic normochromic anemia that is characterized by severely decreased erythrocyte numbers and absence of erythroid precursors in the marrow. The development of red cell aplasia was thought to be secondary to development of anti-Epo antibodies in patients who were receiving rHuEPO for the treatment of anemia of CKD. Most of the cases that were reported in the 1990s occurred outside the USA and after subcutaneous injection. The cases of red pure cell anemia were mainly associated with a specific rHuEPO product, and after removing certain stabilizers of the specific rHuEPO formulation and discontinuing some of the rubber stoppers of prefilled syringes that were thought to have leachates implicated in the development of the anemia, the number of cases significantly decreased [45]. Nowadays, red cell aplasia is considered an exceptionally uncommon side effect of the treatment with rHuEPO.

The first EPO analog that reached the market was epoetin alpha (Procrit/Epogen/Retacrit), produced by DNA technology just 5 years after the EPO gene was cloned. The next analog, darboepoetin alpha (Aranesp), was slightly bigger in structure with five extra amino acids and extra carbohydrate content. The molecular changes made darboepoetin have a two to three times longer half-life than EPO. The latest addition to the EPO analogs, methoxy polyethylene glycol-epoetin beta (Mircera), has an even longer half-life than epoetin alpha (130 hours compared to the 6.8 hour of epoetin alpha after IV administration). Less frequent dosing is believed to be a significant advantage as EPO analogs are given either through intravenous (IV) or subcutaneous (SC) route (Table 13.1).

There are significant differences in the pharmacokinetic properties of epoetin alpha depending on the route of administration. In general, when epoetin alpha is dosed subcutaneously, it is associated with a lower but more persistent peak blood level. This translates clinically in the fact that lower doses of epoetin alpha are needed when SC compared to IV formulation is used to achieve the same Hgb level

Table 13.1 Suggested dose for ESA therapy

	Pre-dialysis CKD	Dialysis
Epo alpha and derivatives	50–100 units/kg × 1 week 10,000–20,000 every other week	50–100 units/kg × 3 week
Darboepoetin alpha	0.45 mcg/kg once every 4 weeks	0.45 mcg/kg × 1 week 0.75 mcg/kg × 1 every other week
Methoxy polyethylene glycol-epoetin beta	0.6 mcg/kg × 1 every other week	0.6 mcg/kg × 1 every other week

[46–49]. Despite this advantage, EPO is mainly used IV in the dialysis population due to convenience and to facilitate compliance [50]. Data from the original darboepoetin trials have shown equivalence between the IV and SC route [51, 52]. Methoxy polyethylene glycol-epoetin beta is also considered equivalent given either IV or SC.

The FDA has suggested the conversion factors between epoetin alpha to darboepoetin and also from epoetin alpha and darboepoetin to methoxy polyethylene glycol-epoetin beta.

The suggested conversion between epoetin and darpoepoetin for adults is based on the weekly epoetin dose. If epoetin is dosed as less than 2500 units a week, the equivalent dose of darboepoetin should be 6.25 mcg/week. If the epoetin dose is between 2500 and 4999 units, the patient should receive 12.5 mcg of darboepoetin. Epoetin dose of 5000–10,999 is equivalent to darboepoetin 25 mcg/week. Doses of 11,000–17,999 units of epoetin a week should be converted to 40 mcg of darboepoetin, 18,000–33,999 units to 60 mcg/week of darboepoetin, 34,000–89,999 units to 100 mcg/week of darboepoetin, and >90,0000 units to 200 mcg of darboepoetin.

The suggested dose of Mircera if the epoetin weekly dose is less than 8000 units or the weekly darboepoetin dose is less than 40 mcg should be 120 mcg a month or 60 mcg every other week. If the dose of epoetin is between 8000 and 16,000 units a week or the dose of darboepoetin is 40–80 mcg/week, the suggested dose of Mircera will be 200 mcg/month or 100 mcg every 2 weeks. If the dose of epoetin is higher than 16,000 units /week or the dose of darboepoetin is more than 80 mcg /week, the suggested does of mircera is 360 mcg/ month or 180 mcg/every 2 weeks.

Despite clear guidelines about the dosing of ESA, there is a tremendous variability in the degree of hemoglobin response. When treatment with epoetin alpha in adult patients is unable to achieve a Hgb >11 g/dL, despite a weekly dose of 500 IU/kg or 30,000 IU/Week (>1.5 μg/kg with darboepoetin), ESA resistance is presumed (Table 13.2) [53].

Recommendations for initial therapy and maintenance therapy with EPO analogs were published by the Kidney Disease Improving Global Outcomes (KDIGO) anemia workgroup in 2012 [54]. The same year Kidney Disease Outcomes Quality Initiative (KDOQI) made a comment on the guidelines published by KDIGO in order to give extra recommendations in certain areas [55].

Table 13.2 Causes of ESA unresponsiveness

Hematological factors	Dialysis-related factors	Inflammatory factors
Blood loss	Severe secondary hyperparathyroidsm	Infection (may be occult)
Iron deficiency anemia, Folate deficiency	Inadequate dialysis	Malnutrition
Pure red cell aplasia	Water contamination	Acute inflammation: e.g., post-surgical
Hematological disorders: Sickle cell anemia, thalassemia, hemolytic anemia, myelodysplastic syndrome		Failed allograft
Cancer with concomitant chemoradiation		

The guidelines acknowledge the risk of utilizing EPO analogs and encourage their use after balancing the patient's specific risks and benefits. The guidelines suggest to consider the use of EPO analogs once the Hgb has been <10 mg/dL in non-dialysis patients and to avoid Hgb decrease lower than 9 mg/dL in dialysis patients. It also acknowledges the fact that anemia symptoms may be present at higher Hgb levels depending on different patient's characteristics and that higher Hgb threshold for treating anemia can be used in certain patients.

The guidelines also proposed to avoid reaching Hgb levels of 13 g/dL with EPO analogs as well as not to maintain levels higher than 11.5 g/dL.

Iron Therapy

Iron deficiency, due to inadequate iron intake as well as increased iron losses, is a major contributor to anemia in chronic kidney disease. Adequate provision of iron is needed before starting therapy with an ESA.

Iron therapy has been in use for the treatment of anemia associated with chronic kidney disease for a long time, but the optimal management of iron therapy in CKD is still unclear due to concerns with safety. These concerns are reflected in the goals of iron repletion published by different organizations. The KDIGO guidelines from 2012 recommended iron repletion with a transferrin saturation (TSAT) $\leq$30% and a serum ferritin $\leq$500 ng/mL [54]. This guideline differs widely from the European Renal Best Practice Guidelines published in 2013 [56], which proposed a more strict threshold for TSAT <20% and a ferritin level <100 ng/mL in order to start iron therapy. Recently, the National Institute for Health and Excellence in 2015 [57] and the Renal Association in 2017 [58] recommended iron therapy up to a ferritin level of 800 ng/mL.

The advances in the understanding of the pathophysiology of anemia in CKD and the role of hepcidin in preventing iron absorption and redistribution from the reticuloendothelial system have facilitated new avenues of research for therapeutic strategies that will improve iron availability.

There also have been updated information about the safety of iron therapy in CKD that we will review briefly.

Oral Iron

Oral iron remains one of the cornerstones of anemia therapy in pre-dialysis CKD. Oral iron is poorly absorbed and associated with significant GI side effects limiting patient compliance and therapeutic success in the general population. Despite these limitations, recent studies continue to demonstrate inferior effectiveness in the treatment of pre-dialysis CKD anemia when compared to IV iron [59, 60].

The most common used form of oral iron continues to be ferrous sulfate as it is inexpensive and widely available. Ferric gluconate, ferric succinate, and iron poly-maltose are less commonly used. Of the most recent additions in the oral iron supplements, ferric citrate deserves special mention. Initially marketed as a non-calcium-containing phosphorus binder, early in its development, it was noticed to be associated with higher ferritins and transferrin saturations reflecting enhanced oral GI absorption [61]. It is currently approved as a phosphate binder in treatment with ESRD but has been recently approved by the FDA for CKD patients with iron-deficiency anemia who are not on dialysis after recent randomized controlled trials have reinforced its efficacy for the treatment of iron deficiency in non-dialysis and dialysis-dependent population [62, 63].

Other oral iron formulations such as ferric maltol, heme iron polypeptide, and oral liposomal iron have limited use in CKD or limited efficacy [64–66].

IV Iron

Most of the literature supports that intravenous iron is superior to oral iron in the treatment of anemia of chronic kidney disease [67, 68]. The literature is even clearer in the dialysis subgroup [69].

The main concern with the use of IV iron has been its potential side effects. The general composition of IV iron products include an iron core surrounded by a carbohydrate shell that will prevent the release of large amounts of labile-free iron that causes significant toxicity including anaphylaxis. The IV formulations marketed in the 1970s and 1980s had a carbohydrate shell that bound poorly to the elemental iron causing frequent reactions. Current formulations are iron carbohydrate complexes or colloids that form a small rounded particle with a larger carbohydrate shells which will release less labile or free iron allowing the administration of higher doses in short periods of time (15–60 minutes).

Iron dextran was the first stable iron formulation to come to the market in the 1940s. The original formulation was a high molecular weight dextran and was associated with rare but serious allergic reactions including anaphylaxis. That led to the development of a low molecular weight iron dextran that was associated with fewer adverse events.

Ferric gluconate (Ferrlecit) and iron sucrose (Venofer) were marketed as new iron formulations without dextran to form the carbohydrate shell around the iron core. Both formulations had lower reports of adverse events. Despite the lower rates of adverse events, the gluconate- or sucrose-based carbohydrate shell is smaller and binds iron less tightly than dextran, limiting the amount of elemental iron that can be infused with every dose.

Ferumoxytol (Feraheme) has an iron oxide core linked to a polyglucose sorbitol carboxymethylether shell. Due to a more stable configuration and a stronger link between the carbohydrate shell and the iron core, a dose of 510 mg of ferrumoxytol can be infused over 15 minutes.

Ferric carboxymaltose's (Injectafer) carbohydrate shell tightly binds elemental iron, allowing a dose of 750 mg or 1.5 g to be infused in a short period of time. It is normally well tolerated but reports of hypophosphatemia most likely secondary to increasing fibroblast growth factor 23 have been reported in some patients.

Ferric derisomaltose or iron isomaloside (Monoferric) was approved in 2020 by the FDA and can be used as a single dose of 1000 mg over 20 minutes. It has an iron core composed of ferric hydroxide and a carbohydrate shell of derisomaltose.

The published evidence suggests that the formulations of parenteral iron currently available, including low molecular weight iron dextran, are all safe and effective and there are no major, clinically important differences among them in terms of either efficacy or safety [70].

Ascorbic acid or vitamin C has been used not only to facilitate gastrointestinal absorption of iron but also to increase iron release form the reticuloendothelial depots. The effectiveness of vitamin C has been proven via intravenous [71] or oral supplementation [72] and could be considered in patients with significant functional iron deficiency characterized by EPO hyporesponsiveness and hyperferritinemia [73].

Besides its anaphylaxis risk, excess iron has been linked with increased oxidative stress. Increased oxidative stress has been associated with higher infection and cardiovascular and hospitalization risks. Two different randomized controlled trials published in 2015 and 2017 tried to shed some light about the safety of IV iron for the treatment of anemia of CKD in non-dialysis patients. Unfortunately, the two trials had dramatically different results. The Find CKD study randomized CKD patients with high and low ferritin to IV and oral iron [74]. The study demonstrated the effectiveness and safety of IV iron when compared to oral iron even in patients who had high ferritin levels. Conversely, the REVOKE study in CKD patients of stages 3–4 had to be terminated early due to concerns with increased cardiovascular and infectious side effects [60]. Two other studies were previously reported in 2013 and 2014 with no significant differences in adverse events in the oral iron versus IV iron groups [75] or between two different IV iron formulation groups [76]. Overall, there is still significant uncertainty in the safety of IV iron versus oral iron use specifically in the CKD population.

In the hemodialysis population, a recent study published in 2019 with more than 2000 patients determined that high IV iron is safe and efficacious when used proactively in dialysis patients with ferritin levels <700 [77].

In sum, limiting iron utilization to ferritin levels less than 500 ng/mL and TSAT <30% may exclude a significant proportion of CKD patients who could respond to treatment. For ferritin levels higher than 800 ng per mL, the clinician should use their judgment and balance the risk of higher EPO doses versus the risk of toxicity.

Hypoxia-Inducible Factor Stabilizers and Anemia of CKD

Agents that inhibit HIF prolyl-hydroxylases can not only improve EPO production but also facilitate iron mobilization from stores and increase iron absorption from the gastrointestinal tract. In comparison to EPO, their route of administration is oral. There are currently six drugs in the HIF prolyl-hydroxylase inhibitor family that are undergoing trials in the USA and other countries: roxadustat, vadadustat, daprodustat, molidustat, enarodustat, and desidustat.

Currently, HIF-1 alpha stabilizers are approved in China for anemia treatment in CKD and dialysis populations and in Japan for the treatment of anemia in the dialysis population. Data on the use of roxadustat in CKD and dialysis patients in China has been published in high-impact journals [78, 79].

In December 2019, data from the three randomized controlled trials on the use of roxadustat that included patients from the USA were presented at the American Society of Nephrology kidney week. The HIMALAYAS and ROCKIES clinical trials included patients receiving dialysis, whereas the OLYMPUS clinical trial focused on the pre-dialysis CKD population. The focus of the HIMALAYAS clinical trial was on the incident dialysis population (subjects were on dialysis for at least 2 weeks but less than 4 months) [80]. The study included over 1000 adult incident hemodialysis (HD) patients who were randomized to roxadustat or epoetin alpha for the treatment of anemia. The primary endpoint was set as changes in Hgb from baseline over week 28–52 of treatment. The study also looked at adverse event profile to assess safety. The mean duration of the study was 1.8 years. At the conclusion of the study, roxadustat was found to be non-inferior and actually reached the superiority margin over epoetin alpha. The safety profile was similar during the study time. In a subgroup analysis of patients with increased inflammation, roxadustat was also non-inferior to EPO. The ROCKIES clinical trial randomized over 2000 patients on HD to roxadustat or epoetin alpha for the treatment of anemia [81]. The primary endpoint was the same as the HIMALAYA clinical trial with change of baseline Hgb over week 28–52. The trial concluded that roxadustat was as effective as EPO for the management of anemia. The study also determined that patients treated with roxadustat had lower hepcidin and ferritin levels and higher serum iron and required less iron repletion than patients treated with EPO. The adverse event profile between the groups was also similar in this study. The OLYMPUS clinical trial focused on non-dialysis CKD patients [82]. Over 2500 patients were randomized to either roxadustat or placebo for the treatment of anemia. Once again in this study, roxadustat showed higher change in Hgb baseline at weeks 28–52. The study also focused on adverse events and found no differences in mortality in the study groups and a similar adverse events profile.

These new drugs will be readily accessible in the next few years and their use will probably change the way we approach the treatment of anemia of CKD. Despite having a new therapeutic class of drugs available for the management of anemia in CKD, further data on the safety of long-term use will be needed, considering the potential for facilitating tumor growth since HIF and PHDs have fundamental roles in cancer progression.

In conclusion, anemia in CKD is very common and more frequent and severe with progression of CKD. Anemia in CKD is multifactorial but erythropoietin deficiency and iron deficiency are very common, especially in patients who are receiving renal replacement therapy. Anemia in CKD is associated with death and morbidity that reduce the quality of life, and hence treatment should be implemented. Treatment includes erythropoietin and iron supplementation but avoiding hemoglobin levels greater than 11.5 g/dL.

References

1. WHO Scientific Group on Nutritional Anaemias & World Health Organization. Nutritional anaemias. Report of a WHO scientific group. World Health Organ Tech Rep Ser. 1968;405:5–37.
2. Beutler E, Waalen J. The definition of anemia: what is the lower limit of normal of the blood hemoglobin concentration? Blood. 2006;107(5):1747–50.
3. Christison R. On granular degeneration of the kidneys, and its connection with dropsy, inflammation, and other diseases. Edinb Med Surg J. 1840;54(144):234–44.
4. Obrador GT, Ruthazer R, Arora P, Kausz AT, Pereira BJ. Prevalence of and factors associated with suboptimal care before initiation of dialysis in the United States. J Am Soc Nephrol. 1999;10(8):1793–800.
5. Stauffer ME, Fan T. Prevalence of anemia in chronic kidney disease in the United States. PLoS One. 2014;9(1):e84943.
6. United States Renal Data System. USRDS annual data report: epidemiology of kidney disease in the United States. Bethesda: National Institutes of Health, National Institute of Diabetes and Digestive and Kidney Diseases; 2017.
7. El-Achkar TM, Ohmit SE, McCullough PA, Crook ED, Brown WW, Grimm R, et al. Higher prevalence of anemia with diabetes mellitus in moderate kidney insufficiency: the kidney early evaluation program. Kidney Int. 2005;67(4):1483–8.
8. Canadian Erythropoietin Study Group. Association between recombinant human erythropoietin and quality of life and exercise capacity of patients receiving haemodialysis. BMJ. 1990;300(6724):573–8.
9. Kliger AS, Fishbane S, Finkelstein FO. Erythropoietic stimulating agents and quality of a patient's life: individualizing anemia treatment. Clin J Am Soc Nephrol. 2012;7(2):354–7.
10. Delano BG. Improvements in quality of life following treatment with r-HuEPO in anemic hemodialysis patients. Am J Kidney Dis. 1989;14(2 Suppl 1):14–8.
11. Moreno F, Lopez Gomez JM, Sanz-Guajardo D, Jofre R, Valderrabano F. Quality of life in dialysis patients. A Spanish multicentre study. Spanish Cooperative Renal Patients Quality of Life Study Group. Nephrol Dial Transplant. 1996;11(Suppl 2):125–9.
12. Xia H, Ebben J, Ma JZ, Collins AJ. Hematocrit levels and hospitalization risks in hemodialysis patients. J Am Soc Nephrol. 1999;10(6):1309–16.
13. Ma JZ, Ebben J, Xia H, Collins AJ. Hematocrit level and associated mortality in hemodialysis patients. J Am Soc Nephrol. 1999;10(3):610–9.
14. Foley RN, Parfrey PS, Harnett JD, Kent GM, Murray DC, Barre PE. The impact of anemia on cardiomyopathy, morbidity, and mortality in end-stage renal disease. Am J Kidney Dis. 1996;28(1):53–61.
15. Locatelli F, Pisoni RL, Combe C, Bommer J, Andreucci VE, Piera L, et al. Anaemia in haemodialysis patients of five European countries: association with morbidity and mortality in the Dialysis Outcomes and Practice Patterns Study (DOPPS). Nephrol Dial Transplant. 2004;19(1):121–32.
16. Levin A, Djurdjev O, Duncan J, Rosenbaum D, Werb R. Haemoglobin at time of referral prior to dialysis predicts survival: an association of haemoglobin with long-term outcomes. Nephrol Dial Transplant. 2006;21(2):370–7.

17. Besarab A, Bolton WK, Browne JK, Egrie JC, Nissenson AR, Okamoto DM, et al. The effects of normal as compared with low hematocrit values in patients with cardiac disease who are receiving hemodialysis and epoetin. N Engl J Med. 1998;339(9):584–90.
18. Singh AK, Szczech L, Tang KL, Barnhart H, Sapp S, Wolfson M, et al. Correction of anemia with epoetin alfa in chronic kidney disease. N Engl J Med. 2006;355(20):2085–98.
19. Drueke TB, Locatelli F, Clyne N, Eckardt KU, Macdougall IC, Tsakiris D, et al. Normalization of hemoglobin level in patients with chronic kidney disease and anemia. N Engl J Med. 2006;355(20):2071–84.
20. Pfeffer MA, Burdmann EA, Chen CY, Cooper ME, de Zeeuw D, Eckardt KU, et al. A trial of darbepoetin alfa in type 2 diabetes and chronic kidney disease. N Engl J Med. 2009;361(21):2019–32.
21. Erslev A. Humoral regulation of red cell production. Blood. 1953;8(4):349–57.
22. Jacobson LO, Goldwasser E, Fried W, Plzak L. Role of the kidney in erythropoiesis. Nature. 1957;179(4560):633–4.
23. Miyake T, Kung CK, Goldwasser E. Purification of human erythropoietin. J Biol Chem. 1977;252(15):5558–64.
24. Lin FK, Suggs S, Lin CH, Browne JK, Smalling R, Egrie JC, et al. Cloning and expression of the human erythropoietin gene. Proc Natl Acad Sci U S A. 1985;82(22):7580–4.
25. Jacobs K, Shoemaker C, Rudersdorf R, Neill SD, Kaufman RJ, Mufson A, et al. Isolation and characterization of genomic and cDNA clones of human erythropoietin. Nature. 1985;313(6005):806–10.
26. Jelkmann W. Molecular biology of erythropoietin. Intern Med. 2004;43(8):649–59.
27. Cotes PM. Immunoreactive erythropoietin in serum. I. Evidence for the validity of the assay method and the physiological relevance of estimates. Br J Haematol. 1982;50(3):427–38.
28. McGonigle RJ, Wallin JD, Shadduck RK, Fisher JW. Erythropoietin deficiency and inhibition of erythropoiesis in renal insufficiency. Kidney Int. 1984;25(2):437–44.
29. Garcia JF, Ebbe SN, Hollander L, Cutting HO, Miller ME, Cronkite EP. Radioimmunoassay of erythropoietin: circulating levels in normal and polycythemic human beings. J Lab Clin Med. 1982;99(5):624–35.
30. Semenza GL. Regulation of tissue perfusion in mammals by hypoxia-inducible factor 1. Exp Physiol. 2007;92(6):988–91.
31. Nangaku M, Rosenberger C, Heyman SN, Eckardt KU. Regulation of hypoxia-inducible factor in kidney disease. Clin Exp Pharmacol Physiol. 2013;40(2):148–57.
32. Wang GL, Jiang BH, Rue EA, Semenza GL. Hypoxia-inducible factor 1 is a basic-helix-loop-helix-PAS heterodimer regulated by cellular O2 tension. Proc Natl Acad Sci U S A. 1995;92(12):5510–4.
33. Wu D, Rastinejad F. Structural characterization of mammalian bHLH-PAS transcription factors. Curr Opin Struct Biol. 2017;43:1–9.
34. Wiesener MS, Turley H, Allen WE, Willam C, Eckardt KU, Talks KL, et al. Induction of endothelial PAS domain protein-1 by hypoxia: characterization and comparison with hypoxia-inducible factor-1alpha. Blood. 1998;92(7):2260–8.
35. Jaakkola P, Mole DR, Tian YM, Wilson MI, Gielbert J, Gaskell SJ, et al. Targeting of HIF-alpha to the von Hippel-Lindau ubiquitylation complex by O2-regulated prolyl hydroxylation. Science. 2001;292(5516):468–72.
36. Ivan M, Kondo K, Yang H, Kim W, Valiando J, Ohh M, et al. HIFalpha targeted for VHL-mediated destruction by proline hydroxylation: implications for O2 sensing. Science. 2001;292(5516):464–8.
37. Hirsila M, Koivunen P, Gunzler V, Kivirikko KI, Myllyharju J. Characterization of the human prolyl 4-hydroxylases that modify the hypoxia-inducible factor. J Biol Chem. 2003;278(33):30772–80.
38. Koury ST, Koury MJ, Bondurant MC, Caro J, Graber SE. Quantitation of erythropoietin-producing cells in kidneys of mice by in situ hybridization: correlation with hematocrit, renal erythropoietin mRNA, and serum erythropoietin concentration. Blood. 1989;74(2):645–51.

39. Maxwell PH, Ferguson DJ, Nicholls LG, Johnson MH, Ratcliffe PJ. The interstitial response to renal injury: fibroblast-like cells show phenotypic changes and have reduced potential for erythropoietin gene expression. Kidney Int. 1997;52(3):715–24.
40. Eschbach JW Jr, Funk D, Adamson J, Kuhn I, Scribner BH, Finch CA. Erythropoiesis in patients with renal failure undergoing chronic dialysis. N Engl J Med. 1967;276(12):653–8.
41. Vos FE, Schollum JB, Coulter CV, Doyle TC, Duffull SB, Walker RJ. Red blood cell survival in long-term dialysis patients. Am J Kidney Dis. 2011;58(4):591–8.
42. Wish JB, Aronoff GR, Bacon BR, Brugnara C, Eckardt KU, Ganz T, et al. Positive iron balance in chronic kidney disease: how much is too much and how to tell? Am J Nephrol. 2018;47(2):72–83.
43. Gotloib L, Silverberg D, Fudin R, Shostak A. Iron deficiency is a common cause of anemia in chronic kidney disease and can often be corrected with intravenous iron. J Nephrol. 2006;19(2):161–7.
44. Bohlius J, Bohlke K, Castelli R, Djulbegovic B, Lustberg MB, Martino M, et al. Management of cancer-associated anemia with erythropoiesis-stimulating agents: ASCO/ASH clinical practice guideline update. J Clin Oncol. 2019;37(15):1336–51.
45. Means RT Jr. Pure red cell aplasia. Blood. 2016;128(21):2504–9.
46. McMahon FG, Vargas R, Ryan M, Jain AK, Abels RI, Perry B, et al. Pharmacokinetics and effects of recombinant human erythropoietin after intravenous and subcutaneous injections in healthy volunteers. Blood. 1990;76(9):1718–22.
47. Kaufman JS, Reda DJ, Fye CL, Goldfarb DS, Henderson WG, Kleinman JG, et al. Subcutaneous compared with intravenous epoetin in patients receiving hemodialysis. Department of Veterans Affairs Cooperative Study Group on Erythropoietin in Hemodialysis Patients. N Engl J Med. 1998;339(9):578–83.
48. Brockmoller J, Kochling J, Weber W, Looby M, Roots I, Neumayer HH. The pharmacokinetics and pharmacodynamics of recombinant human erythropoietin in haemodialysis patients. Br J Clin Pharmacol. 1992;34(6):499–508.
49. Besarab A. Physiological and pharmacodynamic considerations for route of EPO administration. Semin Nephrol. 2000;20(4):364–74.
50. Hynes DM, Stroupe KT, Kaufman JS, Reda DJ, Peterman A, Browning MM, et al. Adherence to guidelines for ESRD anemia management. Am J Kidney Dis. 2006;47(3):455–61.
51. Vanrenterghem Y, Barany P, Mann JF, Kerr PG, Wilson J, Baker NF, et al. Randomized trial of darbepoetin alfa for treatment of renal anemia at a reduced dose frequency compared with rHuEPO in dialysis patients. Kidney Int. 2002;62(6):2167–75.
52. Locatelli F, Canaud B, Giacardy F, Martin-Malo A, Baker N, Wilson J. Treatment of anaemia in dialysis patients with unit dosing of darbepoetin alfa at a reduced dose frequency relative to recombinant human erythropoietin (rHuEpo). Nephrol Dial Transplant. 2003;18(2):362–9.
53. Bamgbola OF. Pattern of resistance to erythropoietin-stimulating agents in chronic kidney disease. Kidney Int. 2011;80(5):464–74.
54. KDIGO. Clinical practice guideline for anemia in chronic kidney disease. Kidney Int Suppl. 2012;2(4):279–335.
55. Kliger AS, Foley RN, Goldfarb DS, Goldstein SL, Johansen K, Singh A, et al. KDOQI US commentary on the 2012 KDIGO clinical practice guideline for anemia in CKD. Am J Kidney Dis. 2013;62(5):849–59.
56. Locatelli F, Barany P, Covic A, De Francisco A, Del Vecchio L, Goldsmith D, et al. Kidney Disease: Improving Global Outcomes guidelines on anaemia management in chronic kidney disease: a European Renal Best Practice position statement. Nephrol Dial Transplant. 2013;28(6):1346–59.
57. National Collaborating Centre for Chronic Conditions. Anaemia management in chronic kidney disease. London: National Institute for Clinical Excellence, Royal College of Physicians; 2015.
58. Mikhail A, Brown C, Williams JA, Mathrani V, Shrivastava R, Evans J, et al. Renal association clinical practice guideline on Anaemia of Chronic Kidney Disease. BMC Nephrol. 2017;18(1):345.

59. Macdougall IC, Bock AH, Carrera F, Eckardt KU, Gaillard C, Van Wyck D, et al. FIND-CKD: a randomized trial of intravenous ferric carboxymaltose versus oral iron in patients with chronic kidney disease and iron deficiency anaemia. Nephrol Dial Transplant. 2014;29(11):2075–84.
60. Agarwal R, Kusek JW, Pappas MK. A randomized trial of intravenous and oral iron in chronic kidney disease. Kidney Int. 2015;88(4):905–14.
61. Yokoyama K, Akiba T, Fukagawa M, Nakayama M, Sawada K, Kumagai Y, et al. Long-term safety and efficacy of a novel iron-containing phosphate binder, JTT-751, in patients receiving hemodialysis. J Ren Nutr. 2014;24(4):261–7.
62. Fishbane S, Block GA, Loram L, Neylan J, Pergola PE, Uhlig K, et al. Effects of ferric citrate in patients with nondialysis-dependent CKD and iron deficiency anemia. J Am Soc Nephrol. 2017;28(6):1851–8.
63. Lewis JB, Sika M, Koury MJ, Chuang P, Schulman G, Smith MT, et al. Ferric citrate controls phosphorus and delivers iron in patients on dialysis. J Am Soc Nephrol. 2015;26(2):493–503.
64. Gasche C, Ahmad T, Tulassay Z, Baumgart DC, Bokemeyer B, Buning C, et al. Ferric maltol is effective in correcting iron deficiency anemia in patients with inflammatory bowel disease: results from a phase-3 clinical trial program. Inflamm Bowel Dis. 2015;21(3):579–88.
65. Dull RB, Davis E. Heme iron polypeptide for the management of anaemia of chronic kidney disease. J Clin Pharm Ther. 2015;40(4):386–90.
66. Pisani A, Riccio E, Sabbatini M, Andreucci M, Del Rio A, Visciano B. Effect of oral liposomal iron versus intravenous iron for treatment of iron deficiency anaemia in CKD patients: a randomized trial. Nephrol Dial Transplant. 2015;30(4):645–52.
67. Kalra PA, Bhandari S, Saxena S, Agarwal D, Wirtz G, Kletzmayr J, et al. A randomized trial of iron isomaltoside 1000 versus oral iron in non-dialysis-dependent chronic kidney disease patients with anaemia. Nephrol Dial Transplant. 2016;31(4):646–55.
68. Spinowitz BS, Kausz AT, Baptista J, Noble SD, Sothinathan R, Bernardo MV, et al. Ferumoxytol for treating iron deficiency anemia in CKD. J Am Soc Nephrol. 2008;19(8):1599–605.
69. Shepshelovich D, Rozen-Zvi B, Avni T, Gafter U, Gafter-Gvili A. Intravenous versus oral iron supplementation for the treatment of anemia in CKD: an updated systematic review and meta-analysis. Am J Kidney Dis. 2016;68(5):677–90.
70. Auerbach M, Macdougall I. The available intravenous iron formulations: history, efficacy, and toxicology. Hemodial Int. 2017;21(Suppl 1):S83–92.
71. Tarng DC, Hung SC, Huang TP. Effect of intravenous ascorbic acid medication on serum levels of soluble transferrin receptor in hemodialysis patients. J Am Soc Nephrol. 2004;15(9):2486–93.
72. Sultana T, DeVita MV, Michelis MF. Oral vitamin C supplementation reduces erythropoietin requirement in hemodialysis patients with functional iron deficiency. Int Urol Nephrol. 2016;48(9):1519–24.
73. Attallah N, Osman-Malik Y, Frinak S, Besarab A. Effect of intravenous ascorbic acid in hemodialysis patients with EPO-hyporesponsive anemia and hyperferritinemia. Am J Kidney Dis. 2006;47(4):644–54.
74. Macdougall IC, Bock AH, Carrera F, Eckardt KU, Gaillard C, Van Wyck D, et al. Renal function in patients with non-dialysis chronic kidney disease receiving intravenous ferric carboxymaltose: an analysis of the randomized FIND-CKD trial. BMC Nephrol. 2017;18(1):24.
75. Charytan C, Bernardo MV, Koch TA, Butcher A, Morris D, Bregman DB. Intravenous ferric carboxymaltose versus standard medical care in the treatment of iron deficiency anemia in patients with chronic kidney disease: a randomized, active-controlled, multi-center study. Nephrol Dial Transplant. 2013;28(4):953–64.
76. Onken JE, Bregman DB, Harrington RA, Morris D, Buerkert J, Hamerski D, et al. Ferric carboxymaltose in patients with iron-deficiency anemia and impaired renal function: the REPAIR-IDA trial. Nephrol Dial Transplant. 2014;29(4):833–42.
77. Macdougall IC, White C, Anker SD, Bhandari S, Farrington K, Kalra PA, et al. Intravenous iron in patients undergoing maintenance hemodialysis. N Engl J Med. 2019;380(5):447–58.

78. Chen N, Hao C, Liu BC, Lin H, Wang C, Xing C, et al. Roxadustat treatment for anemia in patients undergoing long-term dialysis. N Engl J Med. 2019;381(11):1011–22.
79. Chen N, Hao C, Peng X, Lin H, Yin A, Hao L, et al. Roxadustat for anemia in patients with kidney disease not receiving dialysis. N Engl J Med. 2019;381(11):1001–10.
80. Provenzano R, Evgeny S, Liubov E, et al. HIMALAYAS: A phase 3, randomized, open-label, active-controlled study of the efficacy and safety of roxadustat in the treatment of anemia in incident-dialysis patients. Abstract of a presentation at the American Society of Nephrology Kidney Week 2019 (Abstract TH-OR021), November 7, 2019, Washington, DC.
81. Fishbane S, Pollock CA, El-Shahawy MA, et al. ROCKIES: An international, phase 3, randomized, open-label, active-controlled study of roxadustat for anemia in dialysis-dependent CKD patients. Abstract of an oral presentation at the American Society of Nephrology Kidney Week 2019 (TH-OR022), November 7, 2019, Washington, DC.
82. Fishbane S, El-Shahawy MA, Pecoits-Filho R, et al. OLYMPUS: A phase 3, randomized, double-blind, placebo-controlled, international study of roxadustat efficacy in patients with non-dialysis-dependent (NDD) CKD and anemia. Fishbane S, El-Shahawy MA, Pecoits-Filho R, et al. Presented at: American Society of Nephrology Kidney Week 2019, Washington, DC; November 5–10, 2019.

Chapter 14
Chronic Kidney Disease–Mineral and Bone Disorders

Ignacio A. Portales-Castillo, Elaine W. Yu, Harald Jüppner, and Sagar U. Nigwekar

Introduction

Serum levels of calcium are rapidly maintained within a narrow normal range by interactions between the parathyroid gland, bone, kidney, and intestines [1], while serum phosphorus levels are regulated less efficiently. Abnormal function of any of these systems can lead to disorders of calcium and phosphorus. In the renal tubules, reabsorption of calcium and phosphorus is tightly regulated by the actions of parathyroid hormone (PTH) and fibroblast growth factor receptor 23 (FGF-23). With normal renal function, a small reduction in the serum levels of calcium is detected by the calcium sensing receptor (CaSR) within the parathyroid gland to increase PTH production, thus bringing calcium levels back to normal levels [2]. PTH increases the serum calcium by increasing bone resorption, decreasing renal calcium excretion, and elevating the levels of $1,25(OH)_2$ vitamin D by increasing the activity of 1-hydroxylase in the proximal renal

I. A. Portales-Castillo · S. U. Nigwekar (✉)
Division of Nephrology, Department of Medicine, Massachusetts General Hospital, Harvard Medical School, Boston, MA, USA
e-mail: IPORTALESCASTILLO@mgh.harvard.edu; snigwekar@mgh.harvard.edu

E. W. Yu
Endocrine Unit, Department of Medicine, Massachusetts General Hospital, Harvard Medical School, Boston, MA, USA
e-mail: EWYU@mgh.harvard.edu

H. Jüppner
Endocrine Unit, Department of Medicine, Massachusetts General Hospital, Harvard Medical School, Boston, MA, USA

Pediatric Nephrology Unit, Massachusetts General Hospital, Harvard Medical School, Boston, MA, USA
e-mail: HJUEPPNER@mgh.harvard.edu

"""

tubules [3], which results in improved calcium absorption in the intestines. This sensitive response to changes in calcium levels is impaired in patients with chronic kidney disease (CKD), in which the delicate homeostatic balance is disrupted by large shifts in calcium and phosphate handling. In CKD, higher PTH levels are usually required to maintain normal calcium levels by increasing bone resorption and improving $1,25(OH)_2$ vitamin D levels that are reduced, in part, because of increased FGF-23 production. Furthermore, elevated PTH levels as with chronic secondary or tertiary hyperparathyroidism increase bone turnover and resorption, thus affecting bone health [4].

Not surprisingly, patients with advanced CKD have a wide range of abnormalities involving mineral ions and bone. Depending on factors such as the stage of CKD, and medications used, some patients have evidence of pathologically increased PTH action in the bone (osteitis fibrosis cystica), while some others have insufficient PTH action in the bone (adynamic bone disease) [5]. At every stage of CKD, there are clinical manifestations of the disrupted mineral ion homeostasis, namely an increased risk of fractures and adverse cardiovascular events.

In this chapter, we will discuss chronic kidney disease–mineral bone disorders (CKD-MBD), a term coined in 2006, to broadly include any of the above-mentioned abnormalities in CKD patients, with their related clinical manifestations [6]. Dialysis-related amyloidosis, a disease that affects the osteoarticular surfaces of patients in long-term dialysis, has distinct pathophysiology that we will only review briefly in this chapter [7]. To date, there are no validated serum or radiographic markers to accurately predict the specific type of bone disorder that affects a patient with CKD [8]. Thus, understanding the basic pathophysiologic principles of CKD-MBD is critical for interpreting clinical manifestations related to mineral disorders of patients with CKD and providing a rationale for their management.

Important Factors in Bone and Mineral Metabolism

Serum calcium and phosphorus usually remain within normal limits early in CKD, until the glomerular filtration rate (GFR) drops below 40 ml/min/1.73 m^2 [9], by increasing FGF-23 and PTH levels [10] (Fig. 14.1 and Table 14.1). This important regulatory mechanism leads to the so-called "trade-off" hypothesis, originally proposed to explain the abnormally high PTH levels required for maintaining calcium and phosphate levels close to normal. However, this hypothesis applies more to the beneficial phosphaturic actions of FGF-23, which unfortunately reduces $1,25(OH)_2$ vitamin D levels, thus impairing calcium homeostasis and the need for increased PTH secretion. The elevation of both hormones comes at the expense of detrimental effects in other organs including the heart, bone, and vasculature [11, 12].

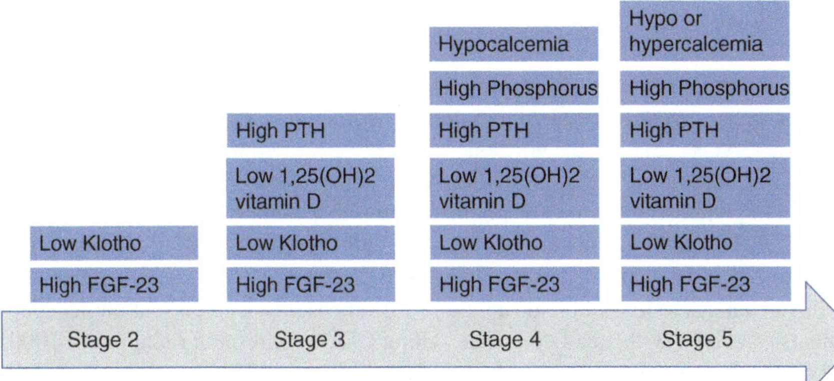

Fig. 14.1 CKD-MBD timeline. General timeline of the abnormalities in CKD-MBD. At every stage, there is increase in the risk of fractures compared to the general population

Table 14.1 Mediators of CKD-MBD

Mediator	Mechanism
Klotho	Decreased levels of Klotho are seen early in CKD and might lead to FGF-23 increase, cardiac fibrosis, and premature senescence features
FGF-23	Increased levels of FGF-23 are seen early in CKD to prevent hyperphosphatemia. Elevated FGF-23 can decrease formation of $1,25(OH)_2$ vitamin D, which lowers intestinal calcium absorption leading to a decline in blood levels of calcium with resultant PTH increase. FGF23 has been implicated in cardiac hypertrophy
PTH	PTH increases to prevent hypocalcemia, caused by reduced $1,25(OH)_2$ vitamin D generation, by increasing osteoclastic bone resorption, which further increases serum phosphate levels. Sustained increases in PTH signaling in the bone lead to high bone turnover, while low PTH or resistance to PTH action in the bone is associated with adynamic bone disease. Later in disease, chronic elevations in PTH can lead to tertiary hyperparathyroidism with accompanying hypercalcemia
Phosphorus	Increased serum phosphorus levels are a stimulus for FGF-23 production. High serum phosphorus levels are associated with increased mortality, CKD progression, and vascular calcification
Calcium	Calcium is vital for cell function. Vitamin D deficiency early in CKD can result in hypocalcemia. On the other hand, hypercalcemia can be seen in tertiary hyperparathyroidism at advanced CKD stages and is synergistic with hyperphosphatemia in extra skeletal calcification
1,25-Dihydroxyvitamin D	FGF-23 increase and loss of functional renal tissue decrease the formation of $1,25(OH)_2D$, thus causing hypocalcemia and elevated PTH levels
Sclerostin	Sclerostin is a negative regulator of the WNT pathway, an important pathway that increases bone density. Elevated levels of sclerostin are prevalent in CKD, but its exact role in CKD-MBD is not completely defined

The pathophysiology of CKD-MBD involves numerous hormones and minerals that increase or decrease as CKD progresses and the principal participants are described
FGF-23 fibroblast growth factor-23, *PTH* parathyroid hormone

FGF-23

FGF-23 was independently discovered by two groups, either as the hormone responsible for severe hypophosphatemia in patients with autosomal dominant hypophosphatemic rickets [13] or as the hormone responsible for tumor-induced osteomalacia (TIO) [14]. Its levels in the circulation were subsequently found to be markedly elevated in patients with severe hypophosphatemia, namely X-linked hypophosphatemia (XLH) and TIO, thus establishing the central role of FGF-23 in phosphate regulation [15]. Elevated serum levels of FGF-23 are one of the earliest detectable adaptive changes to loss of renal function [16]. The rise is seen even at modest decrements of eGFR, with steady increases along CKD progression rising up to 1000-fold above the normal range in end-stage kidney disease (ESKD) patients [17, 18]. FGF-23 is produced in the osteocytes. The primary stimulus for increased FGF-23 production and secretion is elevated serum phosphorus, but recent findings by Simic et al. indicate that glycerol-3-phosphate (G-3-P) is likely to play a prominent role [19]. Other stimuli, such as high $1,25(OH)_2$ vitamin D and iron deficiency, can also increase FGF-23 production [20]. To maintain phosphorus balance, FGF-23 down-regulates expression of the renal sodium-dependent phosphate co-transporters NPT2a (NaPi2a, SLC34A1) and NPT2c (NaPi2c, SLC34A3), with ensuing increase in urinary phosphorus excretion [21]. FGF-23 also inhibits the expression of 1-alpha-hydroxylase enzyme (CYP27B), necessary for the synthesis of active vitamin D [22], and it enhanced the expression of 24-alpha-hydroxylase enzyme (CYP24A), thus reducing the levels of the biologically active vitamin D metabolite through two mechanisms.

FGF-23 levels have been identified as predictive biomarkers of CKD progression and vascular disease. Elevated FGF-23 concentrations are associated with increased mortality [23], earlier need for dialysis initiation in CKD patients, and decrements in renal function in patients not on dialysis [24]. FGF-23 has also been associated with numerous adverse cardiac markers, such as left ventricular mass index (LVMI) and left ventricular hypertrophy (LVH). These epidemiological associations are supported by experimental studies. In the heart, FGF-23 induces hypertrophy of the cardiomyocytes and disrupts calcium trafficking, thereby increasing the risk of arrythmias [25, 26]. It is interesting to note that the actions of FGF-23 in the kidney are mediated by the binding to FGFR1 and the co-receptor Klotho, whereas cardiomyocytes express the receptor FGFR4, which functions independent of Klotho [27].

A human monoclonal antibody anti-FGF-23, burosumab, efficiently binds FGF23 and was therefore developed for the treatment of XLH [28]. XLH is caused by mutations in PHEX, phosphate regulating hormone with homologies to endopeptidase, which lead to excess production of FGF-23 resulting often in severe hypophosphatemia leading to rickets/osteomalacia. Bursoumab dose-dependently improves serum phosphorus levels in patients with XLH, increases $1,25(OH)_2$ vitamin D, and improves bone healing. Although FGF-23 levels are robustly associated with cardiovascular events in CKD, there are currently no animal models in which the negative effects of FGF23 in the heart can be dissociated from its phosphaturic actions. Thus, neutralizing the actions of FGF-23 in a rat model of early CKD increased serum phosphate levels, leading to profound vascular and renal calcifications and much increased mortality [29]. This poor outcome was entirely predictable, given the importance of FGF-23 for promoting phosphate excretion.

Klotho

Klotho was incidentally discovered in transgenic mice that exhibited features of premature aging [30]. These mice were found to be missing a protein encoded by a gene on mouse chromosome 5, which was called Klotho, for the Greek goddess that spins the thread of life. Subsequently, three isoforms of this protein where described (alpha, beta, and gamma). Alpha Klotho is the most common isoform, and we will use its name interchangeably with Klotho in this chapter.

Klotho has dual activity as both a co-receptor for FGF-23 in the kidney and a secreted hormone. Klotho exists as a transmembrane protein with two homologous extracellular domains (KL1 and KL2) and a single transmembrane pass. In this transmembrane state, it serves as a coreceptor (along with FGFR) for FGF-23 and has glucuronidase activity [31]. Its narrow tissue distribution in the renal tubules (distal>proximal), brain, and parathyroid gland suggests that the FGF-23/Klotho complex affects predominantly these organs. Lower levels of Klotho expression are found in other organs. The actions of Klotho as a coreceptor of FGF-23 include downregulation of the renal phosphate transporter, which increases phosphate excretion. In the parathyroid gland, Klotho suppresses PTH transcription and secretion [32].

Klotho also has two soluble forms, which consist of a cleaved portion at the membrane site (i.e., it contains both KL1 and KL2 extracellular domains) and a form that lacks KL2. The soluble form with both extracellular domains is mainly produced in the kidney and circulates in the bloodstream affecting a variety of organs including bone, kidney, heart, brain, and the endothelium. The extracellular domain of Klotho binds to Wnt. Wnt is a conserved cellular signaling pathway, with numerous biological functions, particularly relevant is the regulation of stem cells function [33]. Mice deficient in Klotho die prematurely and are generally infertile. They exhibit hypogonadism, decreased bone mineral density, extra skeletal calcification, among other characteristics of aging. On the contrary, mice over-expressing Klotho have an extended life-span [34].

Lack of Klotho in humans or mice leads to severe hyperphosphatemia and increased 1,25 vitamin D and calcium levels [35]. Decreased serum and urine levels of Klotho have been well documented in CKD, and stem from tissue loss, disordered signaling from activin receptor type IIA [36], and increased serum levels of uremic toxins such as indoxyl sulfate [37]. Similar to the original descriptions of Klotho leading to premature senescence and hyperphosphatemia, patients with CKD suffer from a shorter life span, vascular calcifications, and bone disorders. The contribution of Klotho deficiency to these manifestations has been supported by clinical observations and animal models. For example, low levels of Klotho correlate with cardiac hypertrophy and fibrosis in mice, and supplementation with soluble Klotho protects against these disorders [34].

Molecular Pathways: The Role of Canonic Wnt Pathway

The canonical Wnt pathway has profound effects on the skeleton. In this pathway, Wnt binds the dual receptor complex of frizzled and the low-density lipoprotein receptor-related protein 5 or 6 [38]. Upon activation, this receptor complex leads to β-catenin translocation into the nucleus where it regulates gene transcription with a net effect of enhanced bone formation and reduced bone resorption. This pathway is negatively regulated by sclerostin and Dickkopf-related protein 1 (DKK1). These inhibitors are present in the osteocytes and osteoblasts. The monoclonal antibody romosozumab inhibits sclerostin function, thus allowing the activation of Wnt pathway, and produces remarkable gains in bone mineral density in osteoporotic patients without CKD [39]. In patients with CKD, serum sclerostin levels increase with progression of disease [40]; however, bone expression does not consistently augment [41]. The mechanism for this serum increase has been hypothesized to be related to increased sclerostin production in the bone, because renal elimination of sclerostin is actually increased early in CKD [42]. Given the relation between sclerostin, bone formation, and vascular calcification, sclerostin has emerged as a potentially attractive target in the treatment of CKD-MBD [43].

Phosphorus

Phosphorus is essential for multiple and diverse biological functions. The vast majority of total phosphorus (>80%) is stored in the bone and teeth [16]. The remaining phosphorus has multiple important intracellular roles as an organic compound or as a free anion. Serum phosphorus levels are maintained within 3.5–4.5 mg/dL by regulation of absorption in the intestines by NPT2b, bone formation, and renal excretion, as well as by equilibration between its intracellular and extracellular forms [44]. With a normal glomerular filtration rate (GFR), about 3–6 g of phosphorus get filtered daily [44] and 85% are reabsorbed in the proximal tubule by NPT2a and NPT2c [45]. As GFR declines, less phosphorus is filtered, but this is offset by downregulation of NPT2a and NPT2c expression by FGF23 and PTH, so that serum phosphorus remains usually normal until GFR declines <40 ml/min/1.73.

Elevated phosphorus is a key element of the CKD-MBD pathogenesis [35]. High serum phosphate levels are associated with increased mortality in dialysis patients [46], non-dialysis CKD [47], and even in the general population [48]. High serum phosphorus also correlates with an increase in the risk of CKD progression [49].

Phosphorus can signal the vascular smooth muscle cells (VSMCs) to differentiate to an osteoblast-like phenotype that is able to lay collagen, in which hydroxyapatite crystals can be deposited. High phosphate also increases bone morphogenic protein-2 (BMP-2) expression. BMP-2, a member of the transforming growth factor family, upregulates the osteogenic transcriptional factors Runx-2 and Msx2 and downregulates the expression of the smooth muscle cell marker SM22α [50]. It has also been shown that phosphate has toxic effects on endothelial cells, increasing the production of reactive oxygen species and reducing nitric oxide synthesis, which leads to vasoconstriction [51]. Nevertheless, there are important limitations of the associations of phosphorus levels and adverse clinical outcomes. Serum phosphorus correlates poorly with total body phosphorus balance, and thus might represent a marker of a broader metabolic disorder. In addition, it is important to consider that *in vitro* analysis of the toxic effects of phosphate often relies on supraphysiological amounts of this mineral [52].

Calcium

Similar to phosphorus, most (99%) of the body calcium resides in the bone and teeth, predominantly in the form of hydroxyapatite (Ca_{10} $(PO_4)_6$ $(OH)_2$) [1]. Three forms of calcium circulate in the blood: albumin-bound (40%), ionized (50%), and others complexed with citrate, bicarbonate, and phosphate (10%) [53]. The last two forms of calcium are filtered in the glomerulus. Approximately 10 g of calcium are filtered daily in the glomeruli of which >90% is reabsorbed.

Calcium levels in a CKD patient are usually normal until in advanced stages. Increased PTH levels maintain calcium levels within close-to-normal limits in early CKD, despite the decrease in active vitamin D levels. In advanced CKD, however, hypocalcemia commonly occurs [54]. Further along in disease, persistent activation of the parathyroid glands can lead to hyperplasia and autonomous increase in PTH levels independent of calcium levels, thus leading to tertiary hyperparathyroidism and hypercalcemia. Hypercalcemia is synergistic with hyperphosphatemia in the induction of vascular calcification.

Vitamin-D

Low 1,25(OH)$_2$ vitamin D is common in CKD at all levels of GFR, 13% in those with GFR >80 ml/min1.73 m^2 and >60% in those with GFR <30 ml/min/1.73 m^2 [9]. The nutritional form of vitamin D is obtained from dietary, vegetal (ergocalciferol D$_2$), or animal sources (cholecalciferol D$_3$) and via the skin by exposure to sunlight. In the liver, vitamin D undergoes 25-hydroxylation. An activated form of vitamin D (1,25-dihydroxyvitamin D) is generated by 1-alpha-hydroxylation in the proximal renal tubules. The actions of 1,25(OH)$_2$ vitamin D include increasing intestinal absorption of calcium and phosphorus and decreasing PTH secretion, in addition to other pleiotropic actions that encompass different systems [55].

FGF-23 inhibits the transcription of 1-alpha-hydroxylase. FGF-23 also increases 24-hydroxylase which inactivates $1,25(OH)_2$ vitamin D, thus explaining why even patients with early-stage CKD have lower levels of this biologically active vitamin D analog [11]. With increasing FGF23 levels and a loss of functional renal tissue, the levels of the active vitamin D can decline even further.

PTH

Parathyroid hormone is a 84 amino acid peptide secreted by the parathyroid gland in response to hypocalcemia and possibly hyperphosphatemia [56]. PTH binds to the PTH/PTHrP receptor, a G protein-coupled receptor. Intracellularly, the main pathway activated by the PTH receptor is cyclic AMP generation and subsequently activation of PKA and further downstream signaling [57]. PTH is secreted in a pulsatile form and its effects on the bone depend on whether the PTH secretion and action are transient or sustained. PTH secretion has immediate calcemic and phosphaturic actions. In the bone, PTH actions include bone remodeling with release of stored calcium and phosphorus by increasing osteoclast activity via an increase in osteoblast function. Prolonged PTH signaling favors bone resorption over bone formation [58] and can result in hypercalcemia. PTH also leads to increased transcription of the 1-alpha hydroxylase to generate $1,25(OH)_2$ vitamin D and other less studied effects on the vasculature and the renin, angiotensin, aldosterone system (RAAS) [59]. The critically important synthesis and secretion of PTH are regulated by the calcium-sensing receptor (CaSR) [60], a conserved G protein-coupled receptor that responds to an increase in extracellular calcium with an increase in intracellular free calcium. Acutely, CaSR decreases PTH release, and long-term activation of CaSR suppresses parathyroid hormone gene expression [61]. Calcimimetics are medications that target this CaSR and are frequently used in CKD patients for the treatment of secondary hyperparathyroidism. By mimicking calcium and activating the CaSR, calcimimetics lower PTH levels.

Other Factors Implicated in Renal Osteodystrophy and Vascular Calcification

The bone morphogenic protein 7 (BMP-7) is a regulator of osteoblast differentiation that decreases with renal injury. Treatment with BMP-7 ameliorate renal osteodystrophy in animal models [62]. Deficiency of calcification inhibitors in CKD is common and relevant. These calcification inhibitors include matrix Gla protein (MGP), vitamin K osteopontin, fetuin-A, and pyrophosphate [63]. Vitamin K is a cofactor required for the carboxylation and activation of MGP, and vitamin K deficiency has been shown to be an important risk factor for extra skeletal calcification, including calciphylaxis [64, 65].

Clinical Manifestations of CKD-MBD

Renal Osteodystrophy and Osteoporosis

Renal osteodystrophy, a general term for bone disease in CKD patients, is defined by the KDIGO guidelines as an alteration in bone morphology in a patient with CKD [66]. Osteoporosis, a common diagnosis in the non-CKD population, is defined by the NIH as a "skeletal disorder characterized by compromised bone strength predisposing to an increased risk of fracture" [67]. Bone strength includes bone density (as evaluated by DEXA or CT scan) and bone quality. Bone quality takes into account bone remodeling, collagen cross-linking, bone microarchitecture, and mineralization [68]. In addition to osteoporosis risk factors present in the general aging population, patients with CKD frequently have abnormal turnover and mineralization that further contribute to bone fragility [68]. Thus, most patients with CKD have evidence of both renal osteodystrophy and osteoporosis (Table 14.2).

High Turnover Bone Disorders

The concept of bone disease associated with increased parathyroid hormone secretion has been documented since the 1920s, when the surgical resection of a parathyroid adenoma was performed for the treatment of osteitis fibrosa cystica [69]. In

Table 14.2 Definitions

Terminology	Definition
Renal osteodystrophy	Any alteration in bone morphology in a patient with CKD
Osteoporosis	Skeletal disorder characterized by compromised bone strength predisposing to an increased risk of fracture. Typically associated with low bone density measurement
Osteitis fibrosa cystica	Bone disease resulting from chronically elevated PTH levels and associated with high bone turnover, and increased resorption leading to cyst formation, replaced by fibrous tissue
Adynamic bone disease	Bone disease associated with decreased cellularity and decreased turnover
Osteomalacia	Bone disease characterized by increased osteoid formation that is insufficiently mineralized with normal or low turnover
Mixed uremic osteodystrophy	Bone disease with decreased mineralization and high turnover

1936, Fuller Albright described a patient with osteitis fibrosa cystica and renal disease, which he named "renal osteitis fibrosa cistica" [70], thus linking parathyroid excess in renal disease and bone disease. The bone in patients with osteitis fibrosa cystica from secondary or tertiary hyperparathyroidism shows increased cellularity (osteoblasts and osteoclasts) with disorganized, unmineralized collagen fibers (osteoid) and increased bone erosion. Proof of the association of high serum PTH levels with high turnover was obtained when comparing bone samples labeled with tetracycline in a cohort of CKD patients [71]. High turnover disease is more common in ESKD with very high serum PTH levels (i.e., usually higher than 200–300 pg/mL) [72, 73].

Low Turnover Bone Disorders

The effects of PTH on the bone are attenuated as CKD progresses [74]. The cause for PTH resistance is not completely understood and may involve oxidation of PTH, downregulation of receptor expression, or increased levels of truncated non-functional PTH fragments that compete for PTH receptor (PTHR1) signaling [75]. Indoxyl sulfate, a uremic toxin, can decrease cAMP generation by the PTHR1 in response to PTH [76]. In the late 1970s, it became apparent that some patients with renal disease had a particular form of renal bone disorder that was not responsive to activated vitamin D or calcium. It was soon found that many of these patients had aluminum deposition in the bone and low bone formation, as evaluated by tetracycline-labeled iliac crest bone biopsies, in addition to microcytic anemia and dementia [77]. The associated low turnover bone disease was called adynamic bone disease. Aluminum intoxication was traced to the tap water used in certain geographical areas for hemodialysis treatment and later to the use of aluminum-containing phosphate binders. Around the same time, an increasing number of ESKD patients receiving treatment with calcium and activated vitamin D for PTH suppression were also diagnosed with adynamic bone disease, with the implication that adynamic bone disease was also linked to the use of these medications, without having aluminum toxicity [77].

Histologically, adynamic bone disease is characterized by decreased numbers of osteoblasts and osteoclasts, with few sites of active bone formation. Mineralization is proportional to collagen synthesis, unlike osteomalacia where there is a lag in mineralization with increase in osteoid [73].

Aluminum-associated adynamic bone disease has substantially decreased with improvement in water purification and discontinuation of aluminum phosphate binders. However, iatrogenic suppression of PTH due to overaggressive treatment with Ca and vitamin D1,25 and presence of high calcium in dialysis fluid used for CAPD remain important causes of adynamic bone disease in ESKD patients. Furthermore, diabetes, the most common cause of ESKD in the USA, is associated with decreased secondary hyperparathyroidism and attenuated osteoblastic response to PTH [78, 79].

High turnover disease and adynamic bone disease can occur in the same patient at different stages of CKD. Indeed, adynamic bone disease is more common in pre-dialysis patients (48%), decreasing to 32% in patients on hemodialysis [80]. With progressive PTH increases in advancing CKD, a shift toward woven bone formation is established [77]. This general timeline is dynamic and depends on the risk factors present at each time point.

Disorders of Mineralization

Osteomalacia is a disorder in which there is a failure to mineralize the organic matrix of the bone. Histomorphometry findings consistent with osteomalacia are increased mineralization lag time and excess osteoid [81]. Such mineralization defects are seen in non-CKD patients with vitamin D deficiency, low phosphate, systemic acidosis, among other causes [82]. In CKD, defective mineralization can coexist with any rate of bone turnover. Defective mineralization with normal or low turnover disease is simply called osteomalacia in CKD. "Mixed renal osteodystrophy" indicates findings of high turnover disease combined with decreased mineralization [83].

Fractures

Patients with CKD have more than fourfold higher risk of fracture than the non-CKD population across all stages of CKD [84]. Demographic risk factors include older age, low body mass index, and long dialysis vintage. The increased risk of fracture might also be related to increased risks of falls and frailty, in addition to the bone abnormalities present in CKD [85]. Hip fracture risk has been the most studied. Those patients with CKD who suffer a fracture have worse clinical outcomes, with more prolonged hospitalizations and higher mortality, compared to non-CKD patients with fractures [85–87].

Vascular Calcification and Left Ventricular Hypertrophy

Patients with CKD and biochemical evidence of mineral bone disorders have a higher mortality than those with CKD without these abnormalities [88]. Among patients with CKD-MBD, those with high PTH, calcium, and phosphorus have the highest risk of cardiovascular hospitalization and death [88]. The presence of vascular calcifications, a major risk factor for cardiovascular related outcomes, is dramatically higher in patients with CKD [89]. More than 80% of adults on dialysis, including young adults, have evidence of coronary artery calcification [89, 90]. Vascular calcification consists of two main types: intimal and medial [50]. Patients with CKD have a higher than the average risk for both types of calcification, although medial calcification is more strongly associated with CKD and the underlying mineral disease [91]. Intimal calcification occurs with atherosclerosis, a process in which oxidized cholesterol permeates the arteries and leads to first inflammation [92] and ultimately calcification. The clinical consequences of intimal calcification and atherosclerosis include coronary artery disease, peripheral vascular disease, and cerebrovascular events. Medial calcification, also known as Monckenberg calcification, occurs as an active process from the imbalance of calcification promoters and calcification inhibitors, in which high levels of phosphorus, calcium, and PTH, in addition to low levels of fetuin-A, pyrophosphate, MGP, among others, result in ectopic calcification [47]. Medial calcification results in the loss of normal vessel elasticity, which leads to a higher pulse pressure, end-organ damage, and myocardial hypertrophy [93]. In addition to vascular calcification, the increased levels of FGF-23 and reduced levels of Klotho can independently and synergistically lead to cardiac hypertrophy and fibrosis [20].

Bone Disease After Renal Transplantation

Most patients with CKD have bone abnormalities preceding renal transplant [94]. The effects of renal transplant on bone depend on the pathology prior to transplantation. For most patients, there is a decrease in bone turnover, which is more pronounced in those with the higher turnover pre-transplant [95]. The fracture risk of transplant patients is higher than that of dialysis patients, especially in the first 3 years after transplant and remains higher than the general population even after a decade post-transplant. Three years after the transplant, the risk becomes lower than in dialysis patients [96].

The cause of this excess fracture risk after renal transplant is not well understood. Glucocorticoid use is likely a factor for this, and there is evidence to suggest that contemporary low-dose glucocorticoid has led to decreased bone loss after transplant [97]. Other considerations are the use of immunosuppressive medications [98], patient-specific factors such as age, nutritional status, mobility, and concomitant mineral disorders after transplant such as hypophosphatemia or hypomagnesemia.

Persistent hyperparathyroidism after renal transplant occurs in about 50% of transplant patients, in which the histologic changes that drove secondary or tertiary hyperparathyroidism during CKD fail to resolve after transplant [99]. The most common clinical manifestations include hypercalcemia and hypophosphatemia. Patient with persistently elevated PTH levels months after transplant have increased risk of fractures, and for unclear reasons, such levels are also associated with increased allograft loss and mortality [100].

Tertiary Hyperparathyroidism and Hungry Bone Syndrome

Elevated PTH (>65 pg/ml) becomes very prevalent (~50%) once GFR declines below 60 ml/min/1.73 m^2 [9]. As noted earlier, some patients with ESKD maintain increased PTH secretion despite hypercalcemia or treatment with vitamin D analogs or calcimimetics. This autonomous PTH secretion, i.e., tertiary hyperparathyroidism, is histologically characterized by parathyroid hyperplasia or clonal expansion of parathyroid cells (i.e., parathyroid adenoma) [101], with decreased expression of vitamin D receptors and CaSR in this abnormal parathyroid tissue [102]. CKD patients with preexisting high turnover disease are at particularly high risk for hungry bone syndrome after surgical parathyroidectomy [103]. This occurs when there is a net gain in bone formation over resorption after surgery. Hypocalcemia can be severe and protracted and might be accompanied by hypophosphatemia, hypomagnesemia, and hyperkalemia.

Calciphylaxis

Calciphylaxis is a form of vascular calcification affecting the intima and media of small- and medium-sized arteries of the subcutaneous tissues, leading to tissue ischemia. Patients diagnosed with calciphylaxis have severe morbidity and mortality [104]. The initial lesion of calciphylaxis is often a violaceous or livedo-reticularis like rash located in the thighs or lower-abdomen. This initial rash can be very painful. Later, these areas can become necrotic and lead to ulcers that are indurated. If these lesions become infected, they can lead to sepsis. A high-index of suspicion is important when evaluating any dermatologic disorder, specially ulcers, in patients with CKD, since calciphylaxis can affect non-typical areas such as the distal part of the extremities and penis and is not always painful [105].The disease was traditionally associated with secondary hyperparathyroidism but has more recently been shown that patients have usually PTH within limits for the stage of renal failure [106]. The use of calcium supplements or vitamin D to suppress PTH is a risk factor for calciphylaxis [107].

Dialysis-Related Amyloidosis

Patients living with advanced CKD have ten times higher serum levels of beta-2-microglobulin (B2M), a protein that is part of HLA-1 complexes and 97% renally cleared [108]. Accumulated and modified (i.e., by advanced glycation end products) B2M predominantly deposits in the osteoarticular surfaces and generates corresponding clinical manifestations [109]. Carpal tunnel syndrome is the most prevalent of these manifestations and continues to be a burden for ESKD patients in parts of the world where there is less access to renal transplant [110]. Rotator cuff tendinitis from B2M amyloid can present as unexplained shoulder pain in patients that have been on long-term dialysis (i.e., >10 years) [111]. Destructive spondylo-arthropathy can lead to back pain or weakness due to involvement of the spine or peripheral nerves [112]. The treatment of dialysis-related amyloidosis includes sur-gical correction of the bone lesions, in addition to increased B2M removal by renal transplantation, increased dialysis duration, hemofiltration, or use of an apheresis column that has increased B2M clearance [113].

Other Manifestations

Patients with secondary or tertiary hyperparathyroidism can develop brown tumors (osteoclastomas), which represent cavities inside the bone with necrosis and fibrous tissue accumulation. Uremic leontiasis ossea is a very rare complication of hyper-parathyroidism, resulting from high bone turnover and defective mineralization. Patients exhibit jaw enlargement and protrusion of the mandible [114].

Diagnosis

Biochemistry Diagnosis

Calcium and Phosphorus

Hypocalcemia and hypercalcemia are both common in advanced CKD stages and are associated with greater mortality than corresponding patients with normocalce-mia [5, 115]. Mild hypocalcemia is usually well tolerated, while hypercalcemia can be associated with uncontrolled PTH secretion and carries a higher risk of extra skeletal calcification. This provides the treatment rationale for avoiding hypercalce-mia and hyperphosphatemia by the KDIGO guidelines [6].

PTH and Serologic Markers of Bone Turnover

Circulating PTH includes biologically relevant PTH (1–84), multiple C-terminal fragments, and fewer N-terminal fragments. The kidney is responsible for clearing this C-terminal fragments and thus their proportion is increased in patients with CKD [116]. The biological relevance of this is not clear. However, it is important to note that older, first-generation PTH assays detected these fragments and can lead to diagnosis of hyperparathyroidism when indeed a patient had much lower levels of the intact PTH (1–84) [117, 118]. Third-generation assays use two antibodies that bind to different regions of PTH and detect only the biologically fully active PTH (1–84). It is also possible to detect only the non-oxidized forms of PTH. While oxidized forms might be less active in vitro, the clinical relevance of measuring only non-oxidized PTH has not been proven [119]. Using third-generation assays, the normal range is found to be about 4.6–26.8 pg/ml, which varies between different institutions and assays. Levels <100 pg/ml in dialysis patients are associated with low turnover disease, while levels >500 pg/ml are associated with high turnover disease [66]. The KDIGO guidelines recommend to measure PTH levels every 6–12 months for patients with CKD stage 4 and every 3–6 months in patients with CKD stage 5 [66].

Other markers of bone turnover are bone-specific alkaline phosphatase (BSAP), the amino-terminal propetide, tartrate-resistant acid phosphatase 5b (TRAP5b), and procollagen type 1 N-terminal propeptide (PINP). BSAP and TRAP5b do not accumulate with decreased renal clearance, while PTH fragments (C-truncated) do. Although all these markers are associated with bone turnover, none has the necessary sensitivity or specificity for widespread clinical utilization [120]. Some of the reasons underlying this are that bone formation (measured by PINP) and resorption (measured by TRAP5b) are not adequately coupled in advanced CKD. Thus, it is not possible to consistently predict turnover by measuring only one part of the process. BSAP, which is produced by osteoblast during bone formation, is associated with bone formation rate and is able to discriminate well low turnover disease (AUC >0.80), but it has not been shown to be superior to intact PTH levels in predicting high bone turnover [121].

Vitamin D

Vitamin D can be measured as 25(OH) vitamin D or the active 1,25(OH)$_2$ vitamin D. 25(OH)D concentration is regarded as a biomarker of vitamin D intake from cutaneous synthesis and dietary consumption [122]. KDIGO guidelines endorse the measurement of 25(OH)D to detect deficiency and suggest to correct those with vitamin D deficiency, as in the general population. 1,25(OH)$_2$ vitamin D is not routinely measured in CKD [66].

Imaging

Renal osteodystrophy changes can be seen by X-ray, particularly at advanced stages. The classic findings of osteitis fibrosa cystica include subperiosteal bone resorption, appreciated early in the phalanges, and in advanced stages trabecular reabsorption, which can lead to the classic cranial skull manifestation of "salt and pepper" [123]. Plain X-ray, especially abdominal X-ray, can also be used to detect vascular calcification [124].

Peripheral quantitative computed tomography (pQCT) provides a more detailed bone imaging that is able to discriminate between cortical and trabecular bone. Thinner cortices and trabecular bone loss as analyzed by pQCT have been associated with fractures in CKD patients [125]. This is a useful tool to follow up changes in bone after treatment with medicines for osteoporosis, but it is not established for the diagnosis of osteoporosis [126].

The utility of DXA scan has been well established in the non-CKD population and is endorsed by all society guidelines as a screening method in women more than 65 years old [127] and in other selected population with risk factors.

In CKD patients with stages 3–5, the use of DXA scan for osteoporosis screening, similarly to non-CKD population has been recently recommended by KIDGO guidelines in CKD patients. This recommendation is based on the results of cohort studies that demonstrate that DXA-measured bone mineral density predicts risk of fracture in CKD patients and can help to risk-stratify patients to treatment with new osteoporosis medicines that are now available for patients with reduced GFR [128].

Bone Biopsy

Bone histomorphometry informs bone turnover, mineralization, and volume, and, indirectly, bone quality [77]. Bone biopsy is currently the gold standard for diagnosis of the specific type of renal osteodystrophy and should be considered in patients with high risk for fractures in which knowing the specific type of bone disease can affect management decisions. For example, a bone biopsy could be particularly helpful in a patient with low bone density but near-normal levels of PTH or bone-specific alkaline phosphatase, as it could help distinguish osteoporosis from adynamic bone disease, which have different implications for treatment. However, there are some limitations. First, bone biopsy is an invasive procedure and there are only a limited number of centers that have the sufficient expertise to perform and interpret this. Second, bone biopsy findings reflect skeletal status only at a single time point. Moreover, a biopsy taken from the iliac crest does not necessarily reflect changes at other sites of the skeleton. Despite these limitations, when available bone biopsy can be determinant to inform treatment.

Treatment

Mineral Disorder

The main goal in the treatment of mineral bone disorder is to prevent or delay the development of vascular calcification and its associated morbidity and mortality, while maintaining adequate levels of calcium and phosphorus, both of which are vital for normal cell function. It is recommended to maintain normal levels of phosphorus to avoid hypercalcemia. Phosphate-lowering strategies include dietary interventions, use of phosphate binders, and renal replacement therapy [129].

Dietary counseling is important, especially since highly processed food can have high levels of sodium and phosphorus [130]. However, lowering phosphorus has not demonstrated improvement in clinical outcomes, and there is concern that stringent restrictions in dialysis patients might have detrimental effects [131], so for patients with persistently high phosphorus level despite diet counseling, other measures are frequently needed.

Most patients with CKD stage 5 and dialysis-dependency are prescribed phosphate binders. Types of phosphate binders include aluminum hydroxide, calcium-containing (i.e., calcium acetate), non-calcium-containing (i.e., sevelamer), and iron-based binders (i.e., ferric citrate) [132]. All of them are effective in decreasing phosphate levels. Trials examining phosphate binders have focused on biochemical parameters, in which non-calcium-containing binders have shown superiority to calcium-containing binders [133]. There is no evidence of an impact on cardiovascular mortality or other important clinical outcomes when comparing these medications against placebo [52]. Three recent randomized controlled trials showed that calcium-containing binders were associated with higher cardiovascular mortality than non-calcium-containing binders and there is little doubt that patients with CKD or dialysis tend to have a positive calcium balance when receiving supplemental calcium [134]. These findings support current recommendations of avoiding calcium-containing binders, especially in patients with elevated calcium levels. These studies have several limitations [135], and the off-target effects and costs of specific phosphate binders should be taken into account [136].

Dialysis (hemodialysis or peritoneal dialysis) is effective for treating hyperphosphatemia in advanced renal disease. The dialysis prescription (time and duration) can be adjusted to improve phosphate clearance.

Most patients with CKD do not need specific interventions to maintain serum calcium levels. It is recommended to avoid hypercalcemia, while maintaining normal or even levels slightly below normal in patients with CKD [66].

Secondary and Tertiary Hyperparathyroidism

The optimal level of PTH in patients with CKD is unclear. In patients not on dialysis who have persistently elevated PTH levels, it is important to evaluate for modifiable risk factors such as hyperphosphatemia or vitamin D deficiency. Those who have rising levels (rather than a single level), especially those with >3 times the upper limit, and no modifiable risk factors should be considered for the use of vitamin D agonists, as long as they do not have concomitant hyperphosphatemia or hypercalcemia [137] (Fig. 14.2).

In patients on dialysis, modifiable risk factors should be evaluated, and PTH trends rather than an absolute number should be used when deciding to start medications. Most patients who have PTH levels that are persistently above 4–6 times the upper limit of normal should receive initial treatment with a vitamin D agonist or calcimimetic [66]. This rationale comes from the association of very high PTH levels (i.e., over 6 times normal) and high turnover disease, as well as an association between high PTH levels and mortality. For those who have hypercalcemia or calciphylaxis, a calcimimetic is preferred over vitamin D agonists [138]. The Evaluation of Cinacalcet Hydrochloride Therapy to Lower Cardiovascular Events (EVOLVE) study evaluated the effect of cinacalcet versus placebo in 3883 patients. Patients who received cinacalcet had a non-statistically significant (HR: 0.93; $P = 0.11$) reduction on the primary outcome, a clinical composite which included all-cause mortality and other cardiovascular outcomes [139].

In refractory cases with very high PTH levels, surgical parathyroidectomy should be considered (Fig. 14.2) [66]. Patients who undergo parathyroidectomy are at high risk of hungry bone syndrome [103]. Post-operatively, patients require calcium and vitamin D supplementation, oral and often intravenous. In addition, it is important to supplement magnesium and phosphate and to monitor potassium levels. Patients on dialysis should often be dialyzed the day after surgery for hyperkalemia

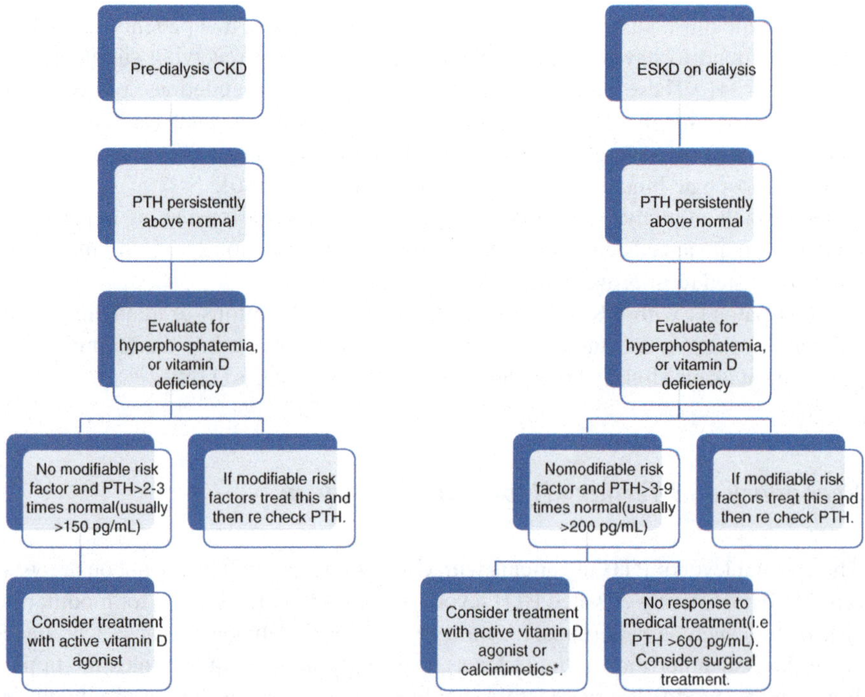

Fig. 14.2 Approach to secondary hyperparathyroidism. No absolute PTH number should be used for decision management. Treatment should be guided by a trend in PTH levels, rather than a single value. *In patients with hypercalcemia or hyperphosphatemia, calcimimetics are preferred over vitamin D agonists

management.

Renal Osteodystrophy

General management of renal osteodystrophy includes mineral management as above and control of metabolic acidosis [140].

Extreme PTH levels are currently used as surrogates for bone turnover status [141]. High turnover disease is managed with PTH suppression. In patients with low turnover disease, calcium supplements, vitamin D, and calcimimetics should be discontinued. The substantial risk of fractures in the CKD population has not been attenuated by treatment of mineral disease or treatment of secondary hyperparathyroidism [84]. Therefore, there is an increased interest in the use of the antiresorptive or anabolic medications, as in the general population. For patients with GFR >30 ml/min, FDA-approved medications include bisphosphonates, denosumab, and teriparatide [84]. *Post-hoc* analysis have shown that risendronate, denosumab, and teriparatide increase bone density in patients with mild to moderate CKD, similar to non-CKD patients [142–144]. Bisphosphonate and denosumab inhibit osteoclast-mediated reabsorption and should be considered for patients with CKD and osteoporosis who do not have evidence of adynamic bone disease. Denosumab can cause severe hypocalcemia, especially in CKD, thus this needs to be monitored [84]. Teriparatide and abaloparatide are PTH and PTHrP analogs, respectively, that have anabolic effects.

While these medicines are promising for patients with CKD and osteoporosis that have high turnover (antiresorptive) or low turnover disease (anabolic), prior studies have excluded patients with abnormal PTH levels, and so there is a need for research that identifies whether these medicines are safe and effective in patients with CKD.

Calciphylaxis

The treatment of calciphylaxis involves local control of established lesions and improving the balance of calcification promoters and calcification inhibitors [104]. Caring for the wounds of calciphylaxis necessitates debridement of non-viable tissues, preferably by a surgeon familiar with these wounds [145]. It is important to minimize trauma to adjacent tissue to avoid precipitating new lesions. Antibiotics should be reserved for wounds with signs of infection.

Hyperphosphatemia should be treated by diet, phosphate binders, and dialysis. The use of non-calcium-containing binders is also preferred for patients with calciphylaxis [146]. Medical treatment of secondary hyperparathyroidism is indicated to maintain PTH levels around 150–300 pg/mL. In the EVOLVE study, cinacalcet use was associated with a reduction in the incidence of calciphylaxis compared to placebo [139]. When medications are insufficient to lower PTH to goal levels, parathyroidectomy is required.

A systematic review of a patient's risk factor and medications should be done [146]. Medications that have been associated with calciphylaxis include warfarin, iron, vitamin D, calcium, and glucocorticoids [104]. Warfarin should be discontinued in all patients with calciphylaxis. If anticoagulation is needed, apixaban may be an option for a select group of ESKD patients [147].

Observational studies suggest that sodium thiosulfate, systemic or intralesional, may provide benefit in the treatment of calciphylaxis [145] and should be considered for all patients. The adverse effects of this include metabolic acidosis, QT prolongation, and hypocalcemia. It is typically prescribed with intermittent hemodialysis sessions 3 times a week in the last hour of dialysis, or 3 times per week in patients on peritoneal dialysis. Other available treatments that are under study and not used routinely are vitamin K and bisphosphonates [105].

Conclusions and Perspectives

Patients with CKD have a substantially increased risk of vascular calcification and fractures, two manifestations linked to the underlying mineral disorder of patients with reduced glomerular filtration. Recognizing a common underlying pathophysiologic process for these clinical manifestations, the acronym CKD-MBD was coined in 2006. Multiple markers exist for CKD-MBD, including high serum phosphorus, PTH, FGF-23, and decreased levels of Klotho, calcium, and active vitamin D. The availability of these markers, bone histomorphometry, and the understanding of the basic pathologic concepts of CKD-MBD have led to progress. Today, extreme effects due to uncontrolled hyperparathyroidism are rare, and aluminum-induced osteomalacia has nearly disappeared. However, effective treatments to prevent and treat vascular calcification, calciphylaxis, and fractures are still lacking. Improving outcomes in this regard will require multiple approaches. For fracture prevention, medicines that have been proven to benefit the non-CKD population should be adequately studied in CKD population. Vascular calcification is a dynamic process where we might need alternative markers of disease and new targets for treatment. While we wait for these advances, a rationale treatment of CKD-MBD can be applied to every patient by integrating each patient's clinical, biochemical, and radiologic parameter.

Conflict of Interest/Financial Disclosure S.U.N. reports grant support from Hope Pharmaceuticals, Laboratories Sanifit, and Inozyme Pharma to his institute and honoraria from Fresenius Renal Therapies, Epizon Pharma, and Laboratoris Sanifit.

References

1. Brown E. Physiology of calcium homeostasis. Parathyroids. 2001;2:167–81.
2. Gardella TJ, Jüppner H, Potts JT Jr. Receptors for parathyroid hormone and parathyroid hormone–related protein. In: Principles of bone biology. Elsevier; 2020. p. 691–712.

3. Wang Y, Zhu J, DeLuca HF. The vitamin D receptor in the proximal renal tubule is a key regulator of serum 1α, 25-dihydroxyvitamin D3. Am J Physiol Endocrinol Metab. 2015;308(3):E201–E5.
4. Tallon S, Berdud I, Hernandez A, Concepcion MT, Almaden Y, Torres A, et al. Relative effects of PTH and dietary phosphorus on calcitriol production in normal and azotemic rats. Kidney Int. 1996;49(5):1441–6.
5. Floege J, Kim J, Ireland E, Chazot C, Drueke T, de Francisco A, et al. Serum iPTH, calcium and phosphate, and the risk of mortality in a European haemodialysis population. Nephrol Dial Transplant. 2011;26(6):1948–55.
6. Isakova T, Nickolas TL, Denburg M, Yarlagadda S, Weiner DE, Gutiérrez OM, et al. KDOQI US commentary on the 2017 KDIGO clinical practice guideline update for the diagnosis, evaluation, prevention, and treatment of chronic kidney disease–mineral and bone disorder (CKD-MBD). Am J Kidney Dis. 2017;70(6):737–51.
7. Labriola L, Jadoul M, editors. Dialysis-related amyloidosis: is it gone or should it be? Semin Dial. 2017;30(3):193–6. Wiley Online Library.
8. Nickolas TL, Chen N, McMahon DJ, Dempster D, Zhou H, Dominguez J, et al. A microRNA approach to discriminate cortical low bone turnover in renal osteodystrophy. JBMR Plus. 2020;4(5):e10353.
9. Rouached M, Boutchich SEK, Al Rifai AM, Garabédian M, Fournier A. Prevalence of abnormal serum vitamin D, PTH, calcium, and phosphorus in patients with chronic kidney disease: results of the study to evaluate early kidney disease. Kidney Int. 2008;74(3):389–90.
10. Block GA, Ix JH, Ketteler M, Martin KJ, Thadhani RI, Tonelli M, et al. Phosphate homeostasis in CKD: report of a scientific symposium sponsored by the National Kidney Foundation. Am J Kidney Dis. 2013;62(3):457–73.
11. Gutiérrez OM. Fibroblast growth factor 23 and disordered vitamin D metabolism in chronic kidney disease: updating the "trade-off" hypothesis. Clin J Am Soc Nephrol. 2010;5(9):1710–6.
12. Bricker NS. On the pathogenesis of the uremic state: an exposition of the trade-off hypothesis. N Engl J Med. 1972;286(20):1093–9.
13. White KE, Evans WE, O'Riordan JL, Speer MC, Econs MJ, Lorenz-Depiereux B, et al. Autosomal dominant hypophosphataemic rickets is associated with mutations in FGF23. Nat Genet. 2000;26(3):345–8.
14. Shimada T, Mizutani S, Muto T, Yoneya T, Hino R, Takeda S, et al. Cloning and characterization of FGF23 as a causative factor of tumor-induced osteomalacia. Proc Natl Acad Sci. 2001;98(11):6500–5.
15. Jonsson KB, Zahradnik R, Larsson T, White KE, Sugimoto T, Imanishi Y, et al. Fibroblast growth factor 23 in oncogenic osteomalacia and X-linked hypophosphatemia. N Engl J Med. 2003;348(17):1656–63.
16. Jüppner H. Phosphate and FGF-23. Kidney Int. 2011;79:S24–S7.
17. Ix JH, Shlipak MG, Wassel CL, Whooley MA. Fibroblast growth factor-23 and early decrements in kidney function: the Heart and Soul Study. Nephrol Dial Transplant. 2010;25(3):993–7.
18. Portale AA, Wolf M, Jüppner H, Messinger S, Kumar J, Wesseling-Perry K, et al. Disordered FGF23 and mineral metabolism in children with CKD. Clin J Am Soc Nephrol. 2014;9(2):344–53.
19. Simic P, Kim W, Zhou W, Pierce KA, Chang W, Sykes DB, et al. Glycerol-3-phosphate is an FGF23 regulator derived from the injured kidney. J Clin Invest. 2020;130(3):1513–26.
20. Gutiérrez OM. Fibroblast growth factor 23 and the last mile. Clin J Am Soc Nephrol. 2020;15(9):1355–7.
21. Gattineni J, Bates C, Twombley K, Dwarakanath V, Robinson ML, Goetz R, et al. FGF23 decreases renal NaPi-2a and NaPi-2c expression and induces hypophosphatemia in vivo predominantly via FGF receptor 1. Am J Physiol Renal Physiol. 2009;297(2):F282–F91.
22. Saito H, Kusano K, Kinosaki M, Ito H, Hirata M, Segawa H, et al. Human fibroblast growth factor-23 mutants suppress Na+−dependent phosphate co-transport activity and 1α, 25-dihydroxyvitamin D3 production. J Biol Chem. 2003;278(4):2206–11.

23. Gutiérrez OM, Mannstadt M, Isakova T, Rauh-Hain JA, Tamez H, Shah A, et al. Fibroblast growth factor 23 and mortality among patients undergoing hemodialysis. N Engl J Med. 2008;359(6):584–92.
24. Smith ER. The use of fibroblast growth factor 23 testing in patients with kidney disease. Clin J Am Soc Nephrol. 2014;9(7):1283–303.
25. Faul C, Amaral AP, Oskouei B, Hu M-C, Sloan A, Isakova T, et al. FGF23 induces left ventricular hypertrophy. J Clin Invest. 2011;121(11):4393–408.
26. Dussold C, Gerber C, White S, Wang X, Qi L, Francis C, et al. DMP1 prevents osteocyte alterations, FGF23 elevation and left ventricular hypertrophy in mice with chronic kidney disease. Bone Res. 2019;7(1):1–12.
27. Faul C. Cardiac actions of fibroblast growth factor 23. Bone. 2017;100:69–79.
28. Carpenter TO, Whyte MP, Imel EA, Boot AM, Högler W, Linglart A, et al. Burosumab therapy in children with X-linked hypophosphatemia. N Engl J Med. 2018;378(21):1987–98.
29. Shalhoub V, Shatzen EM, Ward SC, Davis J, Stevens J, Bi V, et al. FGF23 neutralization improves chronic kidney disease–associated hyperparathyroidism yet increases mortality. J Clin Invest. 2012;122(7):2543–53.
30. Kuro-o M, Matsumura Y, Aizawa H, Kawaguchi H, Suga T, Utsugi T, et al. Mutation of the mouse klotho gene leads to a syndrome resembling ageing. Nature. 1997;390(6655):45–51.
31. Kuro-o M. Klotho as a regulator of oxidative stress and senescence. Biol Chem. 2008;389(3):233–41.
32. Hruska KA, Williams MJ, Sugatani T. Chronic kidney disease–mineral and bone disorders. In: Chronic renal disease. United Kingdom: Elsevier; 2020. p. 551–69.
33. Liu H, Fergusson MM, Castilho RM, Liu J, Cao L, Chen J, et al. Augmented Wnt signaling in a mammalian model of accelerated aging. Science. 2007;317(5839):803–6.
34. Kurosu H, Yamamoto M, Clark JD, Pastor JV, Nandi A, Gurnani P, et al. Suppression of aging in mice by the hormone Klotho. Science. 2005;309(5742):1829–33.
35. Yamada S, Giachelli CM. Vascular calcification in CKD-MBD: roles for phosphate, FGF23, and Klotho. Bone. 2017;100:87–93.
36. Agapova OA, Fang Y, Sugatani T, Seifert ME, Hruska KA. Ligand trap for the activin type IIA receptor protects against vascular disease and renal fibrosis in mice with chronic kidney disease. Kidney Int. 2016;89(6):1231–43.
37. Sun C-Y, Chang S-C, Wu M-S. Suppression of Klotho expression by protein-bound uremic toxins is associated with increased DNA methyltransferase expression and DNA hypermethylation. Kidney Int. 2012;81(7):640–50.
38. Krishnan V, Bryant HU, MacDougald OA. Regulation of bone mass by Wnt signaling. J Clin Invest. 2006;116(5):1202–9.
39. Cosman F, Crittenden DB, Adachi JD, Binkley N, Czerwinski E, Ferrari S, et al. Romosozumab treatment in postmenopausal women with osteoporosis. N Engl J Med. 2016;375(16):1532–43.
40. Pelletier S, Dubourg L, Carlier M-C, Hadj-Aissa A, Fouque D. The relation between renal function and serum sclerostin in adult patients with CKD. Clin J Am Soc Nephrol. 2013;8(5):819–23.
41. Moe SM, Chen NX, Newman CL, Organ JM, Kneissel M, Kramer I, et al. Anti-sclerostin antibody treatment in a rat model of progressive renal osteodystrophy. J Bone Miner Res. 2015;30(3):499–509.
42. Cejka D, Marculescu R, Kozakowski N, Plischke M, Reiter T, Gessl A, et al. Renal elimination of sclerostin increases with declining kidney function. J Clin Endocrinol Metabol. 2014;99(1):248–55.
43. Evenepoel P, D'haese P, Brandenburg V. Sclerostin and DKK1: new players in renal bone and vascular disease. Kidney Int. 2015;88(2):235–40.
44. Blaine J, Chonchol M, Levi M. Renal control of calcium, phosphate, and magnesium homeostasis. Clin J Am Soc Nephrol. 2015;10(7):1257–72.
45. Blumsohn A. What have we learnt about the regulation of phosphate metabolism? Curr Opin Nephrol Hypertens. 2004;13(4):397–401.

46. Fernández-Martín JL, Martínez-Camblor P, Dionisi MP, Floege J, Ketteler M, London G, et al. Improvement of mineral and bone metabolism markers is associated with better survival in haemodialysis patients: the COSMOS study. Nephrol Dial Transplant. 2015;30(9):1542–51.
47. Goodman WG, London G, Amann K, Block GA, Giachelli C, Hruska KA, et al. Vascular calcification in chronic kidney disease. Am J Kidney Dis. 2004;43(3):572–9.
48. Tonelli M, Sacks F, Pfeffer M, Gao Z, Curhan G. Relation between serum phosphate level and cardiovascular event rate in people with coronary disease. Circulation. 2005;112(17):2627–33.
49. Zoccali C, Ruggenenti P, Perna A, Leonardis D, Tripepi R, Tripepi G, et al. Phosphate may promote CKD progression and attenuate renoprotective effect of ACE inhibition. J Am Soc Nephrol. 2011;22(10):1923–30.
50. Moe SM, Chen NX. Mechanisms of vascular calcification in chronic kidney disease. J Am Soc Nephrol. 2008;19(2):213–6.
51. Burger D, Levin A. 'Shedding' light on mechanisms of hyperphosphatemic vascular dysfunction. Kidney Int. 2013;83(2):187–9.
52. Toussaint ND, Pedagogos E, Lioufas NM, Elder GJ, Pascoe EM, Badve SV, et al. A randomized trial on the effect of phosphate reduction on vascular end points in CKD (IMPROVE-CKD). J Am Soc Nephrol. 2020;31(11):2653–66.
53. Felsenfeld AJ, Levine BS, Rodriguez M, editors. Pathophysiology of calcium, phosphorus, and magnesium dysregulation in chronic kidney disease. Semin Dial. 2015;28(6):564–77. Wiley Online Library.
54. Evenepoel P, Wolf M. A balanced view of calcium and phosphate homeostasis in chronic kidney disease. Kidney Int. 2013;83(5):789–91.
55. Pilz S, Iodice S, Zittermann A, Grant WB, Gandini S. Vitamin D status and mortality risk in CKD: a meta-analysis of prospective studies. Am J Kidney Dis. 2011;58(3):374–82.
56. Gardella TJ, Nissenson RA, Jüppner H. Parathyroid hormone. Primer on the metabolic bone diseases and disorders of mineral. Metabolism. 2018;205:205–11
57. Gardella TJ. The parathyroid hormone receptor type 1. Osteoporosis. Switzerland: Springer; 2020. p. 323–47.
58. Hattersley G, Dean T, Corbin BA, Bahar H, Gardella TJ. Binding selectivity of abaloparatide for PTH-type-1-receptor conformations and effects on downstream signaling. Endocrinology. 2016;157(1):141–9.
59. Hulter H, Melby J, Peterson J, Cooke C. Chronic continuous PTH infusion results in hypertension in normal subjects. J Clin Hypertens. 1986;2(4):360.
60. Hofer AM, Brown EM. Extracellular calcium sensing and signalling. Nat Rev Mol Cell Biol. 2003;4(7):530–8.
61. Riccardi D, Kemp PJ. The calcium-sensing receptor beyond extracellular calcium homeostasis: conception, development, adult physiology, and disease. Annu Rev Physiol. 2012;74:271–97.
62. Li T, Surendran K, Zawaideh MA, Mathew S, Hruska KA. Bone morphogenetic protein 7: a novel treatment for chronic renal and bone disease. Curr Opin Nephrol Hypertens. 2004;13(4):417–22.
63. Lomashvili KA, Cobbs S, Hennigar RA, Hardcastle KI, O'Neill WC. Phosphate-induced vascular calcification: role of pyrophosphate and osteopontin. J Am Soc Nephrol. 2004;15(6):1392–401.
64. Levy D, Grewal R, Le TH. Vitamin K deficiency: an emerging player in the pathogenesis of vascular calcification and an iatrogenic consequence of therapies in advanced renal disease. Rockville: American Physiological Society; 2020.
65. Brandenburg VM, Schuh A, Kramann R. Valvular calcification in chronic kidney disease. Adv Chronic Kidney Dis. 2019;26(6):464–71.
66. Update IGOKC-M. KDIGO 2017 clinical practice guideline update for the diagnosis, evaluation, prevention, and treatment of chronic kidney disease–mineral and bone disorder (CKD-MBD). Kidney Int Suppl. 2017;7(1):1.
67. Health NIo. NIH consensus development panel on osteoporosis prevention, diagnosis, and therapy, March 7-29, 2000: highlights of the conference. South Med J. 2001;94(6):569–73.

68. Moe SM. Renal osteodystrophy or kidney-induced osteoporosis? Curr Osteoporos Rep. 2017;15(3):194–7.
69. Mandl F. Therapeutisher Versuch bei Ostitis fibrosa generalisata mittels Exstirpation eines Epithelkorperchentumors. Zentrlbl Chir. 1926;5:260–4.
70. Albright F. Renal osteitis fibrosa cystica: Repot of a case. With dissection of metabolic aspects. Bull Johns Hopkins Hosp. 1937;60:377–99.
71. Ott SM. Renal osteodystrophy—time for common nomenclature. Curr Osteoporos Rep. 2017;15(3):187–93.
72. Evenepoel P, Bover J, Torres PU. Parathyroid hormone metabolism and signaling in health and chronic kidney disease. Kidney Int. 2016;90(6):1184–90.
73. Salusky IB, Goodman WG. Adynamic renal osteodystrophy: is there a problem? J Am Soc Nephrol. 2001;12(9):1978–85.
74. Bover J, Ureña-Torres PA, Evenepoel P, Lloret MJ, Guirado L, Rodríguez M. PTH receptors and skeletal resistance to PTH action. In: Parathyroid glands in chronic kidney disease. Cham: Springer; 2020. p. 51–77.
75. Slatopolsky E, Finch J, Clay P, Martin D, Sicard G, Singer G, et al. A novel mechanism for skeletal resistance in uremia. Kidney Int. 2000;58(2):753–61.
76. Nii-Kono T, Iwasaki Y, Uchida M, Fujieda A, Hosokawa A, Motojima M, et al. Indoxyl sulfate induces skeletal resistance to parathyroid hormone in cultured osteoblastic cells. Kidney Int. 2007;71(8):738–43.
77. Drüeke TB, Massy ZA. Changing bone patterns with progression of chronic kidney disease. Kidney Int. 2016;89(2):289–302.
78. Vincenti F, Hattner R, Amend WJ, Feduska NJ, Duca RM, Salvatierra O. Decreased secondary hyperparathyroidism in diabetic patients receiving hemodialysis. JAMA. 1981;245(9):930–3.
79. Shires R, Teitelbaum S, Bergfeld M, Fallon M, Slatopolsky E, Avioli L. The effect of streptozotocin-induced chronic diabetes mellitus on bone and mineral homeostasis in the rat. J Lab Clin Med. 1981;97(2):231–40.
80. Torres A, Lorenzo V, Hernández D, Rodríguez JC, Concepción MT, Rodríguez AP, et al. Bone disease in predialysis, hemodialysis, and CAPD patients: evidence of a better bone response to PTH. Kidney Int. 1995;47(5):1434–42.
81. Bhan A, Qiu S, Rao SD. Bone histomorphometry in the evaluation of osteomalacia. Bone Rep. 2018;8:125–34.
82. Mankin H. Rickets, osteomalacia, and renal osteodystrophy. An update. Orthop Clin North Am. 1990;21(1):81.
83. Wang M, Hercz G, Sherrard DJ, Maloney NA, Segre GV, Pei Y. Relationship between intact 1–84 parathyroid hormone and bone histomorphometric parameters in dialysis patients without aluminum toxicity. Am J Kidney Dis. 1995;26(5):836–44.
84. Khairallah P, Nickolas TL. Management of osteoporosis in CKD. Clin J Am Soc Nephrol. 2018;13(6):962–9.
85. Kim SM, Long J, Montez-Rath M, Leonard M, Chertow GM. Hip fracture in patients with non-dialysis-requiring chronic kidney disease. J Bone Miner Res. 2016;31(10):1803–9.
86. Maravic M, Ostertag A, Torres P, Cohen-Solal M. Incidence and risk factors for hip fractures in dialysis patients. Osteoporos Int. 2014;25(1):159–65.
87. Tentori F, McCullough K, Kilpatrick RD, Bradbury BD, Robinson BM, Kerr PG, et al. High rates of death and hospitalization follow bone fracture among hemodialysis patients. Kidney Int. 2014;85(1):166–73.
88. Block GA, Kilpatrick RD, Lowe KA, Wang W, Danese MD. CKD–mineral and bone disorder and risk of death and cardiovascular hospitalization in patients on hemodialysis. Clin J Am Soc Nephrol. 2013;8(12):2132–40.
89. Goodman WG, Goldin J, Kuizon BD, Yoon C, Gales B, Sider D, et al. Coronary-artery calcification in young adults with end-stage renal disease who are undergoing dialysis. N Engl J Med. 2000;342(20):1478–83.

90. Merjanian R, Budoff M, Adler S, Berman N, Mehrotra R. Coronary artery, aortic wall, and valvular calcification in nondialyzed individuals with type 2 diabetes and renal disease. Kidney Int. 2003;64(1):263–71.
91. Shanahan CM, Crouthamel MH, Kapustin A, Giachelli CM. Arterial calcification in chronic kidney disease: key roles for calcium and phosphate. Circ Res. 2011;109(6):697–711.
92. Fishbein GA, Fishbein MC. Arteriosclerosis: rethinking the current classification. Arch Pathol Lab Med. 2009;133(8):1309–16.
93. Giachelli CM. Vascular calcification mechanisms. J Am Soc Nephrol. 2004;15(12):2959–64.
94. Drüeke TB, Evenepoel P. The bone after kidney transplantation. Clin J Am Soc Nephrol. 2019;14:795–7.
95. Keronen S, Martola L, Finne P, Burton IS, Kröger H, Honkanen E. Changes in bone histomorphometry after kidney transplantation. Clin J Am Soc Nephrol. 2019;14(6):894–903.
96. Bouquegneau A, Salam S, Delanaye P, Eastell R, Khwaja A. Bone disease after kidney transplantation. Clin J Am Soc Nephrol. 2016;11(7):1282–96.
97. Iyer SP, Nikkel LE, Nishiyama KK, Dworakowski E, Cremers S, Zhang C, et al. Kidney transplantation with early corticosteroid withdrawal: paradoxical effects at the central and peripheral skeleton. J Am Soc Nephrol. 2014;25(6):1331–41.
98. Edwards B, Desai A, Tsai J, Du H, Edwards G, Bunta A, et al. Elevated incidence of fractures in solid-organ transplant recipients on glucocorticoid-sparing immunosuppressive regimens. J Osteoporos. 2011;2011. Article ID: 59179.
99. Wolf M, Weir MR, Kopyt N, Mannon RB, Von Visger J, Deng H, et al. A prospective cohort study of mineral metabolism after kidney transplantation. Transplantation. 2016;100(1):184.
100. Pihlstrøm H, Dahle DO, Mjøen G, Pilz S, März W, Abedini S, et al. Increased risk of all-cause mortality and renal graft loss in stable renal transplant recipients with hyperparathyroidism. Transplantation. 2015;99(2):351–9.
101. Drüeke T. The pathogenesis of parathyroid gland hyperplasia in chronic renal failure. Kidney Int. 1995;48(1):259–72.
102. Grzela T, Chudzinski W, Lasiecka Z, Niderla J, Wilczynski G, Gornicka B, et al. The calcium-sensing receptor and vitamin D receptor expression in tertiary hyperparathyroidism. Int J Mol Med. 2006;17(5):779–83.
103. Ho L-Y, Wong P-N, Sin H-K, Wong Y-Y, Lo K-C, Chan S-F, et al. Risk factors and clinical course of hungry bone syndrome after total parathyroidectomy in dialysis patients with secondary hyperparathyroidism. BMC Nephrol. 2017;18(1):12.
104. Nigwekar SU, Thadhani R, Brandenburg VM. Calciphylaxis. N Engl J Med. 2018;378(18):1704–14.
105. Nigwekar SU. Calciphylaxis. Curr Opin Nephrol Hypertens. 2017;26(4):276–81.
106. Brandenburg VM, Kramann R, Rothe H, Kaesler N, Korbiel J, Specht P, et al. Calcific uraemic arteriolopathy (calciphylaxis): data from a large nationwide registry. Nephrol Dial Transplant. 2016;32(1):126–32.
107. Nigwekar SU, Kroshinsky D, Nazarian RM, Goverman J, Malhotra R, Jackson VA, et al. Calciphylaxis: risk factors, diagnosis, and treatment. Am J Kidney Dis. 2015;66(1):133–46.
108. Jadoul M, Drüeke TB. B2 microglobulin amyloidosis: an update 30 years later. Nephrol Dial Transplant. 2016;31(4):507–9.
109. Dember LM, Jaber BL, editors. Unresolved issues in dialysis: dialysis-related amyloidosis: late finding or hidden epidemic? Semin Dial. 2006;19:105–9. Wiley Online Library.
110. Labriola L, Jadoul M. Dialysis related amyloidosis: is it gone or should it be? Semin Dial. 2017;30(Conference Proceedings):193–6.
111. Jadoul M, Drüeke TB. β2 microglobulin amyloidosis: an update 30 years later. Nephrol Dial Transplant. 2016;31(4):507–9.
112. Maruyama H, Gejyo F, Arakawa M. Clinical studies of destructive spondyloarthropathy in long-term hemodialysis patients. Nephron. 1992;61(1):37–44.

113. Gejyo F, Kawaguchi Y, Hara S, Nakazawa R, Azuma N, Ogawa H, et al. Arresting dialysis related amyloidosis: a prospective multicenter controlled trial of direct hemoperfusion with a B2 microglobulin adsorption column. Artif Organs. 2004;28(4):371–80.
114. Bransky N, Iyer NR, Cannon SM, Tyan AH, Mylavarapu P, Orosco R, et al. Three rare concurrent complications of tertiary hyperparathyroidism: maxillary brown tumor, uremic leontiasis ossea, and hungry bone syndrome. J Bone Metab. 2020;27(3):217–26.
115. Block GA, Hulbert-Shearon TE, Levin NW, Port FK. Association of serum phosphorus and calcium x phosphate product with mortality risk in chronic hemodialysis patients: a national study. Am J Kidney Dis. 1998;31(4):607–17.
116. Donadio C, Ardini M, Lucchesi A, Donadio E, Cantor T. Parathyroid hormone and large related C-terminal fragments increase at different rates with worsening of renal function in chronic kidney disease patients. A possible indicator of bone turnover status? Clin Nephrol. 2007;67(3):131–9.
117. Brossard J-H, Cloutier M, Roy L, Lepage R, Gascon-Barré M, D'Amour P. Accumulation of a non-(1-84) molecular form of parathyroid hormone (PTH) detected by intact PTH assay in renal failure: importance in the interpretation of PTH values. J Clin Endocrinol Metabol. 1996;81(11):3923–9.
118. Brossard J-H, Lepage R, Cardinal H, Roy L, Rousseau L, Dorais C, et al. Influence of glomerular filtration rate on non-(1-84) parathyroid hormone (PTH) detected by intact PTH assays. Clin Chem. 2000;46(5):697–703.
119. Seiler-Mussler S, Limbach AS, Emrich IE, Pickering JW, Roth HJ, Fliser D, et al. Association of nonoxidized parathyroid hormone with cardiovascular and kidney disease outcomes in chronic kidney disease. Clin J Am Soc Nephrol. 2018;13(4):569–76.
120. Vervloet MG, Brandenburg VM. Circulating markers of bone turnover. J Nephrol. 2017;30(5):663–70.
121. Salam S, Gallagher O, Gossiel F, Paggiosi M, Khwaja A, Eastell R. Diagnostic accuracy of biomarkers and imaging for bone turnover in renal osteodystrophy. J Am Soc Nephrol. 2018;29(5):1557–65.
122. Bosworth C, de Boer IH, editors. Impaired vitamin D metabolism in CKD. Semin Nephrol. 2013;33(2):158–68. Elsevier.
123. Jevtic V. Imaging of renal osteodystrophy. Eur J Radiol. 2003;46(2):85–95.
124. Smith ER, Hewitson TD, Holt SG. Diagnostic tests for vascular calcification. Adv Chronic Kidney Dis. 2019;26(6):445–63.
125. Nickolas TL, Stein E, Cohen A, Thomas V, Staron RB, McMahon DJ, et al. Bone mass and microarchitecture in CKD patients with fracture. J Am Soc Nephrol. 2010;21(8):1371–80.
126. Blomquist GA, Davenport DL, Mawad HW, Monier-Faugere M-C, Malluche HH. Diagnosis of low bone mass in CKD-5D patients. Clin Nephrol. 2016;85(2):77.
127. Raisz LG. Screening for osteoporosis. N Engl J Med. 2005;353(2):164–71.
128. Moe SM, Nickolas TL. Fractures in patients with CKD: time for action. Am Soc Nephrol. 2016;11(11):1929–31.
129. Vervloet MG, van Ballegooijen AJ. Prevention and treatment of hyperphosphatemia in chronic kidney disease. Kidney Int. 2018;93(5):1060–72.
130. Montero-Salazar H, Donat-Vargas C, Moreno-Franco B, Sandoval-Insausti H, Civeira F, Laclaustra M, et al. High consumption of ultra-processed food may double the risk of subclinical coronary atherosclerosis: the Aragon Workers' Health Study (AWHS). BMC Med. 2020;18(1):1–11.
131. Lynch KE, Lynch R, Curhan GC, Brunelli SM. Prescribed dietary phosphate restriction and survival among hemodialysis patients. Clin J Am Soc Nephrol. 2011;6(3):620–9.
132. Floege J. Phosphate binders in chronic kidney disease: an updated narrative review of recent data. J Nephrol. 2020;33(3):497–508.
133. Jamal SA, Vandermeer B, Raggi P, Mendelsohn DC, Chatterley T, Dorgan M, et al. Effect of calcium-based versus non-calcium-based phosphate binders on mortality in patients with chronic kidney disease: an updated systematic review and meta-analysis. Lancet. 2013;382(9900):1268–77.

134. Spiegel DM, Brady K. Calcium balance in normal individuals and in patients with chronic kidney disease on low-and high-calcium diets. Kidney Int. 2012;81(11):1116–22.
135. Spoendlin J, Paik JM, Tsacogianis T, Kim SC, Schneeweiss S, Desai RJ. Cardiovascular outcomes of calcium-free vs calcium-based phosphate binders in patients 65 years or older with end-stage renal disease requiring hemodialysis. JAMA Intern Med. 2019;179(6):741–9.
136. Palmer SC, Gardner S, Tonelli M, Mavridis D, Johnson DW, Craig JC, et al. Phosphate-binding agents in adults with CKD: a network meta-analysis of randomized trials. Am J Kidney Dis. 2016;68(5):691–702.
137. Hamdy NA, Kanis JA, Beneton MN, Brown CB, Juttmann JR, Jordans JG, et al. Effect of alfacalcidol on natural course of renal bone disease in mild to moderate renal failure. BMJ. 1995;310(6976):358–63.
138. Xu L, Wan X, Huang Z, Zeng F, Wei G, Fang D, et al. Impact of vitamin D on chronic kidney diseases in non-dialysis patients: a meta-analysis of randomized controlled trials. PLoS One. 2013;8(4):e61387.
139. Investigators ET. Effect of cinacalcet on cardiovascular disease in patients undergoing dialysis. N Engl J Med. 2012;367(26):2482–94.
140. Salam SN, Eastell R, Khwaja A. Fragility fractures and osteoporosis in CKD: pathophysiology and diagnostic methods. Am J Kidney Dis. 2014;63(6):1049–59.
141. Herberth J, Branscum AJ, Mawad H, Cantor T, Monier-Faugere M-C, Malluche HH. Intact PTH combined with the PTH ratio for diagnosis of bone turnover in dialysis patients: a diagnostic test study. Am J Kidney Dis. 2010;55(5):897–906.
142. Shigematsu T, Muraoka R, Sugimoto T, Nishizawa Y. Risedronate therapy in patients with mild-to-moderate chronic kidney disease with osteoporosis: post-hoc analysis of data from the risedronate phase III clinical trials. BMC Nephrol. 2017;18(1):1–8.
143. Jamal SA, Ljunggren Ö, Stehman-Breen C, Cummings SR, McClung MR, Goemaere S, et al. Effects of denosumab on fracture and bone mineral density by level of kidney function. J Bone Miner Res. 2011;26(8):1829–35.
144. Miller P, Schwartz E, Chen P, Misurski D, Krege J. Teriparatide in postmenopausal women with osteoporosis and mild or moderate renal impairment. Osteoporos Int. 2007;18(1):59–68.
145. Seethapathy H, Noureddine L. Calciphylaxis: approach to diagnosis and management. Adv Chronic Kidney Dis. 2019;26(6):484–90.
146. Portales-Castillo I, Kroshinsky D, Malhotra CK, Culber-Costley R, Cozzolino MG, Karparis S, et al. Calciphylaxis-as a drug induced adverse event. Expert Opin Drug Saf. 2019;18(1):29–35.
147. Garza-Mayers AC, Shah R, Sykes DB, Nigwekar SU, Kroshinsky D. The successful use of apixaban in dialysis patients with calciphylaxis who require anticoagulation: a retrospective analysis. Am J Nephrol. 2018;48(3):168–71.

Chapter 15
Hypertension and Cardiovascular Disease in Patients with Chronic Kidney Disease

Seyed Mehrdad Hamrahian

Introduction

Chronic kidney disease (CKD) is a common disorder that is often unrecognized in the early stages and contributes markedly to morbidity and mortality of the patient [1, 2]. It is defined as kidney damage of >3 months, due to structural or functional abnormalities of the kidney, with or without decreased glomerular filtration rate (GFR) or GFR of < 60 ml/min for >3 months without structural abnormality.

The most common causes of CKD are diabetes and hypertension, which are both associated with increased cardiovascular (CV) risk. CKD by itself is an independent risk factor for increased CV disease [3]. The risk is accelerated even when kidney function is only mildly impaired [4]. Studies in various populations have reported that decreased GFR and increased albuminuria are associated with CV disease and all-cause mortality. In contrast to the nonlinear risk relationship for estimated GFR, the association of albuminuria with CV risk has no threshold effect [5, 6].

The interaction between CKD and CV diseases, first reported by Bright in 1836 [7], is called the cardio-renal syndrome. The complex syndrome includes the effect of low cardiac output on renal function and the effects of renal dysfunction (including both pressure and volume overload) on cardiac function [8]. Individuals with CKD have a disproportionately higher risk of CV events compared to age-matched controls and are more likely to die, primarily of CV disease, than to progress to end-stage kidney disease (ESRD) requiring renal-replacement therapy [9]. In addition to traditional risk factors (hypertension, diabetes, smoking, dyslipidemia, and age), the prevalence of CV risk is amplified by non-traditional and novel kidney-specific factors [10, 11]. These include anemia, abnormal metabolism of calcium and

S. M. Hamrahian (✉)
Department of Medicine, Division of Nephrology, Sidney Kimmel School of Medicine, Thomas Jefferson University, Philadelphia, PA, USA
e-mail: seyed.hamrahian@Jefferson.edu

© Springer Nature Switzerland AG 2022
J. McCauley et al. (eds.), *Approaches to Chronic Kidney Disease*,
https://doi.org/10.1007/978-3-030-83082-3_15

phosphorus, proteinuria, inflammation, oxidative stress, activation of renin-angiotensin-aldosterone system (RAAS), and left ventricular hypertrophy (LVH). Traditional risk factors lead to both progression of atherosclerotic heart disease and reduction in GFR.

Impaired kidney function is associated with a variety of specific CV diseases. Cardiovascular co-morbidities in patients with CKD include congestive heart failure (CHF), stroke, peripheral vascular disease (PVD), coronary artery disease (CAD), valvular heart disease, and arrhythmias (specifically atrial fibrillation) [12–14]. CKD patients also develop concentric stiffening of the arterial media, a phenomenon unique in CKD [15]. Moreover, the prevalence of LVH increases with progression of CKD [16]. In addition to hypertension, extracellular fluid volume overload, increased cardiac output secondary to anemia, and bone mineral disease associated vascular calcification play a significant role in the development of LVH that ultimately leads to reduced myocardial perfusion. The histologically characterized myocardial fibrosis and presence of CAD increase the risk of cardiac arrhythmia and the prevalence of sudden cardiac death. Similarly, atherosclerotic and valvular heart diseases (specifically mitral and aortic valves) are frequently seen in patients with kidney failure even at the early stages of CKD [17]. Important modulators include derangement of serum calcium, phosphate, and parathyroid hormone [18].

In summary, individuals with CKD are considered as one of the highest risk groups for CV diseases [19]. Although there are no definitive prospective trials addressing the benefit of lifestyle modification in CKD patients, interventions to slow down the progression of renal insufficiency might not only postpone the need for dialysis or kidney transplantation but also attenuate CV risk (Tables 15.1 and 15.2).

Hypertension, defined as systolic blood pressure (BP) $\geq$130 mmHg and/or diastolic BP $\geq$80 mmHg, is a global public health problem and the leading factor in the global burden of disease [20–22]. It is a strong well-known and most important modifiable risk factor for CV disease and all-cause mortality [23]. There is an

Table 15.1 Lifestyle interventions for patients with chronic kidney disease to prevent progression and cardiovascular disease

Risk factor	Intervention and treatment goal
Dietary sodium restriction	Limit sodium intake to <2 g per day (corresponds to <5 g salt)
Overweight and physical activity	Best goal is ideal body weight Maintain BMI < 25 kg/m². Encourage moderate intensity dynamic exercise of at least 30–60 min, 5 days per week
Dietary protein restriction	Decrease protein intake to 0.8 g/kg of ideal body weight daily
Alcohol consumption	Reduce alcohol consumption to Men: $\leq$2 drinks daily Women: $\leq$1 drink daily
Smoking	Encourage smoking cessation

Table 15.2 Modifiable interventions in patients with chronic kidney disease to prevent progression and cardiovascular disease

Traditional risk factor	Intervention and treatment goal
Hypertension	Reduce blood pressure to <130/80 mmHg Use RAAS blockers in the setting of proteinuria, but avoid combination
Diabetes	Aim for hemoglobin A1c ~ 7.0% Avoid metformin for GFR < 45 ml/min In patients with albuminuria > 300 mg/g, more aggressive glycemic control does not prevent CV events
Hyperlipidemia	Treat in accordance with guidelines for other high-risk population Existing evidence suggests that lowering cholesterol with statins does not decrease risk of CV events in dialysis-dependent patients
Non-traditional risk factor	**Intervention and treatment goal**
Albuminuria	Increases risk of CKD progression and CVD Use RAAS blockers, but avoid combination
Anemia	Consider erythropoiesis-stimulating agents to aim for goal hemoglobin of 10–12 g/dl
Bone mineral disease	Use phosphate binders and low phosphorus diet to maintain serum phosphate concentrations in the normal range
LVH	Control BP and reduce afterload

independent and linear association between BP and the risk of CV disease [24]. Along the same line, large prospective cohort studies have reported that elevated BP is also a strong independent risk factor for CKD and ESRD [25]. Moreover, hypertension is also the most common comorbidity seen in patients with CKD [26]. The relationship between CKD and hypertension is complex and bidirectional. Hypertension, particularly resistant hypertension, can occur not only as the result of CKD, but it also is an important risk factor for CKD progression [27]. At some point, it becomes difficult to determine which disease process precedes the other. The interaction between hypertension and CKD increases the risk of adverse CV events. Randomized clinical trials have demonstrated that BP lowering reduces the risk of CV disease and all-cause mortality. Respectively, treatment of hypertension is even more important for this patient population at substantially higher risk for morbidity and mortality.

Accurate Blood Pressure Measurement

A standardized and accurate BP measurement is important to establish the diagnosis of hypertension and its management [28]. It is important to measure the BP after the patient rests quietly for 5 minutes and use appropriate cuff size. Multiple readings taken at intervals of at least 1–2 minutes and then averaged is a better representation of a patient's BP than a single reading. Significant between-arm BP differences of over 10 mmHg can be seen in patients with advanced CKD due to heavily calcified or atherosclerotic arteries and could indicate an increased risk for vascular disease and death [29]. It is recommended that the higher BP of the two arms be used for management.

Although clinic BP measurements are the most common method of assessment to evaluate hypertension, the ambulatory blood pressure monitoring (ABPM) or home blood pressure monitoring (HBPM) provides useful additional clinical information on a patient's BP pattern, including assessment of nighttime BP, diurnal variation in BP, and diagnostic information, such as white-coat hypertension and/or masked hypertension [30]. White-coat hypertension, defined as persistently elevated clinic BP but normal out-of-office BP values measured by 24-hour ABPM, is a common cause of apparent resistant hypertension [31]. In contrast masked hypertension, defined as normal, or near normal, office BP levels but out-of-office hypertension appears to be remarkably prevalent in CKD patients and is associated with increased risk for target organ damage and CV events [32, 33].

Ambulatory BP monitoring provides additional information of BP variability compared to home and office BP readings. Patients with CKD often have abnormal circadian BP rhythm and lose the physiologic nocturnal fall of 10–20% in systolic and diastolic BP levels [34]. Patients with advanced CKD might even exhibit a rise in nocturnal BP, a phenomenon called riser. There is a strong association between elevated nighttime BP and masked hypertension in CKD [35]. The loss of nocturnal dipping and BP variability are associated with increased risk of CV events and target organ damage, including the progression of CKD [36]. The high prevalence of non-dipping BP, rising BP at night, and/or masked hypertension in patients with CKD reinforces the need to measure out-of-office BP for a full characterization of the burden of hypertension. Additionally, HBPM is prognostically superior to office BP readings, correlates more closely with ABPM, and better predicts adverse CV outcomes [37].

Target Blood Pressure in Chronic Kidney Disease

The goal BP level in the treatment of hypertension in CKD population remains a matter of debate despite recent clinical trial data [38]. In addition to prevention of CV events, the goal is to delay the progression to ESRD and the need for renal transplant or renal replacement therapy [39]. Trials in non-diabetics (e.g., MDRD, AASK, and REIN-2) failed to show benefit from lower BP targets of <130/80 mmHg compared to <140/90 mmHg in slowing the progression of CKD to ESRD and were underpowered for CV events [40–42]. However, the benefit of a lower BP target of <130/80 mm Hg in patients with CKD and proteinuria is supported by post-hoc analyses [43].

The ACCORD and SPRINT trials compared a systolic BP target of 120 vs. 140 mmHg in diabetic and non-diabetic participants, respectively [38, 44]. The ACCORD trial excluded patients with a serum creatinine >1.5 mg/dL, but 36% of

Table 15.3 Recommended blood pressure targets in CKD

Guideline	CKD without proteinuria	CKD with proteinuria
AHA	<130/80 mmHg	<130/80 mmHg
JNC8	<140/90 mmHg	<140/90 mmHg
KDIGO	<140/90 mmHg	<130/80 mmHg
NICE	<140/90 mmHg	<130/80 mmHg
CHEP	<140/90 mmHg	<140/90 mmHg
ESC/ESH	<140 mmHg	<130 mmHg
ASH/ISH	<140/90 mmHg	<140/90 mmHg
ADA	<140/80 mmHg	

Abbreviations: *AHA* American Heart Association, *ADA* American Diabetes Association, *ASH/ISH* American Society of Hypertension/International Society of Hypertension, *CHEP* Canadian Hypertension Education Program, *ESC/ESH* European Society of Cardiology/European Society of Hypertension, *KDIGO* Kidney Disease: Improving Global Outcomes, *NICE* National Institute for Heath and Care Excellence, *JNC8* USA Eighth Joint National Committee

participants had CKD defined by albuminuria. Results indicated that lower BP did not reduce CV events except for stroke and were associated with more serious adverse events. The SPRINT trial included 28% non-diabetic CKD participants. The subgroup analysis of participants with CKD found that intensive BP treatment resulted in significant reductions in the risk of CV disease and death compared with standard BP [45]. Although there was an increased rate of estimated GFR decline and more instances of acute kidney injury, hyperkalemia, and hypokalemia in the intensive BP control group, there was no difference in doubling of creatinine and ESRD. These findings suggest that the observed estimated GFR decline seen in the intensive treatment group predominantly reflects hemodynamic changes rather than intrinsic damage to the kidney. Based on current knowledge from the two major studies and the CKD subgroup analyses, intensive BP control is associated with an increase in some adverse events, but there is mortality and possibly CV event reduction with intensive BP control. Respectively, the latest guidelines from the American Heart Association recommend lower BP target of <130/80 mm Hg for all CKD patients (Table 15.3).

Pathogenesis of Hypertension in Chronic Kidney Disease

The pathophysiology of CKD-associated hypertension is complex since the kidney is both the contributing and the target organ of the hypertensive processes [46]. Four main pathways contribute to hypertension in CKD: abnormal sodium regulation, increased sympathetic nervous system (SNS) activity, active humoral system–renin angiotensin aldosterone system (RAAS), and impairment of auto-regulatory system [47]. These pathways could have independent or interdependent effects on BP regulation. Additional exogenous factors, including diet and drugs, can influence BP and its management in patients with CKD.

Auto-Regulatory System and Sodium Regulation

Hypertension can cause and accelerate renal injury when impaired auto-regulation allows the transmission of high systemic pressures to the glomeruli, resulting in glomerulosclerosis [48]. Epidemiological studies have demonstrated a causal relationship between sodium intake, hypertension, and risk of CV disease [49]. Renal injury and loss of GFR in turn can cause hypertension due to impairment in sodium excretion. The kidneys filter over 25,000 mmol of sodium per day excreting only less than 1% of the filtered sodium load. Inadequate sodium excretion in the setting of CKD over time can result in volume-mediated hypertension resulting in increased cardiac filling and cardiac output. Loss of sodium regulation leads to the increased prevalence of salt-sensitive hypertension, commonly seen in CKD [50]. In addition, increased sodium intake results in arterial vessel stiffness, decreased nitric oxide release, and the promotion of inflammatory processes, all of which contribute to BP elevation and increased risk of development of systolic hypertension in CKD [51]. Moreover, excessive salt intake blunts the BP lowering effect of most classes of antihypertensive agents, particularly in patients with CKD, thus favoring development of resistant hypertension [52, 53]. Similarly, non-steroidal anti-inflammatory drugs (NSAIDs) have an inhibitory effect on renal prostaglandin production, especially prostaglandin E2 and prostaglandin I2. This effect can lead to sodium and fluid retention, effects that are more pronounced in salt-sensitive patients including individuals with CKD [54]. In conclusion, dietary sodium reduction is recommended to decrease risk of hypertension and prevent CV diseases and increased mortality. Moreover, diuretics are the key component of antihypertensive management in CKD.

Sympathetic Nervous System Regulation

SNS activity is increased in CKD [47]. The renal artery is highly innervated, with efferent renal nerves that originate from the central nervous system and afferent renal nerves that originate from the kidneys. Stimulation of efferent renal nerves via β-1 adrenoreceptor stimulates renin secretion and activates the RAAS resulting in decreased urinary sodium excretion. Maximal stimulation of the efferent nerves can lead to an increase in renal vascular resistance [55]. Accordingly, β-1 adrenergic blockers and RAAS blockers (e.g., ACE inhibitors, ARBs) are among the most effective antihypertensive agents in conditions of high SNS activity status, including CKD, obesity, and obstructive sleep apnea (OSA).

Humoral System–Renin Angiotensin Aldosterone Regulation

Renin is secreted from the juxtaglomerular apparatus, which is the nephron site wherein there is contact between the afferent arteriole and the distal convoluted tubule. The secretion of renin is highly volume regulated and is stimulated by SNS through the efferent renal nerves as well [56]. In response to renin secretion, subsequent activation of RAAS causes vasoconstriction via the angiotensin II effect, in which sodium reabsorption is increased by both angiotensin II in the proximal tubule and aldosterone in the distal nephron in exchange for the secretion of potassium. In addition to mineralocorticoid receptor stimulation in the distal nephron, aldosterone has a direct effect on the vasculature, increasing the risk of arterial stiffness that promotes hypertension [57].

Chronic Kidney Disease and Resistant Hypertension

There is a strong association between CKD and resistant hypertension. The increased prevalence of resistant hypertension in CKD results from impaired sodium excretion and excess salt intake leading to subclinical volume overload. Therefore, salt restriction can have a synergistic effect on antihypertensive drugs [58]. The presence of significant proteinuria may have an accentuating effect. Aberrant filtration of plasminogen and its conversion within the urinary space to plasmin by urokinase-type plasminogen activator increase sodium retention by activating the epithelial sodium channel (ENaC), contributing further to volume overload status [59].

Evaluation of Hypertension in Chronic Kidney Disease

Medical history and physical examination can provide information on duration, course, severity of the hypertension, and if possible the chronologic relation to the established CKD diagnosis. It is important to inquire about prior medication regimens used, the presence of orthostatic symptoms, and any other experienced side effects. History of snoring, witnessed apnea, and excessive daytime sleepiness indicate the need for further evaluation for OSA. Presence of between the arms BP discrepancy or abdominal bruits in an elderly patient with known atherosclerotic disease increases the possibility of reno-vascular hypertension.

When evaluating a patient with CKD and difficult-to-treat hypertension, it is important to confirm the diagnosis of true treatment resistance hypertension and exclude pseudo-resistance [60] (Fig. 15.1). These include inaccurate blood pressure measurement technique; non-adherence to treatment regimen secondary to polypharmacy, drug costs, dosing inconvenience, or drug adverse effects; lifestyle factors such as obesity, physical inactivity, high dietary salt intake, excessive alcohol ingestion, and use of substances with potential interference with antihypertensive medications; and secondary causes of hypertension such as obstructive sleep apnea and/or possibly hyperaldosteronism.

It is essential to screen for the extent of target-organ damage, including LVH, retinopathy, degree of albuminuria, and CKD stage, by estimated GFR to assess the overall increased risk of CV complications. The risk increases with both the degree and duration of uncontrolled BP and CKD [61]. Hence, in accordance with the US Preventive Services Task Force statement and evidence-based data, it is

Fig. 15.1 Algorithm for
evaluation of patient with
chronic kidney disease and
difficult-to-treat
hypertension (see text for
details)

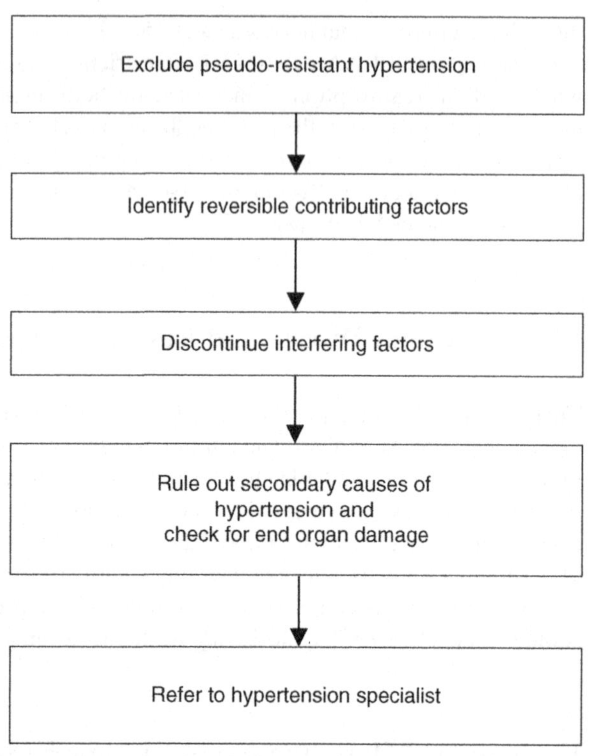

recommended to confirm a diagnosis of hypertension or resistant hypertension with
ABPM [62].

Basic laboratory evaluation of a hypertensive individual with CKD includes a
routine metabolic profile and urinalysis. A duplex renal ultrasound study evaluation
to rule out renal artery stenosis should be considered in patients at increased risk of
atherosclerotic disease, particularly with recent deterioration in renal function following therapy with ACE-inhibitors or ARBs, or history of flash pulmonary edema
[63]. This modality is preferred over computer tomographic angiography in patients
with CKD in view of increased risk of contrast induced acute kidney injury. The
presence of persistent and otherwise unexplained hypokalemia requires measurement of both plasma aldosterone concentration and plasma renin activity to rule out
hyperaldosteronism. Suppressed renin level without elevated aldosterone concentration is suggestive of inappropriate volume expansion commonly seen in patients
with CKD. Echocardiography provides valuable information on target organ damage, LVH, and valvular disease, but is not routinely recommended.

Non-pharmacologic Therapy

The modification of lifestyle factors—restriction of dietary salt, regular exercise,
weight loss, decreased alcohol ingestion, smoking cessation, and discontinuation of
any potentially interfering substances, like NSAIDs—is highly important in the

treatment of resistant hypertension commonly seen in CKD [64]. A high-salt diet blunts the effect of ACE inhibitors, whereas sodium reduction enhances the anti-proteinuric effect of ARBs [27, 65]. Accordingly, a low sodium diet of <2000 mg per day is recommended by most clinical practice guidelines.

Additionally, ingestion of a potassium-rich diet (e.g., fruits and vegetables) and close monitoring of the potassium levels in CKD patients reduce systolic and diastolic BP compared to a usual diet in hypertensive patients [66]. Caution is advised for this recommendation since hyperkalemia, a common electrolyte abnormality encountered in patients with advanced CKD with or without intake of RAAS blockers or mineralocorticoid receptor antagonist (MRA), increases the risk of death from any cause, particularly cardiovascular events.

Finally, regular aerobic exercise and weight loss are clearly associated with modest improvement of BP level and can lead to a reduction in the number of antihypertensive medications [67]. High alcohol consumption is associated with increased risk of resistant hypertension. Limited alcohol consumption to no more than 28 g of ethanol per day for men and 14 g per day for women significantly improves BP control [68].

Pharmacologic Therapy

The goal of pharmacologic therapy should be to achieve and maintain BP control by maximizing patient's adherence to prescribed medications with use of a drug combination that considers its effect on renal and CV outcomes. It is important to avoid complex dosing regimens, high out-of-pocket costs and drugs with significant adverse effects. Individualization of treatment should consider pathophysiology and comorbidities that commonly co-exist with CKD [69]. The medication regimen should be simplified by using long-acting drugs and include drugs from different classes with synergistic effects that act on different BP regulatory systems to increase renal sodium excretion and inhibit both the RAAS and the SNS activities. The standard recommended medical treatment regimen for hypertension of A + C + D (A = angiotensin-converting enzyme inhibitor or angiotensin-receptor blocker, C = calcium channel blocker, D = thiazide-like diuretic) is well tolerated [70]. There is a strong evidence that combination regimens reduce cardiovascular events in hypertensive individuals [71].

Diuretics are essential to enhance sodium excretion in the setting of avid sodium retention due to low GFR and to maintain euvolemic status. Lack or underuse of diuretics in patients with CKD is a common cause of treatment-resistant hypertension. Appropriate diuretic choice, based on estimated GFR, is the cornerstone of hypertension management in CKD patients [72, 73]. Thiazides or thiazide-type diuretics are the generally preferred drug of choice when the GFR is ≥ 30 ml/min/1.73 m^2; loop diuretics, which are more potent natriuretic agents, are recommended when GFR is lower, although a few small studies have reported on the efficacy of thiazide-type diuretics even at GFR < 30 ml/min/1.73 m^2 [74]. To avoid counter-regulatory rebound sodium reabsorption and volume retention in patients with CKD, diuretics should be given at higher doses and more frequently if long-acting diuretics such as chlorthalidone or torsemide are not used. Moreover, the sequential blockade of sodium channels along the nephron with both a loop and thiazide diuretic is very effective, but this combination of diuretics requires frequent serum creatinine and electrolytes monitoring [75].

ACE inhibitors and ARBs, if tolerated, are the most important class of drugs recommended for CKD patients because of their efficacy, relatively low side effect profile, reno-protective effects, and reduced risk for CV and renal events [76]. RAAS blockers exert their reno-protective effect by reducing intraglomerular pressure, thereby decreasing proteinuria. Reduction in GFR and associated rise in serum creatinine of up to 30% is acceptable and physiologic [77]. Unless there is complication of persistent hyperkalemia refractory to treatment, the RAAS blockade should not be discontinued. The approval of two new and safer potassium-binding agents, patiromer and sodium zirconium cyclosilicate (ZS-9), has increased the armature of the nephrologist in management of hyperkalemia tendency in patient with advanced CKD on RAAS blockade if continuation of the drug outweighs the risk associated with discontinuation of the drug. Patiromer is a non-absorbed polymer that binds K^+ in exchange for Ca^{2+}, and the most common side effect is dose-dependent hypomagnesemia. Because of significant drug-drug interaction, patiromer needs to be taken 3–6 hours apart from other oral medications. ZS-9 is an inorganic, non-absorbable crystalline compound that exchanges both sodium and hydrogen ions for K^+ and $NH4^+$ in the intestine [78, 79]. A rise in serum creatinine of more than 30% after initiation of RAAS blockade could be due to volume contraction, use of NSAIDs, or bilateral renal artery stenosis that requires further investigation.

The combination of RAAS blockers should be avoided because it is associated with significant adverse effects, including risk of severe hyperkalemia, hypotension, and acute renal failure [80]. The combination of calcium channel blockers (CCBs) with ACE inhibitors might be more effective in slowing the progression of CKD, particularly in black patients [81]. Dihydropyridine CCBs, in contrast to non-dihydropyridine CCBs, do not have anti-proteinuric effect, but are more potent anti-hypertensive drugs. A common side effect of this drug class, lower extremity edema due to higher precapillary arterial dilatation effect of the drug, is refractory to diuretics but improves or resolves with the use of an ACE inhibitor or ARB.

Uncontrolled BP, despite a combination regimen of A + C + D, requires a search for the pathogenic mechanism. For patients uncontrolled on multidrug regimens and low-renin status, mineralocorticoid receptor antagonist (MRA) or aldosterone antagonists are the most important recommended fourth drug of choice [82]. The most common adverse effect of spironolactone, breast tenderness with or without breast enlargement, is particularly seen in men and at higher doses (e.g., 50–100 mg/day). Eplerenone, a nonsteroidal selective MRA is less associated with this side effect. Combination of MRA with an ACE inhibitor or ARB, although not contraindicated, requires careful monitoring of serum potassium and creatinine levels. The risk of hyperkalemia is increased in patients taking NSAIDs or having co-morbidities like diabetes or low GFR of <30 mL/min/1.73 m^2 and plasma potassium concentrations of >4.5 mmol/L. In patients with uncontrolled hypertension and significant proteinuria, amiloride, an indirect aldosterone antagonist that blocks the epithelial sodium channel, has been shown to be an effective add-on therapy [59].

Beta-blockers are more often used when there is a coexisting cardiac disease, such as ischemic heart disease or heart failure [83]. If indicated, the more effective drugs are the non-selective combined alpha and beta antagonists. Clonidine, a centrally acting agent, is very effective but requires frequent dosing. The drug is also associated with a significant adverse effect profile, and using a dose of over 0.6 mg/day is associated with rebound hypertension if a dose is missed. Potent vasodilators, such as hydralazine or minoxidil, have a high incidence of adverse effects including lower extremity edema and tachycardia. Finally, in the setting of increased SNS activity and/or arterial stiffness, use of an alpha-blocker such as doxazosin may have a favorable effect on BP and vascular remodeling. The main side effect of this drug is dizziness.

An important factor in the management of hypertension in CKD is the concept of chronotherapy. For example, intake of at least one of the hypertensive agents at bedtime may be associated with better 24-hour mean BP control and could induce the desired nocturnal dip in non-dippers, reducing cardiovascular event risk [84]. Patients with CKD and resistant hypertension have an unfavorable prognosis [27]. They are more likely to experience the combined outcome of death, myocardial infarction, congestive heart failure, stroke, or worsening of CKD over time compared to those who have achieved goal blood pressure [85].

In Summary

Hypertension is the major modifiable risk factor for CV disease. CKD is both a common cause and complication of uncontrolled hypertension. It is also an independent risk factor for CV disease. The interaction between hypertension and CKD is complex and bidirectional. It increases the risk of adverse CV outcomes. This is particularly significant in the setting of resistant hypertension commonly seen in CKD. Key pathogenic mechanisms of CKD-associated hypertension include sodium dysregulation, increased SNS activity, and alterations in RAAS, all of which play an important role in determining the pharmacological approach (i.e., antihypertensive medication) in addition to the non-pharmacological approaches. Out-of-office BP measurements, including ABPM, provide a better assessment of diurnal BP variation commonly seen in CKD. In the setting of resistant hypertension, evaluation by a hypertension specialist may be required to exclude pseudo-resistance and treatable secondary causes.

References

1. National Kidney Foundation. K/DOQI clinical practice guidelines for chronic kidney disease: evaluation, classification, and stratification. Am J Kidney Dis. 2002;39(2 Suppl. 1):S1–S266.
2. Kidney Disease: Improving Global Outcomes (KDIGO) CKD Work Group. KDIGO 2012 clinical practice guideline for the evaluation and management of chronic kidney disease. Kidney Int Suppl. 2013;3:1–150.

3. Ggg Levey AS, et al. National Kidney Foundation practice guidelines for chronic kidney disease: evaluation, classification, and stratification. Ann Intern Med. 2003;139:137–47.
4. Weiner DE, et al. Chronic kidney disease as a risk factor for cardiovascular disease and all-cause mortality: a pooled analysis of community-based studies. J Am Soc Nephrol. 2004;15:1307–15.
5. Van der Velde M, Matsushita K, Coresh J, Astor BC, Woodward M, Levey A, de Jong P, Gansevoort RT, Chronic Kidney Disease Prognosis Consortium, et al. Lower estimated glomerular filtration rate and higher albuminuria are associated with all-cause and cardiovascular mortality. A collaborative meta-analysis of high-risk population cohorts. Kidney Int. 2011;79:1341–52.
6. Garg AX, Clark WF, Haynes RB, House AA. Moderate renal insufficiency and the risk of cardiovascular mortality: results from the NHANES I. Kidney Int. 2002;61:1486–94.
7. Bright R. Cases and observations illustrative of renal disease accompanied with the secretion of albuminous urine. Guy's Hosp Trans. 1836;1:338–79.
8. Ronco C, Haapio M, House AA, Anavekar N, Bellomo R. Cardiorenal syndrome. J Am Coll Cardiol. 2008;52:1527–39.
9. United States Renal Data System. USRDS annual data report: epidemiology of kidney disease in the United States. Bethesda: National Institutes of Health, National Institute of Diabetes and Digestive and Kidney Diseases; 2016. p. 2016.
10. Goff DC Jr, Lloyd-Jones DM, Bennett G, et al. 2013 ACC/AHA guideline on the assessment of cardiovascular risk: a report of the American College of Cardiology/American Heart Association Task Force on Practice Guidelines. J Am Coll Cardiol. 2014;63(25 Pt B):2935–59.
11. van der Zee S, Baber U, Elmariah S, Winston J, Fuster V. Cardiovascular risk factors in patients with chronic kidney disease. Nat Rev Cardiol. 2009;6:580–9.
12. Kottgen A, Russell SD, Loehr LR, et al. Reduced kidney function as a risk factor for incident heart failure: the Atherosclerosis Risk In Communities (ARIC) study. J Am Soc Nephrol. 2007;18:1307–15.
13. Abramson JL, Jurkovitz CT, Vaccarino V, Weintraub WS, McClellan W. Chronic kidney disease, anemia, and incident stroke in a middle-aged, community-based population: the ARIC study. Kidney Int. 2003;64:610–5.
14. Wattanakit K, Folsom AR, Selvin E, Coresh J, Hirsch AT, Weatherley BD. Kidney function and risk of peripheral arterial disease: results from the Atherosclerosis Risk In Communities (ARIC) study. J Am Soc Nephrol. 2007;18:629–36.
15. Mathew RO, Bangalore S, Lavelle MP, et al. Diagnosis and management of atherosclerotic cardiovascular disease in chronic kidney disease: a review. Kidney Int. 2016;91(4):797–807.
16. Levin A, Singer J, Thompson CR, Ross H, Lewis M. Prevalent LVH in the predialysis population: identifying opportunities for intervention. Am J Kidney Dis. 1996;27:347–54.
17. Moe SM, Chen NX. Mechanisms of vascular calcification in chronic kidney disease. J Am Soc Nephrol. 2008;19:213–6.
18. Kestenbaum B, et al. Serum phosphate levels and mortality risk among people with chronic kidney disease. J Am Soc Nephrol. 2005;16:520–8.
19. Wen CP, Cheng TYD, Tsai MK. All-cause mortality attributable to chronic kidney disease: a prospective cohort study based on 462 293 adults in Taiwan. Lancet. 2008;371:2173–82.
20. Whelton PK, et al. 2017 ACC/AHA/AAPA/ABC/ACPM/AGS/APhA/ASH/ASPC/NMA/PCNA guideline for the prevention, detection, evaluation, and management of high blood pressure in adults: a report of the American College of Cardiology/ American Heart Association Task Force on clinical practice guidelines. Circulation. 2018;138:e484–594.
21. World Health Organization. A global brief on hypertension: silent killer, global public health crisis. World Health Day 2013. Geneva: World Health Organization; 2013. p. 1–39.
22. Murray CJ, Lopez AD. Measuring the global burden of disease. N Engl J Med. 2013;369:448–57.
23. GBD 2017 Causes of Death Collaborators, G. A, et al. Global, regional, and national age-sex-specific mortality for 282 causes of death in 195 countries and territories, 1980-2017: a systematic analysis for the global burden of disease study 2017. Lancet. 2018;392:1736–88.

24. Ettehad D, et al. Blood pressure lowering for prevention of cardiovascular disease and death: a systematic review and meta-analysis. Lancet. 2016;387:957–67.
25. Anderson AH, et al. Time-updated systolic blood pressure and the progression of chronic kidney disease: a cohort study. Ann Intern Med. 2015;162:258–65.
26. Muntner P, Anderson A, Charleston J, Chen Z, Ford V, Makos G, et al. Hypertension awareness, treatment, and control in adults with CKD: results from the Chronic Renal Insufficiency Cohort (CRIC) study. Am J Kidney Dis. 2010;55:441–51.
27. De Nicola L, Gabbai FB, Agarwal R, Chiodini P, Borrelli S, Bellizzi V, et al. Prevalence and prognostic role of resistant hypertension in chronic kidney disease patients. J Am Coll Cardiol. 2013;61:2461–7.
28. Pickering TG, Hall JE, Appel LJ, Falkner BE, Graves J, Hill MN, et al. Recommendations of blood pressure measurement in humans and experimental animals. Part 1: blood pressure measurement in humans. A statement for professionals from the Subcommittee of Professional and Public Education of the American Heart Association Council on High Blood Pressure Research. Circulation. 2005;111:697–716.
29. Clark CE, Taylor RS, Shore AC, Ukoumunne OC, Campbell JL. Association of a difference in systolic blood pressure between arms with vascular disease and mortality: a systematic review and metaanalysis. Lancet. 2012;379:905–14.
30. Drawz PE, Abdalla M, Rahman M. Blood pressure measurement: clinic, home, ambulatory, and beyond. Am J Kidney Dis. 2012;60:449–62.
31. de la Sierra A, Segura J, Banegas JR, Gorostidi M, de la Cruz JJ, Armario P, et al. Clinical features of 8295 patients with resistant hypertension classified on the basis of ambulatory blood pressure monitoring. Hypertension. 2011;57:898–902.
32. Agarwal R, Pappas MK, Sinha AD. Masked uncontrolled hypertension in CKD. J Am Soc Nephrol. 2016;27:924–32.
33. Fagard RH, Cornelissen VA. Incidence of cardiovascular events in white-coat, masked and sustained hypertension versus true normotension: a meta-analysis. J Hypertens. 2007;25:2193–8.
34. Kanno A, Kikuya M, Asayama K, Satoh M, Inoue R, Hosaka M, et al. Night-time blood pressure is associated with the development of chronic kidney disease in a general population: the Ohasama Study. J Hypertens. 2013;31:2410–7.
35. Drawz PE, Alper AB, Anderson AH, Brecklin CS, Charleston J, Chen J, et al. Masked hypertension and elevated nighttime blood pressure in CKD: prevalence and association with target organ damage. Clin J Am Soc Nephrol. 2016;11:642–52.
36. Ciobanu AO, Gherghinescu CL, Dulgheru R, Magda S, Dragoi Galrinho R, Florescu M, et al. The impact of blood pressure variability on subclinical ventricular, renal and vascular dysfunction, in patients with hypertension and diabetes. Maedica (Bucur). 2013;8:129–36.
37. Niiranen TJ, Hänninen MR, Johansson J, Reunanen A, Jula AM. Home measured blood pressure is a stronger predictor of cardiovascular risk than office blood pressure: the Finn-Home study. Hypertension. 2010;55:1346–51.
38. SPRINT Research Group, Wright JT Jr, Williamson JD, Whelton PK, Snyder JK, Sink KM, et al. A randomized trial of intensive versus standard blood-pressure control. N Engl J Med. 2015;373:2103–16.
39. McCullough PA, Steigerwalt S, Tolia K, Chen SC, Li S, Norris KC, et al. Cardiovascular disease in chronic kidney disease: data from the Kidney Early Evaluation Program (KEEP). Curr Diab Rep. 2011;11:47–55.
40. Klahr S, Levey AS, Beck GJ, Caggiula AW, Hunsicker L, Kusek JW, et al. The effects of dietary protein restriction and blood-pressure control on the progression of chronic renal disease. Modification of Diet in Renal Disease Study Group. N Engl J Med. 1994;330:877–84.
41. Wright JT Jr, Bakris G, Greene T, Agodoa LY, Appel LJ, Charleston J, et al. Effect of blood pressure lowering and antihypertensive drug class on progression of hypertensive kidney disease: results from the AASK trial. JAMA. 2002;288:2421–31.
42. Ruggenenti P, Perna A, Loriga G, Ganeva M, Ene-Iordache B, Turturro M, et al. Blood-pressure control for renoprotection in patients with non-diabetic chronic renal disease (REIN-2): multicentre, randomised controlled trial. Lancet. 2005;365:939–46.

43. Upadhyay A, Earley A, Haynes SM, Uhlig K. Systematic review: blood pressure target in chronic kidney disease and proteinuria as an effect modifier. Ann Intern Med. 2011;154:541–8.
44. Margolis KL, O'Connor PJ, Morgan TM, et al. Outcomes of combined cardiovascular risk factor management strategies in type 2 diabetes: the ACCORD randomized trial. Diabetes Care. 2014;37(6):1721–8.
45. Cheung AK, Rahman M, Reboussin DM, et al. Effects of intensive BP control in CKD. J Am Soc Nephrol. 2017;28(9):2812–23.
46. Hamrahian SM. Management of hypertension in patients with chronic kidney disease. Curr Hypertens Rep. 2017;19:43.
47. Klein IH, Ligtenberg G, Neumann J, Oey PL, Koomans HA, Blankestijn PJ. Sympathetic nerve activity is inappropriately increased in chronic renal disease. J Am Soc Nephrol. 2003;14:3239–44.
48. Bidani AK, Polichnowski AJ, Loutzenhiser R, Griffin KA. Renal microvascular dysfunction, hypertension and CKD progression. Curr Opin Nephrol Hypertens. 2013;22:1–9.
49. He J, Whelton PK. Salt intake, hypertension and risk of cardiovascular disease: an important public health challenge. Int J Epidemiol. 2002;31:322–7.
50. Koomans HA, Roos JC, Boer P, Geyskes GG, Mees EJ. Salt sensitivity of blood pressure in chronic renal failure. Evidence for renal control of body fluid distribution in man. Hypertension. 1982;4:190–7.
51. Briet M, Boutouyrie P, Laurent S, London GM. Arterial stiffness and pulse pressure in CKD and ESRD. Kidney Int. 2012;82:388–400.
52. Luft FC, Weinberger MH. Review of salt restriction and the response to antihypertensive drugs: satellite symposium on calcium antagonists. Hypertension. 1988;11:I-229–32.
53. Boudville N, Ward S, Benaroia M, House AA. Increased sodium intake correlates with greater use of antihypertensive agents by subjects with chronic kidney disease. Am J Hypertens. 2005;18:1300–5.
54. Johnson AG, Nguyen TV, Day RO. Do nonsteroidal anti-inflammatory drugs affect blood pressure? A meta-analysis. Ann Intern Med. 1994;121:289–300.
55. DiBona GF, Kopp UC. Neural control of renal function. Physiol Rev. 1997;77:75–197.
56. Davis JO, Freeman RH. Mechanisms regulating renin release. Physiol Rev. 1976;56:1–56.
57. Briet M, Schiffrin EL. Vascular actions of aldosterone. J Vasc Res. 2013;50:89–99.
58. Kwakernaak AJ, Krikken JA, Binnenmars SH, Visser FW, Hemmelder MH, Woittiez AJ, et al. Effects of sodium restriction and hydrochlorothiazide on RAAS blockade efficacy in diabetic nephropathy: a randomised clinical trial. Lancet Diabetes Endocrinol. 2014;2:385–95.
59. Svenningsen P, Friis UG, Versland JB, Buhl KB, Møller Frederiksen B, Andersen H, et al. Mechanisms of renal NaCl retention in proteinuric disease. Acta Physiol (Oxf). 2013;207:536–45.
60. Burnier M, Wuerzner G, Struijker-Boudier H, Urquhart J. Measuring, analyzing, and managing drug adherence in resistant hypertension. Hypertension. 2013;62:218–25.
61. Muiesan ML, Salvetti M, Rizzoni D, Paini A, Agabiti-Rosei C, Aggiusti C, et al. Resistant hypertension and target organ damage. Hypertens Res. 2013;36:485–91.
62. Siu AL, U.S. Preventive Services Task Force. Screening for high blood pressure in adults: U.S. preventive services task force recommendation statement. Ann Intern Med. 2015;163:778–86.
63. Rimoldi SF, Scherrer U, Messerli FH. Secondary arterial hypertension: when, who, and how to screen? Eur Heart J. 2014;35:1245–54.
64. Vollmer WM, Sacks FM, Ard J, Appel LJ, Bray GA, Simons-Morton DG, et al. Effects of diet and sodium intake on blood pressure: subgroup analysis of the DASH-sodium trial. Ann Intern Med. 2001;135:1019–28.
65. Singer DR, Markandu ND, Sugden AL, Miller MA, MacGregor GA. Sodium restriction in hypertensive patients treated with a converting enzyme inhibitor and a thiazide. Hypertension. 1991;17:798–803.
66. Appel LJ, Moore TJ, Obarzanek E, Vollmer WM, Svetkey LP, Sacks FM, et al. A clinical trial of the effects of dietary patterns on blood pressure. DASH Collaborative Research Group. N Engl J Med. 1997;336:1117–24.

67. Aucott L, Poobalan A, Smith WC, Avenell A, Jung R, Broom J. Effects of weight loss in overweight/obese individuals and long-term hypertension outcomes: a systematic review. Hypertension. 2005;45:1035–41.
68. Aguilera MT, de la Sierra A, Coca A, Estruch R, Fernandez-Sola J, Urbano-Marquez A. Effect of alcohol abstinence on blood pressure: assessment by 24-hour ambulatory blood pressure monitoring. Hypertension. 1999;33:653–7.
69. Sica DA. The kidney and hypertension: causes and treatment. J Clin Hypertens (Greenwich). 2008;10:541–8.
70. Weber MA, Schiffrin EL, White WB, Mann S, Lindholm LH, Kenerson JG, et al. Clinical practice guidelines for the management of hypertension in the community: a statement by the American Society of Hypertension and the International Society of Hypertension. J Clin Hypertens (Greenwich). 2014;16:14–26.
71. Chalmers J, Arima H, Woodward M, Mancia G, Poulter N, Hirakawa Y, et al. Effects of combination of perindopril, indapamide, and calcium channel blockers in patients with type 2 diabetes mellitus: results from the Action in Diabetes and Vascular Disease: Preterax and Diamicron Controlled Evaluation (ADVANCE) trial. Hypertension. 2014;63:259–64.
72. Tamargo J, Segura J, Ruilope LM. Diuretics in the treatment of hypertension. Part 1: thiazide and thiazide-like diuretics. Expert Opin Pharmacother. 2014;15:527–47.
73. Tamargo J, Segura J, Ruilope LM. Diuretics in the treatment of hypertension. Part 2: loop diuretics and potassium-sparing agents. Expert Opin Pharmacother. 2014;15:605–21.
74. Cirillo M, Marcarelli F, Mele AA, Romano M, Lombardi C, Bilancio G. Parallel-group 8-week study on chlorthalidone effects in hypertensives with low kidney function. Hypertension. 2014;63:692–7.
75. Izzo JL. Value of combined thiazide-loop diuretic therapy in chronic kidney disease: heart failure and reninangiotensin-aldosterone blockade. J Clin Hypertens. 2012;14:344.
76. Maione A, Navaneethan SD, Graziano G, Mitchell R, Johnson D, Mann JF, et al. Angiotensin-converting enzyme inhibitors, angiotensin receptor blockers and combined therapy in patients with micro- and macroalbuminuria and other cardiovascular risk factors: a systematic review of randomized controlled trials. Nephrol Dial Transplant. 2011;26:2827–47.
77. Holtkamp FA, de Zeeuw D, Thomas MC, Cooper ME, de Graeff PA, Hillege HJ, et al. An acute fall in estimated glomerular filtration rate during treatment with losartan predicts a slower decrease in long-term renal function. Kidney Int. 2011;80:282–7.
78. Li L, Harrison SD, Cope MJ, et al. Mechanism of action and pharmacology of patiromer, a nonabsorbed cross-linked polymer that lowers serum potassium concentration in patients with hyperkalemia. J Cardiovasc Pharmacol Ther. 2016;21(5):456–65.
79. Stavros F, Yang A, Leon A, Nuttall M, Rasmussen HS. Characterization of structure and function of ZS-9, a K+ selective ion trap. PLoS One. 2014;9(12):e114686.
80. ONTARGET Investigators, Yusuf S, Teo KK, Pogue J, Dyal L, Copland I, et al. Telmisartan, ramipril, or both in patients at high risk for vascular events. N Engl J Med. 2008;358:1547–59.
81. Weir MR, Bakris GL, Weber MA, Dahlof B, Devereux RB, Kjeldsen SE, et al. Renal outcomes in hypertensive Black patients at high cardiovascular risk. Kidney Int. 2012;81:568–76.
82. Williams B, MacDonald TM, Morant S, Webb DJ, Sever P, McInnes G, et al. Spironolactone versus placebo, bisoprolol, and doxazosin to determine the optimal treatment for drug-resistant hypertension (PATHWAY-2): a randomised, double-blind, crossover trial. Lancet. 2015;386:2059–68.
83. Rosendorff C, Lackland DT, Allison M, Aronow WS, Black HR, Blumenthal RS, et al. Treatment of hypertension in patients with coronary artery disease: a scientific statement from the American Heart Association, American College of Cardiology, and American Society of Hypertension. Hypertension. 2015;65:1372–407.
84. Hermida RC, Diana E, Ayala DE, Mojón A, Fernández JR. Bedtime dosing of antihypertensive medications reduces cardiovascular risk in CKD. J Am Soc Nephrol. 2011;22:2313–21.
85. Daugherty SL, Powers JD, Magid DJ, Tavel HM, Masoudi FA, Margolis KL, et al. Incidence and prognosis of resistant hypertension in hypertensive patients. Circulation. 2012;125:1635–42.

Chapter 16
Chronic Kidney Disease in Elderly: Do Kidneys Behave Differently as we age?

Anju Yadav

Introduction

With better medical care and recent advances, we have increasing number of aging elderly population. According to the data of National Health and Nutrition Examination Survey (NHANES), approximately 11% of the US population has chronic kidney disease (CKD), and this may be as high as 30% in the older population [1]. However, data from US renal data system (USRDS) show that incidence of CKD steadily increases with advancing age (Table 16.1) [2, 3]. Age group above 65 years is rapidly rising and is reported to rise to 53 million by the end of 2020 (Fig. 16.1) [3].

It is important that physicians familiarize themselves in health care related issues with elderly so that this population can be taken care of appropriately. Evaluation of this age group includes assessment of cognitive, affective, functional, social, economic, and environmental status. The average 75-year-old suffers from 3.5 chronic diseases as per US Census Bureau (www.census.gov/). Most common co-morbid conditions associated with CKD in addition to aging are hypertension, diabetes, hyperlipidemia, smoking, alcohol use, and liver disease.

Since automatic reporting of estimated glomerular filtration fraction (eGFR) using Modification of Diet in Renal Disease (MDRD) formula has started, many patients have been reported to have impaired kidney function. Most of these patients are elderly due to age used in the MDRD equation. These patients usually get referred to nephrology for decreased eGFR seen on lab reports. However, over-referral is probably preferable to under-referral [4]. Signs of ongoing active renal disease such as an active urine sediment or significant proteinuria are reason for a

A. Yadav (✉)
Division of Nephrology, Hypertension and Transplantation, Thomas Jefferson University Hospital, Philadelphia, PA, USA
e-mail: anju.yadav@jefferson.edu

© Springer Nature Switzerland AG 2022
J. McCauley et al. (eds.), *Approaches to Chronic Kidney Disease*,
https://doi.org/10.1007/978-3-030-83082-3_16

Table 16.1 Age-adjusted percentages (with standard errors) of selected diseases and conditions among adults aged 18 and above based on selected characteristics: United States, 2018

	Selected characteristic	Diabetes	Uloers	Kidney disease	Liver disease	Arthritis diagnosis	Chronic joint symptoms
Total		9.5 (021)	5.6 (0.17)	2.2 (0.10)	1.7 (0.10)	21.4 (0.28)	28.4 (0.37)
	Sex						
Male		10.2 (0.31)	5.0 (0.23)	2.2 (0.15)	2.0 (0.16)	18.9 (0.36)	28.2 (0.54)
Female		8.9 (0.27)	6.1 (0.24)	2.1 (0.13)	1.4 (0.11)	23.7 (0.38)	28.6 (0.45)
	Age (years)						
18–44		3.3 (0.23)	3.4 (0.21)	0.6 (0.09)	1.0 (0.12)	7.0 (0.31)	16.5 (0.48)
45–64		12.9 (0.47)	6.9 (0.35)	2.4 (0.20)	2.6 (0.22)	30.3 (0.59)	37.6 (0.68)
85–74		22.2 (0.79)	10.3 (0.55)	5.4 (0.41)	3.0 (0.31)	48.3 (0.93)	48.2 (0.90)
75 and over		22.8 (0.99)	9.4 (0.62)	8.0 (0.60)	1.4 (0.26)	53.7 (1.06)	51.2 (1.13)

Ref: https://ftp.cdc.gov/pub/Health_Statistics/NCHS/NHIS/SHS/2017_SHS_Table_A-4.pdf

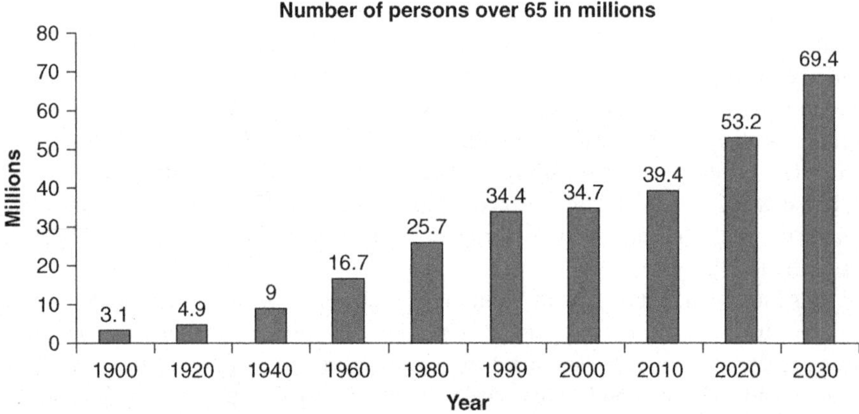

Fig. 16.1 Projected population over age 65 years from the US census Bureau. (Source: Jocelyn Wiggins. Chap. 2, ASN curriculum for geriatric nephrology)

nephrologist's care. However, eGFR values between 45 and 59 ml/min/1.73 m^2 in those who are 70 years of age and older should be interpreted with caution. If other signs of kidney damage (e.g., proteinuria and hematuria) and an absence of CKD-related complications are observed, a stable eGFR in this range may be consistent with typical GFR for this age. Patients showing complications of decreased renal function such as anemia, bone-mineral disorders, and hyperkalemia need nephrology management.

Other medical conditions seen frequently in CKD/end-stage kidney disease (ESKD) populations include the following:

- 70% of dialysis patients 55 years of age and older have chronic cognitive impairment of a level severe enough to impact on their compliance and ability to make informed decisions [5].

Table 16.2 Common geriatric conditions that impact nephrology care

Visual/ hearing impairment
Malnutrition/weight loss
Urinary incontinence
Balance/gait impairment/falls
Polypharmacy
Cognitive impairment; affective disorders
Functional limitations
Lack of social support
Economic hardship
Home environment/safety

- Prevalence of depression is reported to be as high as 45% in the older dialysis population [6–8].
- Metabolic bone disease is complicated by age-related osteoporosis. The cardiovascular consequences of CKD are complicated by structural heart disease such as valvular insufficiency and atrial fibrillation [9, 10].
- Neurodegenerative disease impacts on the patient's mobility and cognitive function. Osteoarthritis and neuropathy limit their physical activity. As age and disease advance, frailty becomes an issue [5]. Other conditions in this population that can impact effective nephrology care are listed in Table 16.2.

CKD and ESKD are huge financial burdens to our medical system. In 2005, Medicare costs for CKD were $42 billion and for ESKD were $20 billion. The cost of ESKD was one half that of CKD, although only a small percentage of patients with CKD progress to ESKD. According to NHANES data, about 11% of the US population has CKD, whereas 0.2% of the US population has ESKD. Despite this low prevalence, ESKD was responsible for 6.4% of the entire Medicare budget [5].

Prevalence of Chronic Kidney Disease in Elderly

Patients 75 years and older currently represent one of the fastest growing contingents of the ESKD population, most likely reflecting both an aging population and the high overall prevalence of CKD in the elderly as shown in Table 16.1. Thus, a critical challenge for health systems and providers caring for older patients with CKD lies in identifying the relatively small proportion, but large absolute number, of older patients with CKD who are at greatest risk for progressive loss of renal function and ultimate need for dialysis. Around half of the patients start dialysis without nephrology care and this needs to change [11]. Male gender, African-American race (mostly in middle age), diabetes, and presence of micro- or macroalbuminuria are high risk factors for CKD progression in elderly [12].

Age-Related Decline in Kidney Function

In humans and some animals [13], the number of glomeruli present in adulthood are predetermined between weeks 32 and 36 of gestation [13–15]. In humans, the superficial cortex glomeruli differ in size from the juxta-arcuate glomeruli until age 2. At this age, the size of all of the glomeruli is the same and the kidney is functioning at adult capacity. The number of glomeruli among individuals is quite variable, ranging from 247,652 to 1,825,380 per kidney. Renal mass increases from 50 g at birth to 400 g during the third and fourth decades of life before decreasing to 300 g by the ninth decade [13–15]. The latter decrease correlates with the loss of the renal cortex. Radiographically, the size of the kidney has been shown to decrease in size by 10% after age 40 to 30% by age 80.

Cross-sectional and longitudinal studies have looked at the natural progression of the kidney with aging. A linear relationship between aging and a decline in the renal function were noted [16, 17], but elderly persons who had no underlying disease had adequate renal reserves [15, 18–20]. The overall rate of decline in creatinine clearance was 0.87 ml/min per year beginning at age 40 and was inversely related to age.

Reductions of estimated GFR to 50–59 ml/min/1.73 m^2 do not increase mortality risk among patients aged 65 years or older compared with patients with eGFR of more than 60 ml/min [21]. These observations have sparked debate that whether the decrease in GFR that occurs with aging should really be considered unhealthy [22] and whether term "chronic kidney disease" in such cases should be replaced with "age-related reduced kidney function or age-related decline in renal function" [23].

Assessment of Renal Function

There are no consensus or guidelines on optimal approach to estimate GFR assessment in elderly populations. MDRD and Cockcroft- Gault formula have age in their calculations, but none have been validated in estimating GFR for patients over 70 years of age with standard techniques such as isotope clearance. Serum cystatin C equation, independent of muscle mass, may be superior to both and is an independent risk factor for mortality in elderly [24–27].

Not many studies have been done to perform risk assessment in this population. Co-morbid conditions like high blood pressure, diabetes are more prevalent in elderly population, which further contribute to development of CKD. Hence, course of CKD depends on patient's past medical history, overall health, and renal reserves more than with actual disease process. Depending on acuity and rate of progression, presence of proteinuria, and active sediment, diagnosis of CKD can be made. Obstructive uropathy, renal artery stenosis, and medication-associated side effects should also be considered.

In general, older patients are more likely to have a low eGFR than their younger counterparts but are less likely to experience progression to ESKD. Most older patients who meet CKD criteria are much more likely to die before they reach ESKD; this is true even for older patients with severe reduction in eGFR. It is often difficult to know which subset of older patients with CKD will progress to ESKD. The importance of interventions to slow progression of CKD should be weighed against other, perhaps competing, physical, and mental health priorities.

Histologic Change in the Aging Kidney

The four compartments in kidney change with age in the following manner [28]:

- Glomerulus: thickening of basement membrane, increase in mesangial matrix, focal global sclerosis, hypertrophy progressive loss of capillary loops, atubular glomeruli
- Podocytes: fusion intermittent, detachment, vacuoles
- Interstitium: tubular dilatation/atrophy, tubular cast, monocytes infiltrates, interstitial fibrosis
- Vessels: atrophy of afferent and efferent vessels, hyalinosis of vessels, glomerulus vessels

Mechanisms associated with age-associated renal disease are mainly factors leading to oxidative stress, increased transforming growth factor-beta (TGF-β) expression, accumulation of advanced glycation products, renal ischemia, loss of nitric oxide leading to endothelial dysfunction, intrarenal renin angiotensin system activation, glomerular hypertension and hyperfiltration, senescence, and chronic effect of uric acid.

Functional Changes in an Aging Kidney

With aging, renal blood flow decreases in both human and animal populations. The lower renal plasma blood flow and the decrease in GFR contribute to the increase in the filtration fraction (ratio of the glomerular filtration rate to the renal plasma flow) found in elderly persons. Elderly people are hence more susceptible to acute kidney injury in a low perfusion state because of attenuated responses to vasodilators and an increase in response to vasoconstrictors in presence of decreased renal reserve. Table 16.3 shows fluid and electrolytes in aging [29–38].

Endocrine function and renal hormones: Erythropoietin (EPO) levels increase with age due to increased EPO resistance but show a poor response to low hemoglobin [39]. Elderly women with eGFR below 60 ml/min have lower calcium absorption and lower 1,25-hydroxyvitamin D levels, probably due to diminished conversion of 25-hydroxyvitamin D to 1,25-dihydroxyvitamin D by the aging kidney [36]. Kidney removes about 50% of insulin in the peripheral circulation by filtration and proximal tubular uptake and degradation. The decline of renal function in the elderly

Table 16.3 Fluid and electrolytes in aging [29–38]

Sodium	Impaired sodium excretion after salt load and defective conservation in sodium restriction[a] Proximal sodium reabsorption increased Distal sodium reabsorption maybe reduced	Development of systolic hypertension Salt sensitivity in 85% of population and hence sodium restriction results in >10 mmHg decline in mean arterial pressure
Potassium	Impaired potassium excretion due to reduction in tubules Decline in eGFR, lower basal rate of aldosterone, and tubulointerstitial scarring impairs $Na^+K^+ATPase$[b] transporters	More incidence of hyperkalemia especially if on potassium-sparing medications
Acid-base homeostasis	Impaired distal tubular function Impaired acid excretion Low serum renin, renin activity, and aldosterone	Acid-base disturbance Impaired response to hypovolemia
Calcium	More incidence of institutionalized patients with malignancy, hyperparathyroidism, immobilization, thiazide diuretic use	Hypercalcemia occurs in 2–3% of these patients
	Chronic kidney disease, chronic malabsorption, and malnourishment	Hypocalcemia
Magnesium	Malnutrition, laxatives, PPI, diuretics	7–10% elderly population has hypomagnesemia
	Magnesium-containing laxatives, chronic kidney disease	Hypermagnesemia
Uric acid	Impaired excretion and increased incidence of kidney disease	Gout and hyperuricemia
Osmoregulation and water handling	Impaired water handling Defective concentration and diluting function Decreased maximal urine osmolality and thirst response to hyperosmolarity Blunted response to anti-diuretic hormone	Hypernatremia

[a]Yanomamo Indians of South Venezuela who ingest low-sodium diets do not show an increase in blood pressure with age
[b]Sodium-potassium ATPase

leads to a decrease in insulin clearance. This is in part offset by diminished glucose tolerance, which may relate to the increasing frequency of obesity observed in aging individuals [40].

Clinical Manifestations of Chronic Kidney Disease

Given the limitation and changes in glomerular and tubular function in elderly people, even the slightest change in homeostasis impact elderly much more drastically. Fluid balance, intravenous fluids, ischemic injury, hypoxemia, and medication toxicity affect more severely the elderly due to loss of renal reserve and lack of adequate compensation. Hence, there is an increased risk of hyponatremia, hyperkalemia, hypertension, and acute kidney injury.

Glomerular Diseases Except for some glomerular disease, prevalence is same in general population. It is common to have a combination of different glomerulonephritis (GN) in elderly, like diabetic kidney disease in combination with hypertensive nephrosclerosis, atherosclerosis etc. Several other commonly seen glomerulonephritis in this population are membranous nephropathy (MN), granulomatous polyangiitis, (GPA)/antineutrophilic cytoplasmic antibody (ANCA)-related vasculitis, membranoproliferative glomerulonephritis (MPGN), and amyloidosis [41] (Fig. 16.2). Only 2% of patients with systemic lupus erythematosus present after age of 60% [41].

Renovascular and Atherosclerotic Diseases There is increased risk of hypertension in patients with CKD and vice versa. As we all know, there is increased frequency of renovascular and atherosclerotic disease with aging for obvious reasons. Magnetic renal arteriogram and renal artery duplex scanning are recommended in patients with history of vascular disease with hypertension and elevated serum creatinine [42, 43].

Acute Kidney Injury There is an increased risk in elderly population, especially during peri-operative time, due to reduction in functional renal reserve, impaired autoregulation, defective fluid hemostasis, and increased susceptibility to drug nephrotoxicity [44]. Proteinuria and sudden changes in GFR indicate presence of kidney disease or glomerulonephritis. Early detection of potential GN should be prioritized and should be managed as would be in a younger population.

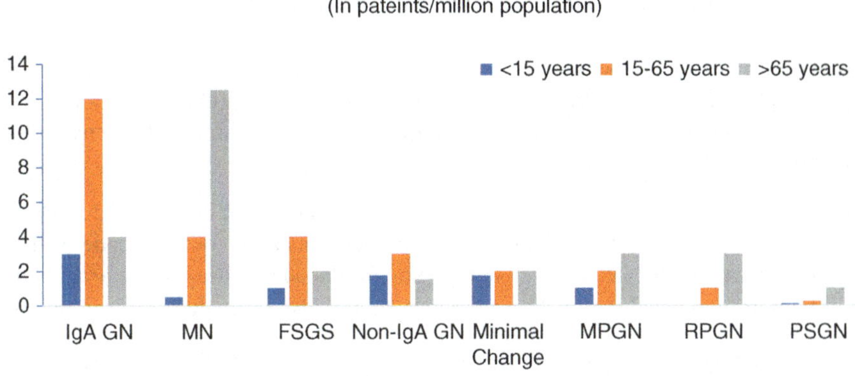

Fig. 16.2 Epidemiology of primary glomerulonephritis by age. *IgA GN* IgA nephropathy, *MN* membranous nephropathy, *FSGS* focal segmental glomerulosclerosis, *Non-IgA GN* other mesangio-proliferative glomerulonephritis, *MPGN* membrano-proliferative glomerulonephritis, *RPGN* rapidly progressive glomerulonephritis, *PSGN* post-streptococcal glomerulonephritis. (Adapted from 5th edition: Comprehensive Textbook of Nephrology)

Pauci-immune GN, immunoglobulin A (IgA) nephropathy, and minimal change disease (MCD) are disease of elderly [41].

Urinary Tract Infections (UTI) There is increased risk of asymptomatic bacteriuria and symptomatic UTI with aging. This might be due to benign prostatic hypertrophy (BPH) and increased risk of kidney stones. Chronic use of indwelling catheters might put them at higher risk as well. Treatment should be based on symptoms and guidelines regarding high-risk patients and immunocompromised status.

Obstructive Uropathy Obstructive uropathy is common in elderly men due to BPH, cancer, and strictures. In women, the incidence is one-third compared to men and is mainly due to malignancy in the GU tract. Ultrasound is the modality of evaluation for suspected obstruction. Management is based on etiology and complexity. Multi-specialty approach involving urology and nutrition is often needed.

Urinary Incontinence In case of urinary incontinence, bladder capacity decreases and postvoid residual bladder volume increases by about 50–100 ml with age. Elderly people also have a higher frequency of nocturia, due in part to the decrease in renal concentrating capacity, BPH, and perhaps also due to disordered sleep. Transient urinary incontinence is common in the elderly with multiple potentially treatable causes, which are best recalled by a mnemonic, DIAPPERS (delirium/confusional state; infection – urinary; atrophic urethritis/vaginitis; pharmaceuticals like diuretics; psychological- depression; endocrine– hypercalcemia, hypokalemia, glycosuria; restricted mobility; stool impaction) [28]. In men, the most common cause is overflow incontinence from prostatic obstruction, whereas in women, a prolapsed uterus is frequently the cause. If a reversible cause is not promptly identified, referral to a neurologist (to rule out conditions such as normal-pressure hydrocephalus) or urologist is recommended.

In the absence of an easily reversible cause, nonsurgical therapeutic options for urinary incontinence include behavioral therapy and biofeedback, pelvic floor exercises, pharmacologic therapy (e.g., α-adrenergic antagonists to reduce prostatic hypertrophy), and, if it is unavoidable, long-term catheterization. Surgery may be required for large cystoceles, vaginal vault prolapse, and postprostatectomy stress incontinence [28].

Hematuria In men, hematuria is most commonly, and might be, related to malignancy, stones, infections. Bladder cancer risk increases after fourth decade of life. Renal cell carcinoma (RCC) is noted in 6th–7th decade of life. Hematuria needs thorough urologic evaluation. These patients should also be evaluated for glomerular diseases.

Nephrotoxicity and Drug Dosing Polypharmacy is unfortunately extremely common in elderly population due to medical comorbidities. Altered pharmacokinetics can be related to age, drugs/interactions, and disease. Medications such as angiotensin-converting enzyme inhibitor (ACE-I), antibiotics, antifungals, antivirals, anticoagulants, digoxin, sotalol, opioids, non-steroidal anti-inflammatory drugs, NSAIDs, proton pump inhibitors, PPIs, COX2 inhibitors, radiocontrast, chemotherapy, psychotropic and anti-convulsant, hypoglycemics especially biguanides, gout medication, etc., should be carefully instituted and monitored. Medication list should always be reviewed for potential drug-srug interactions. Dose of medications should be adjusted for renal function. Modification in dosages means either reducing the actual dose or reducing dosing interval. Elderly patients are more prone to drug-related nephrotoxicity as their creatinine is seemingly normal, and normal renal function is assumed. They need to be adjusted based on age, renal function, and presence of comorbid conditions. Special mention to aminoglycosides, digoxin, procainamide, tetracycline, vancomycin, etc. Drugs like thiazides, diuretics, and SSRI can lead to dysnatremia as well. GN can be also due to NSAIDs, bisphosphonates, etc.

Mineral Bone Diseases Renal osteodystrophy and osteoporosis may coexist in elderly. Choice of therapy should be based on each patient's personal past medical history. DEXA scan for osteoporosis is an ideal study. Calcium, phosphorus, parathyroid hormone, and vitamin D levels should be routinely measured. Appropriate therapy based on levels should be offered. Lifestyle changes like exercise, smoking cessation, weight management are equally important. Calcium, vitamin D supplements, bisphosphonates, calcimimetic, hormonal replacement therapy, etc., are available options.

End-Stage Kidney Disease and Renal Replacement Therapy

Data collected by USRDS show that ESKD is a disease of the older population, with numbers starting to rise significantly after the age of 50. Mean age at the start of renal replacement therapy is 62.3 years for men and 63.4 years for women. Peak incident counts of treated ESKD occur in the 70- to 79-year age group at 15,000 patients per year or 1543 patients per million population (Fig. 16.3) (USRDS 2018 data).

1-year survival probabilities in incident ESKD patients based on age shows a drop off after 79 years of age. This probably reflects the tendency of older patients, with significant burden of disease refusing dialysis. The incident rates have been rising steadily over the last 25 years with a narrowing gap between rates in the 70- to 79-year-old age group compared with the 80-year age group (Fig. 16.4) (USRDS 2018 data).

However, dialysis is associated with poor quality of life, loss of independence, and longer post-dialysis fatigue [45–47]. Home dialysis therapy like peritoneal dialysis, daily short home hemodialysis, and nocturnal dialysis are better tolerated modalities and have better outcomes with less post-HD fatigue [48, 49]. For some patients, in-center hemodialysis gives them a sense of community where important (sometimes the only) social interactions take place. So, modality should be decided based on patients' lifestyle and social situation. No pre-dialysis nephrology care

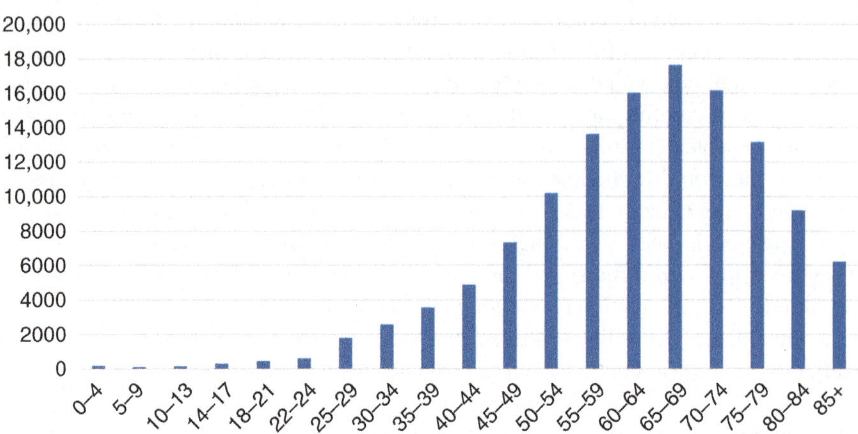

Fig. 16.3 Incidence rate of end-stage renal disease (ESRD) patient per million based on USRDS data 2018. (Data from: https://adr.usrds.org/2020/end-stage-renal-disease/5-mortality)

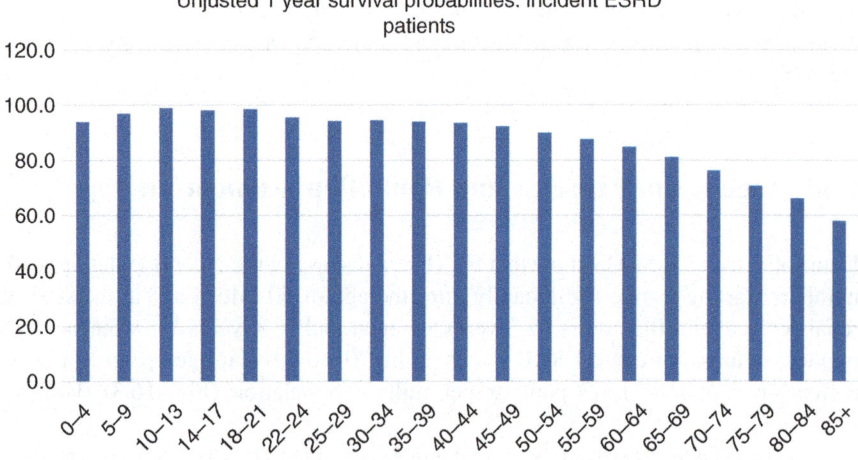

Fig. 16.4 Unadjusted 1 year survival probabilities in incident ESRD patients. (Data from: https://adr.usrds.org/2020/end-stage-renal-disease/5-mortality)

and poor socioeconomic status and education status are some of the factors associated with suboptimal care before dialysis initiation. Even today, 50% of patients undergo dialysis with a dialysis catheter [50].

A higher occurrence of ESRD in older subjects is due to either diabetes or hypertension. Despite the frequency of CKD among elderly patients, ESRD is far less common than cardiovascular morbidity or mortality [42]. Older patients with CKD stage 3 are more likely to die and less likely to reach ESRD than their younger counterparts [51].

The rapid growth of this population will presumably be accompanied by a rise in per-patient dialysis expenditures because costs for HD in a person over 65 years average 10–35% more than for a person under 65 year.

For example, the actuarial life expectancy of a 75-year-old patient on dialysis is approximately 3 years, as opposed to 11 years for one not on dialysis [52]. For those 90 years and older when starting dialysis, survival is 50% at 1 year [53].

The decision to offer renal replacement therapy is no longer based on the age of the individual. Patients often do very well with either hemodialysis or peritoneal dialysis unless there are comorbid conditions such as cardiovascular disease. As with younger subjects, vascular access remains the Achilles heel of hemodialysis. Even in this population, the survival of arteriovenous fistulas is significantly greater than that of arteriovenous grafts. Transplantation should be considered in the management of elderly patients with ESRD because studies have clearly shown that the elderly recipient benefits from renal transplantation by a significant reduction in mortality (41%) compared with waitlisted ESRD patients [54]. Increasing number of elderly patients are being managed with dialysis, and some of these may benefit from a kidney transplant. There is no consensus about age limit for transplant. Some data show benefit of transplant in septuagenarians [55]. However, in some transplant centers, the cutoff age is 70 years.

Elderly subjects are at a lower immunological risk and receive basiliximab for induction. They require overall lesser immunosuppression. However, because they have a higher rate of death with functioning grafts, overall graft survival is similar to that in younger population.

Palliative Care

Based on CMS data, median time from discontinuation of dialysis to death as reported in CMS death notification form was 6 days (IQR 3–12 days). The percentage of patients who discontinued dialysis before death increased from 19.3% in 2000 to 24.9% in 2012. This number was highest for patients aged 85+ years (34.2%) and lowest for those aged 20–44 years (10.9%). White race was associated with highest number of dialysis discontinuation (27.3%) compared to other races (10.2%). These trends coincide with patients utilizing palliative care and hospice options at the end of life care, with Caucasian using more hospice care compared to other races. Utilization of hospice care has steadily increased from 11.4% in 2000 to 25.4% in 2012. Again 85+ year patients used hospice option 28.9% of the time compared to 20 to 44-year age group who utilized hospice option only 7% of the time.

The time to expire from discontinuation of dialysis depends on the patient's residual renal function, comorbid conditions, and other lifestyle choices. Every patient should be encouraged to have end-of-life and advance directive discussion. Living wills are equally important. Various conservative measures can be considered depending on patient's choice of level of palliative or hospice care.

References

1. Razzaque MS. Does renal aging affect survival? Ageing Res Rev. 2007;6:211–22.
2. Coresh J, Astor BC, Greene T, Eknoyan G, Levey AS. Prevalence of chronic kidney disease and decreased kidney function in the adult US population: Third National health and Nutrition Examination Survey. Am J Kidney Dis. 2003;41:1–12.
3. Wiggona J. Chapter 2. Why Do We Need a Geriatric Nephrology Curriculum? JASN Curriculum for geritraic nephrology. https://www.asnonline.org/education/distancelearning/curricula/geriatrics/Chapter2.pdf.
4. Lindeman RD, Tobin J, Shock NW. Longitudinal studies on the rate of decline in renal function with age. J Am Geriatr Soc. 1985;33:278–85.
5. American Society of Nephrology. American Society of Nephrology kidney disease populations: an occult burden. Adv Chronic Kidney Dis. 2008;15:123–32.
6. Murray AM, Tupper DE, Knopman DS, Gilbertson DT, Pederson SL, Li S, Smith GE, Hochhalter AK, Collins AJ, Kane RL. Cognitive impairment in hemodialysis patients is common. Neurology. 2006;67:216–23.
7. Madero M, Gul A, Sarnak MJ. Cognitive function in chronic kidney disease. Semin Dial. 2008;21:29–37.
8. Kimmel PL, Cohen SD, Peterson RA. Depression in patients with chronic renal disease: where are we going? J Ren Nutr. 2008;18:99–103.
9. Kimmel PL. Depression in patients with chronic renal disease: what we know and what we need to know. J Psychosom Res. 2002;53:951–6.
10. Watnick S, Kirwin P, Mahnensmith R, Concato J. The prevalence and treatment of depression among patients starting dialysis. Am J Kidney Dis. 2003;41:105–10.
11. Collins AJ, Foley R, Herzog C, Chavers B, Gilbertson D, Ishani A, Kasiske B, Liu J, Mau LW, McBean M, Murray A, St Peter W, Xue J, Fan Q, Guo H, Li Q, Li S, Li S, Peng Y, Qiu Y, Roberts T, Skeans M, Snyder J, Solid C, Wang C, Weinhandl E, Zaun D, Zhang R, Arko C, Chen SC, Dalleska F, Daniels F, Dunning S, Ebben J, Frazier E, Hanzlik C, Johnson R, Sheets D, Wang X, Forrest B, Constantini E, Everson S, Eggers P, Agodoa L. Excerpts from the United States Renal Data System 2007 annual data report. Am J Kidney Dis. 2008;51:S1–S320.
12. Baggio B, Budakovic A, Perissinotto E, Maggi S, Cantaro S, Enzi G, Grigoletto F. ILSA working group: atherosclerotic risk factors and renal function in the elderly: the role of hyperfibrinogenaemia and smoking. Results from the Italian Longitudinal Study on Ageing (ILSA). Nephrol Dial Transplant. 2005;20:114–23.
13. Hoy WE, Douglas-Denton RN, Hughson MD, Cass A, Johnson K, Bertram JF. A stereological study of the glomerular number and volume: preliminary findings in a multiracial study of kidneys at autopsy. Kidney Int. 2003;63:S31–7.
14. Manalich R, Reyes L, Herrera M, Melendi C, Fundora I. Relationship between weight and the number and size of renal glomeruli in humans: a histomorphometric study. Kidney Int. 2000;58:770–3. American Society of Nephrology Geriatric Nephrology Curriculum 5.
15. Epstein M. Aging and the kidney. J Am Soc Nephrol. 1996;7:1106–22. [PMID: 8866401].
16. Wesson LG Jr. Renal hemodynamics in physiological states. New York: Grune & Stratton; 1969.
17. Esposito C, Plati A, Mazzullo T, et al. Renal function and functional reserve in healthy elderly individuals. J Nephrol. 2007;20:617–25. [PMID: 17918149].
18. Jones CA, Francis ME, Eberhardt MS, et al. Microalbuminuria in the U.S. population: Third National Health and Nutrition Examination Survey. Am J Kidney Dis. 2002;39:445–59. [PMID: 11877563].
19. Rowe JW, Andres R, Tobin JD, et al. The effect of age on creatinine clearance in men: a cross-sectional and longitudinal study. J Gerontol. 1976;31:155–63.
20. Danziger RS, Tobin JD, Becker LC, Lakatta EE, Fleg JL. The age associated decline in glomerular filtration in healthy normotensive volunteers lack of relationship no cardiovascular performance. J Am Geriatr Soc. 1990;38:1127–32.

21. O'Hare AM, Bertenthal D, Covinsky KE, et al. Mortality risk stratification in chronic kidney disease: one size for all ages? J Am Soc Nephrol. 2006;17:846–53. [PMID: 16452492].
22. Glassock RJ. Glomerular disease in the elderly population. Geriatr Nephrol Urol. 1998;8:149–54. [PMID: 10221173].
23. Glassock RJ, Winnearls C. CKD in the elderly. Am J Kidney Dis. 2008;52:803–4. [PMID: 18805350].
24. Verhave JC, Fesler P, Ribstein J, et al. Estimation of renal function in subjects with normal serum creatinine levels: influence of age and body mass index. Am J Kidney Dis. 2005;46:233–41. [PMID: 16112041].
25. Shlipak MG, Wassel Fyr CL, Chertow GM, et al. Cystatin C and mortality risk in the elderly: the health, aging, and body composition study. J Am Soc Nephrol. 2006;17:254–61. [PMID: 16267155].
26. Schaeffner ES, Ebert N, Delanaye P, et al. Two novel equations to estimate kidney function in persons aged 70 years or older. Ann Intern Med. 2012;157:471–81. [PMID: 23027318].
27. Fehrman- Ekholm I, Skeppholm L. Renal function in the elderly(70 year old) measured by means of iohexol clearance, serum creatinine, serum urea and estimated clearance. Scand J Urol Nephrol. 2004;38:73–7.
28. Rosner MH, Lerma EV, Swaminathan S. Chapter 67. Geriatric nephrology. Comprehensive textbook of nephrology. 5th ed. Elsevier Publication.
29. Fliser D, Franek E, Joest M, et al. Renal function in the elderly: impact of hypertension and cardiac function. Kidney Int. 1997;51:1196–204. [PMID: 9083286].
30. Burt VL, Whelton P, Roccella EJ, et al. Prevalence of hypertension in the US adult population. Results from the Third National Health and Nutrition Examination Survey, 1988–1991. Hypertension. 1995;25:305–13. [PMID: 7875754].
31. Weinberger MH, Fineberg NS. Sodium and volume sensitivity of blood pressure. Age and pressure change over time. Hypertension. 1991;18:67–71. [PMID: 1860713].
32. Oliver WJ, Cohen EL, Neel JV. Blood pressure, sodium intake, and sodium related hormones in the Yanomamo Indians, a "no-salt" culture. Circulation. 1975;52:146–51. [PMID: 1132118].
33. Streeten DH, Anderson GH Jr, Wagner S. Effect of age on response of secondary hypertension to specific treatment. Am J Hypertens. 1990;3:360–5. [PMID: 2350475].
34. Stachenfeld NS, Mack GW, Takamata MA, et al. Thirst and fluid regulatory responses to hypertonicity in older adults. Am J Phys. 1996;271:R757–65. [PMID: 8853401].
35. Kishore BK, Krane CM, Reif M. Molecular physiology of urinary concentration defects in elderly population. Int Urol Nephrol. 2001;33:235–48.
36. Jacob S, Spinler SA. Hyponatremia associated with selective serotonin-reuptake inhibitors in older adults. Ann Pharmacother. 2006;40:1618–22. [PMID: 16896026].
37. Musso CG, Miguel R, Algranati L, Dos Ramos Farias E. Renal potassium excretion: comparison between chronic renal disease patients and old people. Int Urol Nephrol. 2005;37:167–70. [PMID: 16132781].
38. Agarwal BN, Cabebe FG. Renal acidification in elderly subjects. Nephron. 1980;26:219–95.
39. Carpenter MA, Kendall RG, O'Brien AE, et al. Reduced erythropoietin response to anaemia in elderly patients with normocytic anaemia. Eur J Haematol. 1992;49:119–21. [PMID: 1446724].
40. Ershler WB, Sheng S, McKelvey J, et al. Serum erythropoietin and aging: a longitudinal analysis. J Am Geriatr Soc. 2005;53:1360–5. [PMID: 16078962].
41. National Institute of Diabetes and Digestive and Kidney Diseases. Kidney disease statistics for the United States. NIH publication No. 12–3895; 2012. http://kidney.niddk.nih.gov.proxy1.lib.tju.edu/kudiseases/pubs/kustats/#4; Accessed 5 January 2013.
42. Weiner DE, Tighiouart H, Elsayed EF, Griffith JL, Salem DN, Levey AS, Sarnak MJ. Inflammation and cardiovascular events in individuals with and without chronic kidney disease. Kidney Int. 2008;73:1406–12.

43. Lindeman RD, Tobin JD, Shock NW. Association between blood pressure and the rate of decline in the renal function with age. Kidney Int. 1984;26:861–8.
44. Chronopoulos A, Rosner MH, Cruz DN, Ronco C. Acute kidney injury in elderly intensive care patients: a review. Intensive Care Med. 2010;36:1454–64. [PMID: 20631983].
45. Kurella Tamura M, Covinsky KE, Chertow GM, et al. Functional status of elderly adults before and after initiation of dialysis. N Engl J Med. 2009;361:1539–47. [PMID: 19828531].
46. Jassal SV, Chiu E, Hladunewich M. Loss of independence in patients starting dialysis at 80 years of age or older. N Engl J Med. 2009;361:1612–3. [PMID: 19828543].
47. Lazarides MK, Georgiadis GS, Antoniou GA, Staramos DN. A meta-analysis of dialysis access outcome in elderly patients. J Vasc Surg. 2007;45:420–6.
48. Brown EA, Johansson L, Farrington K, et al. Broadening Options for Long-term Dialysis in the Elderly (BOLDE): differences in quality of life on peritoneal dialysis compared to haemodialysis for older patients. Nephrol Dial Transplant. 2010;25:3755–63. [PMID: 20400451].
49. Couchoud C, Moranne O, Frimat L, et al. Associations between comorbidities, treatment choice and outcome in the elderly with end-stage renal disease. Nephrol Dial Transplant. 2007;22:3246–54. [PMID: 17616533].
50. DE Obrador GT, Ruthazer R, Arora P, Kausz AT, Pereira BJ. Prevalence of and factors associated with suboptimal care before initiation of dialysis in the United States. J Am Soc Nephrol. 1999;10:1793–800.
51. Gallagher JC, Rapuri P, Smith L. Falls are associated with decreased renal function and insufficient calcitriol production by the kidney. J Steroid Biochem Mol Biol. 2007;103:610–3. [PMID: 17236758].
52. U.S. Renal Data System. USRDS 2008 annual data report: atlas of chronic kidney disease and end-stage renal disease in the United States. Bethesda: National Institute of Diabetes and Digestive and Kidney Diseases; 2008.
53. Kurella M, Covinsky KE, Collins AJ, Chertow GM. Octogenarians and nonagenarians starting dialysis in the United States. Ann Intern Med. 2007;146:177–83.
54. Segall L, Nistor I, Pascual J, Mucsi I, Guirado L, Higgins R, Van Laecke S, Oberbauer R, Van Biesen W, Abramowicz D, Gavrilovici C, Farrington K, Covic A. Criteria for and appropriateness of renal transplantation in elderly patients with end-stage renal disease. Transplantation. 2016;100(10):e55–e65.
55. Katz G, Yadav A, Martinez PM, Singh P. Patient and kidney allograft outcomes in septuagenarians - a single Center experience. ATC abstract. Am J Transplant. 2020;20(suppl 3) https://atcmeetingabstracts.com/abstract/patient-and-kidney-allograft-outcomes-in-septuagenarians-a-single-center-experience/.

Chapter 17
Chronic Kidney Disease in Non-renal Solid Organ Transplantation

Christina Mejia and Anju Yadav

Introduction

As of 2019, more than 110,000 people are waiting for an organ transplant [1]. Almost half of transplants performed in the United States are kidney transplants. Around 20% of cases are orthotopic liver transplants and the remaining 30% include heart, lung, pancreas, intestine, and combined organ transplants (i.e., heart-lung, kidney-pancreas, liver-kidney). Acute and chronic kidney dysfunctions are frequently seen in non-renal solid organ transplantation (NR-SOT). Similar to other medical and surgical settings, acute kidney injury (AKI) is associated with increased morbidity and mortality in NR-SOT recipients. In one retrospective cohort of 519 liver, heart, and lung recipients, development of AKI after transplant was associated with a four- to ninefold increase in the risk of mortality, with an even higher risk for those who required renal replacement therapy [2]. AKI was also associated with longer hospital stay of around 3 weeks and increased health care cost. Meanwhile, Ojo et al. reported that chronic kidney disease (CKD) after NR-SOT was associated with 4.5-fold increased risk of death [3]. Because of the consequences of kidney dysfunction in this population, recognition, surveillance, and timely treatment of AKI and CKD in NR-SOT recipients are of great importance.

C. Mejia
Medicine-Nephrology, Johns Hopkins University, Baltimore, MD, USA
e-mail: cmejia5@jh.edu

A. Yadav (✉)
Division of Nephrology, Hypertension and Transplantation, Thomas Jefferson University Hospital, Philadelphia, PA, USA
e-mail: anju.yadav@jefferson.edu

© Springer Nature Switzerland AG 2022
J. McCauley et al. (eds.), *Approaches to Chronic Kidney Disease*,
https://doi.org/10.1007/978-3-030-83082-3_17

Kidney Disease in NR-SOT: Definitions and Prevalence

In the non-transplant population, Kidney Disease: Improving Global Outcomes (KDIGO) guidelines define CKD as abnormalities of kidney structure and function present for more than 3 months and is classified based on estimated glomerular function rate (eGFR) and level of albuminuria (Fig. 17.1) [4]. A GFR <60 ml/min/1.73 m^2 is generally regarded as decreased eGFR, while an eGFR <15 ml/min/1.73 m^2 is considered kidney failure. GFR is estimated by equations using serum creatinine (SCr), with the newer CKD-EPI equation generally being favored over the Modification of Diet in Renal Disease Study (MDRD) and the Cockroft-Gault equations. Screening for albuminuria is performed using a random albumin-to-creatinine ratio or a urine protein dipstick. Meanwhile, multiple definitions of acute kidney injury (AKI) exist, but all include acute increases in SCr from baseline or the development of oliguria as part of the criteria (Table 17.1) [5].

Among NR-SOT recipients, CKD and AKI are not well defined. Creatinine-based equations that estimate GFR have not been well validated in this population. Due to the chronicity of their underlying illness and a higher catabolic state from infections or inflammation, transplant candidates and recipients generally have

Prognosis of CKD by GFR and albuminuria category

Prognosis of CKD by GFR and albuminuria categories: KDIGO 2012				Persistent albuminuria categories Description and range		
				A1	A2	A3
				Normal to mildly increased	Moderately increased	Severely increased
				<30 mg/g <3 mg/mmol	30-300 mg/g 3-30 mg/mmol	>300 mg/g >30 mg/mmol
GFR categories (ml/min/1.73 m^2) Description and range	G1	Normal or high	≥90			
	G2	Mildly decreased	60-89			
	G3a	Mildly to moderately decreased	45-59			
	G3b	Moderately to severely decreased	30-44			
	G4	Severely decreased	15-29			
	G5	Kidney failure	<15			

Fig. 17.1 KDIGO classification of CKD based on eGFR and albuminuria. Green: low risk (if no other markers of kidney disease, no CKD); yellow: moderately increased risk; orange: high risk; red: very high risk

Table 17.1 Definitions of acute kidney injury [5]

Definitions	Serum creatinine (SCr) criteria	Urine output criteria
RIFLE	Increase in SCr 1.5-fold of baseline or decrease in eGFR by 25% in 48 hours	<0.5 ml/kg/h for 6 hours
AKIN	Increase in SCr 1.5-fold of baseline or $\geq$ 0.3 mg/dl in 48 hours	<0.5 ml/kg/h for 6 hours
KDIGO[a]	SCr $\geq$ 0.3 mg/dl in 48 hours SCr $\geq$1.5-fold of known baseline or has occurred within the prior 7 days	<0.5 ml/kg/h for 6 hours

RIFLE Risk, Injury, Failure, Loss of Kidney function, and End-stage kidney disease, *AKIN* Acute Kidney Injury Network, *KDIGO* Kidney Disease Improving Global Outcomes
[a]Further classified into Stage 1–3 based on severity

lower muscle mass or sarcopenia resulting in decreased creatinine generation. Hemodynamic changes like volume overload and/or volume depletion, especially among heart and liver transplant candidates and recipients, may also result in fluctuations in SCr. Medications like calcineurin inhibitors, renin-angiotensin-aldosterone system (RAAS) blockers, and sulfamethoxazole-trimethoprim (SMX-TMP) are commonly used in NR-SOT recipients and may result in physiologic elevations in SCr or alterations in renal tubular creatinine secretion. Broekroelofs et al. found that creatinine-based estimates of GFR underestimated the degree of GFR loss among heart transplant recipients and likely holds true for other NR-SOT recipients as well [6]. Among liver transplant recipients, Gonwa et al. found that the MDRD equation correlated better than the Cockroft-Gault and Nankivell equations with measured GFR using ^{125}I-iothalamate clearance as the gold standard [7]. Most of these studies pre-dated the CKD-EPI equation, and in the absence of higher-quality data, both MDRD and EPI equations can likely be used among NR-SOT keeping in mind their limitations [8]. Using the CKD-EPI cystatin-C-based equation can address the shortcomings of SCr, but may be costly and not readily available. In addition to estimating GFR, clinical correlation with history and physical examination and assessment of proteinuria should always be part of the renal evaluation in this population.

The reported prevalence of CKD among NR-SOT patients ranges from 8% to 83% over median follow-up durations of 1–6 years [3, 9–13]. This wide range is due to the different criteria used by authors to define a reduced eGFR and CKD. Using data from the Scientific Registry of Transplant Recipients (SRTR), Ojo et al. performed a population-based cohort analysis of more than 69,000 NR-SOT recipients [3]. Using an eGFR < 30 ml/min/1.73 m^2 to define CKD or the onset of end-stage renal disese (ESRD) requiring dialysis or preemptive renal transplant, the cumulative incidence of CKD was 1.9% for heart, 1.7% for heart-lung, 9.6% for intestine, 8.0% for liver, and 2.9% for lung recipients after the first post-transplant year. The cumulative incidences at 5-years post-transplant were 10.9% for heart, 6.9% for heart-lung, 21.3% for intestine, 18.1% for liver, and 15.8% for lung recipients. ESRD developed in 28% of their patients and 46% of those were eventually listed for kidney transplant. Also using SRTR data, Srinivas et al. reported that the number of NR-SOT recipients listed for a kidney transplant has tripled from 1995 to 2008, composing around 3% of all those on the wait-list [14]. Compared to other kidney transplant candidates, more NR-SOT recipients were listed preemptively [14].

Risk Factors for Chronic Kidney Disease in NR-SOT

Multiple risk factors for developing CKD exist among NR-SOT recipients and can be viewed as those present prior to transplant and those that result from transplantation itself (Table 17.2). Pre-existing CKD is an obvious risk factor for developing progressive kidney dysfunction after transplant. As discussed earlier, SCr usually overestimates renal function among NR-SOT candidates. This results in an under-appreciation of the degree of underlying kidney disease in this population. Ojo et al. noted that around 20% of their population had an eGFR of <60 ml/min/1.73 m^2 and around 5% had an eGFR <30 ml/min/1.73 m^2 prior to NR-SOT [3]. They also noted that 1–18% of their recipients had underlying hypertension and 3–9% had diabetes prior to transplant, both common causes of nephropathy. Older age at the time of transplant and female gender are non-modifiable risk factors found to be associated with doubling of SCr after NR-SOT [15, 16]. Other risk factors are hepatitis B and C infections which can cause glomerulonephritis (GN) and may remain undetected among liver candidates in the absence of a kidney biopsy. The apolipoprotein L1 (APOL-1) high-risk genotype was found to be associated with an increased risk of end-stage kidney disease from conditions like focal segmental glomerulosclerosis among patients with African ancestry [17]. Its impact among kidney transplant donors and recipients is currently being studied but has not yet been explored in the setting of CKD in NR-SOT recipients.

Past and recurrent episodes of AKI are established risk factors for later development of kidney dysfunction. In the general population, AKI results in an eightfold increased risk of developing CKD and a threefold increased risk of developing ESRD [5]. In the study by Wyatt et al. on 519 NR-SOT recipients, 25% developed post-transplant AKI with 8% requiring renal replacement therapy [2]. In patients awaiting transplant, AKI may develop as they decompensate, leading to worsening

Table 17.2 Risk factors for CKD in NRSOT

Pre-transplant	Perioperative	Post-transplant
Pre-existing CKD	Acute kidney injury	CNI toxicity
Hypertension	Cardiorenal syndrome	BKPVAN
Diabetes	Hepatorenal syndrome	Hypertension
Hyperlipidemia	Cardiopulmonary bypass	Post-transplant diabetes
Older age	Hypotension/hypovolemia	Exposure to nephrotoxins
Female	Sepsis	
Hepatitis B & C	Atheroembolic events	
	Exposure to nephrotoxins	

BKPVAN BK polyoma virus associated nephropathy, *CNI* calcineurin inhibitors cardiorenal and hepatorenal syndromes observed in heart and liver transplant candidates, respectively. Hyperbilirubinemia can also result in pigment nephropathy as liver dysfunction worsens. During the peri-operative period, additional risk factors for developing AKI include hypotension, hypovolemia, sepsis, atheroembolic events, and exposure to nephrotoxins like iodinated contrast, antibiotics, and nonsteroidal anti-inflammatory medications [8]. Among NR-SOT recipients, it is important to acknowledge that AKI may not immediately or completely reverse after transplantation of a new organ [18]. Furthermore, more medically complex patients are now being transplanted which may explain the increasing number of AKI observed among NR-SOT in recent years [19].

Unique to post-transplant patients is the effect of immunosuppression on kidney function. The discovery of calcineurin inhibitors (CNI) has revolutionized transplant medicine but has resulted in dose- and duration-dependent CNI nephrotoxicity. Cyclosporine and to a lesser extent, tacrolimus, lead to renal vasoconstriction and ischemic injury resulting in acute and chronic kidney dysfunction. Acute depression of eGFR may occur as CNI levels increase to supratherapeutic levels [20] or with concomitant use of RAAS blockers. Chronic CNI nephrotoxicity results from prolonged exposure. Steep declines in eGFR may be observed within the first 6 months of transplant, corresponding to higher CNI doses, followed by a slower decline and non-nephrotic-range albuminuria. The diagnosis of CNI nephrotoxicity is confirmed through kidney biopsy. However, it is rarely perfomed for this purpose alone and is usually considered to rule out other causes of kidney dysfunction. The typical histopathologic finding in chronic CNI nephrotoxicity is that of a "stripped" or "zebra" appearance of interstitial fibrosis. In addition to recurrent vasoconstriction and ischemia, oxidative stress and chronic thrombotic microangiopathy (TMA) are other proposed mechanisms for CNI nephrotoxicity [8]. BK polyomavirus associated nephropathy (BK-PVAN) is a consequence of over-immunosuppression and is better described among kidney transplant recipients. The reported prevalence of BK viremia among NR-SOT ranges from 7–32% while only a few cases of BV-PVAN have been reported among NR-SOT recipients [21–23]. BK-PVAN usually presents with asymptomatic increases in SCr, but hemorrhagic cystitis can be a rare presentation. The mainstay of treatment for BK-PVAN is reduction in immunosuppression.

Hypertension and diabetes may develop after NR-SOT or may worsen in those with these diseases prior to transplant. CNI use likely contributes to post-transplant hypertension [8]. New-onset diabetes after transplantation, also referred to as post-transplant diabetes mellitus (PTDM), develops in 2–53% of all SOT recipients [24]. Risk factors for developing PTDM include African-American and Hispanic ethnicities, obesity, older age, family history of diabetes, history of hepatitis C, and impaired glucose tolerance prior to transplant [24]. Glucocorticoids are commonly part of induction and maintenance immunosuppression regimens and result in hyperglycemia. The risk of PTDM was found to increase by 5% for every 0.1 mg/kg/day increase in prednisolone dose [25]. Although most of the studies are on kidney transplant recipients, tacrolimus, more than cyclosporine, is known to be diabetogenic and is thought to be due to CNI-induced impairment in insulin secretion

[26]. Among pancreas recipients, CNIs are also thought to result in direct reversible toxicity to pancreatic islet cells [27]. Similar to its effects in the general population, post-transplant hypertension and diabetes contribute to the development of CKD in NR-SOT recipients as well as to cardiovascular morbidity and mortality in this population.

The risk of developing CKD after NR-SOT varies depending on the organ transplanted, with certain factors unique to specific organ transplantations. Heart and lung transplant recipients are subjected to cardiopulmonary bypass and aortic cross-clamping [18], which even in non-transplant surgeries is associated with post-operative AKI [28]. In addition, heart and lung recipients are usually kept in a volume-depleted state with more aggressive diuresis resulting in more episodes of pre-renal AKI [18]. Heart, lung, and intestines are also thought to be more immunogenic organs than the liver and kidneys and require higher CNI trough levels to prevent rejection. Lung transplant recipients are more prone to develop fungal infections, and exposure to amphotericin was associated with increased risk of post-transplant AKI [29]. As already mentioned, due to hepatitis B and C, liver transplant patients may have underlying GN predisposing them to worsening kidney function. Ojo et al. reported varying relative risks (RR) for developing CKD based on the organ transplanted, with a RR of 0.48 (95% CI 0.36–0. 65) for combined heart-lung, RR 0.63 (95% CI 0.61–0.66) for heart alone, 0.99 (95% CI 0.93–1.06) for lung alone, and 1.36 (95% CI 1.0–1.86) for intestine recipients using liver translant as the reference group [3].

Prevention and Management of Kidney Disease in NRSOT

Pre-, peri-, and post-transplant renal protection strategies among NR-SOT recipients are similar to those that are performed in other clinical settings. Avoiding hypotension, maintaining euvolemia, and limiting exposure to nephrotoxic agents like NSAIDs, iodinated contrast, and other nephrotoxic medications are important [8]. Optimal blood pressure, lipid, and glucose control all contribute to delaying progression of renal disease. Recommendations of expert groups regarding the prevention, screening, and treatment goals for hypertension, dyslipidemia, and diabetes for the general population should also apply to NR-SOT recipients.

Angiotensin-converting enzyme inhibitors (ACEI) or angiotensin receptor blockers (ARB) should be initiated when indicated for hypertension and proteinuria. In addition to its well-established renoprotective effects in the non-transplant CKD population, RAAS blockade is also thought to slow down kidney fibrinogenesis and may lower the risk for CNI-related nephropathy [30, 31]. The timing of initiation of ACEI or ARBs should be balanced against their hemodynamic effects on the kidneys, especially in patients who are recovering from an episode of AKI. SGLT-2 inhibitors which have been shown to lower the risk of cardiovascular events and renal failure among type 2 diabetics with CKD [32] have not been well-studied in transplant cohorts and in PTDM. The use of CNI-sparing strategies should be an open discussion between the nephrologist and the transplant teams. Increasing the dose of the anti-metabolite mycophenolate and the use of mTOR inhibitors like sirolimus can allow for lower doses of CNIs and less nephrotoxicity but should be balanced against the risk of rejection [8]. Lastly, drug-drug interactions should always be monitored among transplant recipients. Commonly prescribed medications like non-dihydropyridine calcium channel blockers and other CYP3A inhibitors may lead to supratherapeutic levels of CNI.

For NR-SOT recipients who progress to CKD, monitoring and management of the complications associated with CKD should follow KDIGO and Kidney Disease Outcomes Quality Initiative (KDOQI) recommendations for non-transplant CKD patients. Physicians should perform careful cardiovascular examination looking for signs of end-organ damage and volume overload. Subtle uremic symptoms like fatigue and dysgeusia should be part of the review of systems. In addition to a complete metabolic panel, screening for proteinuria should be routinely performed. Renal ultrasound will reveal signs of chronicity and help rule out structural abnormalities or obstruction that may contribute to renal dysfunction. The need for a kidney biopsy will depend on whether certain diagnoses other the CNI-nephrotoxicity are being considered, keeping in mind that primary kidney disease can concomitantly occur in NR-SOT recipients. Attention should be given to CKD-related anemia, electrolyte and acid-base abnormalities, and bone-mineral disease. Involvement of a nephrologist should be considered early on as the development of CKD can be anticipated especially with prolonged CNI exposure.

With medical and surgical advancements in treating transplant-related complications, the lifespan of NR-SOT recipients has improved with the consequence of more recipients reaching ESRD. Timely discussion regarding renal replacement therapy (RRT) is crucial so that patients can be prepared for dialysis or referred for kidney transplant evaluation. Kidney transplant remains the preferred RRT as it confers a survival benefit over remaining on dialysis [33]. As these patients are under close follow-up with transplant teams, early referral for kidney transplant evaluation and preemptive transplant should be the goal. Both hemodialysis and peritoneal dialysis can be considered in NR-SOT recipients. The choice of dialysis modality usually depends on individual patient factors and preference, similar to non-transplant ESRD patients.

Simultaneous solid-organ-kidney transplant may be considered in certain patients. In the US, majority of multi-organ transplants are simultaneous liver-kidney transplant (SLKT), with few heart-kidney, lung-kidney, and pancreas-kidney transplantations being performed each year. Transplant centers carefully consider who should qualify for simultaneous solid organ-kidney, as this takes away from the deceased-donor kidney transplant pool with close to 100,000 candidates waiting for a kidney transplant alone. Based on the United Network for Organ Sharing (UNOS) policy, SLKT can be considered for patients with GFR < 60ml/min for at least 90 days prior to transplant or in patients with sustained AKI with a GFR < 25ml/min or are dialysis-dependent for at least six consecutive weeks [34]. Criteria for simultaneous kidney transplant with other solid organs are not as well defined.

Conclusion

Acute and chronic kidney diseases are frequently seen in NR-SOT recipients. Defining and detecting kidney dysfunction in this population remain a challenge as estimates of GFR are based on serum creatinine and based on studies on non-transplant populations. Calcineurin inhibitor use leads to chronic nephrotoxicity, but various pre-, peri-, and post-transplant factors also contribute to the development of AKI and CKD among NR-SOT recipients. Renoprotective strategies and management of CKD and its complications among NR-SOT recipients should follow general expert guidelines applied to non-transplant populations. Kidney transplant remains the RRT of choice among NR-SOT recipients who progress to ESRD. A multidisciplinary approach involving the transplant teams and the nephrologist is important in caring for NR-SOT with kidney dysfunction.

References

1. Transplant trends. UNOS. Accessed 3 Dec 2019. https://unos.org/data/transplant-trends/.
2. Wyatt CM, Arons RR. The burden of acute renal failure in nonrenal solid organ transplantation. Transplantation. 2004;78(9):1351–5. https://doi.org/10.1097/01.tp.0000140848.05002.b8.
3. Ojo AO, Held PJ, Port FK, Wolfe RA, Leichtman AB, Young EW, Arndorfer J, Christensen L, Merion RM. Chronic renal failure after transplantation of a nonrenal organ. N Engl J Med. 2003;349(26):2563–5. https://doi.org/10.1056/nejm200312253492617.
4. Kidney Disease: Improving Global Outcomes (KDIGO). Clinical practice guideline for the evaluation and management of the chronic kidney disease (CKD). 2012. https://kdigo.org/guidelines/ckd-evaluation-and-management/.
5. Feehally J. Comprehensive clinical nephrology. Edinburgh: Elsevier; 2019.
6. Broekroelofs J, Stegeman C, Navis G, Haan JD, Bij WVD, Boer WD, de Zeeuw D, Jong PD. Creatinine-based estimation of rate of long-term renal function loss in lung transplant recipients. Which method is preferable? J Heart Lung Transplant. 2000;19(3):256–62. https://doi.org/10.1016/s1053-2498(99)00133-3.
7. Gonwa TA, Jennings L, Mai ML, Stark PC, Levey AS, Klintmalm GB. Estimation of glomerular filtration rates before and after orthotopic liver transplantation: evaluation of current equations. Liver Transpl. 2004;10(2):301–9. https://doi.org/10.1002/lt.20017.
8. Bloom RD, Reese PP. Chronic kidney disease after nonrenal solid-organ transplantation. J Am Soc Nephrol. 2007;18(12):3031–41. https://doi.org/10.1681/asn.2007040394.
9. Ishani A, Erturk S, Hertz MI, Matas AJ, Savik K, Rosenberg ME. Predictors of renal function following lung or heart-lung transplantation. Kidney Int. 2002;61(6):2228–34. https://doi.org/10.1046/j.1523-1755.2002.00361.x.
10. Myers BD, Newton L. Cyclosporine-induced chronic nephropathy: an obliterative microvascular renal injury. J Am Soc Nephrol. 1991;2(Suppl):S45–52.
11. O'Riordan A, Wong V, McCormick PA, Hegarty JE, Watson AJ. Chronic kidney disease post-liver transplantation. Nephrol Dial Transplant. 2006;21:2630–6.
12. Platz K-P, Mueller AR, Blumhardt G, Bachmann S, Bechstein WO, Kahl A, Neuhaus P. Nephrotoxicity following orthotopic liver transplantation: a comparison between cy- closporine and FK506. Transplantation. 1994;58:170–8.
13. Mccauley J, Thiel DHV, Starzl TE, Puschett JB. Acute and chronic renal failure in liver transplantation. Nephron. 1990;55(2):121–8. https://doi.org/10.1159/000185938.

14. Srinivas TR, Stephany BR, Budev M, Mason DP, Starling RC, Miller C, Goldfarb DA, Flechner SM, Poggio ED, Schold JD. An emerging population: kidney transplant candidates who are placed on the waiting list after liver, heart, and lung transplantation. Clin J Am Soc Nephrol. 2010;5(10):1881–6. https://doi.org/10.2215/cjn.02950410.

15. Guitard J, Ribes D, Kamar N, Cointault O, Lavayssiere L, Esposito L, Rostaing L, Muscari F, Suc B, Peron JM. Predictive factors for chronic renal failure one year after orthotopic liver transplantation. Ren Fail. 2006;28:419–25.

16. Canales M, Youssef P, Spong R, Ishani A, Savik K, Hertz M, Ibrahim HN. Predictors of chronic kidney disease in long-term survivors of lung and heart-lung transplantation. Am J Transplant. 2006;6:2157–63.

17. Freedman BI, Moxey-Mims M. The APOL1 long-term kidney transplantation outcomes network—APOLLO. Clin J Am Soc Nephrol. 2018;13(6):940–2. https://doi.org/10.2215/cjn.01510218.

18. Bloom R, Doyle A. Kidney disease after heart and lung transplantation. Am J Transplant. 2006;6(4):671–9. https://doi.org/10.1111/j.1600-6143.2006.01248.x.

19. Nadkarni GN, Chauhan K, Patel A, Saha A, Poojary P, Kamat S, Patel S, Ferrandino R, Konstantinidis I, Garimella PS, Menon MC, Thakar CV. Temporal trends of dialysis requiring acute kidney injury after orthotopic cardiac and liver transplant hospitalizations. BMC Nephrol. 2017;18(1) https://doi.org/10.1186/s12882-017-0657-8.

20. Ruggenenti P, Perico N, Mosconi L, Gaspari F, Benigni A, Amuchastegui CS, Bruzzi I, Remuzzi G. Calcium channel blockers protect transplant patients from cyclosporine-induced daily renal hypoperfusion. Kidney Int. 1993;43(3):706–11. https://doi.org/10.1038/ki.1993.101.

21. Thomas LD, Vilchez RA, White ZS, Zanwar P, Milstone AP, Butel JS, Dummer S. A prospective longitudinal study of polyomavirus shedding in lung transplant recipients. J Infect Dis. 2007;195:442–9.

22. Randhawa P, Uhrmacher J, Pasculle W, Vats A, Shapiro R, Eghtsead B, Weck K. A comparative study of BK and JC virus infections in organ transplant recipients. J Med Virol. 2005;77:238–43.

23. Muñoz P, Fogeda M, Bouza E, Verde E, Palomo J, Bañares R. Prevalence of BK virus replication among recipients of solid organ transplants. Clin Infect Dis. 2005;41(12):1720–5. https://doi.org/10.1086/498118.

24. Pham P-T, Pham P-M, Pham P-C. New onset diabetes after transplantation (NODAT): an overview. Diabetes Metab Syndr Obes. 2011:175. https://doi.org/10.2147/dmso.s19027.

25. Hjelmesth J, Hartmann A, Kofstad J, Stenstrm J, Leivestad T, Egeland T, Fauchald P. Glucose intolerance after renal transplantation depends upon prednisolone dose and recipient age 1. Transplantation. 1997;64(7):979–83. https://doi.org/10.1097/00007890-199710150-00008.

26. Bloom RD, Crutchlow MF. New-onset diabetes mellitus in the kidney recipient: diagnosis and management strategies. Clin J Am Soc Nephrol. 2008;3(Supplement 2) https://doi.org/10.2215/cjn.02650707.

27. Drachenberg CB, Klassen DK, Wiland A, Weir MR, Fink JC, Cangro CB, Blahut S, Papadimitriou JC. Islet cell damage associated with tacrolimus and cyclosporine: morphological features in pancreas allograft biopsies and clinical correlation. Transplantation. 1999;67(7) https://doi.org/10.1097/00007890-199904150-00834.

28. Nadim MK, Forni LG, Bihorac A, Hobson C, Koyner JL, Shaw A, Arnaoutakis GJ, Ding X, Engelman DT, Gasparovic H, Gasparovic V, Herzog CA, Kashani K, Katz N, Liu KD, Mehta RL, Ostermann M, Pannu N, Pickkers P, Price S, Ricci Z, Rich JB, Sajja LR, Weaver FA, Zarbock A, Ronco C, Kellum JA. Cardiac and vascular surgery–associated acute kidney injury: the 20th international consensus conference of the ADQI (Acute Disease Quality Initiative) group. J Am Heart Assoc. 2018;7(11) https://doi.org/10.1161/jaha.118.008834.

29. Rocha PN, Rocha AT, Palmer SM, Davis RD, Smith SR. Acute renal failure after lung transplantation: incidence, predictors and impact on perioperative morbidity and mortality. Am J Transplant. 2005;5(6):1469–76. https://doi.org/10.1111/j.1600-6143.2005.00867.x.

30. Lin J, Valeri AM, Markowitz GS, Dagati VD, Cohen DJ, Radhakrishnan J. Angiotensin converting enzyme inhibition in chronic allograft nephropathy. Transplantation. 2002;73(5):783–8. https://doi.org/10.1097/00007890-200203150-00022.

31. Artz MA. Blockade of the renin-angiotensin system increases graft survival in patients with chronic allograft nephropathy. Nephrol Dial Transpl. 2004;19(11):2852–7. https://doi.org/10.1093/ndt/gfh462.
32. Gogia A, Kakar A, Gangwani A. Canagliflozin and renal outcomes in type 2 diabetes and nephropathy. Curr Med Res Pract. 2019;9(4):164. https://doi.org/10.1016/j.cmrp.2019.07.012.
33. Cassuto JR, Reese PP, Sonnad S, Bloom RD, Levine MH, Olthoff KM, Shaked A, Abt P. Wait list death and survival benefit of kidney transplantation among nonrenal transplant recipients. Am J Transplant. 2010;10(11):2502–11. https://doi.org/10.1111/j.1600-6143.2010.03292.x.
34. Simultaneous Liver-Kidney Allocation (SLK) policy changes now in effect. UNOS, June 6, 2019. https://unos.org/news/simultaneous-liver-kidney-allocation-slk-policy-changes-now-in-effect/.

Chapter 18
Chronic Kidney Disease and Pregnancy

Seyed Mehrdad Hamrahian

Introduction

During normal pregnancy, maternal anatomic and physiologic adaptations alter systemic and renal hemodynamics [1, 2] (Table 18.1). Awareness of these adaptive pregnancy-associated renal physiologic changes is necessary in order to identify and interpret the unique disorders that may result in de novo or worsening of existing renal disease [3]. Moreover, pregnancy in patients with underlying renal disease has important implications for maternal and fetal morbidity and mortality [4]. It is important to understand these adaptive changes for appropriate risk assessment before conception and to provide close monitoring during pregnancy to identify early the maternal and fetal compromise. Similarly, availability of pre-pregnancy baseline renal function, urinalysis, and blood pressure recordings can avoid misclassification of any abnormalities encountered during pregnancy.

Anatomic and Physiologic Adaptations

During pregnancy, kidneys increase in size by about 1–1.5 cm in length secondary to an increase in renal volume by up to 30%. A physiologic hydronephrosis occurs due to the influence of progesterone hormone inhibiting ureteral peristalsis and to the mechanical obstruction of the ureter (right > left) due to dextrorotation of the uterus by the sigmoid colon. These physiologic changes typically peak by the 20th week of gestation and resolve within 48 hours after delivery, but they may persist for up to 12 weeks postpartum [5].

S. M. Hamrahian (✉)
Department of Medicine, Division of Nephrology, Sidney Kimmel School of Medicine,
Thomas Jefferson University, Philadelphia, PA, USA
e-mail: seyed.hamrahian@Jefferson.edu

© Springer Nature Switzerland AG 2022
J. McCauley et al. (eds.), *Approaches to Chronic Kidney Disease*,
https://doi.org/10.1007/978-3-030-83082-3_18

Table 18.1 Anatomic and physiologic renal adaptations in pregnancy

Anatomic changes	Clinical implications
Dilatation of the collecting system and increase in renal size	Increases risk of pyelonephritis in asymptomatic bacteriuria Makes diagnosis of true obstruction difficult

Physiologic changes	Clinical implications
Systemic and renal vasodilatation	Decreases blood pressure
Increases blood volume	Physiologic edema and anemia
Increases renal blood flow rate and glomerular filtration rate	Decreases serum creatinine, BUN Mildly increases proteinuria
Altered tubular function	Causes glucosuria, hypercalciuria, hypouricosuria

Blood pressure (BP) falls shortly after conception and returns to normal at term. This decrease is due to peripheral vasodilatation and insensitivity to angiotensin II secondary to high prostacyclin and prolactin levels, increased nitric oxide synthesis, and relaxin produced by the placenta and corpus luteum [6]. The hemodynamic changes that result in a rapid fall in preload and afterload lead to a compensatory increase in heart rate and activation of volume-restoring mechanisms, including the renin-angiotensin-aldosterone system (RAAS). The circulating blood volume increases by 50% in part due to cumulative sodium retention (500–900 mEq) in the proximal tubule stimulated by angiotensin II and in the distal portion of nephrons secondary to elevated aldosterone levels. The resultant rise in stroke volume increases cardiac output (CO) by about 40% above the non-pregnant level at mid-gestation. This could lead further to increased extracellular fluid volume, weight gain, and "benign" edema of lower extremities. The increased CO and renal vasodi-latation increases renal blood flow by as much as 85% in the second trimester. This results in renal hyperfiltration and increased glomerular filtration rate (GFR) of about 50% and, respectively, blood urea nitrogen (BUN) and creatinine levels fall [7]. Therefore, as GFR equations commonly overestimate or underestimate the true renal function, trends in serum creatinine levels, even small increases, provide bet-ter assessment of kidney function deterioration [8]. These changes return to prepar-tum levels within 3 months of delivery. Interestingly, despite highly RAAS activity, in part secondary to increased angiotensinogen production by estrogen, there is resistance to hypertensive action of angiotensin II due to increased synthesis of prostaglandins by the placenta. Similarly, aldosterone-associated kaliuresis is blunted by progesterone, which competes for mineralocorticoid receptor [9].

A range of other physiologic changes occurs with pregnancy. Hypo-osmolar hyponatremia occur due to a downward resetting of the osmotic threshold for both AVP secretion and thirst. Transient diabetes insipidus occurs due to high placental vasopressinase activity. It usually occurs at term and is short lived, and it responds to synthetic AVP analog desmopressin (DDAVP), which is not metabolized by vaso-pressinase [10]. Physiologic anemia of pregnancy is secondary to lower red blood cell mass rise of 30% compared to 50% rise in plasma volume. There is an increased calciuria secondary to high 1,25 (OH)$_2$ vitamin D$_3$ production without increased risk of nephrolithiasis.

Hyperfiltration can result in microalbuminuria due to an increase in fractional excretion of albumin, but significant proteinuria of over 300 mg in a 24-hour period or hematuria always indicates unmasked kidney disease and worsening of pre-existing or de novo development of renal disease. Uric acid levels decrease secondary to increased GFR. Glycosuria secondary to inefficient tubular reabsorption in the setting of increased filtered load of glucose is a common normal finding. The early-morning urine is more alkaline due to mild chronic respiratory alkalosis secondary to progesterone-induced hyperventilation. Respectively, serum bicarbonate levels are generally lower. Asymptomatic bacteriuria warrants treatment due to dilatation of the renal collecting system that can result in pyelonephritis, bacteremia, septic shock, renal failure, or mid-trimester abortions.

Acute Kidney Injury in Normal Pregnancy

Pregnancy-associated acute kidney injury (AKI) is a rare but serious complication and has significant adverse outcomes for both maternal and fetal well-being [11, 12]. Unfortunately, there is no standardized definition of pregnancy-associated AKI. Unfortunately, early and accurate diagnosis and classification of pregnancy-associated AKI are difficult due to the increase in GFR related to renal hyperfiltration and the reduction of the serum creatinine. Although AKI could be reversible, affected women are at increased risk of developing CKD [13]. Acute kidney injury could occur during pregnancy in early pregnancy, late pregnancy, or postpartum period or result from other causes [14] (Table 18.2).

Pregnancy in Women with Underlying Chronic Kidney Disease

Chronic kidney disease represents a heterogeneous group of disorders characterized by changes in the structure or function of the kidney. Low GFR, hypertension, and proteinuria are the typical clinical manifestations, with the severity depending on underlying cause of renal disease. Progression of CKD results in diminished fertility, and women on long-term dialysis get pregnant rarely. Moreover, human chorionic gonadotropin levels are inversely related to GFR and therefore results must be interpreted with caution. Pregnancy in women with underlying CKD is associated with a significant risk factor for adverse outcome [15]. Women with CKD planning pregnancy should ideally have pre-conception baseline renal function testing, including serum creatinine, BUN, creatinine clearance, and proteinuria; complete blood cell count; uric acid; and liver enzymes in view of being potentially at high risk for progression of underlying kidney disease or development of preeclampsia later in pregnancy. The degree of renal insufficiency, even in the early stages, is a critical determinant of pregnancy outcome. There is a stepwise increase in risks

Table 18.2 Acute kidney injury in pregnancy

Early pregnancy	Late pregnancy	Postpartum	Other causes
Pre-renal azotemia due to hyperemesis gravidarum or hemorrhage of spontaneous abortion. In severe cases, this could lead to ATN	Acute fatty liver of pregnancy that typically presents with jaundice and abdominal pain and possible fulminant hepatic failure in severe cases	Days to weeks after normal pregnancy, secondary to thrombotic thrombocytopenic purpura/hemolytic uremic syndrome	Obstructive uropathy secondary to gravid uterus, polyhydramnios, nephrolithiasis, or enlarged uterine fibroids
ATN secondary to septic abortion in the first trimester or pigment induced secondary to myoglobulinuria in the setting of Clostridium induced myonecrosis of the uterus	Preeclampsia, eclampsia, and HELLP syndrome		
Renal cortical necrosis secondary to obstetric catastrophes: abruption placentae, septic abortion, severe preeclampsia, amniotic fluid embolism, and retained fetus			

ATN acute tubular necrosis, *HELLP* hemolysis, elevated liver enzymes, low platelets

both for maternal and fetal outcomes from stage 1 to stage 5 with the highest risk in patients on dialysis [16, 17]. Respectively, women with stage 1 CKD and hypertension and/or proteinuria should be followed closely during pregnancy due to an increased risk of preeclampsia, intrauterine growth retardation, preterm delivery, prematurity, small for gestation age, fetal loss, or neonatal death compared to women with normal renal function. Moreover, pregnancy can accelerate the renal disease progression, such as development of hypertension, increase in proteinuria, and decrease in GFR, either reversible or irreversible, leading to the so-called CKD shift and the need to start dialysis earlier than anticipated. The likelihood of disease progression depends on the severity of underlying kidney disease rather than the type. In addition to the degree of renal dysfunction, the risk of disease progression increases in the setting of coexisting hypertension, chronic diseases like diabetes or lupus, and nephrotic syndrome. Currently, there are no means to predict which women will experience renal deterioration during or immediately after pregnancy. Similarly, pregnancy termination does not reliably reverse the decline in renal function [18–23]. Finally, optimization of pre-existing diseases significantly affects the pregnancy outcome [24, 25].

Women with CKD are likely to have concomitant hypertension, as the relationship is bidirectional. Hypertension during pregnancy with characteristic dilated afferent arteriole of glomerulus may play a detrimental role in underlying disease due to high intraglomerular capillary pressure induced by transmission of systemic BP into glomerulus. Women with CKD and hypertension are at an increased risk for preeclampsia. The maternal and fetal outcomes depend on maternal renal function/GFR at the beginning of pregnancy, underlying hypertension, and proteinuria. Any persistent renal damage, even in the setting of preserved GFR and in the absence of uncontrolled hypertension or significant proteinuria, increases the risk for adverse pregnancy outcomes. High maternal BUN levels can act as osmotic diuresis within the fetal renal system resulting in polyhydramnios, early labor, and or even fetal loss.

In summary, pregnancy in the setting of underlying CKD does not only increase the risk of pregnancy-associated complications, but also influences the quality of life of the mother and child. In general, women with preserved kidney function before pregnancy are unlikely to have significant renal function loss as long as BP and proteinuria are managed prior to conception. Respectively, strategies to optimize outcomes need to begin preconception and continue through delivery and the postpartum period.

Shared decision-making in a multi-disciplinary setting is of paramount importance. Pre-pregnancy counseling and risk stratification are crucial for optimal maternal and fetal outcomes and should be provided by a multi-disciplinary care provider team, including a nephrologist, high-risk obstetrician, and maternal–fetal medicine specialist for pregnancy-associated complications. Special care includes management of hypertension and any proteinuria or CKD deterioration, prevention of preeclampsia, avoidance of nephrotoxic or teratogenic medications, and renal dosing of all medications. Ideally, one should discuss the pregnancy planning while the patient is still in the lower stages of CKD or postpone pregnancy until after kidney transplantation secondary to relatively lower risk [26–28].

Proteinuria Treatment

Proteinuria should be addressed and minimized preconception, because the degree of proteinuria is associated with adverse pregnancy outcomes. Renal biopsy should preferably be performed before conception or, in case of new-onset nephrotic syndrome, in early gestation if definitive diagnosis will affect treatment options [29]. Use of RAAS blockers to suppress proteinuria is contraindicated, but diuretics can be used cautiously for peripheral edema [30]. Safe immunosuppression regimen during pregnancy and breastfeeding include prednisone, azathioprine, and calcineurin inhibitors. In contrast, mycophenolate mofetil and cyclophosphamide are contraindicated during pregnancy and breast-feeding.

Hypertension Management

Chronic hypertension is a risk factor for maternal and fetal outcomes [31]. Respectively, preconception intensive BP control decreases the risk of adverse pregnancy outcomes. Patients should ideally be switched to antihypertensive medications compatible with pregnancy, such as nifedipine, labetalol, hydralazine, or methyldopa before conception. Angiotensin-converting enzyme inhibitors and angiotensin receptor blockers are teratogenic in the second and third trimesters and ideally should be discontinued preconception or no later than the eighth week of gestation with careful fetal imaging and monitoring [32].

There is no definite consensus on the diagnosis and definition of hypertension in pregnancy. Hypertensive disorders of pregnancy are classified as outlined in (Tables 18.3 and 18.4) [33]. In general, hypertension is defined as systolic BP > 140 mm Hg and diastolic BP > 90 mm Hg [34]. Moreover, currently there is no optimal BP target for pregnant patients with or without CKD. Data from the CHIPS (Control of Hypertension in Pregnancy Study) trial, which randomized women to a target diastolic BP of 85 mm Hg (tight control) or 100 mm Hg (less tight control) found no significant difference in risks of adverse pregnancy outcomes between the groups. However, more individuals developed severe hypertension (>160/110 mm Hg) in the less tight group [35]. Further, the International Society for the Study of

Table 18.3 ISSHP classification for hypertensive disorders in pregnancy

1. Chronic hypertension	Hypertension that predates the pregnancy or is recognized at <20 weeks' gestation
2. Transient gestational hypertension	De novo hypertension that develops at any gestation and that resolves without treatment during the pregnancy
3. Gestational hypertension	De novo hypertension that develops at or after 20 weeks' gestation without any features of pre-eclampsia
4. Preeclampsia	Gestational hypertension developed at or after 20 weeks' gestation and the coexistence of one or more of the new onset conditions listed in Table 18.4
5. Preeclampsia superimposed upon chronic hypertension	Chronic hypertension with signs and symptoms of preeclampsia as defined above
6. White coat hypertension	Elevated BP in the office/clinic, but normal BP in the out-of-office setting
7. Masked hypertension	Elevated BP in the out-of-office setting, but normal BP in the office/clinic

BP blood pressure, *ISSHP* International Society for the Study of Hypertension in Pregnancy

Table 18.4 ISSHP definition of preeclampsia

1. Proteinuria: spot urine protein/creatinine > 30 mg/g or >300 mg/day
2. Other maternal organ dysfunction:
   Renal insufficiency (creatinine > 1 mg/dL)
   Liver involvement (elevated transaminases with or without right upper quadrant or epigastric pain)
   Neurological complications (eclampsia, altered mental status, blindness, stroke, or more commonly hyperreflexia when accompanied by clonus, severe headaches, persistent visual scotomata)
   Hematological complications (thrombocytopenia, DIC, hemolysis)
3. Uteroplacental dysfunction (fetal growth restriction, abnormal umbilical artery Doppler wave form analysis, stillbirth)

Hypertension in Pregnancy (ISSHP) recommends maintaining BP in the range 110–140/80–85 mm Hg. Regardless of the hypertensive disorder of pregnancy, BP requires urgent treatment in a monitored setting when ≥160/110 mm Hg.

Because uncontrolled hypertension increases the risk of preeclampsia in pregnant women with CKD, home BP monitoring and adequate BP control are even more critical for these patients. They should be monitored for developing signs of preeclampsia using urinalysis at each visit along with clinical assessment, and blood tests should include hemoglobin, platelet count, liver transaminases, uric acid, and creatinine levels. Other recommended measures to prevent preeclampsia include supplementation with low-dose aspirin (preferably 150 mg/day started before 16th week of gestation) and calcium of 1.2 g/day in the setting of low calcium intake (<600 mg/day) [36, 37]. Delivery should be dependent on gestational age and maternal and fetal status. All women with chronic hypertension, gestational hypertension, or preeclampsia require lifelong follow-up because of their increased cardiovascular risk.

Pre-conception Medication and Contraception Use in Chronic Kidney Disease

Use of commonly prescribed teratogenic medications (e.g., RAAS blockers, statins, and certain immunosuppressors [mycophenolate mofetil, cyclophosphamide, rituximab]) should be preceded by a negative pregnancy test or discontinued ideally preconception in patients with CKD. It is also important to review effective contraceptive options. The choice of contraceptive may have an effect on underlying hypertension and proteinuria as the potential associated side effects of the drug. Both estrogen/progesterone combinations and exogenous progesterone upregulate RAAS, causing an increase in BP and development of albuminuria. Therefore, patient should be closely monitored for worsening hypertension and proteinuria. Progestin-only options do not significantly affect BP, and they do not worsen proteinuria. Due to the anti-mineralocorticoid activity of drosipernone, women with advanced CKD should be monitored for risk of hyperkalemia [38, 39].

Management of Chronic Kidney Disease in Pregnancy

Patients need regular monitoring of their renal function including BUN, creatinine, bicarbonate and electrolyte levels, complete blood cell count, urinalysis with spot urine protein to creatinine ratio, and parathyroid hormone as indicated. In general, nephrotoxic medications, including NSAIDs, and tocolytic agents, such as indomethacin, should be avoided. Teratogenic medications should be discontinued ideally preconception or as soon as a pregnancy test is confirmed positive. All other medications are to be dose-adjusted appropriately for estimated GFR.

Anemia associated with CKD should be treated early with appropriate iron replacement and/or initiation of erythropoietin-stimulating agent (ESA) as indicated. Due to relative erythropoietin deficiency secondary to high demand for red blood cell production as well as erythropoietin resistance from inflammatory cytokine production associated with the pregnant state, higher doses of ESA are usually required. Secondary hyperparathyroidism and the associated hyperphosphatemia can be treated with calcium-based phosphate binders and vitamin-D analogs despite limited safety data. Sodium bicarbonate therapy may be required in case of significant metabolic acidosis (pH < 7.2).

In the setting of advanced CKD or disease progression without evidence of fetal deterioration, dialysis should be initiated earlier to prevent significant metabolic disorder and elevated BUN levels. Inadequate clearance of uremic toxins (elevated BUN) results in fetal osmotic diuresis and polyhydramnios, requiring frequent assessment for intensification of dialysis dose or an increase in ultrafiltration volume with close monitoring of intra hemodialysis BP [40–42]. In general, outcomes are significantly improved with an intensified dialysis regimen. Hemodialysis should be performed almost daily to prevent significant fluid and metabolic shifts. There is a positive relationship between the number of hours on dialysis and fetal outcome. Longer and more frequent hemodialysis sessions increase the live birth rate from 48% in those dialyzed <20 hours/week compared to 85% in those dialyzed >36 hours/week [43, 44]. The spontaneous abortion rate is as high as 50% in women on dialysis, but in pregnancies that continue, overall fetal survival has been reported as high as 80%. Despite significant improvement in outcomes with intensified dialysis, patients are at high risk for complications (e.g., preeclampsia, preterm birth, fetal growth restriction, low birth weight for gestational age) and require a multidisciplinary team care approach. Infant survival is higher when pregnancies are conceived before dialysis is initiated [45].

Nutritional support and proper weight gain assessment are essential for successful pregnancy with recommended weight gain of 0.3–0.5 kg/week in second and third trimesters. Recommended daily intake of protein during pregnancy in the setting of ESRD requiring dialysis is approximately 1.5–1.8 g/kg/day [46]. Blood pressure is to be monitored closely due to increased risk of worsening hypertension or superimposed preeclampsia. Simultaneously, intra-dialytic hypotension is to be avoided to lessen the risk of placental hypoperfusion and fetal distress. Peritoneal dialysis with small volume and frequent exchanges can be used successfully to prevent intermittent hypotension episodes.

Pregnancy and Renal Transplantation

Kidney transplantation restores fertility in women with ESRD. Pregnancies are typically successful, especially in living-related donor transplant recipients and in patients with stable allograft function as evidenced by serum creatinine <1.5 mg/dL without an episode of rejection within the past year, with no or minimal proteinuria, and with use of a minimal antihypertensive regimen. In general, in patients with stable non-impaired allograft function, pregnancy does not significantly affect long-term graft function. The recommended immunosuppression regimen during pregnancy is prednisone, azathioprine, and calcineurin inhibitors (CNIs). Calcineurin inhibitor levels should be monitored closely due to an increase in volume of distribution. Mycophenolate mofetil and sirolimus are contraindicated and should be stopped 6 weeks before conception is attempted. Despite better outcomes compared to women undergoing dialysis, patients with renal transplantation are still at higher risk for complications compared to the general population [47–49].

In Summary

Management of pregnant women with CKD is difficult and challenging. To improve both maternal and fetal outcomes, a multidisciplinary approach should be taken, including appropriate pre-pregnancy counseling on risk stratification, optimization of maternal health prior to conception, and management of potential pregnancy-associated complications.

References

1. Krane NK, Hamrahian SM. Pregnancy: kidney diseases and hypertension. Am J Kidney Dis. 2007;49(2):336–45.
2. Odutayo A, Hladunewich M. Obstetric nephrology: renal hemodynamic and metabolic physiology in normal pregnancy. Clin J Am Soc Nephrol. 2012;7:2073–80.
3. Hou SH, Grossman SD, Madias NE. Pregnancy in women with renal and moderate renal insufficiency. Am J Med. 1985;78:185–94.
4. Imbasciati E, Ponticelli C. Pregnancy and renal disease: predictors for fetal and maternal outcome. Am J Nephrol. 1991;11:353–62.
5. Christensen T, Klebe JG, Bertelsen V, Hansen HE. Changes in renal volume during normal pregnancy. Acta Obstet Gynecol Scand. 1989;68:541–3.
6. Duvekot JJ, Cheriex EC, Pieters FA, Menheere PP, Peeters LH. Early pregnancy changes in hemodynamics and volume homeostasis are consecutive adjustments triggered by a primary fall in systemic vascular tone. Am J Obstet Gynecol. 1993;169:1382–92.
7. Davison JM, Dunlop W. Renal hemodynamics and tubular function in normal human pregnancy. Kidney Int. 1980;18:152–61.
8. Koetje PM, Spaan JJ, Kooman JP, Spaanderman ME, Peeters LL. Pregnancy reduces the accuracy of the estimated glomerular filtration rate based on Cockroft-Gault and MDRD formulas. Reprod Sci. 2011;18:456–62.
9. Lindheimer MD, Davison JM, Katz AI. The kidney and hypertension in pregnancy: twenty exciting years. Semin Nephrol. 2001;21:173–89.
10. Lindheimer MD, Barron WM, Davison JM. Osmoregulation of thirst and vasopressin release in pregnancy. Am J Phys. 1989;257(2 Pt 2):F159–69.
11. Krane NK. Acute renal failure in pregnancy. Arch Intern Med. 1988;148:2347–57.
12. Nwoko R, Plecas D, Garovic VD. Acute kidney injury in the pregnant patient. Clin Nephrol. 2012;78:478–86.

13. Greenberg JH, Coca S, Parikh CR. Long-term risk of chronic kidney disease and mortality in children after acute kidney injury: a systematic review. BMC Nephrol. 2014;15:184.
14. Hayslett JP. Current concepts: Postpartum renal failure. N Engl J Med. 1985;312:1556–9.
15. Piccoli GB, Cabiddu G, Attini R, Vigotti FN, Maxia S, Lepori N, et al. Risk of adverse pregnancy outcomes in women with CKD. J Am Soc Nephrol. 2015;26(8):2011–22.
16. Piccoli GB, Attini R, Vasario E, Conijn A, Biolcati M, D'Amico F, Consiglio V, Bontempo S, Todros T. Pregnancy and chronic kidney disease: a challenge in all CKD stages. Clin J Am Soc Nephrol. 2010;5:844–55.
17. Hou S. Pregnancy in chronic renal insufficiency and end-stage renal disease. Am J Kidney Dis. 1999;33:235–52.
18. Williams D, Davison J. Chronic kidney disease in pregnancy. BMJ. 2008;336:211–5.
19. Piccoli GB, Fassio F, Attini R, et al. Pregnancy in CKD: whom should we follow and why? Nephrol Dial Transplant. 2012;27(suppl 3):iii111–8.
20. Jones DC, Hayslett JP. Outcome of pregnancy in women with moderate or severe renal insufficiency. N Engl J Med. 1985;335:226–32.
21. Holley JL, Bernardini J, Quadri KHM, Greenberg A, Laifer SA. Pregnancy outcomes in a prospective matched control study of pregnancy and renal disease. Clin Nephrol. 1996;45:77–82.
22. Piccoli GB, Cabiddu G, Attini R, Vigotti FN, Maxia S, Lepori N, et al. Risk of adverse pregnancy outcomes in women with CKD. J Am Soc Nephrol. 2015;26:2011–22.
23. Chapman AB, Johnson AM, Gabow PA. Pregnancy outcome and its relationship to progression of renal failure in autosomal dominant polycystic kidney disease. J Am Soc Nephrol. 1994;5:1178–85.
24. Smyth A, Oliveira GH, Lahr BD, et al. A systematic review and metaanalysis of pregnancy outcomes in patients with systemic lupus erythematosus and lupus nephritis. Clin J Am Soc Nephrol. 2010;5:2060–8.
25. Purdy LP, Hantsch CE, Molitch ME, et al. Effect of pregnancy on renal function in patients with moderate-to-severe diabetic renal insufficiency. Diabetes Care. 1996;19:1067–74.
26. Counseling, Bramham K, Lightstone L. Pre-pregnancy counseling for women with chronic kidney disease. J Nephrol. 2012;25:450–9.
27. Wiles KS, Bramham K, Vais A, Harding KR, Chowdhury P, Taylor CJ, et al. Pre-pregnancy counselling for women with chronic kidney disease: a retrospective analysis of nine years' experience. BMC Nephrol. 2015;16:28.
28. Piccoli GB, Attini R, Cabiddu G. Kidney diseases and pregnancy: a multidisciplinary approach for improving care by involving nephrology, obstetrics, neonatology, urology, diabetology, bioethics, and internal medicine. J Clin Med. 2018;7:E135.
29. Kuller JA, D'Andrea NM, McMahon MJ. Renal biopsy and pregnancy. Am J Obstet Gynecol. 2001;184:1093–6.
30. Bullo M, Tschumi S, Bucher BS, Bianchetti MG, Simonetti GD. Pregnancy outcome following exposure to angiotensin converting enzyme inhibitors or angiotensin receptor antagonists: a systematic review. Hypertension. 2012;60:444–50.
31. Bramham K, Parnell B, Nelson-Piercy C, et al. Chronic hypertension and pregnancy outcomes: systematic review and meta-analysis. BMJ. 2014;g2301:348.
32. Diav-Citrin O, Shechtman S, Halberstadt Y, et al. Pregnancy outcome after in utero exposure to angiotensin converting enzyme inhibitors or angiotensin receptor blockers. Reprod Toxicol. 2011;31:540–5.
33. Brown MA, et al. The hypertensive disorders of pregnancy: ISSHP classification, diagnosis & management recommendations for international practice. Pregnancy Hypertens. 2018;13:291–310.
34. Report of the National High Blood Pressure Education Program Working Group on high blood pressure in pregnancy. Am J Obstet Gynecol. 2000;183:S1–S22.
35. Magee LA, von Dadelszen P, Rey E, Ross S, Asztalos E, Murphy KE, et al. Less-tight versus tight control of hypertension in pregnancy. N Engl J Med. 2015;372:407–17.

36. Rolnik DL, Wright D, Poon LC, O'Gorman N, Syngelaki A, de Paco Matallana C, et al. Aspirin versus placebo in pregnancies at high risk for preterm preeclampsia. N Engl J Med. 2017;377:613–22.
37. Hofmeyr GJ, Duley L, Atallah A. Dietary calcium supplementation for prevention of pre-eclampsia and related problems: a systematic review and commentary. BJOG. 2007;114:933–43.
38. ACOG practice bulletin no. 206: use of hormonal contraception in women with coexisting medical conditions. Obstet Gynecol. 2019;133:e128–50.
39. Burgner A, Hladunewich MA. Contraception and chronic kidney disease. Clin J Am Soc Nephrol. 2020;15(4):563–5.
40. Krane NK. Hemodialysis and peritoneal dialysis in pregnancy. Hemodial Int. 2001;5:96–100.
41. BUN, Asamiya Y, Otsubo S, Matsuda Y, Kimata N, Kikuchi K, Miwa N, et al. The importance of low blood urea nitrogen levels in pregnant patients undergoing hemodialysis to optimize birth weight and gestational age. Kidney Int. 2009;75:1217–22.
42. Intensive hemodialysis, Hladunewich MA, Hou S, Odutayo A, Cornelis T, Pierratos A, Goldstein M, et al. Intensive hemodialysis associates with improved pregnancy outcomes: a Canadian and United States cohort comparison. J Am Soc Nephrol. 2014;25:1103–9.
43. Piccoli GB, Minelli F, Versino E, Cabiddu G, Attini R, Vigotti FN, et al. Pregnancy in dialysis patients in the new millennium: a systematic review and meta-regression analysis correlating dialysis schedules and pregnancy outcomes. Nephrol Dial Transpl. 2015;31:1905–34.
44. Piccoli GB, Cabiddu G, Daidone G, Guzzo G, Maxia S, Ciniglio I, et al. The children of dialy-sis: live-born babies from on-dialysis mothers in Italy – an epidemiological perspective com-paring dialysis, kidney transplantation and the overall population. Nephrol Dial Transplant. 2014;29(8):1578–86.
45. Jesudason S, Grace BS, McDonald SP. Pregnancy outcomes according to dialysis commencing before or after conception in women with ESRD. Clin J Am Soc Nephrol. 2014;9:143–9.
46. Ikizler TA, Pupim LB, Brouillette JR, Levenhagen DK, Farmer K, Hakim RM, et al. Hemodialysis stimulates muscle and whole body protein loss and alters substrate oxidation. Am J Physiol Endocrinol Metab. 2002;282:E107–16.
47. McKay DB, Josephson MA, Armenti VT, et al. Reproduction and transplantation: report on the AST consensus conference on reproductive issues and transplantation. Am J Transplant. 2005;5:1592–9.
48. Davison JM, Bailey DJ. Pregnancy following renal transplantation. J Obstet Gynaecol Res. 2003;29:227–33.
49. Levidiotis V, Chang S, McDonald S. Pregnancy and maternal outcomes among kidney trans-plant recipients. J Am Soc Nephrol. 2009;20:2433–40.

Chapter 19
CKD in Minorities: Non-Hispanic Blacks, Hispanics, Asians, and Indian Americans

Xiaoying Deng and Jingjing Zhang

Chronic kidney disease (CKD) is a global public health problem that carries significant premature morbidity and mortality. The prevalence and incidence of CKD have increased in the past several decades, particularly in the minority/ethnic population. Despite similar rates of early-stage CKD across different racial/ethnic groups [1–3], the prevalence of end-stage renal disease (ESRD) is greater for minorities than for non-Hispanic whites [1, 4–6]. Some racial/ethnic groups are more susceptible to kidney damage but have better survival rates once they progress to ESRD and require hemodialysis (HD) [7–9].

In 2006, 14.7% of the US population declared themselves as Hispanic, 12.3% as black, 0.8% as American Indian or Alaskan Native, 4.3% as Asian, and 66.5% as white. Projections suggest that 50% of the US population will be comprised of minority groups by the year 2050 [10]. Knowing the characteristics of CKD in minorities is crucial for providers, especially for primary care physicians.

We review recent data on the disparity of CKD in the US population and focus on risk factors in the development and progression of CKD in minorities.

X. Deng
Department of Medicine, Division of Nephrology, Sanford Clinic North, North Fargo, ND, USA
e-mail: Xiaoying.deng@sanfordhealth.org

J. Zhang (✉)
Department of Medicine, Division of Nephrology, Thomas Jefferson University Hospital, Philadelphia, PA, USA
e-mail: Jingjing.zhang@jefferson.edu

© Springer Nature Switzerland AG 2022

J. McCauley et al. (eds.), *Approaches to Chronic Kidney Disease*,
https://doi.org/10.1007/978-3-030-83082-3_19

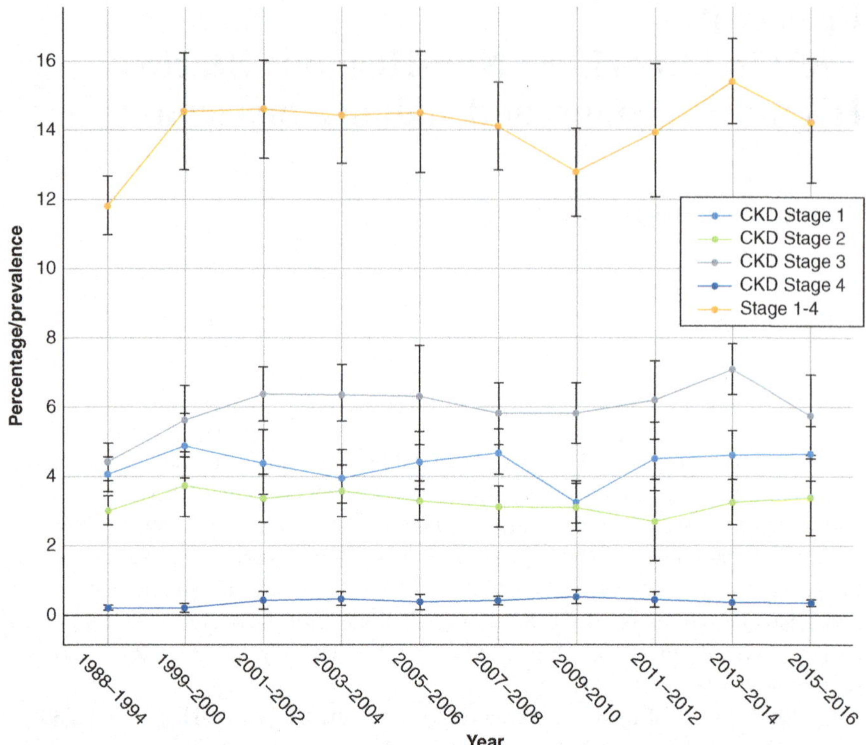

Fig. 19.1 The Centers for Disease Control and Prevention Chronic Kidney Disease Surveillance System – United States. https://nccd.cdc.gov/ckd. (Derived from CDC website: https://nccd.cdc.gov/CKD/detail.aspx?Qnum=Q372#refreshPosition [11])

Incidence and Prevalence of CKD in Different Racial/ Ethnic Groups

The crude yearly prevalence of CKD stages 1–4 was 12.8–15.5% in the United States over the past three decades (Fig. 19.1) [11]. The percentage of adults with stage 1–4 CKD from 1999 to 2016 has remained relatively unchanged. The most recent updated data of earlier stages of CKD was at 14.8% in 2017 (Table 19.1) (United States Renal Data System, USRDS) [12]. The estimated prevalence of CKD varies by racial/ethnic group and geographic location [13]. According to data from the National Health and Nutrition Examination Survey (NHANES) 2009–2012, 16.3% of non-Hispanic blacks had CKD, while 11.9% Mexican Americans and 13.6% non-Hispanic whites had CKD (Table 19.2) [14]. The prevalence was similar after adjustment for age and sex.

In addition to the prevalence being similar, a large national data analysis found that mortality risks after adjusting for age and risk factors are no longer different for whites and African American patients in the territories versus the 50 states but

Table 19.1 Number and percentage of incident ESRD patients receiving hemodialysis (HD), peritoneal dialysis (PD), and a transplant, by age, sex, race, and ethnicity, in the US population, 2017

	Total	HD		PD		Transplant	
	n	n	%	n	%	n	%
Age							
0–21	1,319	677	51.3	367	27.8	275	20.8
22–44	13,454	10,533	78.2	2,011	14.9	920	6.8
45–64	47,191	40,232	85.3	5,213	11.0	1,746	3.7
65–74	33,735	30,075	89.0	3,055	9.0	655	1.9
75+	28,610	26,614	93.0	1,926	6.7	70	0.2
Sex							
Male	72,403	62,927	86.9	7,394	10.2	2,082	2.9
Female	51,966	45,204	87.0	5,178	10.0	1,584	3.0
Rate							
White	83,368	71,379	86.2	8,789	10.5	2,700	3.2
Black/African American	31,965	28,975	90.6	2,657	8.3	333	1.0
American Indian or Alaska Native	1,151	1,038	90.2	72	6.3	41	3.6
Asian	5,570	4,394	78.9	808	14.5	368	6.6
Native Hawaiian or Pacific Islander	1,548	1,351	87.3	178	11.5	19	1.2
Other or Multiracial	426	344	80.8	54	12.7	28	6.6
Unknown	341	150	44.0	14	4.1	177	51.9
Ethnicity							
Hispanic	18,361	16,260	88.6	1,769	9.6	332	1.8
Non-Hispanic	104,620	91,263	87.2	10,734	10.3	2,623	2.5
Unknown	1,388	608	43.8	69	5.0	711	51.2

Derived from USRDS 2019 [12]

Table 19.2 Prevalence (%) of CKD in NHANES population within age, sex, race/ethnicity, and categories, 2001–2016

	All CKD			
	2001–2004	2005–2008	2009–2012	2013–2016
Age				
20–39	5.4	6.1	5.5	6.3
40–59	9.7	10.1	8.3	10.4
60+	38.8	34.5	33.1	32.2
Sex				
Male	12.7	12.1	12.3	12.9
Female	15.5	16.3	14.6	16.7
Race/ethnicity				
Non-Hispanic White	14.3	14.4	13.6	15.6
Non-Hispanic Black/African American	14.7	16.3	16.1	15.9
Mexican American	11.4	11.8	11.9	12.6
Other Hispanic	13.0	14.9	11.5	11.4
Other non-Hispanic	15.9	11.4	11.7	12.6

Derived from USRDS annual report 2018 [14]

remain much greater for territory-indwelling Hispanics and Asians [15]. It has long been known that African Americans experience a much higher prevalence of ESRD in the United States compared with whites [16]. Whether the cause is a high prevalence of CKD has been brought up by researchers. Another question is whether CKD prevalence is different in other minorities in the United States compared with non-Hispanic white individuals.

When studying the CKD in African Americans, we need to know that there are important differences in renal function measurements in African Americans compared with non-African Americans. Studies have found that African Americans have higher serum creatinine levels and urinary creatinine excretion rates for a given glomerular filtration rate (GFR) [17]. Therefore, the eGFR in African American will be 20% higher than that in non-African Americans who have the same level of serum creatinine.

The prevalence of CKD in the United States has been stable since early 2000. From NHANES in 1988–1994 and every 2 years from 1999 to 2012, the adjusted prevalence of disease among non-Hispanic blacks still showed a continued increase through 2012, differing from the pattern in other race/ethnicity subgroups, but it was not statistically significantly different. Even though CKD prevalence is similar within African Americans and other minorities, ESRD is disproportionately higher in African Americans. In the United States, black individuals shoulder a disproportionate burden of ESRD, comprising to 32% of the ESRD population, but only 13% of the general population [2].

By using a birth cohort analysis with data from the NHANES and the USRDS, the study showed similar results. For each 100 African Americans with CKD in 1991, 5 new cases of ESRD developed in 1996, whereas only 1 case of ESRD developed per 100 whites with CKD (risk ratio, 4.8; 95% confidence interval, 2.9–8.4). The higher incidence of ESRD is not due to a greater prevalence of CKD among African Americans [1]. The disproportionately higher rate of ESRD in African American compared with white patients was also shown in a national sample of veterans between 2001 and 2005 [2]. The study from Mehtra provides some insight into the reasons for the higher risk for death among younger black individuals with CKD, relative to white individuals, which excludes the possibility that more white individuals died before reaching ESRD [18].

In addition to African American, Hispanics also account for large minority population. Over 90,000 US Hispanics/Latinos with ESRD were treated by HD in 2011, and the rate of incident ESRD among Hispanics/Latinos is 50% greater than in non-Hispanics whites [19].

In a recent large diverse contemporary cohort of Hispanic/Latino studies, the overall prevalence of age-adjusted CKD among Hispanics/Latinos was 13.7% [20]. The study also found the overall prevalence of CKD to be similar between Hispanic and non-Hispanic white groups. This suggests that Hispanics/Latinos may be at increased risk for CKD progression or, alternatively, that the mortality rate before the onset of ESRD is higher in non-Hispanic whites than that in with Hispanics/Latinos [20]. However, no significant differences in outcomes between Mexican Americans and white individuals with CKD were identified [18]. Even though there was a higher all-cause and cardiovascular mortality among Mexican Americans, none of the trends reached statistical significance.

Interestingly, among US Hispanic/Latino adults, there was significant variation in CKD prevalence among different background groups. The overall prevalence of CKD was 13.0%, and it was lowest in persons with a South American background (7.4%) and highest (16.6%) in persons with a Puerto Rican background. In men, the prevalence of CKD was 15.3%, and it was lowest (11.2%) in persons with South American backgrounds and highest in those who identified their Hispanic background as "other" (16.0%) [20].

As the fastest-growing race or ethnic group in the United States, the Asian population surged by 12.5–13.5 million (which includes Asian and Pacific Islander ethnicities) from April 1, 2000, to July 1, 2003. The US Asian population is an ethnically diverse group representing different Asian ancestries and socioeconomic backgrounds. The Asian population accounts for 5.6% of the total US population by estimation in 2019 [21]. Compared to whites, the prevalence of ESRD is 1.5 times greater for American Asians. However, the first large US population-based studies of American Asians have shown a comparatively higher risk of elevated albumin-to-creatinine ratio (ACR) >300 mg/g levels (A3) but a lower risk of CKD. Of course, the prevalence of CKD is similar to that of other races/ethnicities [22].

American Indians (AIs) have their own health services, but the information on their rate of CKD is still scant. The CRIC study is planning to recruit 500 AIs to enrich the study on this minority. From the Indian Health Service database, the AI/Alaska natives (AN) include at least 3.3 million individuals in 2008, representing a diverse collection of 560 tribes and nations. These tribes range from small villages in Alaska encompassing several hundred individuals to large tribes in the Southwestern United States, with 250,000 members [23].

Several studies have shown that AI/AN populations have an increasing rate of CKD, such as the Strong Heart Study, which is a longitudinal study that measures risk factors for cardiovascular disease among AI/AN. It has shown high rates of abnormal albumin excretion (20–50%) in all tribes studied [24]. Even persons without diabetes also had high rates (10–20%) of abnormal albuminuria. Another study showed that CKD in AI/AN is more than 2.5 times higher than the composite US population in that area, including an eightfold higher burden of stage 5 CKD [25].

Both the prevalence and incidence of ESRD among AI/AN populations are twice those observed among white Americans. Nearly three quarters of all incident ESRD cases among AI/AN are attributable to diabetes (primarily type 2), compared with only 40% for other racial groups [23].

Progression of CKD to ESRD in Different Racial/Ethnic Groups

CKD incidence is similar within all ethnic minority patients, and ESRD incidence is higher in all minority patients than white patients (Table 19.1). The likely explanation is that progression from CKD to ESRD is more rapid in ethnic minority patients [26, 27], and this rapid progression is closely associated with GFR decline.

There are no available data on the timeline of mild CKD progression to ESRD, but there is significant racial disparity in the progression from CKD to ESRD [20, 26–28].

African Americans comprise only 13.4% of the US population, Asians comprise 5.9%, and Hispanics comprise 18.3% [29]. Compared to whites, ESRD prevalence in 2014 was approximately 3.7 times greater in blacks, 1.5 times greater in AI/AN, 1.3 times greater in Asians, and 9.5 times greater in Native Hawaiians/Pacific Islanders [30].

In the United States, faster rates of decline among black groups have been observed, which may be related to social deprivation or differences in access to healthcare [31, 32]. A study from a population in northern California showed a higher ESRD prevalence in Asians and blacks than in whites, even after sociodemographic and comorbidity status justification [33]. However, Netherlands data showed that healthcare system factors have a less influential role than previously thought in explaining black-white differences [34]. The UK data also showed that health system is not a factor in the Asian population. A recent large UK-based community-managed diabetic cohort studied three geographically contiguous East London clinical commissioning groups. The results showed that while South Asian patients, particularly of Bangladeshi ethnicity, had the greatest annual loss of eGFR and significantly reduced risk of death relative to white groups, black groups were most at risk of rapid CKD progression and had the highest risk of developing ESRD [28]. However, some studies did not show a difference in eGFR decline between Asian and white populations.

The Causes of Disparity of CKD Progress to ESRD in Minorities

Severe renal disease requiring renal replacement therapy disproportionately impacts black and Hispanic patients. There are some explanations for these disparities that have included biological differences, access to care, comorbid illnesses, socioeconomic status (SES), and lifestyle habits.

Risk Factors for CKD

The main risk factors for CKD in the United States and worldwide are diabetes mellitus (DM), hypertension (HTN), and obesity. DM and HTN are the main contributors to CKD in minorities in the United States and many Asian countries as well [4]. Glomerulonephritis and unknown causes are the most common etiologies in South Asia [35]. The prevalence of HTN in non-Hispanic whites was 29.1%, non-Hispanic blacks 42.5%, and Mexican Americans 26.1% according to NHANES survey from 1999 to 2000 [36]. Adequate BP control was lower in the minority population, only 17.7% as compared to 33.4% in whites [37].

Hypertensive kidney disease is the predominant cause of ESRD for African Americans [15]. African American ESRD patients had a more than 17-fold greater rate of HTN as the etiology of ESRD than whites [38].

Minorities also have a higher incidence of DM in the United States. The incidence is 8.3% in whites, 14.6% in African American, and 15.3% in Mexican Americans in 2006 [36]. The greatest increase in the prevalence of DM was among Hispanics (38.5%) and Asians (68.0%) [39].

Obesity is an independent risk factor for CKD progression, and it is associated with HTN, DM, and proteinuria. The incidence and prevalence of obesity are steadily increasing in developed and developing countries [40], which increases the obesity prevalence in Asian minorities in the United States.

Since the incidence and prevalence of CKD are similar in minorities, the difference in DM, HTN, and obesity prevalence is unlikely the culprit for fast progression to ESRD for minorities.

Albuminuria is a known independent risk factor for the progression of CKD [41, 42].

From NHANES III data, blacks had 2.18-fold (95% CI, 1.44–3.30) and Mexican Americans had 1.81-fold (95% CI, 1.08–3.02) greater odds of microalbuminuria or macroalbuminuria than whites after adjustment for potential confounding factors. Minorities with DM did not have a statistically significant increase in adjusted odds of albuminuria compared with whites [43]. In a study from northern California, blacks with DM had a 22% higher incidence of albuminuria than white patients. In the same study, Asians with DM were found to have a 35% higher incidence of albuminuria compared with whites [44].

Decreasing albuminuria could delay the progression of CKD. However, racial disparity exists in the application of the treatments targeting to improving albuminuria/proteinuria. In previous hypertension guidelines, the first-line treatment for HTN in African Americans was calcium channel blockers, while renin-angiotensin II-aldosterone system (RAAS) blockers were used for white Americans, leading to less African American patients being on RAAS blockade [45]. In addition, improved blood pressure control and improved glucose control could delay the eGFR decline [46, 47]. There were also differences in terms of sodium restriction in HTN patients and glucose control in diabetes patients among different ethnic/minority patients [48].

Genetics

Genetics might be responsible for the rapid progression of CKD into ESRD in minority patients. Genes predicting kidney disease in blacks have been described [49–51], adding credence to the hypothesis that there may be genetic differences that account for different proportions of patients on dialysis. Several risk factors have been studied vigorously including apolipoprotein 1 (APOL1) and non-muscle myosin heavy chain 9 (MYH9) [52]. These two genes are located on chromosome 22 [51]. Research found that two variants of G1 and G2 in the last exon of APOL1 increased risks for HIV nephropathy [51, 53, 54], focal segmental glomerulosclerosis (FSGS) [53], CKD secondary to HTN [51], and ESRD secondary to non-DM etiology [49] among African Americans. The G1 and G2 of APOL1 confer resistance to lethal *Trypanosoma brucei* infections, which are rarely seen in other populations [55]. It is perplexing that approximately 40% of patients who had two copies of APOL1 high-risk variants did not progress to the composite renal outcome and APOL1 variants are not associated with mortality in AASK and CRIC studies [51]. APO L1 high-risk variants have also been associated with an increased risk of progression to ESRD in Hispanics since there is a greater degree of African ancestry [56].

Socioeconomic Status (SES)

The incidence and prevalence of CKD and the progression of CKD to ESRD vary by SES [57]. Poverty and less than high school education are associated with microalbuminuria in multiple epidemiology studies in the United States and other countries [58–60]. The prevalence of CKD was seen more frequently in African Americans who had less than 12 grades education, lower income, and unemployment [59, 61]. Lower income was also associated with microalbuminuria [62] and lower eGFR of <60 ml/min/1.73 m^2 [61], especially in African American CKD patients.

Low birth weight is more common among African American infants than white infants [63]. Low birth weight is associated with increased risks in adults for CKD [64], HTN [65, 66], DM [67], and cardiovascular diseases [68, 69]. The reason for lower birth weight with increased CKD risks is likely from reduced nephron numbers/body mass index ratio, a primary mechanism of prenatally programmed CKD [70].

In addition to strong association of established risk factors (e.g., HTN and DM) with prevalent CKD in the Hispanic/Latino population, lower annual household income was reported to be associated with prevalent CKD [20].

Access to Healthcare

The earlier onset and more severe CKD might be partly due to poor SES and worse access to healthcare [15]. Minority groups have worse access to healthcare and later referral to nephrology [26, 27]. Social deprivation and differences in access to healthcare are ascribed to the rapid progression of CKD in the United States [31, 32] and some other countries. However, in the countries where access to healthcare is universal, such as the United Kingdom, the Netherlands, and Canada, a faster decline in eGFR in nonwhite people is reported [34, 71, 72]. Equivalent declines between ethnic groups [73–75] are noted and reported as well. Rapid renal decline was defined as eGFR decreases more than 5 ml/min/1.73 m^2 in 1 year in a small study [75].

African American CKD patients are more likely to have delayed [76] or no nephrology referral [77] as compared to their white counterparts. The Agency for Healthcare Research and Quality found that African Americans had less access to care than white Americans across 10 of 21 measures, including insurance, usual source of care, and timeline of care [78]. Lack of insurance and a usual source of care might be responsible for the 10% disparity in ESRD incidence seen between African American and white Americans [79].

A single payer system was noted to have fewer cardiovascular procedures in women and minorities with CKD when coverage was dispensed among multiple providers [10]. Furthermore, a single payer system is associated with racial/ethnic equity for KDOQI CKD recommended targets [80] and a survival advantage for African American chronic diabetic nephropathy patients at the Veterans Administration [81].

Other psychosocial factors such as stress, depression, and social support have also been studied in the disparity of CKD patients, but data are very limited. Unemployment and lower income are strongly associated with increased depression in African American patients with hypertensive CKD [82].

Only 2% of African American patients had proficient health literacy compared with 14% of white Americans. Poor health literacy is associated with decreased CKD knowledge and kidney function [83, 84]. The neighborhoods of lower-income communities have less access to resources that are important to health. These communities have poor air quality, more toxic waste sites, few areas that are walkable and safe for exercise, few healthy food stores, and more fast food restaurants and convenience stores than healthy food supermarkets. The unhealthy food has high sodium and phosphorus, which could exacerbate CKD progression; lack of fresh fruits and vegetables could increase dietary acid load, leading to decreased eGFR, albuminuria, and progression of CKD to ESRD [85].

Dialysis is not the final goal for ESRD patients. The kidney transplant candidate should receive transplant to prolong life expectancy and improve quality of life.

Racial disparities in the use of renal transplantation were discussed 20 years ago. The authors found evidence of both underuse of transplantation among blacks and overuse among whites from data of five states and the District of Columbia [86].

The more markedly improved outcomes of post-kidney transplant for blacks were reported in the 2012 cohort; there were no statistically significant differences in 1-year or 3-year graft loss after living donor or deceased donor kidney transplant between black and white kidney transplant recipients [87]. The results should encourage nephrologists and patients to aggressively promote access to transplantation in the black community. However, a quarter of dialysis units across the United States still showed racial disparity in the waiting list, which means a lower prevalence for black patients than white patients in consecutive 3 years is reported [88].

Summary

Over 30 million American adults may already have CKD, and the incidence of CKD and ESRD by 2050 will be even higher given the increased prevalence of CKD and increased CKD risk factors in the minority population [89]. As ethnic minorities are highly heterogeneous groups, culturally intelligent approaches are needed to understand the barriers and enablers of access within individual country systems and to learn from international comparisons [27].

The World Health Organization (WHO) proposed three key tenets to improve health globally in 2007 [90]: (1) improve the conditions of daily life; (2) tackle the inequitable distribution of power, money, and resources – the structural drivers of those conditions of daily life; and (3) develop a workforce trained in the social determinants of health and raise public awareness about the social determinants of health. It will be a long battle for all renal care providers to reach this goal in the coming decades.

References

1. Hsu CY, Lin F, Vittinghoff E, Shlipak MG. Racial differences in the progression from chronic renal insufficiency to end-stage renal disease in the United States. J Am Soc Nephrol. 2003;14(11):2902–7.
2. Choi AI, Rodriguez RA, Bacchetti P, Bertenthal D, Hernandez GT, O'Hare AM. White/black racial differences in risk of end-stage renal disease and death. Am J Med. 2009;122(7):672–8.
3. McClellan W, Warnock DG, McClure L, Campbell RC, Newsome BB, Howard V, et al. Racial differences in the prevalence of chronic kidney disease among participants in the Reasons for Geographic and Racial Differences in Stroke (REGARDS) Cohort Study. J Am Soc Nephrol. 2006;17(6):1710–5.
4. Saran R, Robinson B, Abbott KC, Agodoa LYC, Bhave N, Bragg-Gresham J, et al. US renal data system 2017 annual data report: epidemiology of kidney disease in the United States. Am J Kidney Dis. 2018;71(3 Suppl 1):A7.
5. Saran R, Robinson B, Abbott KC, Agodoa LYC, Bragg-Gresham J, Balkrishnan R, et al. US renal data system 2018 annual data report: epidemiology of kidney disease in the United States. Am J Kidney Dis. 2019;73(3S1):A7–8.
6. Grams ME, Chow EK, Segev DL, Coresh J. Lifetime incidence of CKD stages 3-5 in the United States. Am J Kidney Dis. 2013;62(2):245–52.
7. Streja E, Molnar MZ, Kovesdy CP. Race, age, and mortality among patients undergoing dialysis. JAMA. 2011;306(20):2215; author reply -6.
8. Kalantar-Zadeh K, Streja E, Kovesdy CP, Oreopoulos A, Noori N, Jing J, et al. The obesity paradox and mortality associated with surrogates of body size and muscle mass in patients receiving hemodialysis. Mayo Clin Proc. 2010;85(11):991–1001.
9. Miller JE, Kovesdy CP, Nissenson AR, Mehrotra R, Streja E, Van Wyck D, et al. Association of hemodialysis treatment time and dose with mortality and the role of race and sex. Am J Kidney Dis. 2010;55(1):100–12.
10. Powe NR. Let's get serious about racial and ethnic disparities. J Am Soc Nephrol. 2008;19(7):1271–5.
11. Prevention CfDCa. Chronic kidney disease (CKD) surveillance system 2020. [cited 2020]. Available from: https://nccd.cdc.gov/CKD/detail.aspx?Qnum=Q372#refreshPosition.

12. System USRD. US renal data system 2019 annual data report: epidemiology of kidney disease in the United States 2019. [cited 2020]. Available from: https://www.usrds.org/annual-data-report/previous-adrs/.
13. Murphy D, McCulloch CE, Lin F, Banerjee T, Bragg-Gresham JL, Eberhardt MS, et al. Trends in prevalence of chronic kidney disease in the United States. Ann Intern Med. 2016;165(7):473–81.
14. USRDS. CKD in the general population. 2018.
15. Yan G, Shen JI, Harford R, Yu W, Nee R, Clark MJ, et al. Racial and ethnic variations in mortality rates for patients undergoing maintenance dialysis treated in US territories compared with the US 50 states. Clin J Am Soc Nephrol. 2020;15(1):101–8.
16. Xue JL, Ma JZ, Louis TA, Collins AJ. Forecast of the number of patients with end-stage renal disease in the United States to the year 2010. J Am Soc Nephrol. 2001;12(12):2753–8.
17. Lewis J, Agodoa L, Cheek D, Greene T, Middleton J, O'Connor D, et al. Comparison of cross-sectional renal function measurements in African Americans with hypertensive nephrosclerosis and of primary formulas to estimate glomerular filtration rate. Am J Kidney Dis. 2001;38(4):744–53.
18. Mehrotra R, Kermah D, Fried L, Adler S, Norris K. Racial differences in mortality among those with CKD. J Am Soc Nephrol. 2008;19(7):1403–10.
19. Collins AJ, Foley RN, Herzog C, Chavers B, Gilbertson D, Herzog C, et al. US Renal Data System 2012 Annual Data Report. Am J Kidney Dis. 2013;61(1 Suppl 1):A7, e1–476.
20. Ricardo AC, Flessner MF, Eckfeldt JH, Eggers PW, Franceschini N, Go AS, et al. Prevalence and correlates of CKD in Hispanics/Latinos in the United States. Clin J Am Soc Nephrol. 2015;10(10):1757–66.
21. Asian-American and Pacific Islander Heritage Month: May 2019. Available from: https://www.census.gov/newsroom/facts-for-features/2019/asian-american-pacific-islander.html.
22. Kataoka-Yahiro M, Davis J, Gandhi K, Rhee CM, Page V. Asian Americans & chronic kidney disease in a nationally representative cohort. BMC Nephrol. 2019;20(1):10.
23. Narva AS, Sequist TD. Reducing health disparities in American Indians with chronic kidney disease. Semin Nephrol. 2010;30(1):19–25.
24. Robbins DC, Knowler WC, Lee ET, Yeh J, Go OT, Welty T, et al. Regional differences in albuminuria among American Indians: an epidemic of renal disease. Kidney Int. 1996;49(2):557–63.
25. Scavini M, Stidley CA, Paine SS, Shah VO, Tentori F, Bobelu A, et al. The burden of chronic kidney disease among the Zuni Indians: the Zuni Kidney Project. Clin J Am Soc Nephrol. 2007;2(3):509–16.
26. Young BA, Katz R, Boulware LE, Kestenbaum B, de Boer IH, Wang W, et al. Risk factors for rapid kidney function decline among African Americans: The Jackson Heart Study (JHS). Am J Kidney Dis. 2016;68(2):229–39.
27. Wilkinson E, Brettle A, Waqar M, Randhawa G. Inequalities and outcomes: end stage kidney disease in ethnic minorities. BMC Nephrol. 2019;20(1):234.
28. Barbour SJ, Lee E, Djurdjev O, Karim M, Levin A. Differences in progression of CKD and mortality amongst Caucasian, Oriental Asian and South Asian CKD patients. Nephrol Dial Transplant. 2010;25(11):3663–72.
29. Breau USC. Quick facts United States 2019 [cited 20 Jan 2020]. Available from: https://www.census.gov/quickfacts/fact/table/US/IPE120218.
30. System USRD. 2016 ADR Chapters 2016 [cited 20 Jan 2020]. Available from: https://www.usrds.org/2016/view/Default.aspx.
31. Fedewa SA, McClellan WM, Judd S, Gutiérrez OM, Crews DC. The association between race and income on risk of mortality in patients with moderate chronic kidney disease. BMC Nephrol. 2014;15:136.
32. Lewis EF, Claggett B, Parfrey PS, Burdmann EA, McMurray JJ, Solomon SD, et al. Race and ethnicity influences on cardiovascular and renal events in patients with diabetes mellitus. Am Heart J. 2015;170(2):322–9.

33. Hall YN, Hsu CY, Iribarren C, Darbinian J, McCulloch CE, Go AS. The conundrum of increased burden of end-stage renal disease in Asians. Kidney Int. 2005;68(5):2310–6.
34. van den Beukel TF, de Goeij MC, Dekker FW, Siegert CE, Halbesma N. Differences in progression to ESRD between black and white patients receiving predialysis care in a universal health care system. Clin J Am Soc Nephrol. 2013;8(9):1540–7.
35. Jha V, Garcia-Garcia G, Iseki K, Li Z, Naicker S, Plattner B, et al. Chronic kidney disease: global dimension and perspectives. Lancet (London, England). 2013;382(9888):260–72.
36. Fryar CD, Hirsch R, Eberhardt MS, Yoon SS, Wright JD. Hypertension, high serum total cholesterol, and diabetes: racial and ethnic prevalence differences in U.S. adults, 1999-2006. NCHS Data Brief. 2010;36:1–8.
37. Hajjar I, Kotchen TA. Trends in prevalence, awareness, treatment, and control of hypertension in the United States, 1988-2000. JAMA. 2003;290(2):199–206.
38. Qualheim RE, Rostand SG, Kirk KA, Rutsky EA, Luke RG. Changing patterns of end-stage renal disease due to hypertension. Am J Kidney Dis. 1991;18(3):336–43.
39. McBean AM, Li S, Gilbertson DT, Collins AJ. Differences in diabetes prevalence, incidence, and mortality among the elderly of four racial/ethnic groups: whites, blacks, hispanics, and asians. Diabetes Care. 2004;27(10):2317–24.
40. Dinsa GD, Goryakin Y, Fumagalli E, Suhrcke M. Obesity and socioeconomic status in developing countries: a systematic review. Obes Rev. 2012;13(11):1067–79.
41. Astor BC, Matsushita K, Gansevoort RT, van der Velde M, Woodward M, Levey AS, et al. Lower estimated glomerular filtration rate and higher albuminuria are associated with mortality and end-stage renal disease. A collaborative meta-analysis of kidney disease population cohorts. Kidney Int. 2011;79(12):1331–40.
42. Gansevoort RT, Matsushita K, van der Velde M, Astor BC, Woodward M, Levey AS, et al. Lower estimated GFR and higher albuminuria are associated with adverse kidney outcomes. A collaborative meta-analysis of general and high-risk population cohorts. Kidney Int. 2011;80(1):93–104.
43. Bryson CL, Ross HJ, Boyko EJ, Young BA. Racial and ethnic variations in albuminuria in the US Third National Health and Nutrition Examination Survey (NHANES III) population: associations with diabetes and level of CKD. Am J Kidney Dis. 2006;48(5):720–6.
44. Choi AI, Karter AJ, Liu JY, Young BA, Go AS, Schillinger D. Ethnic differences in the development of albuminuria: the distance study. Am J Manag Care. 2011;17(11):737–45.
45. Norris KC, Agodoa LY. Unraveling the racial disparities associated with kidney disease. Kidney Int. 2005;68(3):914–24.
46. Humalda JK, Navis G. Dietary sodium restriction: a neglected therapeutic opportunity in chronic kidney disease. Curr Opin Nephrol Hypertens. 2014;23(6):533–40.
47. Herget-Rosenthal S, Dehnen D, Kribben A, Quellmann T. Progressive chronic kidney disease in primary care: modifiable risk factors and predictive model. Prev Med. 2013;57(4):357–62.
48. Powe NR, Melamed ML. Racial disparities in the optimal delivery of chronic kidney disease care. Med Clin North Am. 2005;89(3):475–88.
49. Kao WH, Klag MJ, Meoni LA, Reich D, Berthier-Schaad Y, Li M, et al. MYH9 is associated with nondiabetic end-stage renal disease in African Americans. Nat Genet. 2008;40(10):1185–92.
50. McDonough CW, Hicks PJ, Lu L, Langefeld CD, Freedman BI, Bowden DW. The influence of carnosinase gene polymorphisms on diabetic nephropathy risk in African-Americans. Hum Genet. 2009;126(2):265–75.
51. Parsa A, Kao WH, Xie D, Astor BC, Li M, Hsu CY, et al. APOL1 risk variants, race, and progression of chronic kidney disease. N Engl J Med. 2013;369(23):2183–96.
52. Kopp JB, Winkler CA, Nelson GW. MYH9 genetic variants associated with glomerular disease: what is the role for genetic testing? Semin Nephrol. 2010;30(4):409–17.
53. Kopp JB, Nelson GW, Sampath K, Johnson RC, Genovese G, An P, et al. APOL1 genetic variants in focal segmental glomerulosclerosis and HIV-associated nephropathy. J Am Soc Nephrol. 2011;22(11):2129–37.

54. Atta MG, Estrella MM, Kuperman M, Foy MC, Fine DM, Racusen LC, et al. HIV-associated nephropathy patients with and without apolipoprotein L1 gene variants have similar clinical and pathological characteristics. Kidney Int. 2012;82(3):338–43.
55. Abecasis GR, Auton A, Brooks LD, DePristo MA, Durbin RM, Handsaker RE, et al. An integrated map of genetic variation from 1,092 human genomes. Nature. 2012;491(7422):56–65.
56. Tzur S, Rosset S, Skorecki K, Wasser WG. APOL1 allelic variants are associated with lower age of dialysis initiation and thereby increased dialysis vintage in African and Hispanic Americans with non-diabetic end-stage kidney disease. Nephrol Dial Transplant. 2012;27(4):1498–505.
57. Patzer RE, McClellan WM. Influence of race, ethnicity and socioeconomic status on kidney disease. Nat Rev Nephrol. 2012;8(9):533–41.
58. Martins D, Tareen N, Zadshir A, Pan D, Vargas R, Nissenson A, et al. The association of poverty with the prevalence of albuminuria: data from the Third National Health and Nutrition Examination Survey (NHANES III). Am J Kidney Dis. 2006;47(6):965–71.
59. White SL, McGeechan K, Jones M, Cass A, Chadban SJ, Polkinghorne KR, et al. Socioeconomic disadvantage and kidney disease in the United States, Australia, and Thailand. Am J Public Health. 2008;98(7):1306–13.
60. Bruce MA, Beech BM, Crook ED, Sims M, Wyatt SB, Flessner MF, et al. Association of socioeconomic status and CKD among African Americans: the Jackson heart study. Am J Kidney Dis. 2010;55(6):1001–8.
61. McClellan WM, Newsome BB, McClure LA, Howard G, Volkova N, Audhya P, et al. Poverty and racial disparities in kidney disease: the REGARDS study. Am J Nephrol. 2010;32(1):38–46.
62. Crews DC, McClellan WM, Shoham DA, Gao L, Warnock DG, Judd S, et al. Low income and albuminuria among REGARDS (Reasons for Geographic and Racial Differences in Stroke) study participants. Am J Kidney Dis. 2012;60(5):779–86.
63. Wise PH. The anatomy of a disparity in infant mortality. Annu Rev Public Health. 2003;24:341–62.
64. White SL, Perkovic V, Cass A, Chang CL, Poulter NR, Spector T, et al. Is low birth weight an antecedent of CKD in later life? A systematic review of observational studies. Am J Kidney Dis. 2009;54(2):248–61.
65. Barker DJ, Forsen T, Eriksson JG, Osmond C. Growth and living conditions in childhood and hypertension in adult life: a longitudinal study. J Hypertens. 2002;20(10):1951–6.
66. Sandboge S, Osmond C, Kajantie E, Eriksson JG. Early growth and changes in blood pressure during adult life. J Dev Orig Health Dis. 2016;7(3):306–13.
67. Eriksson JG, Osmond C, Kajantie E, Forsen TJ, Barker DJ. Patterns of growth among children who later develop type 2 diabetes or its risk factors. Diabetologia. 2006;49(12):2853–8.
68. Osmond C, Kajantie E, Forsen TJ, Eriksson JG, Barker DJ. Infant growth and stroke in adult life: the Helsinki birth cohort study. Stroke. 2007;38(2):264–70.
69. Barker DJ, Forsen T, Uutela A, Osmond C, Eriksson JG. Size at birth and resilience to effects of poor living conditions in adult life: longitudinal study. BMJ (Clin Res Ed). 2001;323(7324):1273–6.
70. Luyckx VA, Brenner BM. Birth weight, malnutrition and kidney-associated outcomes--a global concern. Nat Rev Nephrol. 2015;11(3):135–49.
71. Dreyer G, Hull S, Mathur R, Chesser A, Yaqoob MM. Progression of chronic kidney disease in a multi-ethnic community cohort of patients with diabetes mellitus. Diabet Med. 2013;30(8):956–63.
72. Earle KK, Porter KA, Ostberg J, Yudkin JS. Variation in the progression of diabetic nephropathy according to racial origin. Nephrol Dial Transplant. 2001;16(2):286–90.
73. Ali O, Mohiuddin A, Mathur R, Dreyer G, Hull S, Yaqoob MM. A cohort study on the rate of progression of diabetic chronic kidney disease in different ethnic groups. BMJ Open. 2013;3(2):e001855.
74. Pallayova M, Mohammed A, Langman G, Taheri S, Dasgupta I. Predicting non-diabetic renal disease in type 2 diabetic adults: the value of glycated hemoglobin. J Diabetes Complicat. 2015;29(5):718–23.

75. Koppiker N, Feehally J, Raymond N, Abrams KR, Burden AC. Rate of decline in renal function in Indo-Asians and Whites with diabetic nephropathy. Diabet Med. 1998;15(1):60–5.
76. Navaneethan SD, Aloudat S, Singh S. A systematic review of patient and health system characteristics associated with late referral in chronic kidney disease. BMC Nephrol. 2008;9:3.
77. Navaneethan SD, Kandula P, Jeevanantham V, Nally JV Jr, Liebman SE. Referral patterns of primary care physicians for chronic kidney disease in general population and geriatric patients. Clin Nephrol. 2010;73(4):260–7.
78. Quality AfHRa. 2014 National Healthcare Quality and Disparities Report 05/2015 [cited 20 Jan 2020]. Available from: https://www.rootcausecoalition.org/wp-content/uploads/2017/07/2014-National-Healthcare-Quality-and-Disparities-Report.pdf.
79. Evans K, Coresh J, Bash LD, Gary-Webb T, Köttgen A, Carson K, et al. Race differences in access to health care and disparities in incident chronic kidney disease in the US. Nephrol Dial Transplant. 2011;26(3):899–908.
80. Gao SW, Oliver DK, Das N, Hurst FP, Lentine KL, Agodoa LY, et al. Assessment of racial disparities in chronic kidney disease stage 3 and 4 care in the department of defense health system. Clin J Am Soc Nephrol. 2008;3(2):442–9.
81. Young BA, Maynard C, Boyko EJ. Racial differences in diabetic nephropathy, cardiovascular disease, and mortality in a national population of veterans. Diabetes Care. 2003;26(8):2392–9.
82. Fischer MJ, Kimmel PL, Greene T, Gassman JJ, Wang X, Brooks DH, et al. Sociodemographic factors contribute to the depressive affect among African Americans with chronic kidney disease. Kidney Int. 2010;77(11):1010–9.
83. Ricardo AC, Yang W, Lora CM, Gordon EJ, Diamantidis CJ, Ford V, et al. Limited health literacy is associated with low glomerular filtration in the Chronic Renal Insufficiency Cohort (CRIC) study. Clin Nephrol. 2014;81(1):30–7.
84. Devraj R, Borrego M, Vilay AM, Gordon EJ, Pailden J, Horowitz B. Relationship between health literacy and kidney function. Nephrology (Carlton). 2015;20(5):360–7.
85. Banerjee T, Crews DC, Wesson DE, Tilea AM, Saran R, Rios-Burrows N, et al. High dietary acid load predicts ESRD among adults with CKD. J Am Soc Nephrol. 2015;26(7):1693–700.
86. Epstein AM, Ayanian JZ, Keogh JH, Noonan SJ, Armistead N, Cleary PD, et al. Racial disparities in access to renal transplantation--clinically appropriate or due to underuse or overuse? N Engl J Med. 2000;343(21):1537–44, 2 p preceding.
87. Purnell TS, Luo X, Kucirka LM, Cooper LA, Crews DC, Massie AB, et al. Reduced racial disparity in kidney transplant outcomes in the United States from 1990 to 2012. J Am Soc Nephrol. 2016;27(8):2511–8.
88. Gander JC, Plantinga L, Zhang R, Mohan S, Pastan SO, Patzer RE. United States dialysis facilities with a racial disparity in kidney transplant waitlisting. Kidney Int Rep. 2017;2(5):963–8.
89. Collins AJ, Foley RN, Gilbertson DT, Chen SC. United States renal data system public health surveillance of chronic kidney disease and end-stage renal disease. Kidney Int Suppl (2011). 2015;5(1):2–7.
90. Hawkes CCM, Friel S, Thow AM. Achieving health equity: from root causes to fair outcomes. Lancet. 2007;370(9593):1153–63.

Chapter 20
Nutrition in Chronic Kidney Disease

Kelsey Pawson, Monica Salas, and Lea Borgi

Incidence and Prevention of Chronic Kidney Disease

Chronic kidney disease (CKD) is a global public health crisis affecting ~10% of the population worldwide and 15% of the general US population [1]; one in every nine US adults has CKD [2]. Kidney disease was included in the top ten leading causes of death in 2017 according to a CDC report. The largest percentage of patients with CKD is in the early stages; as a result, early recognition and interventions against factors involved in disease progression are crucial to improving the outcomes of these individuals [3]. Comorbid conditions associated with CKD and its progression include cardiovascular disease, hypertension, diabetes, malnutrition, and others [4]. CKD is responsible for an overwhelming amount of health problems in the United States, as well as an increasing economic burden. Treatment for CKD is likely to exceed $48 billion per year in the United States alone [5]. Because of the expansive and alarming health and financial issues related to kidney disease, maximizing prevention and optimizing treatment are of utmost importance.

CKD, a decline in renal function overtime, is defined as kidney damage for more than 3 months, characterized by structural and functional kidney abnormalities [6]. CKD, as opposed to acute kidney injury (AKI), is progressive and irreversible; it is classified by stages, according to the estimated glomerular filtration rate (eGFR) (below 60 mL/min/1.73m^2, stages 3–5 CKD) and albuminuria. As the disease progresses and eGFR declines, nitrogen-containing products from both dietary and

K. Pawson · M. Salas
Friedman School of Nutrition Science and Policy, Tufts University, Dietetic Intern, Frances
Stern Nutrition Center, Tufts Medical Center, Boston, MA, USA
e-mail: Kelsey.Pawson@tufts.edu; Monica.Salas@tufts.edu

L. Borgi (✉)
Brigham and Women's Hospital, Boston, MA, USA
e-mail: lborgi@bwh.harvard.edu

© Springer Nature Switzerland AG 2022
J. McCauley et al. (eds.), *Approaches to Chronic Kidney Disease*,
https://doi.org/10.1007/978-3-030-83082-3_20

Table 20.1 Stages of chronic kidney disease

National Institute of Diabetes and Digestive and Kidney Diseases	
Stage 1: Kidney damage with normal kidney function	GFR ≥ 90 mL/min and persistent (≥3 months) proteinuria as defined by ACR > 70 mg/mmol or PCR > 100 mg/mmol unless known to be due to diabetes
Stage 2: Kidney damage with mild loss of kidney function	GFR = 60–89 mL/min and persistent (≥3 months) proteinuria as defined by ACR > 70 mg/mmol or PCR > 100 mg/mmol unless known to be due to diabetes
Stage 3A: Mild to severe loss of kidney function	GFR = 45–59 mL/min
Stage 3: Mild to severe loss of kidney function	GFR = 30–44 mL/min
Stage 4: Severe loss of kidney function	GFR = 15–29 mL/min
Stage 5: Could require renal replacement therapy, such as dialysis or transplant	GFR < 15 mL/min

intrinsic protein catabolism accumulate, resulting in different symptoms, such as distorted taste and smell and decreased appetite. Dietary adjustments are therefore required, as CKD patients are at a higher risk of diminished nutritional status, protein-energy wasting, and malnutrition [7].

Medical nutrition therapy provided by a registered dietitian (RD) has been shown to be effective in the treatment and prevention of malnutrition and mineral and electrolyte disorders, as well as minimizing the impact of comorbid conditions in CKD patients [8]. Referral to a dietitian should begin during CKD stage 3 when the eGFR is <60 mL/min/1.73m^2 or at the patient's earliest request. Nutrition therapy offers many benefits addressing the management of uremia, electrolyte and acid-base imbalances, water and salt retention, mineral and bone disorders, anemia due to low iron stores and impaired erythropoiesis, and failure to thrive. In addition, nutrition therapy can delay the initiation of dialysis therapy by slowing disease progression [7, 8]. Because CKD is usually an indolent disease, early interventions are important to slow the disease's progression and prevent renal replacement therapy.

As mentioned above, CKD is categorized by various disease stages. Table 20.1 below provides a description of each of the stages as defined by GFR.

Role of Nutrition Therapy

Individuals with CKD that receive nutrition therapy have slower disease progression, fewer hospital admissions, and decreased incidence of sudden death [8]. Nutrition management in CKD patients involves complex diet therapies, including maintaining a balanced intake of protein, calories, sodium, fluid, phosphorus, and potassium. Patients must also adhere to the dietary recommendations of their other conditions if applicable. For instance, those with diabetes must also integrate methods of maintaining a balanced carbohydrate intake.

To effectively plan nutrition interventions, factors beyond dietary intake need to be considered, such as patients' knowledge, beliefs, medications, behavior, and access to food [7]. Nutritional therapy requires behavioral changes that involve education regarding lifestyle management. One form of lifestyle management, self-management, is an approach that has been successful in CKD patients, as it helps them recognize the central role their involvement plays in their own health and illness management [9, 10]. Dietitians are instrumental in teaching CKD patients self-management skills to promote lifestyle changes.

Treating patients with CKD requires an interdisciplinary approach and coordinated care that involves frequent assessments of the patient's dietary intake. To estimate the dietary intake of protein, sodium, and potassium, a 24-hour urine collection and a 24-hour dietary recall or food diary assessment should be conducted. This will allow for accurate measurements and assessments of an individual's compliance with dietary recommendations. The RD can then provide insight and help patients overcome barriers impacting adherence to dietary restrictions.

The patient's nutrition needs will change throughout the disease course, progressing from earlier stages of CKD to the posttransplant period [7]. Nutrition assessment should be repeated when the patient receives renal replacement therapy, dialysis (peritoneal or hemodialysis), and/or transplant [7]. The Kidney Disease Outcomes Quality Initiative (KDOQI) guidelines recommend that nutrition assessments be conducted every 6–12 months for stage 3 CKD patients and every 1–3 months in advanced CKD stages [7].

Recommended dietary adjustments need to be feasible, sustainable, and suited for patients' food preferences and clinical needs to ensure patient success. This chapter will address treatment recommendations and nutrition therapies for patients with CKD.

Dietary Factors Contributing to CKD

Effect of Specific Nutrients

Some factors that influence risk for CKD development are not modifiable. These include factors such as age, gender, race, and family history. Diet, on the other hand, is a known modifiable CKD risk factor. There is an inverse association between a healthy diet pattern and development of CKD-related conditions including type 2 diabetes, hypertension, cardiovascular disease, etc. An overall healthy dietary pattern that emphasizes a variety of nutrients while restricting others can play a role in CKD development.

Sodium is notable because of its role in blood pressure control. Hypertension is considered both a cause and consequence of CKD due to damage it causes to blood

Table 20.2 Sample plant-based protein sources

US Department of Agriculture's Food Data Central		
Food	Serving	Amount of protein per serving (g)
Lentils	½ cup	26
Soybeans	½ cup	22
Black beans	½ cup	8
Almonds	1.5 ounce	9
Quinoa	1 cup	8
Tofu	¾ cup	15

vessels in the kidneys and throughout the body. Therefore, reduction of dietary sodium in hypertensive individuals is of utmost importance to improve blood pressure control and, ultimately, prevent CKD development and progression [11]. The typical Western diet is high in sodium as it emphasizes packaged and processed foods instead of fruit and vegetable intake. Looking from a preventative perspective, intake of potassium and sodium can be considered concurrently because consuming adequate potassium-containing foods could potentially blunt the effect of excessive dietary sodium on hypertension. Alternatively, decreased potassium intake can augment the consequences of increased dietary sodium [12]. Analysis of diet patterns in the United States shows that about 90% of the population consume above the daily recommendation of sodium, at an average of 3440 mg of sodium per day [13]. The American Heart Association recommends no more than 2300 mg of sodium per day, but this value can vary individually. The average potassium intake for adults in the United States is ≤2000 mg per day [12], while the recommended daily intake for most adults is 4700 mg (Dietary Guidelines for Americans 2015–2020).

Restricting protein in early stages of CKD (e.g., in individuals with diabetes and albuminuria) has been shown to decrease CKD development. Decreased albuminuria is associated with slower progression of CKD [11]. Limiting dietary protein could help activate adaptive responses and decrease albuminuria while increasing serum albumin [11]. Also, the types of protein consumed have been linked with the risk of CKD development. Indeed, red and processed meat are associated with an increased CKD risk [14], while higher intake of plant-based protein such as nuts, legumes, and low-fat dairy products is associated with a lower CKD risk [14]. Specific examples of plant-based protein sources are depicted in Table 20.2.

Dietary Patterns

While a Western diet has been associated with an increased risk of CKD, a plant-based diet has been linked with a lower risk of developing CKD. A plant-based diet is described as a dietary pattern that emphasizes nutrient-dense plant foods and reduces/eliminates the amount of animal-derived foods consumed. There are a few mechanisms that could help explain this association.

Consumption of a plant-based dietary pattern can lower dietary acid load [15]. The kidneys help in maintaining the body's acid-base balance. Metabolic acidosis contributes to rapid kidney disease progression, increasing the overall risk of death [16]. Certain foods such as cheese, meat, eggs, and grain produce acid, while others, such as fruit and vegetables, produce base [17]. The net dietary acid load is a balance between both. A lower dietary acid load, such as that seen in a plant-based diet pattern, is beneficial because of its association with lower risk of CKD [15].

A plant-based diet also increases the intake of fiber, which has been found to decrease the incidence of CKD [15]. Inadequate intake of fiber in the Western diet is common, with <3% of Americans meeting the recommended intake of about 25–30 grams per day [18]. Adequate fiber intake is important to add bulk to stool to prevent constipation. Constipation can lead to a higher retention of uremic toxins and the development of hyperkalemia; however, increasing fiber intake will lead to looser stools, which, in turn, increases fluid loss and removal of nitrogenous waste [19]. In addition, vegetarian diets have a higher fiber content and less fermentable protein, which enhances peristalsis and the frequency of bowel movements that is associated with less uremic toxin production, exposure, and, therefore, absorption [20]. Fiber reduces the risk of CKD by lessening risk factors of CKD, especially hypertension and type 2 diabetes [18]. In addition, fiber has been shown to improve glycemic control and insulin secretion, both associated with a lower risk of proteinuria.

An increased consumption of fruits and vegetables is associated with reduced inflammation and oxidative stress [15] and improved endothelial function [12], both factors positively linked with kidney health.

Dietary patterns that emphasize a higher intake of fresh fruits, vegetables, and legumes, such as the Mediterranean and the Dietary Approaches to Stop Hypertension (DASH), have been shown to decrease CKD incidence [21–23]. Frequently, the DASH diet is used to manage hypertension, because it emphasizes the importance of limiting saturated and hydrogenated fats while encouraging the consumption of fresh fruits, vegetables, whole grains, low-fat dairy, and omega-3 fatty acids. Of note, a diet high in potassium is not appropriate for CKD patients with hyperkalemia. An RD can help in modifying the DASH diet to fit the needs of patients with CKD (discussed separately).

Dietary Recommendations for Individuals with Chronic Kidney Disease

Protein

For individuals with CKD who are not undergoing renal replacement therapy, KDOQI recommends protein intake of 0.6–0.75 g protein/kg/day. Increased dietary protein dilates the afferent arterioles, increasing glomerular filtration and further damaging the glomeruli [24]. In contrast, lower consumption of dietary protein has a preglomerular effect which enhances the post-glomerular effect of angiotensin pathway mediators that dilate efferent arterioles, resulting in lower intraglomerular pressure. Protein intake also influences urea generation, which explains the relationship between dietary protein restriction and the reduction in urea, an important factor in the development of uremic symptoms.

Protein catabolism and nitrogen balance in CKD are also connected to overall energy intake. Insufficient energy intake can accelerate protein catabolism, as protein will be used for energy supply, leading to a negative nitrogen balance. Clinical judgment and personalized nutrition recommendation by an RD should be applied when considering protein restriction so as to prevent protein malnutrition.

Adequate protein intake is crucial in preventing lean body mass wasting. A variety of protein recommendations are in place ranging from 0.28 g/kg/day for individuals receiving keto acid analogs to 0.9 g/kg/day for those who have diabetes. While varying ranges of protein intake have been studied, KDOQI recommends 0.6–0.75 g/kg/day for patients with CKD [7]. Greatly restricting protein intake is not ideal; providing sufficient energy intake (25–35 kcal/kg/day) and slightly reduced protein (0.6–0.75 g/kg/day) intake is appropriate for the majority of CKD patients. An intake of 0.6–0.75 g/kg is sufficient to meet energy needs and prevent protein-energy wasting. Recommendations provided should be based on the patient's ideal body weight (HAMWI: IBW (females) = 100lbs + 5lbs/inch over 5 feet and IBW (males) = 106lbs + 6lbs/inch over 5 feet).

The Modification of Diet in Renal Disease (MDRD) study showed increased mortality rates in patients with a very low-protein intake of 0.3 g/kg [25]. Very low-protein restrictions pose many challenges and concerns, the greatest of which are patient safety, feasibility, adherence, weight loss, and protein-energy wasting. In order to improve patient safety when on a low-protein diet, adequate energy intake (30–35 kcal/kg/day) by means of adjusting intake of carbohydrate and fat should be encouraged. This should be paired with continuing education, monitoring, and guidance to ensure that estimated needs are met. When an individual limits the intake of certain types of foods, they replace it with alternate foods. Individuals with diabetes can face challenges with worsening glycemic control and insulin response on low-protein diets, because they will often replace protein foods with foods high in fat and carbohydrates. An RD can work with the patient to create a personalized dietary plan that appropriately meets his or her needs.

With a low-protein diet, fat and carbohydrate combined should account for ~90% of the daily total energy intake to prevent protein-energy wasting [26]. Patients with diabetes need to ensure appropriate glycemic control while still maintaining adequate energy intake to mitigate the risk of protein-energy wasting and hypoglycemia, which increases with worsening kidney function. As kidney function declines, insulin and other diabetic medications remain in the system for longer periods due to decreased kidney clearance. In a diabetic patient, insulin and other diabetes medications will require continuous adjustments.

One important behavior change that typically needs to be addressed is portion size. Advising patients to consume the recommended portion size will help them

Table 20.3 Comparison of animal vs. plant protein

4 ounces of ground beef	3.5 ounces of red kidney beans
21.9 g protein	8.12 g protein
224 calories	121 calories
14.4 g total fat	0.93 g total fat
327 mg potassium	118 mg phosphorus
198 mg phosphorus	250 mg potassium
76.8 mg sodium	208 mg sodium

stay within their target goals. Also, selecting plant proteins over animal proteins may help patients adhere to the recommended ranges. Table 20.3 helps visualize the nutritional differences between an animal source of protein, such as ground beef, and a plant-based source of protein, such a red kidney beans. Plant-based foods are low in saturated fat and bioavailable phosphorus and lead to less acid production. Also, they are a great source of fiber, poly- and monounsaturated fat, magnesium, and iron. Consuming a plant-based diet has been associated with better outcomes among people with CKD [27].

Energy

The baseline recommended energy intake is calculated using resting energy expenditure (REE). Overall, individuals with CKD and end-stage renal disease (ESRD) have increased REE when compared to individuals without kidney disease [28]. REE is even more elevated in individuals receiving dialysis. Recommendations for energy intake also take into consideration weight status, age, gender, level of physical activity, and metabolic stressors (KDOQI guidelines). Therefore, patients with CKD and ESRD can be susceptible to insufficient energy intake. A minimal caloric intake of 23–35 kcal/kg/day is advised for CKD patients to prevent malnutrition [8]. For patients in CKD stages 4–5, KDOQI recommends a higher intake of 30–35 kcal/kg/day for those younger than 60 years of age and 35 kcal/kg/day for patients older than 60 [7, 8].

Sodium and Fluid

Dietary sodium intake should be considered in all stages of CKD because of its potential direct and indirect outcomes on kidney disease. Indirect mechanisms involve increased blood pressure and proteinuria [29]. These factors can result in vascular and renal injury leading to CKD progression (Fig. 20.1). In addition, dietary sodium intake can affect the kidneys and vascular system directly, independently of blood pressure [29]. Increased intake of sodium increases oxidative stress in the kidney by increasing generation and decreasing breakdown of reactive

Fig. 20.1 Relationship
between sodium load,
blood pressure, and
proteinuria

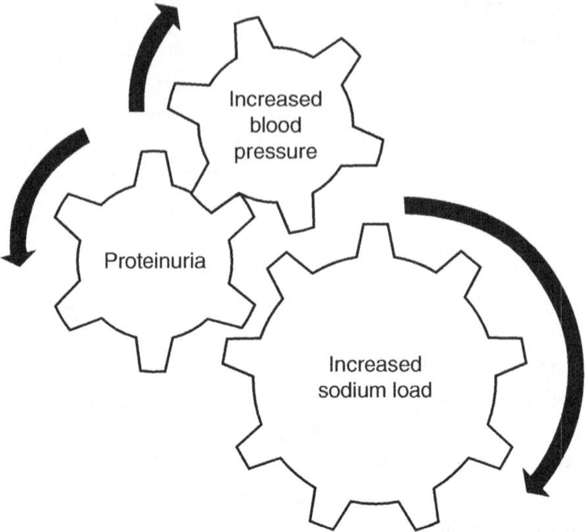

oxygen species [29]. Sodium intake can also have an effect on endothelium, modulating the production of TGFβ1 and nitric oxide, resulting in vascular and glomerular fibrosis [29]. Overall, these physiological effects can lead to a decline in kidney function.

In patients with established CKD, and especially in those with concomitant hypertension and/or proteinuria, a dietary sodium restriction should be implemented [24]. Increased sodium intake can augment urinary albumin excretion and diminish anti-proteinuric effects of angiotensin-converting enzyme (ACE) inhibitor therapies [29]. In contrast, reducing sodium intake can enhance the effects of a diet lower in protein, by decreasing intraglomerular pressure and potentially decreasing proteinuria (NJEM 2017). For individuals with ESRD and on dialysis, increased sodium intake can also impact volume homeostasis.

Although sodium restriction in CKD patients is recommended, patients are met with a variety of barriers: limited knowledge about sodium content of foods, difficulty in reading food labels, taste preferences, public policy modifications, etc. [29]. A 2006 cross-sectional study showed that even though most people reported using food labels, many individuals had difficulties in understanding them, regardless of literacy status [30]. Figure 20.2 depicts a nutrition facts label, highlighting what an individual needs to identify in order to determine sodium content of the product.

Managing sodium and fluid balance can be challenging for individuals with CKD; therefore, these patients should focus on limiting or eliminating high-sodium foods. The recommended daily intake of sodium for CKD patients is <2.3 g/day [7, 8]. Prepared and packaged foods, as well as meals consumed in restaurants, tend to have the largest amounts of sodium per serving [31]. Some examples of what to look for when purchasing low-sodium products are listed in Table 20.4. For example, a turkey sandwich with a side salad and pickle at a restaurant contains ~1935 mg sodium vs. ~668 mg sodium in a similar sandwich made at home [31]. It is

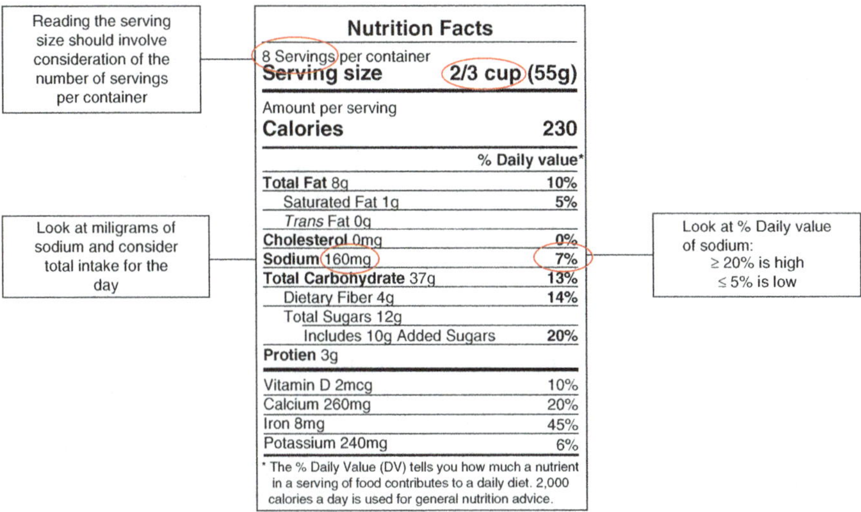

Fig. 20.2 Nutrition facts label from FDA

Table 20.4 Low-salt and low-sodium packaged foods will say: (look for the label to say less than 20% daily value)

Sodium/salt free	No salt added
Very low/low sodium	Unsalted
Reduced or less sodium	Lightly salted
Light in sodium	

recommended that individuals with CKD avoid packaged foods and prepare most meals at home to avoid excess sodium intake.

Fluid is not routinely restricted in all CKD patients. Patients can have difficulty regulating fluid balance at different times during CKD; as such, fluid recommendations need to be individualized based on patient needs and CKD stage.

Potassium

Potassium is the main intracellular cation that acts as a mediator for cellular electrophysiology, vascular function, neuromuscular function, and blood pressure. An imbalance of potassium level can result in muscular weakness, ventricular arrhythmias, and even death [32]. While patients with CKD can experience low levels of potassium (especially those on a diuretic, which leads to an increased potassium removal in urine), high levels of potassium is more common in CKD. It is essential to address hyperkalemia in CKD patients because of its serious or even fatal outcomes. Caution is imperative because there are no warning signs when serum potassium levels are elevated to dangerous levels [33].

For prevention of CKD, adequate potassium is encouraged. Once CKD has developed, potassium restriction should be implemented in patients with documented hyperkalemia only. Serum potassium level increases in CKD patients because the kidneys are unable to excrete potassium. Additionally, patients might be on medications that inhibit potassium excretion (such as ACE inhibitors), therefore increasing and/or worsening serum potassium levels.

Hyperkalemia is especially dangerous in advanced CKD because it is one of the reasons patients are started on dialysis. It is recommended that patients with hyperkalemia restrict potassium intake to <2.4 g/day, yet the importance of incorporating high-fiber fruits and vegetables still needs to be emphasized. Hidden sources of potassium are important to identify. Salt substitutes (including "low-salt" foods), chocolate, granola, and peanut butter are all high-potassium foods. Table 20.5 provides some examples of potassium content of various foods.

One of the challenges patients face when restricting dietary potassium intake is that patients are then encouraged to make more atherogenic selections [8, 34]. Frequently, these choices tend to be lower in fiber, increasing the incidence of constipation, which, in turn, results in greater potassium absorption in the gut and, subsequently, higher serum potassium levels [35]. As such, patient education is crucial in ensuring that appropriate selections are made.

Phosphorus

Hyperphosphatemia can be seen in advanced stages of CKD. Restriction of phosphorus should be considered when levels are above target as recommended by the KDOQI guidelines. Hyperphosphatemia in CKD patients is associated with greater mortality and worse cardiovascular outcomes [36]. Biochemical alterations observed in mineral bone disorder include elevated fibroblast growth factor-23 and parathyroid hormone (PTH), decreased 1,25-dihydroxyvitamin D, increased serum phosphate, and decreased serum calcium [37]. Control of phosphorus intake is the cornerstone for prevention and treatment of these CKD-related complications such as renal bone disease, soft tissue calcification, and secondary hyperparathyroidism (KDOQI 2013). Treatment of hyperphosphatemia can involve decreasing ingestion of phosphorus, as well as increasing renal phosphorus removal with phosphate binders.

The two main sources of dietary phosphorus are organic (animal- and plant-based protein-rich foods) and inorganic (mostly food additives). Organic and inorganic phosphorus are absorbed at different rates, with plant-based organic phosphorus being lower than inorganic phosphorus [38]. Table 20.6 lists commonly consumed foods that are high in organic phosphorus. Certain medications can also contain phosphorus because of its role in pharmaceutical preparations [39]. Although phosphorus content may not be particularly high in one medication alone, patients with CKD or ESRD, especially those on dialysis, could be taking multiple phosphorus-containing medications.

Table 20.5 Potassium content of foods

Food	Serving size	Mg/serving
Foods higher in potassium		
Potato, baked, with skin	1 medium	925
Beans, white, navy, lima, lentils, soybeans	½ cup	355–500
Fish: swordfish, walleye, snapper, halibut, tuna	3 ounces	425–450
Banana	1 medium	420
Raisin bran	1 cup	380
Tomato sauce	½ cup	365
Salmon	3 oz	375
Avocados, sliced	½ cup	355
Raisins	¼ cup	350
Quinoa, cooked	1 cup	320
Yogurt, plain, skim milk	½ cup	310
Kale, cooked	½ cup	295
Beef, roast or ground (85% lean)	3 ounces	280
Nuts: Brazil, mixed nuts, peanuts, almonds	¼ cup	210–260
Zucchini, cooked	½ cup	240
Chicken, light or dark meat	3 ounces	205–230
Cantaloupe	½ cup	210
Turkey, light or dark meat	3 ounces	210
Foods lower in potassium		
Beans, green, cooked	½ cup	90
Cauliflower, cooked	½ cup	90
Apricots	1	90
Peas, sugar, snap	½ cup	85
Watermelon, diced	½ cup	85
Bread, whole wheat	1 slice	80
Cucumbers, sliced	½ cup	75
Egg	1 large	65
Hummus	2 tbsp	70
Cheese: cheddar, Swiss, provolone, mozzarella	1 oz	20–55
Blueberries	½ cup	55
Pasta	1 cup	55
Rice, white, cooked	1 cup	55
Shrimp, steamed or boiled	4 large	35

Additionally, there can be various sources of hidden phosphorus in the diet. Phosphorus additives are sometimes added to food products to modify texture and taste, as well as to act as a preservative. A method to help identify hidden phosphorus is to look in the ingredient list found near the nutrition facts label on food products. Phosphorus additives can be listed under a variety of names, so they are not always easily recognizable as a source of phosphorus intake. Phosphorus additives

Table 20.6 Foods high in phosphorus (>100 mg per serving)

Food	Serving size	Mg/serving
Sardines	3 oz	420
Plain yogurt, low-fat	8 oz	327
Fish: cod, halibut, salmon tuna	3 oz	200–280
Milk, all kinds	1 cup	240
Beef	3 oz	200
Turkey	3 oz	180
Oatmeal	½ cup	160
Chicken, white meat	3 oz	150
Cheese: American, cheddar, mozzarella, Swiss, provolone	1 oz	150
Potato, baked with skin	1 medium/6 oz	120

Table 20.7 Common phosphorus additives found in foods

Disodium phosphate	Dicalcium phosphate
Monosodium phosphate	Trisodium phosphate
Phosphoric acid	Sodium tripolyphosphate
Sodium hexametaphosphate	Tetrasodium pyrophosphate

Fig. 20.3 Ingredient list with phosphorus additive identified

are increasingly added to processed and fast foods as preservatives; Table 20.7 lists commonly used phosphorus additives. However, they contain inorganic phosphorus which is about 100% absorbed [7]. Such additives have been found in meat and poultry products creating a higher than average phosphorus to protein ratio, much greater than additive-free products [7]. Phosphorus additives are most commonly found in bakery products, enhanced meats, and processed cheeses [7]. In addition, Fig. 20.3 gives an example of a food product label with a phosphorus additive.

Phosphorus homeostasis is central in the treatment and prevention of renal osteodystrophy, secondary hyperparathyroidism, and soft tissue calcification in CKD patients [8]. Serum phosphorus levels are used as a biomarker for phosphorus homeostasis and have been reported as an important risk factor for all-cause cardiovascular mortality in individuals with CKD [8]. Recommendations must be individualized, including dietary restriction, phosphate binders, and calcium and vitamin D supplementation [8].

KDOQI recommends that dietary phosphorus should be restricted in CKD patients to 800–1000 mg/day when serum levels are greater than 5.5 mg/dL [8]. An individualized dietary approach can be used to maintain adequate levels [40]. Even in conjunction with a low-protein diet, the quantity and bioavailability of phosphorus vary depending on the type of protein consumed since the absorption of phosphorus from plants is lower than that of animal protein (30–50% compared to 50–70%) [41]. Processed foods and food additives contain readily absorbable phosphorus, increasing phosphorus load. Therefore, intake of these foods should be kept minimal [42].

Typically, foods with organic phosphorus are more nutrient dense and have a greater nutritional value compared to processed foods that are phosphate additives. Those foods are usually lower in nutritional value and are often paired with sodium and potassium additives [7].

Calcium and Vitamin D

For patients with CKD, both negative and positive calcium balance can have negative consequences. Negative calcium balance can result in osteoporosis and fractures in the setting of mineral and bone disorder, and a positive balance can increase risk for extraskeletal calcification, as well as cardiovascular events [37]. Calcium balance is difficult to determine because serum calcium levels do not reflect overall body calcium balance; in addition, maintenance can be altered by factors such as bone turnover, degree of kidney function, hormones, use of vitamin D supplementation, and calcium intake. This is why the patient's medical and nutrition history must be reviewed and considered.

Once a patient has stage 3–5 CKD, calcium restriction could be recommended if the individual has persistent or recurrent hypercalcemia and if serum PTH levels are consistently low [32]. This includes calcium from calcium-based phosphate binders. Serum calcium concentration is an important factor in regulating PTH secretion and has an effect on soft tissue calcification and bone integrity (KDOQI). In advanced CKD, the kidneys are not as efficient in increasing urine calcium excretion. As 1,25-dihydroxyvitamin D levels decrease, the absorption of calcium in the gastrointestinal tract is altered. Calcium absorption becomes dependent on a positive gradient to maintain adequate levels [37].

The kidneys play a crucial role in metabolism and regulation of vitamin D. In CKD and ESRD patients, vitamin D insufficiency/deficiency is commonly observed [15]. Current recommendations are to utilize treatment of active vitamin D or its analogues in the setting of secondary hyperparathyroidism and vitamin D insufficiency/deficiency [15].

Total elemental calcium, including dietary sources, supplements, and calcium-based phosphate binders, should not exceed 2000 mg/day in patients with moderate to advanced CKD [8]. Vitamin D supplementation is recommended in order to maintain adequate calcium levels, if serum 25-hydroxyvitamin D falls below 30 ng/ml.

Kidney disease patients with serum levels of 25(OH)-D > 30 ng/ml and PTH above the target range can be supplemented with active vitamin D (calcitriol, alfacalcidol, or doxercalciferol) [8].

Supplements

Many patients report taking supplements in the United States. However, there is insufficient evidence to indicate whether micronutrients or multivitamin supplementation is beneficial or detrimental in the CKD population. Over-the-counter supplements contain many pharmacologically active compounds that can interact with prescription drugs or other supplements and can therefore be harmful for individuals with kidney disease. Patients should be encouraged to share any nutrition concerns they have with their physician, including the disclosure of any over-the-counter supplements. The patient's current intake needs to be considered when recommending any nutrition supplements, fortified foods, and nutrient-enhanced products.

Conclusion

CKD is a complex and progressive condition, with treatment mostly focused on slowing its progression. In this chapter, we have explored the significant impact nutrition can have on an individual with CKD. With the instrumental help of an RD, nutrition therapy can help prevent the development of CKD in patients with known risk factors (such as diabetes and hypertension) and delay the progression of kidney disease from one stage to another.

While nutrition in kidney disease is being recognized as an important tool in treating CKD patients, it is important for nutrition research to continue to assess the intricate link between diet and CKD.

References

1. Centers for Disease Control and Prevention. Chronic kidney disease in the United States, 2019. Atlanta: US Department of Health and Human Services, Centers for Disease Control and Prevention; 2019.
2. Coresh J, Selvin E, Stevens LA, Manzi J, Kusek JW, Eggers P, Van Lente F, Levey AS. Prevalence of chronic kidney disease in the United States. JAMA. 2007;298(17):2038–47.
3. Palmer SC, Hayen A, Macaskill P, Pellegrini F, Craig JC, Elder GJ, Strippoli GF. Serum levels of phosphorus, parathyroid hormone, and calcium and risks of death and cardiovascular disease in individuals with chronic kidney disease: a systematic review and meta-analysis. JAMA. 2011;305(11):1119–27.

4. Bolton WK. Renal physicians association clinical practice guideline: appropriate patient preparation for renal replacement therapy: guideline number 3. J Am Soc Nephrol. 2003;14(5):1406–10.

5. Global Facts: About Kidney Disease. National Kidney Foundation, 11 Mar 2015, www.kidney. org/kidneydisease/global-facts-about-kidney-disease.

6. Vassalotti JA, Centor R, Turner BJ, Greer RC, Choi M, Sequist TD, Initiative NKFKDOQ. Practical approach to detection and management of chronic kidney disease for the primary care clinician. Am J Med. 2016;129(2):153–62. E7.

7. Ikizler TA, Burrowes JD, Byham-Gray LD, Campbell KL, Carrero JJ, Chan W, et al. KDOQI clinical practice guideline for nutrition in CKD: 2020 update. Am J Kidney Dis. 2020;76(3 Suppl 1):S1–S107. https://doi.org/10.1053/j.ajkd.2020.05.006. Erratum in: Am J Kidney Dis. 2021 Feb;77(2):308.

8. Handu D, Rozga M, Steiber, A. Executive Summary of the 2020 Academy of Nutrition and Dietetics and National Kidney Foundation Clinical Practice Guideline for Nutrition in CKD. Journal of the Academy of Nutrition and Dietetics 2021;121(9):1881–1893.

9. Gillis BP, Caggiula AW, Chiavacci AT, Coyne T, Doroshenko L, Milas NC, Nowalk MP, Scherch LK. Nutrition intervention program of the modification of diet in renal disease study: a self-management approach. J Am Diet Assoc. 1995;95(11):1288–94.

10. Milas NC, Nowalk MP, Akpele L, Castaldo L, Coyne T, Doroshenko L, Kigawa L, Korzec-Ramirez D, Scherch LK, Snetselaar L. Factors associated with adherence to the dietary protein intervention in the modification of diet in renal disease study. J Am Diet Assoc. 1995;95(11):1295–300.

11. Chronic Kidney Disease and Diet: Assessment, Management and Treatment. An Overview Guide for Dietitians. National Kidney Disease Education Program. April 2015.

12. DuBose TD Jr. Inadequate dietary potassium and progression of CKD. Clin J Am Soc Nephrol. 2019;14(3):319–20. https://doi.org/10.2215/CJN.01020119. Epub 2019 Feb 14.

13. Centers for Disease Control and Prevention (CDC). Usual sodium intakes compared with dietary guidelines. MMWR Morb Mortal Wkly Rep. 2011;60(41):1413–7.

14. Haring B, Selvin E, Liang M, Coresh J, Grams M, Petruski-Ivleva N, Steffen LM, Rebholz CM. Dietary protein sources and risk for incident chronic kidney disease: results from the Atherosclerosis Risk in Communities (ARIC) Study. J Ren Nutr. 2017;27(4):233–42.

15. Kim H, Caulfield LE, Garcia-Larsen V, Steffen LM, Grams ME, Coresh J, Rebholz CM. Plant-based diets and incident CKD and kidney function. Clin J Am Soc Nephrol. 2019;14:682–91.

16. Goraya N, Simoni J, Jo C, Wesson DE. Dietary acid reduction with fruits and vegetables or bicarbonate attenuates kidney injury in patients with a moderately reduced glomerular filtration rate due to hypertensive nephropathy. Kidney Int. 2012;81(1):86–93.

17. Scialla J, Anderson C. Dietary acid load: a novel nutritional target in chronic kidney disease? Adv Chronic Kidney Dis. 2013;20(2):141–9. https://doi.org/10.1053/j.ackd.2012.11.001.

18. Clemens R, Kranz S, Mobley A, Nicklas T, Raimondi MP, Rodriguez JC, Slavin JL, Warshaw H. Filling America's fiber intake gap: summary of a roundtable to probe realistic solutions with a focus on grain-based foods. J Nutr. 2012;142(7):1390S–401S. https://doi.org/10.3945/jn.112.160176. Epub 2012 May 30

19. Sumida K, Molnar MZ, Potukuchi PK, Thomas F, Lu JL, Matsushita K, Yamagata K, Kalantar-Zadeh K, Kovesdy CP. Constipation and incident CKD. J Am Soc Nephrol. 2017;28(4):1248–58.

20. David LA, Maurice CF, Carmody RN, Gootenberg DB, Button JE, Wolfe BE, Ling AV, Devlin AS, Varma Y, Fischbach MA. Diet rapidly and reproducibly alters the human gut microbiome. Nature. 2014;505(7484):559–63.

21. Khatri M, Moon YP, Scarmeas N, Gu Y, Gardener H, Cheung K, Wright CB, Sacco RL, Nickolas TL, Elkind MS. The association between a Mediterranean-style diet and kidney function in the Northern Manhattan Study cohort. Clin J Am Soc Nephrol. 2014;9(11):1868–75.

22. Rebholz CM, Crews DC, Grams ME, Steffen LM, Levey AS, Miller ER III, Appel LJ, Coresh J. DASH (Dietary Approaches to Stop Hypertension) diet and risk of subsequent kidney disease. Am J Kidney Dis. 2016;68(6):853–61.

23. Chang A, Van Horn L, Jacobs DR Jr, Liu K, Muntner P, Newsome B, Shoham DA, Durazo-Arvizu R, Bibbins-Domingo K, Reis J. Lifestyle-related factors, obesity, and incident microalbuminuria: the CARDIA (Coronary Artery Risk Development in Young Adults) study. Am J Kidney Dis. 2013;62(2):267–75.

24. Kalantar-Zadeh K, Fouque D. Nutrition management of chronic kidney disease. N Engl J Med. 2017;377:1765–76.

25. Klahr S, Levey AS, Beck GJ, Caggiula AW, Hunsicker L, Kusek JW, Striker G. The effects of dietary protein restriction and blood-pressure control on the progression of chronic renal disease. N Engl J Med. 1994;330(13):877–84.

26. Kovesdy CP, Kopple JD, Kalantar-Zadeh K. Management of protein-energy wasting in non-dialysis-dependent chronic kidney disease: reconciling low protein intake with nutritional therapy. Am J Clin Nutr. 2013;97(6):1163–77.

27. Chen X, Wei G, Jalili T, Metos J, Giri A, Cho ME, Boucher R, Greene T, Beddhu S. The associations of plant protein intake with all-cause mortality in CKD. Am J Kidney Dis. 2016;67(3):423–30.

28. Zha Y, Qian Q. Protein nutrition and malnutrition in CKD and ESRD. Nutrients. 2017;9:208. https://doi.org/10.3390/nu9030208.

29. Wright J, Cavanaugh K. Dietary sodium in chronic kidney disease: a comprehensive approach. Semin Dial. 2010;23(4):415–21. https://doi.org/10.1111/j.1525-139X.2010.00752.x.

30. Rothman RL, Housam R, Weiss H, Davis D, Gregory R, Gebretsadik T, Shintani A, Elasy TA. Patient understanding of food labels: the role of literacy and numeracy. Am J Prev Med. 2006;31(5):391–8.

31. American Heart Association. "Sodium sources: Where does all that sodium come from?" Heart.org, www.heart.org/en/healthy-living/healthyeating/eat-smart/sodium/sodium-sources.

32. KDIGO clinical practice guideline for the evaluation and management of chronic kidney disease. Kidney Int Suppl. 2013;3:1–150.

33. Cuppari L, Nerbass FB, Avesani CM, Kamimura MA. A practical approach to dietary interventions for nondialysis-dependent CKD patients: the experience of a reference nephrology center in Brazil. BMC Nephrol. 2016;17:85.

34. Khoueiry G, Waked A, Goldman M, El-Charabaty E, Dunne E, Smith M, Kleiner M, Lafferty J, Kalantar-Zadeh K, El-Sayegh S. Dietary intake in hemodialysis patients does not reflect a heart healthy diet. J Ren Nutr. 2011;21(6):438–47.

35. St-Jules DE, Goldfarb DS, Sevick MA. Nutrient non-equivalence: does restricting high-potassium plant foods help to prevent hyperkalemia in hemodialysis patients? J Ren Nutr. 2016;26(5):282–7.

36. Sim JJ, Bhandari SK, Smith N, Chung J, Liu IL, Jacobsen SJ, Kalanter-Zadeh K. Phosphorus and risk of renal failure in subjects with normal renal function. Am J Med. 2013;126(4):311–8.

37. Gallant K, Spiegel D. Calcium balance in chronic kidney disease. Curr Osteoporos Rep. 2017;15:214–21.

38. Noori N, Sims JJ, Kopple JD, Shah A, Colman S, Shinaberger CS, Bross R, Mehrotra R, Kovesdy CP, Kalantar-Zadeh K. Organic and inorganic dietary phosphorus and its management in chronic kidney disease. Iran J Kidney Dis. 2010;4(2):89–100.

39. Li J, Wang L, Han M, Xiong Y, Liao R, Li y, Sun S, Maharjan A, Su B. The role of phosphate-containing medications and low dietary phosphorus-protein ratio in reducing intestinal phosphorus load in patients with chronic kidney disease. Nutr Diabet. 2019;9:14.

40. Morey B, Walker R, Davenport A. More dietetic time, better outcome? A randomized prospective study investigating the effect of more dietetic time on phosphate control in end-stage kidney failure haemodialysis patients. Nephron Clin Pract 2008;109:c173–c180.

41. Moorthi RN, Armstrong CL, Janda K, Ponsler-Sipes K, Asplin JR, Moe SM. The effect of a diet containing 70% protein from plants on mineral metabolism and musculoskeletal health in chronic kidney disease. Am J Nephrol. 2014;40(6):582–91.
42. Sullivan C, Sayre SS, Leon JB, Machekano R, Love TE, Porter D, Marbury M, Sehgal AR. Effect of food additives on hyperphosphatemia among patients with end-stage renal disease: a randomized controlled trial. JAMA. 2009;301(6):629–35.

Chapter 21
Drug Dosing in CKD Polypharmacy and Nephrotoxicity

Olivia Marchionda and Andrew Moyer

Background

Many medications and other pharmaceutical agents are renally excreted. Therefore, the dose or frequency of a prescribed medication may need to be reduced in patients with acute kidney injury (AKI) or chronic kidney disease (CKD) in order to optimize medication therapies and reduce the risk of toxicity. The KDIGO 2012 Clinical Practice guidelines recommend that prescribers should take glomerular filtration rate (GFR) into account when dosing medications [1]. This chapter will review pharmacokinetic and pharmacodynamics considerations in medication prescribing, dose selection, and monitoring to optimize medication therapy and avoid toxicity. It will also review the types of kidney injury caused by select medications, considerations for medication selection and dosing, and the most common renal function equations that are applied to medication dose adjustments. Finally, this chapter will provide recommended medication dosing based on the degree of renal impairment for commonly prescribed medications based on the best-known available data. It is important to note that renal function calculations using estimated glomerular filtration rate (eGFR) and creatinine clearance (CrCl) are based on stable renal function, and more selective analysis of medication therapies and doses is needed when patients have a progressing AKI.

O. Marchionda (✉)
Department of Pharmacy, Thomas Jefferson University Hospital, Philadelphia, PA, USA
e-mail: olivia.marchionda@jefferson.edu

A. Moyer
Department of Pharmacy, Augusta Health, Fishersville, VA, USA
e-mail: AM5880719@augustahealth.com

© Springer Nature Switzerland AG 2022
J. McCauley et al. (eds.), *Approaches to Chronic Kidney Disease*,
https://doi.org/10.1007/978-3-030-83082-3_21

Effects of Drug Pharmacology in Kidney Disease

A patient's response to a medication is dependent on both the medication's pharmacokinetics and pharmacodynamics. Pharmacodynamics represents the effect of the medication on the body, including interactions between the medication, its target site of action, and downstream biochemical effects. Pharmacokinetics describes the effect of the body on the medication which relates to the physiologic processes of absorption, distribution, metabolism, and excretion [2]. A change in pharmacokinetics can alter medication exposure and predispose patients to either over- or underdosing as compared to the anticipated, or standard, dose response. Chronic kidney disease is characterized by multiple physiologic effects, which induce clinically significant changes in pharmacokinetics [3]. Understanding these changes is essential to rational medication use and optimization of treatment regimens. In this section, the pharmacologic parameters that are altered by renal dysfunction are summarized, and an approach to appropriate medication use and recommended dosage adjustments is described.

Bioavailability

Absolute bioavailability is the fraction of medication that reaches systemic circulation following administration, most commonly considered in association with oral administration [2]. Oral bioavailability depends on the extent of gastrointestinal absorption and intestinal and hepatic first-pass metabolism. The effect of CKD on absorption and overall bioavailability is not well understood. For most medications that have been evaluated, gastrointestinal absorption is largely unchanged. However, there are several factors to consider that may alter drug absorption.

Many patients with CKD are prescribed proton pump inhibitors and histamine-2 receptor antagonists, leading to an increased gastric pH. For medications that are best absorbed in an acidic environment (furosemide, ketoconazole, ferrous sulfate), drug dissolution and ionization are often reduced in the setting of increased gastric pH, resulting in reduced bioavailability [4]. The absorption of certain medications such as digoxin, iron, levothyroxine, tetracyclines, and fluoroquinolones may be reduced with concomitant use of phosphate binders [5–7]. Many patients with CKD, particularly those with comorbid diabetes, suffer from gastroparesis, which results in delayed gastric emptying, prolonging the time to reach maximum drug concentration [8]. This should be considered when rapid onset is needed following oral administration of a medication (e.g., sulfonylureas). Gut edema has also been attributed to reduced oral absorption, particularly in CKD patients with concomitant cirrhosis, congestive heart failure (CHF), or nephrotic syndrome, but it is uncertain how to best manage medication prescribing for these secondary complications [9].

An often-overlooked component of drug bioavailability is intestinal first-pass metabolism. Several medications undergo significant metabolism in the gastrointestinal tract, including cyclosporine and tacrolimus. Renal insufficiency is associated with decreased activity of CYP450 enzymes, likely due to reduced gene expression.

CKD-induced reductions in intestinal CYP450 metabolism result in an increase in overall oral bioavailability [10]. In general, estimation and evaluation of oral absorption is a difficult task in the CKD population, and it is important to consider patient-specific factors that may alter drug absorption.

Distribution

The volume of distribution (Vd) of a medication can be used to calculate the dose required to achieve a desired systemic level. Generally, there is an inverse correlation between the serum concentration of a medication and its Vd. Several factors related to medication distribution are influenced by renal function. Proposed mechanisms of changes in Vd seen in CKD include alterations in body composition due to fluid overload, decreased plasma protein binding due to hypoalbuminemia, competitive binding interactions with uremic toxins, and altered tissue binding [2]. Plasma drug concentrations are a representation of both a drug bound to plasma proteins and unbound (free) drug. Only free drug, however, can cross cellular membranes and exert a pharmacologic effect.

Acidic medications, which have a high plasma protein binding ratio, such as barbiturates, penicillins, cephalosporins, furosemide, phenytoin, salicylates, valproate, and warfarin, are significantly affected by reduced protein binding in CKD [11]. Decreased plasma protein binding due to competition at binding sites may result in displacement of medications from these binding sites and thus increase the concentration of free drug. The volume of distribution may also be affected by altered tissue binding, particularly with digoxin. Digoxin's Vd is reduced by half in patients with CKD stage 5, which results in increased serum concentrations if the loading and maintenance doses are not reduced [12].

CKD-induced changes in body composition can have a variable impact on Vd of hydrophilic medications. One factor that leads to an increase in Vd is an increase in total body water, manifested as increased extracellular fluid volume, ascites, or peripheral edema. This will lead to a decrease in plasma levels of water-soluble and protein-bound drugs, such as pravastatin, fluvastatin, morphine, and codeine [13]. Contrarily, muscle wasting and fluid removal by hemodialysis may reduce Vd and increase serum concentrations of hydrophilic medications, leading to significant shifts in serum concentrations if significant volume changes occur in an end-stage renal patient in a short time period.

Metabolism

The majority of drug metabolism takes place in the liver; however, cells in the intestine, lungs, and kidney may also contain enzymes that produce these metabolic reactions [12]. Drug metabolism is classified as either a phase I or phase II reaction. Phase I reactions are affected mostly by the CYP450 system and include oxidation,

Table 21.1 Medication metabolites impacted by CKD

Parent drug	Metabolite	Pharmacologic activity of metabolite
Allopurinol	Oxipurinol	Suppresses xanthine oxidase (primary activity)
Azathioprine	Mercaptopurine	Immunosuppressant (metabolite only)
Morphine	Morphine-6-glucuronide (M-6G)	More active than the parent compound; prolonged narcotic effect in ESRD
Mycophenolic acid	Mycophenolic acid glucuronide	GI side effects
Sulfonamides	Acetylated metabolites	Increased toxicity (bone marrow suppression)
Theophylline	1,3-dimethyl uric acid	Cardiotoxicity
Zidovudine	Zidovudine triphosphate	Antiretroviral activity (primary activity)

reduction, and hydrolysis. In general, phase I hydrolysis and reduction reactions are slowed in CKD [14]. This is largely due to nonspecific inhibition of the liver enzymes and to the fact that a small portion of CYP450 reactions takes place in renal tissues. Phase II reactions act primarily to transform a parent drug or metabolite of a phase I reaction into a water-soluble compound that can be easily excreted in the urine or bile [15].

Phase II metabolic processes are most affected by CKD, including glucuronidation reactions [10]. By inhibiting glucuronidation, the amount of parent drug available is increased, leading to potential toxicities. Examples of medications with metabolites affected by CKD are listed below (Table 21.1).

While many of these metabolic reactions result in the formation of inactive compounds, there are several medications that undergo metabolism to a pharmacologically active compound. For example, meperidine is metabolized to normeperidine, which is dependent on renal elimination. Although normeperidine has little opioid receptor effect compared to the parent compound, it is a central nervous system irritant that lowers the seizure threshold and can accumulate in patients with impaired renal function. Meperidine should be avoided in late stage and end-stage renal disease [16].

In addition to phase I and phase II reactions in the liver, the brush border of the kidney metabolizes some medications. An example of this is insulin [17]. Insulin is filtered at the glomerulus and metabolized in the proximal tubule. In patients with CKD, this process is inhibited, which results in a prolonged duration of action of insulin. Overall, it is difficult to predict the clinical impact of CKD on medication metabolism. As a patient's kidney disease progresses, the effectiveness and potential adverse effects of each medication should be evaluated due to the complexities of the pharmacokinetic changes associated with renal dysfunction.

Elimination

Kidney function is the most predictable and quantifiable determinant of medication clearance. For many medications, total clearance consists of additive renal and nonrenal components. Renal excretion of medications is dependent on glomerular filtration rate, renal tubular secretion, and reabsorption. The glomerular filtration rate depends on the molecular weight and protein binding characteristics of the medication. An albumin-bound medication is not filtered, resulting in a filtration rate that is directly proportional to the medication's free plasma concentration. In CKD, medication elimination by glomerular filtration is decreased, resulting in a prolonged free drug elimination half-life [2]. This is a result of a decreased number of functioning nephrons, reduced renal blood flow, reduced glomerular filtration rate, and reduced tubular secretion. The significance of altered kidney function on medication elimination depends primarily on two variables. These include the fraction of medication normally eliminated by the kidney unchanged or the fraction of active metabolites eliminated by the kidney in addition to the degree of functional impairment [18].

Assessment of Kidney Function in Relation to Medication Dosing

In patients with CKD stages 1 through 5, the Cockcroft-Gault (CG) equation is commonly used to estimate creatinine clearance (CrCl) as a composite index of renal function. As creatinine is excreted by glomerular filtration and tubular secretion, CrCl has been strongly associated with the total and renal clearance of many medications that are eliminated by the kidney and is the primary estimate used for medication dosing in US Food and Drug Administration (FDA) product labeling. Newer equations that estimate GFR such as the CKD-EPI and the Modification of Diet in Renal Disease (MDRD) equations have not consistently demonstrated utility in drug dosing for patients with renal impairment. Recent studies have shown that eGFR equations yield higher estimates of kidney function resulting in different dose calculations when compared to the CG equation [19–22]. The variation in estimated renal function varies more significantly based on the CKD class, with the CG equation estimating a lower renal function than the MDRD or CKD-EPI equations as renal function worsens [23]. It is important to note that each of the equations used to estimate GFR was done in patients with stable renal function and is not reliable to use when a patient has acute kidney injury [24]. Renal dosing practices should be consistent with the original pharmacokinetic studies evaluating the use of the specific drug in patients with CKD, which most often involves an estimation of CrCl. The CG, MDRD, and CKD-EPI equations are described below (Table 21.2).

The CG equation is the most readily utilized equation incorporated in the design of pharmacokinetic studies and the development of drug dosing guidelines by manufacturers based on the FDA 1998 publication, *Guidance for Industry: Pharmacokinetics in Patients with Impaired Renal Function – Study Design, Data Analysis, and Impact on Dosing and Labeling*, which recommended the CG equation be used to estimate kidney function [23]. Most clinical laboratories now report eGFR using alternate equations such as the MDRD or CKD-EPI based on the National Kidney Disease Education Program (NKDEP) recommendation [25].

Table 21.2 Renal function estimate equations

Cockcroft-Gault (CG) equation is as follows:

If male:

$$\mathrm{CrCl}\left(\mathrm{mL}\,/\,\mathrm{min}\right)=\frac{\left(140-\mathrm{age}\right)\times\mathrm{IBW}}{72\times\mathrm{SCr}}$$

If female:

$$\mathrm{CrCl}\left(\mathrm{mL}\,/\,\mathrm{min}\right)=\frac{\left(140-\mathrm{age}\right)\times\mathrm{weight}}{72\times\mathrm{SCr}}\times0.85$$

Ideal body weight (males): 50 kg + 2.3 kg [height (inches) − 60]

Ideal body weight (females): 45.5 + 2.3 kg [height (inches) − 60]

Modification of Diet in Renal Disease (MDRD) equation:

$$\mathrm{GFR}\left(\mathrm{mL}\,/\,\mathrm{min}/\,1.73\,\mathrm{m}^{2}\right)=175\times\left(\mathrm{SCr}\right)^{-1.154}\times\left(\mathrm{Age}\right)^{-0.203}\times\left(0.742\text{ if female}\right)$$
$$\times\left(1.212\text{ if African American}\right)$$

CKD-EPI equation is as follows:

$$\mathrm{GFR}\left(\mathrm{mL}\,/\,\mathrm{min}/\,1.73\,\mathrm{m}^{2}\right)=141\times\min\left(\mathrm{SCr}\,/\,\kappa,\,1\right)^{\alpha}\times\max\left(\mathrm{SCr}\,/\,\kappa,\,1\right)^{-1.209}\times0.993^{\mathrm{Age}}$$
$$\times1.018\left[\text{if female}\right]\times1.159\left[\text{if black}\right]$$

SCr is serum creatinine in mg/dL

κ is 0.7 for females and 0.9 for males

α is −0.329 for females and −0.411 for males

min indicates the minimum of SCr/κ or 1

max indicates the maximum of SCr/κ or 1

The utilization of different equations to estimate renal function has led to confusion and debate about which equations to use when making medication dose modifications for CKD, and this is especially confusing since the KDIGO 2012 guidelines define CKD categories using the CKD-EPI creatinine equation, and the majority of medications have dosing recommendations based on the CG equation [26]. The FDA has updated the *Guidance for Industry* to recommend that drug manufacturers report dosing adjustments utilizing either CrCl (mL/min) as estimated by CG or eGFR (mL/min/1.73 m²) as estimated by MDRD [27]. For the purposes of this chapter, medication dose adjustment recommendations will be based off of the manufacturer labeling and will be listed as either CrCl, i.e., most all medications except metformin, or eGFR, for metformin.

Medications That Can Alter Renal Function or Cause Renal Injury

Drug-induced nephrotoxicity is a significant contributor to kidney disease, including acute kidney injury and CKD. In addition to a medication's nephrotoxic effects, patients with CKD are also susceptible to other adverse effects with agents routinely used in the management of comorbid conditions [28]. This section will focus on the most common mechanisms of drug-induced nephrotoxicity.

There are three main types of renal injury: prerenal, intrinsic, and postrenal, which are classified based on the underlying cause. While there are multiple pathophysiologic causes for each type of renal injury, drugs are common precipitating factors for each category [29]. See previous chapters for additional information on the differential diagnosis of acute renal injury. Table 21.3 lists medications associated with renal injury and an increased risk of developing CKD.

Prerenal injury accounts for 40–70% of cases and results from decreased perfusion to the kidney [30]. This may be due to decreased intravascular volume from blood loss, dehydration, or decreased effective blood volume with disease states such as congestive heart failure, hypoalbuminemia, nephrotic syndrome, hypotension, and liver failure.

Intrinsic kidney injury is characterized according to the structural component of the kidney that is affected. Acute interstitial nephritis (AIN), a form of intrinsic AKI, results from lymphocytic infiltration of the interstitium. The classic triad of fever, rash, and eosinophilia may be present in patients with AIN and may aid in distinguishing AIN from acute tubular necrosis, which is the most common cause of intrinsic AKI [31].

Another mechanism by which medications can cause kidney injury is through postrenal injury. This can occur from malignancy, precipitation of drug or metabolite crystals within the renal tubules, or urethral strictures [24]. This not only causes obstruction to tubular outflow but also can damage the renal tubular cells. Examples of medications that contribute to kidney injury according to their mechanism are listed below (Table 21.3).

Table 21.3 Medications associated with acute renal injury

Drugs associated with acute renal injury				
	Intrinsic		Postrenal	
Prerenal	Acute interstitial nephritis	Acute tubular necrosis	Glomerular injury	Obstructive nephropathy
Diuretics	Penicillins	Cisplatin	Captopril	Acyclovir
ACE inhibitors	Rifampin	Methotrexate	Foscarnet	Foscarnet
ARBs	Proton pump inhibitors	Lithium	Lithium	Ganciclovir
NSAIDs	NSAIDs	Radiocontrast	NSAIDs	Methotrexate
COX-2 inhibitors	Lithium	media		Sulfonamides
Cyclosporine	Acyclovir	Aminoglycosides		Triamterene
Tacrolimus	Tetracyclines			
Vasodilators	Phenytoin			
Radiocontrast media	Cimetidine			
	Statins			
	Cidofovir			
	Pentamidine			
	Fluoroquinolones			
	Allopurinol			
	Cephalosporins			
	Thiazide diuretics			
	Mesalamine			

Nonsteroidal Anti-inflammatory Drugs

Nonsteroidal anti-inflammatory drugs (NSAIDs) are among the most common pre-scription and over-the-counter medications used in the United States. While patients may reach for NSAIDs because they are effective and seemingly benign, they have been identified as nephrotoxic agents with both acute and chronic effects on kidney function. Risk factors for NSAID-induced renal injury include CKD, volume deple-tion from aggressive diuresis, or arterial volume depletion due to heart failure, nephrotic syndrome, or cirrhosis [28]. Concomitant use of other medications such as angiotensin-converting enzyme (ACE) inhibitors, angiotensin II receptor block-ers (ARBs), or calcineurin inhibitors may increase the risk of NSAID-induced injury. The pathogenesis involves an imbalance with prostaglandin-mediated vaso-dilation [28]. NSAID inhibition of cyclooxygenase (COX) enzymes with subse-quent reduction in prostaglandin synthesis can lead to reversible renal ischemia and a decline in glomerular hydraulic pressure, which is the major driving force for glomerular filtration [28]. Prostaglandin synthesis is increased in the setting of pro-longed renal vasoconstriction among patients with CKD and serves to protect the glomerular filtration rate. This is accomplished by decreasing pre-glomerular resis-tance, thus preserving renal blood flow. By inhibiting prostaglandin-mediated affer-ent vasodilation and reducing peritubular blood flow, NSAIDs cause an acute decrease in GFR.

Angiotensin-Converting Enzyme Inhibitors and Angiotensin II Receptor Blockers

Current guidelines recommend ACE inhibitors (ACE-Is) or angiotensin II receptor blockers (ARBs) as first-line antihypertensives for patients with CKD stage 3 and higher or for patients with stage 1–2 with albuminuria ≥300 mg/dL. In addition to lowering blood pressure, ACE-Is and ARBs also lower glomerular capillary pres-sure and protein filtration, which may contribute to their beneficial effect in slowing progression of CKD [28]. However, under certain clinical circumstances, they have the potential for harm. This is most often the case in conditions where the kidney is autoregulation-dependent, including CHF, active diuresis, and other illnesses with attendant volume depletion.

Upon initiation of an ACE-I or ARB, an increase in serum creatinine of up to 30% above baseline within the first week is expected due to altered glomerular hemodynamics caused by relaxation of the efferent arteriole [28]. A follow-up serum creatinine (SCr) level should be obtained within 1 week of initiating an ACE-I or ARB to confirm that the SCr has stabilized and does not continue to increase.

Hyperkalemia is another adverse effect of ACE-Is and ARBs, caused by the decreased secretion of aldosterone. A moderate increase in potassium level is gener-ally acceptable if the patient understands the need for dietary potassium restriction and is not exposed to additional medications, such as spironolactone, that may exacerbate hyperkalemia. It is important to avoid dehydration and excessive use of diuretics and NSAIDs with ACE-Is or ARBS due to the potentiation of renal injury. In patients with an increase in serum creatinine of more than 30% or those with uncontrollable hyperkalemia, the ACE-I or ARB should be discontinued or titrated to a lower dose [28].

Diuretics

Thiazide and loop diuretics are commonly used for natriuresis and blood pressure control with a reduced GFR. Loop diuretics can cause kidney injury in the setting of prerenal or intrinsic causes [24]. Although no specific guidelines exist, special care should be given to balance the need of maintaining euvolemia with the risk of kidney injury in the ambulatory setting.

Combination of NSAIDs, ACE-I/ARBs, and Diuretics

Although NSAIDs, ACE-I/ARBs, and diuretics can cause renal injury on their own, the risk significantly increases when these medications are used in combination. Each class of medications affects kidney function differently. Diuretics could lead to hypoperfusion due to hypovolemia, NSAIDs constrict the afferent arterioles, and ACE-I/ARBs cause dilation of efferent arterioles [24]. Regulation of the tone of the renal afferent and efferent arterioles is necessary to maintain perfusion pressure, particularly in the setting of reduced blood flow [24].

Calcineurin Inhibitors (Tacrolimus/Cyclosporine)

Calcineurin inhibitors (CNIs), specifically cyclosporine and tacrolimus, are essential medications in many posttransplant immunosuppressive regimens. One of the most common dose-limiting toxicities associated with these medications is nephrotoxicity. The mechanism of renal injury involves hemodynamic changes that are reversible and typically classified as prerenal. These changes are mediated by vasoconstriction of the afferent arterioles, resulting in reduced renal blood flow [28]. Long-term CNI use can contribute to irreversible and progressive tubule-interstitial injury and glomerulosclerosis, labeled as chronic CNI-induced nephrotoxicity [28]. Risk factors for CNI-induced nephrotoxicity include supra-therapeutic concentration of the medication, concomitant NSAID, and diuretic use. A strategy for preventing CNI nephrotoxicity should aim to reduce excessive medication exposure through therapeutic serum drug level monitoring. Additionally, dihydropyridine calcium channel blockers play a protective role in minimizing CNI nephrotoxicity as their intrarenal vasodilatory effects offset the vasoconstrictive effects of the CNIs at the afferent arteriole [28].

Oral Antimicrobials

Beta-lactams

Penicillins and cephalosporins are among the most common antimicrobials implicated in acute interstitial nephritis. The presentation often includes a "classic" triad of symptoms: eosinophilia, rash, and fever. AIN is idiosyncratic, and therefore, there are no preventative measures. Patients on prolonged courses of beta-lactam antibiotics of more than 7–10 days should consider routine evaluation of renal function or if a patient is reported to have symptoms of AKI.

Fluoroquinolones

Of the fluoroquinolones, ciprofloxacin is most commonly implicated in AIN and crystal nephropathy. Fluoroquinolones can precipitate crystals in alkaline urine. Preventative measures include ensuring adequate hydration and using appropriate doses based on the calculated CrCl and again monitoring renal function when a patient is prescribed a prolonged course of therapy.

Sulfonamides

The mechanisms by which trimethoprim/sulfamethoxazole causes kidney injury include AIN, acute tubular necrosis (ATN), and crystal nephropathy. The sulfa component of this antibiotic causes an idiosyncratic cell-mediated immune reaction, leading to AIN. There is no dose relationship with sulfonamides and AIN. ATN and crystal nephropathy may be potentially preventable by ensuring adequate fluid intake (>3 L per day) and monitoring urine for crystals. If crystals are seen in the urine, alkalinization of the urine is recommended to maintain pH > 7.15.

Pseudo-AKI

While an elevation in serum creatinine usually reflects a reduction in GFR, there are medications that can cause SCr to increase independent of decreasing GFR [32]. Factors that may artificially increase SCr include increased production of creatinine, interference with the assay, and decreased tubular secretion.

Table 21.4 Medications associated with pseudo-AKI

	Mechanism		
	Decreased secretion of creatinine	Interference with the serum assay	Increased creatinine production
Drug-induced causes	Trimethoprim Cimetidine Famotidine Ranitidine	Cefoxitin Flucytosine	Fenofibrates

Creatinine is produced in the muscle, and therefore the creatinine generated is proportional to muscle mass and is relatively constant. An increase in serum creatinine can result from increased intake of meat or protein and ingestion of creatine supplements. Fenofibrates have been shown to increase metabolic production of creatinine, particularly in patients with mild to moderate renal failure [33]. The mechanism underlying this is poorly understood; however fenofibrates are not thought to impair GFR. The antibiotic cefoxitin can falsely increase the serum creatinine level by interfering with the colorimetric assay used to measure serum creatinine levels [34]. The antibiotic trimethoprim-sulfamethoxazole and cimetidine, an H2-blocker, are two commonly used medications that decrease the secretion of creatinine [35, 36]. This can result in a self-limited and reversible increase in the serum creatinine level by as much as 0.4–0.5 mg/dL. Famotidine and ranitidine can similarly cause an increase but to a lesser extent [36]. In each of these cases, the blood urea nitrogen (BUN) typically does not change. Therefore, an increase in creatinine level suggests a true decrease in GFR only if accompanied by a corresponding increase in BUN level. However, patients with an AKI on a low-protein diet may have a falsely low BUN, so this must also be considered in order to distinguish between true AKI and pseudo-AKI. Medications associated with pseudo-AKI due to alteration in serum creatinine levels is listed below (Table 21.4).

Therapeutic Drug Monitoring in CKD

Some medications have a narrow therapeutic range, and routine medication level monitoring is recommended. Even when a medication dose is adjusted for the estimated renal insufficiency, it is beneficial to monitor medication levels for these agents. Select times to consider obtaining a medication levels are after starting the medication, when changes in renal function occur, and when there is addition or elimination of another agent with potential interaction or nephrotoxicity [13]. Examples of medications that should be routinely monitored in CKD are listed below (Table 21.5).

Table 21.5 Narrow therapeutic range medications requiring monitoring

Medication	Timing of level	Therapeutic range[a]	Frequency of level[b]
Aminoglycosides: gentamicin, tobramycin, amikacin	Conventional dosing: Trough: 0–30 minutes prior to giving dose Peak: 30 minutes after dose is complete	Gentamicin and tobramycin: Trough: 0.5–2 mg/L Peak: 5–8 mg/L	Obtain peak and trough around third dose For therapy <72 hours (h), levels may not be necessary
		Amikacin: Peak: 20–30 mg/L Trough: 8–10 mg/L	Repeat drug levels at least weekly or if renal function changes
Carbamazepine	Trough: immediately prior to dose	4–12 g/mL	Check 2–4 days after starting or with change in dose
Cyclosporine	Trough: immediately prior to dose	150–400 ng/mL (based on indication)	Daily for the first week, then weekly until consistent level maintained, then routinely with follow-up
Digoxin	12 h after maintenance dose and prior to the next dose	0.6–2.0 ng/mL	2–5 days after the first dose and then routinely with follow-up
Enoxaparin	4 h after the second or third dose	Anti-Xa: 0.7–1.1 units/mL	Weekly and as needed
Lithium	Trough: before morning dose at least 12 h since last dose	Acute: 0.8–1.2 mM Chronic: 0.6–0.8 mM	Routinely with follow-up
Phenobarbital	Trough: immediately prior to the dose	15–40 g/mL	Check within 2 weeks after the first dose or change in dose follow-up level in 1–2 months
Phenytoin Free phenytoin	Trough: immediately prior to the dose	10–20 g/mL 1–2 g/mL	5–7 days after the first dose or after change in dose
Procainamide	Trough: immediately prior to next dose or 12–18 h after starting or changing the dose	4–10 g/mL Trough: 4 g/mL Peak: 8 g/mL	Routinely with follow-up
NAPA (n-acetyl procainamide)	Draw with procainamide sample	Procainamide + NAPA level: 10–30 g/mL	
Sirolimus	Trough: immediately prior to the dose	10–20 ng/dL 4–12 ng/dL (when administered concurrently with cyclosporine or tacrolimus)	Daily for the first week, then weekly for first month, then routinely with follow-up
Tacrolimus	Trough: immediately prior to the dose	5–10 ng/mL	Daily for the first week, then weekly for the first month, then routinely with follow-up

Table 21.5 (continued)

Medication	Timing of level	Therapeutic range[a]	Frequency of level[b]
Valproic acid (divalproex sodium)	Trough: immediately prior to the dose	50–100 g/mL	Check 2–4 days after the first dose or change in dose
Vancomycin	Trough: 0–30 minutes prior to the third or fourth dose	Trough: 10–20 mg/L (based on site of infection and minimum inhibitory concentration of culture)	With third or fourth dose. For therapy <72 h, levels not necessary. Repeat drug levels at least weekly or if renal function changes

Derived from: Olyaei and Steffl [13]

[a]Therapeutic ranges are based on general dosing recommendations. Individualized ranges may be needed based on the disease state being treated, patient tolerance, and clinical response to therapy

[b]Frequency of monitoring levels is based on general recommendations. The need for more or less frequent monitoring may be warranted based on the clinical situations, overall patient status, tolerance of therapy, disease state being treated, and clinical response to therapy

Considerations in Patients on Dialysis

The optimization of pharmacotherapy for patients receiving intermittent hemodialysis (iHD) is dependent on several factors including drug characteristics and the type of dialyzer. Medication-related factors affecting clearance in dialysis include the size of the drug molecule, the degree of protein binding, and volume of distribution [13]. During iHD, the majority of medications are removed primarily by the process of diffusion across the dialysis membrane [13]. Conventional or low-flux dialyzers are relatively impermeable to medications with a molecular weight greater than 1000 Da [13]. The utilization of high-flux iHD is more common, with the ability to remove medications with a molecular weight of about 10,000 daltons (Da) from the plasma to the dialysate through the filter membrane [37]. With regard to protein binding, only free, or unbound, medication can be removed during dialysis. Therefore, medications that are highly protein bound have a low proportion of free drug to pass through the dialysis membrane, while medications with low-protein binding may cross dialysis membranes much readily [33]. Additionally, medications with large volumes of distribution have a lower proportion of medication that is removed by dialysis compared to those with a small Vd, as medications with a large Vd are dispersed into extravascular spaces and tissue and are not present in the bloodstream for filtration [33].

In the inpatient setting, medication dosage regimens for patients receiving intermittent hemodialysis are often individualized based on therapeutic drug monitoring [33]. However, given the time associated with measurement and reporting of serum concentrations, patients in the ambulatory setting benefit from implementation of practical dosage regimens based on data derived from previous studies.

Conclusion

The impact of chronic kidney disease and acute renal injury on medication pharmacokinetics is a complex process of physiologic changes in the body. A comprehensive approach to evaluating a patient's medications to determine both the impact of each medication on the patient's kidney function and the effect of kidney injury on medication dosing should occur with each patient encounter (Fig. 21.1).

Dose adjustments or selection of an alternate medication should occur if a medication is suspected to cause kidney injury. Jointly, medication selection or dose adjustment must take place when kidney injury impacts elimination, possibly leading to toxicity or other adverse effects. Numerous references are readily available, and medication package labeling often described dose considerations in patients with impaired renal function. The last section of this chapter provides recommended dosing for routinely prescribed medications.

Review of Commonly Used Drugs and Dose Adjustments

Dose adjustment recommendations are listed in the below tables based on medication class (Tables 21.6, 21.7, 21.8, 21.9, 21.10, and 21.11). These lists are not comprehensive but intended to guide the clinician for optimal dosing in commonly prescribed medications. The clinician must not rely solely on the tables provided but rather should use them as a reference to select the best dosing based on predicted renal function and indication for use. Patient-specific comorbid conditions, age, and weight, and risk of drug interactions also must be considered. FDA-approved package inserts can be downloaded from the National Library of Medicine website, dailymed.nlm.nih.gov, or by going directly to the manufacturer's websites and are good sources to consider the proper selection and dosing of medications in CKD.

Fig. 21.1 Approach to drug dosing in CKD

1. Obtain history and relevant clinical information
2. Estimate GFR
3. Review current medications
4. Determine individual treatment regimen
5. Monitor
6. Revise Regimen

Table 21.6 Antimicrobials

Drug	Normal dose	Dosage adjustment in CKD (CrCl = mL/min)	Intermittent hemodialysis
Acyclovir (oral) [38]	HSV treatment: 800 mg q4h	CrCl 10–25: 800 mg q8h CrCl <10: 200 mg q12h	If usual dose 800 mg q4h: 400 mg load followed by 200 mg q12h Supplement with single 400 mg dose after each dialysis session
	Chronic suppressive therapy: 400 mg q12h	CrCl <10: 200 mg q12h	
	Genital herpes: 200 mg q4h	CrCl <10: 200 mg q12h	If usual dose 200 mg q4h or 400 mg q12: 200 mg q12h
Amoxicillin [39]	500 mg q8h	CrCl 10–30: 500 mg q12h CrCl <10: 500 mg q24h	500 mg q24h
Amoxicillin/clavulanate [40]	875 mg q12h or 500 mg q8h	CrCl 10–30: 500 mg q12h CrCl <10: 500 mg q24n	500 mg q24h
Ampicillin (IV) [41]	1–2 g q6–8h	CrCl 10–50: 1–2 g q6–12h CrCl <10: 1–2 g q12–24 h	1–2 g q12h
Ampicillin/sulbactam (IV) [42]	1.5–3 g q6–8h	CrCl 15–30: 1.5–3 g q12h CrCl 5–14: 1.5–3 g q24h	3 g q24h
Cefazolin (IV) [43]	1–2 g q8h	CrCl 11–34: 1 g q12h CrCl <10: 1 g q24h	20 mg/kg after each iHD session; no dose on non-dialysis days
Cefdinir [44]	300 mg q12h	CrCl < 30: 300 mg q24h	300 mg q24h
Cefepime (IV) [45]	2 g q8h	CrCl 30–60: 2 g q12h CrCl 11–29: 2 g q24h CrCl < 10: 1 g q24h	1 g q24h

(continued)

Table 21.6 (continued)

Drug	Normal dose	Dosage adjustment in CKD (CrCl = mL/min)	Intermittent hemodialysis
Cefuroxime axetil [46]	250–500 mg q12h	CrCl 29–10: 250–500 mg q24h CrCl < 10: 250–500 mg q48h	250–500 mg after each iHD session; no dose on non-dialysis days
Cephalexin [47]	500 mg q6h	CrCl 10–50: 500 mg q12h CrCl < 10: 250 mg q12h	250 mg q12h
Ciprofloxacin (PO) [48]	250–750 mg q12h	CrCl < 30: 250 mg q12h or 750–500 mg q24h	500 mg q24h
Daptomycin [49]	4–10 mg/kg q24h	CrCl < 30: 4–10 mg/kg/q48h	4–10 mg/kg after each iHD session; no dose on non-dialysis days
Ertapenem [50]	1 g q24h	CrCl < 30: 500 mg q24h	500 mg q24h
Fluconazole (IV,PO) [51]	200–400 mg q24h	CrCl < 50: 100–200 mg q24h	100–200 mg q24h
Levofloxacin (IV, PO) [52]	500–750 mg q24h	CrCl 20–49: 750 mg q48h or 250 mg q24h	250–500 mg q48h
Meropenem [53]	1–2 g q8h	CrCl 26–50: 1–2 g q12h CrCl 10–25: 1 g q12h CrCl < 10: 500 mg q24h	500 mg q24h
Nitrofurantoin [54]	50–100 mg q6h	CrCl < 60: avoid	Avoid
Oseltamivir [55]	75 mg q12h	CrCl 30–60: 30 mg q12h CrCl 10–30: 30 mg q24h	30 mg after each iHD session; no dose on non-dialysis days
Piperacillin/tazobactam [56]	3.375 g q8h	CrCl < 20: 3.375 g q12h	3.375 g q12h
Trimethoprim/sulfamethoxazole (800 mg/160 mg) DS [57]	1 DS tab q12h, 2 DS tab q12h	CrCl 15–30: 1 DS tab q24h CrCl < 15: avoid	Avoid

Table 21.6 (continued)

Drug	Normal dose	Dosage adjustment in CKD (CrCl = mL/min)	Intermittent hemodialysis
Valacyclovir [58]	HSV treatment: 1 g q8h	CrCl 30–49: 1 g q12h	
		CrCl < 10: 500 mg q24h	
	Genital herpes, initial episode: 1 g q12h	CrCl 10–20: 1 g q24h	
	Genital herpes, recurrent episode: 500 mg q12h	CrCl < 10: 500 mg q24h	
	Genital herpes, suppressive therapy: 1 g q24h	CrCl < 30: 500 mg q24h	
	Cold sores: 2gm q12h	CrCl < 30: 500 mg q24h	
		CrCl 30–49: 1 g q12h CrCl 10–20: 500 mg q12h CrCl < 10: 500 mg q24h	
Tenofovir alafenamide [59]	25 mg daily	CrCl < 15 and not on dialysis: not recommended	25 mg on dialysis days Give dose after dialysis
Tenofovir disoproxil fumarate [60]	300 mg q24h	CrCl ≥ 50: 300 mg q24h CrCl 30–49: 300 mg q48h CrCl 10–29: 300 mg q72–96h CrCl < 10 and not on dialysis: no data	300 mg q 7 days Give dose after dialysis

Table 21.7 Antiarrhythmics

Drug	Normal dose	Dosage adjustment in CKD (CrCl = mL/min)	Intermittent hemodialysis
Disopyramide [61]	200–800 mg/day in divided doses	CrCl > 40–80: 400 mg/day in divided doses CrCl 30–40: 100 mg q8h CrCl 15–30: 100 mg q12h CrCl < 15: 100 mg q24h	A maintenance dose after dialysis sessions is recommended
Dofetilide [62]	500 mcg q12h	CrCl 40–60 and QTc or QT ≤ 440 msec: 250 mcg q12h If QTc or QT increases by more than 15% or > 500 msec: reduce dose to 125 mcg q12h. CrCl 20–39 and QTc or QT ≤ 440 msec: 125 mcg q12h If QTc or QT increases by more than 15% or > 500 msec: reduce dose to 125 mcg daily. CrCl < 20: Use contraindicated	Use contraindicated
Flecainide [63]	*Paroxysmal atrial fibrillation/flutter*: 50–150 mg q12h	CrCl ≤ 35: 50 mg q12h or 100 mg daily. Monitor plasma levels frequently	No dose adjustment necessary
	Paroxysmal supraventricular tachycardia: 50–150 mg q12h	CrCl ≤ 35: 50 mg q12h or 100 mg daily. Monitor plasma levels frequently	
	Ventricular arrhythmia: 100–200 mg q12h	CrCl ≤ 35: 100 mg q12h. Monitor plasma levels frequently	
Sotalol (PO) [64]	*Afib*: 80 mg q12h	CrCl 40–60: 80 mg q24h CrCl < 40: avoid	40 mg q24h (use with extreme caution)
	Ventricular arrhythmia: 160 mg q12h	CrCl 30–60: 160 mg q24h CrCl 10–29: 160 mg q36–48h CrCl < 10: use with caution	40 mg q24h (use with extreme caution)

Table 21.8 Anticoagulant/antiplatelet agents

Drug	Normal dose	Dosage adjustment in CKD (CrCl = mL/min)	Intermittent hemodialysis
Apixaban [65]	*Acute DVT/PE*: 10 mg q12h × 7 days followed by 5 mg q12h	Avoid use if CrCl < 25	Use may be permissible for patients on iHD in carefully selected individuals who do not have a low BMI and are not on concomitant strong CYP3A4 and P-gp inhibitors[a]
	NVAF: 5 mg q12h	Presence of two or more of the following: age ≥ 80 years, wt ≤ 60 kg or SCr ≥ 1.5 mg/dL: reduce dose to 2.5 mg q12h	Age ≥ 80 years, wt ≤ 60 kg, reduce to 2.5 mg q12h
Edoxaban [66]	*NVAF*: CrCL > 50 - ≤ 95: 60 mg once daily Do not use in patients with CrCL > 95 mL/min	*NVAF*: CrCl 15–50: 30 mg once daily	Avoid use – no data available
	DVT and PE: 60 mg once daily	*DVT and PE*: CrCl 15–50 (or weight < 60 kg): 30 mg once daily	
Dabigatran [67]	*Acute DVT/PE*: 150 mg q12h	CrCl < 30: avoid, not studied	Avoid
	NVAF: 150 mg q12h	CrCl 15–30: 75 mg q12h CrCl < 15: avoid CrCl < 30: avoid	
	Ortho VTE prophylaxis: 110 mg × 1 followed by 220 mg q24h		
Enoxaparin (clot treatment) [68]	1 mg/kg (actual BW) SC q12h	CrCl 15–30: 1 mg/kg SC q24h	Avoid
	1.5 mg/kg (actual BW) SC q24h	CrCl < 15: avoid	

(continued)

Table 21.8 (continued)

Drug	Normal dose	Dosage adjustment in CKD (CrCl = mL/min)	Intermittent hemodialysis
Rivaroxaban [69]	*NVAF*: 20 mg q24h with evening meal	CrCl 15–50: 15 mg q24h with evening meal CrCl < 15: avoid	15 mg q24h
	Acute DVT/PE; or prevention of recurrent DVT/PE: 15 mg q12h × 21 days followed by 20 mg q24h with meals	CrCl < 30: avoid	
	Post-op DVT Prophylaxis – knee Arthroplasty: 10 mg q24h		

[a]No dose adjustment necessary

Additional Resources

A. McEvoy G. AHFS Drug Information®. Bethesda, MD: American Society of Health-System Pharmacists, Inc.; 2014.

B. Aronoff G, Bennett W, Berns J, al. e. Drug Prescribing in Renal Failure: Dosing Guidelines for Adults American College of Physicians. 2007

C. DrugPoints Summary. Micromedex 2.0. Truven Health Analytics Inc.; 2015. http://www.micromedexsolutions.com/micromedex2/librarian. Accessed 14 April 2015.

D. Drug Facts and Comparisons. Facts & Comparisons eAnswers. Wolters Kluwer Health, Inc.; 2015. http://online.factsandcomparisons.com/index.aspx? Accessed 14 April 2015.

E. Bailie G, Mason N. 2012 Dialysis of Drugs. Saline, MI: Renal Pharmacy Consultants. LLC2012.

F. Lexi-Drugs. Lexicomp. Wolters Kluwer Health, Inc.; 2015. https://online.lexi.com/lco/action/home/switch. Accessed 14 April 2015.

G. Panel on Antiretroviral Guidelines for Adults and Adolescents. Guidelines for the use of antiretroviral agents in HIV-1-infected adults and adolescents. http://www.aidsinfo.nih.gov/ContentFiles/AdultandAdolescentGL.pdf.

H. Package inserts

Table 21.9 Diabetic management agents

Drug	Normal dose	Dosage adjustment in CKD (CrCl = mL/min)	Intermittent hemodialysis
Glipizide [70]	Initial: 5 mg before breakfast Divide doses above 15 mg before breakfast and dinner Max: 40 mg daily in divided doses	No specific dose adjustment recommended Use lowest effective dose	Evaluate dose based on patient response
Glyburide [71]	Initial: 2.5–5 mg daily Maintenance: max 20 mg daily	Initial: 1.25 mg daily Maintenance: conservative dosing to avoid hypoglycemia	Avoid use
Micronized glyburide [72]	Initial: 1.5–3 mg daily Maintenance: max 12 mg daily	Initial: 0.75 mg daily Maintenance: conservative dosing to avoid hypoglycemia	Evaluate dose based on patient response
Metformin [73]	500 mg q12h before breakfast/dinner	eGFR 30–40: initiation not recommended Continuation: assess risk and benefits	Avoid use
	Increase by 500 mg weekly to max of 2500 mg/day	eGFR < 30: contraindicated	
Canagliflozin [74]	100–300 mg daily with first meal of day	eGFR 45–60: 100 mg daily eGFR 30–45: 100 mg daily	Contraindicated
Dapagliflozin [75]	5–10 mg daily with or without food	eGFR < 60: do not use	Do not use
Empagliflozin [76]	10–25 mg daily with or without food	eGFR < 45: do not use	Do not use
Linagliptin [77]	5 mg daily	No dose adjustment needed	No dose adjustment needed
Saxagliptin [78]	2.5–5 mg daily	CrCl ≤ 50: 2.5 mg daily	2.5 mg daily
Sitagliptin [79]	100 mg q24h	CrCl 30–49: 50 mg q24h CrCl < 30: 25 mg q24h	25 mg q24h

Combination products exist. Refer to specific medication FDA-approved product label for specific dosing recommendations

Table 21.10 Anticonvulsants

Drug	Normal dose	Dosage adjustment in CKD (CrCl = mL/min)	Intermittent hemodialysis
Brivaracetam (IV,PO) [80]	25–100 mg BID	No dose adjustment needed	Use not recommended
Eslicarbazepine [81]	Initial: 400 mg daily Maintenance: 800–1600 mg daily	CrCl < 50: Reduce initial, titrating, and maintenance dose by 50%	No data
Felbamate [82]	1200–3600 mg daily in 3–4 divided doses	Renal impairment (no CrCl designation). Initial and maintenance doses should be reduced by 50%	No data
Gabapentin [83]	300–1200 mg q8h (max 3600 mg/day)	CrCl 30–59: 200–700 mg q12h CrCl 15–29: 200–700 mg q24h CrCl 15: 100–300 mg q24h CrCl < 15: proportionate dose decrease	Based on CrCl; supplemental dose 100–300 mg post-HD may be necessary
Lacosamide [84]	100–200 mg q12h	CrCl ≤ 30: maximum 300 mg q24h	Maximum: 300 mg q24h Supplemental dose of up to 50% is recommended post each HD session
Levetiracetam [85]	500–1500 mg q12h	CrCl 50–80: 500–1000 mg q12h CrCl 30–50: 250–750 mg q12h CrCl < 30: 250–500 mg q12h	50% removed by dialysis; dose q12h, add 50% of AM dose to PM dose post each HD session
Perampanel [86]	2–12 mg daily at bedtime	Severe impairment (no CrCl designation): use not recommended	Use not recommended
Pregabalin [87]	150–600 mg q12h or q8h	CrCl 30–60: 75–300 mg q12h or q8h CrCl 15–30 mg: 25–150 mg q12h or q24h CrCl < 15: 25–75 mg q24h	25–75 mg q24h plus supplemental dose of 25–150 mg post-hemodialysis

Table 21.10 (continued)

Drug	Normal dose	Dosage adjustment in CKD (CrCl = mL/min)	Intermittent hemodialysis
Primidone [88]	100 mg daily to 250 mg TID to QID	CrCl > 50–80: increase dosing interval to q8h CrCl 10–50: increase dosing interval to q8h-q12h CrCl < 10: increase dosing interval to q12h-q24h	Administer 1/3 of normal dose after hemodialysis
Rufinamide [89]	200–1600 mg BID	No dose adjustment necessary	Hemodialysis may reduce drug levels about 30%. Consider dose adjustment
Stiripentol [90]	50 mg/kg/day divided in 2–3 doses. Max: 3000 mg daily	Moderate to severe: use not recommended	Use not recommended
Topiramate [91]	25–400 mg/day. Divided doses may be needed based on prescribed formulation	CrCl < 70: use 50% of dose	Supplemental dose may be required. Topiramate is cleared 4–6 times greater than a normal individual
Vigabatrin [92]	500–1500 mg BID	CrCl > 50–80: reduce dose by 25% CrCl > 30–50: reduce dose by 50% CrCl 10–30: reduce dose by 75%	No data
Zonisamide [93]	100–600 mg daily	Metabolized by the liver and excreted by the kidneys Renal impairment (no CrCl designated) may require slower dose titration and more monitoring	Metabolized by the liver and excreted by the kidneys Renal impairment (no CrCl designated) may require slower dose titration and more monitoring

Table 21.11 Miscellaneous medications

Drug	Normal dose	Dosage adjustment in CKD (CrCl = mL/min)	Intermittent hemodialysis
Allopurinol [94]	Initial: 100 mg q24h	CrCl < 30: Initial 50 mg q24h	Initial: 100 mg q48h; dose after dialysis
	Titrate in 100 mg increments every 2–4 weeks to achieve desired serum acid level; doses up to 800 mg q24h may be required	Maintenance: increase cautiously to achieve desired serum uric acid level	Maintenance: increase cautiously to 300 mg q24h based on response
Colchicine [95]	*Gout flare treatment*: day 1: 1.2 mg followed in 1 h by single dose of 0.6 mg	No dose reduction required but may be considered	0.6 mg as a single dose
	Day 2 and thereafter: 0.6 mg q12–24h		
	Gout prophylaxis: 0.6 mg q12–24h	CrCl < 30: initial 0.3 mg q24h	0.3 mg twice weekly
Metoclopramide [96]	10 mg q6h	CrCl 10–50: 75% of usual dose CrCl < 10: 50% of usual dose	50% of usual dose
Cimetidine [97]	300 mg QID – 800 mg once daily	CrCl < 30: 300 mg q12h	Take the lowest effective dose after each dialysis
Famotidine [98]	40 mg q24h or 20 mg q12h	CrCl < 50: 20 mg q24h	20 mg q24h
Nizatidine [99]	150 mg BID or 300 mg at bedtime	CrCl 20–50: 150 mg daily CrCl < 20: 150 mg every other day	150 mg every other day
Ranitidine [100]	75–150 mg q12h	CrCl < 50: 150 mg q24h	150 mg q24h

Administer dose after iHD

Combination products exist. Refer to specific medication FDA-approved product label for specific dosing recommendations

References

1. Chapter 4: other complications of CKD: CVD, medication dosage, patient safety, infections, hospitalizations, and caveats for investigating complications of CKD. Kidney Int Suppl. 2013;3:91–111. https://doi.org/10.1038/kisup.2012.67.
2. Lea-Henry TN, Carland JE, Stocker SL, Sevastos J, Roberts DM. Clinical pharmacokinetics in kidney disease. Clin J Am Soc Nephrol. 2018;13:1085–95. https://doi.org/10.2215/CJN.00340118.
3. Roberts DM, Sevastos J, Carland JE, Stocker SL, Lea-Henry TN. Clinical pharmacokinetics in kidney disease: application to rational design of dosing regimens. Clin J Am Soc Nephrol. 2018;13:1254–63. https://doi.org/10.2215/CJN.05150418.
4. Hassan Y, Al-Ramahi R, Abd Aziz N, Ghazali R. Drug use and dosing in chronic kidney disease. Ann Acad Med Singap. 2009;38:1095–103.

5. Aronson JK. Clinical pharmacokinetics of digoxin 1980. Clin Pharmacokinet. 1980;5:137–49. https://doi.org/10.2165/00003088-198005020-00002.

6. Fish DN. Fluoroquinolone adverse effects and drug interactions. Pharmacotherapy. 2001;21(Pt 2):253S–72S.

7. Greig SL, Plosker GL. Sucroferric oxyhydroxide: a review in hyperphosphataemia in chronic kidney disease patients undergoing dialysis. Drugs. 2015;75:533–42. https://doi.org/10.1007/s40265-015-0366-1.

8. Krishnasamy S, Abell TL. Diabetic gastroparesis: principles and current trends in management. Diabetes Ther. 2018;9(Supple 1):1–42. https://doi.org/10.1007/s13300-018-0454-9.

9. Wagner LA, Tata AL, Fink JC. Patient safety issues in CKD: core curriculum 2015. Am J Kidney Dis. 2015;66:159–69. https://doi.org/10.1053/j.ajkd.2015.02.343.

10. Dreisbach AW, Lertora JJ. The effect of chronic renal failure on drug metabolism and transport. Expert Opin Drug Metab Toxicol. 2008;4:1065–74. https://doi.org/10.1517/17425255.4.8.1065.

11. Vanholder R, De Smet R, Ringoir S. Factors influencing drug protein binding in patients with end stage renal failure. Eur J Clin Pharmacol. 1993;44(Suppl 1):17–21.

12. Verbeeck RK, Musuamba FT. Pharmacokinetics and dosage adjustment in patients with renal dysfunction. Eur J Clin Pharmacol. 2009;65:757–73. https://doi.org/10.1007/s00228-009-0678-8.

13. Olyaei AJ, Steffl JL. A quantitative approach to drug dosing in chronic kidney disease. Blood Purif. 2011;31:138–45. https://doi.org/10.1159/000321857.

14. Leblond FA, Petrucci M, Dube P, Bernier G, Bonnardeaux A, Pichette V. Downregulation of intestinal cytochrome P450 in chronic renal failure. J Am Soc Nephrol. 2002;13:1579–85.

15. Dowling TC, Matzke GR, Murphy JE, Burckart GJ. Evaluation of renal drug dosing: prescribing information and clinical pharmacist approaches. Pharmacotherapy. 2010;30:776–86. https://doi.org/10.1592/phco.30.8.776.

16. O'Connor NR, Corcoran AM. End-stage renal disease: symptom management and advance care planning. Am Fam Physician. 2012;85:705–10.

17. Rabkin R, Ryan MP, Duckworth WC. The renal metabolism of insulin. Diabetologia. 1984;27:351–7.

18. Perazella MA, Tonelli M, Gipson DS, Gilbert SJ, Weiner DE, National Kidney Foundation. National Kidney Foundation primer on kidney diseases [Internet]. 6th ed. Philadelphia: Saunders; 2013. [cited 2019 Nov 17]

19. Stevens LA, Padala S, Levey AS. Advances in glomerular filtration rate-estimating equations. Curr Opin Nephrol Hypertens. 2010;19(3):298–307. https://doi.org/10.1097/MNH.0b013e32833893e2.

20. Melloni C, Peterson ED, Chen AY, Szczech LA, Newby LK, Harrington RA, et al. Cockcroft-Gault versus modification of diet in renal disease: importance of glomerular filtration rate formula for classification of chronic kidney disease in patients with non-ST-segment elevation acute coronary syndromes. J Am Coll Cardiol. 2008;51:991–6. https://doi.org/10.1016/j.jacc.2007.11.045.

21. Gill J, Malyuk R, Djurdjev O, Levin A. Use of GFR equations to adjust drug doses in an elderly multi-ethnic group—a cautionary tale. Nephrol Dial Transplant. 2007;22:2894–9.

22. Golik MV, Lawrence KR. Comparison of dosing recommendations for antimicrobial drugs based on two methods for assessing kidney function: Cockcroft-Gault and Modification of Diet in Renal Disease. Pharmacotherapy. 2008;28:1125–32. https://doi.org/10.1592/phco.28.9.1125.

23. Stevens LA, Nolin TD, Richardson MM, Feldman HI, Lewis JB, Rodby R, Townsend R, et al. Comparison of drug dosing recommendations based on measured GFR and kidney function estimating equations. Am J Kidney Dis. 2009;54:33–42. https://doi.org/10.1053/j.ajkd.2009.03.008.

24. Sifontis NM, Miklich MA. Nephrologic/geriatric care. In: Dong BJ, Elliott DP, editors. Ambulatory care self-assessment program. Book. Lenexa: ACCP; 2018. p. 3.

25. National Institute of Diabetes and Digestive and Kidney Diseases: The National Institute of Health. https://www.niddk.nih.gov/health-information/communication-programs/nkdep/laboratory-evaluation/glomerular-filtration-rate/estimating (2019). Accessed 17 Oct 2019.

26. KDIGO. Chapter 1: definition and classification of CKD. In: KDIGO 2012 clinical practice guideline for the evaluation and management of chronic kidney disease; 2013. https://kdigo.org/wp-content/uploads/2017/02/KDIGO_2012_CKD_GL.pdf. Accessed 17 Oct 2019.

27. Center for Drug Evaluation and Research (CDER) at the Food and Drug Administration Guidance for industry: pharmacokinetics in patients with impaired renal function — study design, data analysis, and impact on dosing and labeling. Renal Impairment Guidance Working Group. 2010. https://www.fda.gov/media/78573/download. Accessed 18 Oct 2019.

28. Pazhayattil GS, Shirali AC. Drug-induced impairment of renal function. Int J Nephrol Renovasc Dis. 2014;7:457–68. https://doi.org/10.2147/IJNRD.S39747.

29. Awdishu L, Mehta RL. The 6R's of drug induced nephrotoxicity. BMC Nephrol. 2017;18:1–12.

30. Mueller BA. Acute renal failure. In: Pharmacotherapy. 6th ed. New York: McGraw-Hill; 2005. p. 781–90.

31. Nolin TD, Himmelfarb J, Matzke GR. Drug-induced kidney disease. In: Pharmacotherapy. 6th ed. New York, NY: McGraw-Hill; 2005. p. 871–87.

32. Samra M, Abcar A. False estimates of elevated creatinine. Perm J. 2012;16:51–2.

33. Hottelart C, El Esper C, Rose F, Achard JM, Fournier A. Fenofibrate increases creatininemia by increasing metabolic production of creatinine. Nephron. 2002;92:536–41. https://doi.org/10.1159/000064083.

34. Saah AJ, Koch TR, Drusano GL. Cefoxitin falsely elevates creatinine levels. JAMA. 1982;247:205–6.

35. Berg KJ, Gjellestad A, Nordby G, et al. Renal effects of trimethoprim in ciclosporin-and azathioprine-treated kidney-allografted patients. Nephron. 1989;53:218.

36. Rocci ML, Vlasses PH, Ferguson RK. Creatinine serum concentrations and H2-receptor antagonists. Clin Nephrol. 1984;22:214.

37. Haroon S, Davenport A. Choosing a dialyzer: what clinicians need to know. Hemodial Int. 2018;22:S65–74.

38. Zovirax® [package insert on the Internet]. Research Triangle Park: GlaxoSmithKline; 2005 [Accessed 18 Nov 2019]. Available from: https://www.accessdata.fda.gov/drugsatfda_docs/label/2005/018828s030%2C020089s019%2C019909s020lbl.pdf.

39. Amoxil® [package insert on the Internet]. Research Triangle Park: GlaxoSmithKline; 2006 [Accessed 18 Nov 2019]. Available from: https://www.accessdata.fda.gov/drugsatfda_docs/label/2008/050760s11,050761s11,050754s12,050542s25lbl.pdf.

40. Amoxicillin Clavulanate Potassium [package insert on the Internet]. Sellersville: Teva Pharmaceuticals USA; 2008 [Accessed 18 Nov 2019]. Available from: https://www.accessdata.fda.gov/drugsatfda_docs/label/2009/065162s021lbl.pdf.

41. Ampicillin [package insert on the Internet]. New York: Pfizer; 2010 [Accessed 18 Nov 2019]. Available from: https://www.pfizer.com/files/products/uspi_ampicillin_10g_bulk.pdf.

42. Unasyn® [package insert on the Internet]. New York: Pfizer; 2007 [Accessed 18 Nov 2019]. Available from: https://www.accessdata.fda.gov/drugsatfda_docs/label/2008/050608s029lbl.pdf.

43. Cefazolin [package insert on the Internet]. Irungattukottai: Hospira Healthcare India; 2010 [Accessed 18 Nov 2019]. Available from: https://www1.apotex.com/products/us/downloads/pil/cefo_sinj_10gm_ins.pdf.

44. Omnicef® [package insert on the Internet]. Carolina: CEPH International Corporation; 2005 [Accessed 18 Nov 2019]. Available from: https://medlibrary.org/lib/rx/meds/omnicef/page/7/.

45. Cefepime [package insert on the Internet]. Lake Forest: Hospira; 2012 [Accessed 18 Nov 2019]. Available from: https://www.accessdata.fda.gov/drugsatfda_docs/label/2013/050679s034lbl.pdf.

46. Ceftin® [package insert on the Internet]. Research Triangle Park: GlaxoSmithKline; 2017 [Accessed 18 Nov 2019]. Available from: https://www.gsksource.com/pharma/content/dam/GlaxoSmithKline/US/en/Prescribing_Information/Ceftin/pdf/CEFTIN.PDF.

47. Keflex® [package insert on the Internet]. Carolina: CEPH International Corporation; 2006 [Accessed 18 Nov 2019]. Available from: https://www.accessdata.fda.gov/drugsatfda_docs/label/2006/050405s097lbl.pdf.

48. Cipro® [package insert on the Internet]. Whippany: Bayer HealthCare Pharmaceuticals; 2016 [Accessed 18 Nov 2019]. Available from: https://www.accessdata.fda.gov/drugsatfda_docs/label/2016/019537s086lbl.pdf.

49. Cubicin® [package insert on the Internet]. Whitehouse Station: Merck & Co.; 2015 [Accessed 18 Nov 2019]. Available from: https://www.merck.com/product/usa/pi_circulars/c/cubicin/cubicin_pi.pdf.

50. Invanz® [package insert on the Internet]. Whitehouse Station: Merck & Co.; 2011 [Accessed 18 Nov 2019]. Available from: https://www.accessdata.fda.gov/drugsatfda_docs/label/2012/021337s038lbl.pdf.

51. Diflucan® [package insert on the Internet]. New York: Pfizer; 2011 [Accessed 18 Nov 2019]. Available from: https://www.accessdata.fda.gov/drugsatfda_docs/label/2011/019949s051lbl.pdf.

52. Levaquin® [package insert on the Internet]. Gurabo: Janssen Ortho; 2018 [Accessed 18 Nov 2019]. Available from: https://www.accessdata.fda.gov/drugsatfda_docs/label/2018/020634s069lbl.pdf.

53. Merrem® [package insert on the Internet]. Wilmington: AstraZeneca; 2006 [Accessed 18 Nov 2019]. Available from: https://www.accessdata.fda.gov/drugsatfda_docs/label/2008/050706s022lbl.pdf.

54. Macrobid® [package insert on the Internet]. North Norwich: Norwich Pharmaceuticals; 2009 [Accessed 18 Nov 2019]. Available from: https://www.accessdata.fda.gov/drugsatfda_docs/label/2009/020064s019lbl.pdf.

55. Tamiflu® [package insert on the Internet]. South San Francisco: Genentech; 2019 [Accessed 18 Nov 2019]. Available from: https://www.gene.com/download/pdf/tamiflu_prescribing.pdf.

56. Zosyn® [package insert on the Internet]. Philadelphia: Wyeth Pharmaceuticals; 2017 [Accessed 18 Nov 2019]. Available from: https://www.accessdata.fda.gov/drugsatfda_docs/label/2017/050684s88s89s90_050750s37s38s39lbl.pdf.

57. Bactrim® [package insert on the Internet]. Philadelphia: Mutual Pharmaceutical Company; 2013 [Accessed 18 Nov 2019]. Available from: https://www.accessdata.fda.gov/drugsatfda_docs/label/2013/017377s068s073lbl.pdf.

58. Valtrex® [package insert on the Internet]. Research Triangle Park: GlaxoSmithKline; 2008 [Accessed 18 Nov 2019]. Available from: https://www.accessdata.fda.gov/drugsatfda_docs/label/2008/020487s014lbl.pdf.

59. Vemlidy® [package insert on the Internet]. Foster City: Gilead Sciences; 2019 [Accessed 18 Nov 2019]. Available from: https://www.gilead.com/~/media/files/pdfs/medicines/liver-disease/vemlidy/vemlidy_pi.pdf?la=en.

60. Viread® [package insert on the Internet]. Foster City: Gilead Sciences; 2012 [Accessed 18 Nov 2019]. Available from: https://www.accessdata.fda.gov/drugsatfda_docs/label/2012/021356s042,022577s002lbl.pdf.

61. Norpace® [package insert on the Internet]. New York: Pfizer; 2016 [Accessed 18 Nov 2019]. Available from: https://www.pfizer.com/files/products/uspi_norpace.pdf.

62. Tikosyn® [package insert on the Internet]. New York: Pfizer; 2014 [Accessed 18 Nov 2019]. Available from: http://labeling.pfizer.com/showlabeling.aspx?id=639.

63. Rythmol® [package insert on the Internet]. Research Triangle Park: GlaxoSmithKline; 2013 [Accessed 18 Nov 2019]. Available from: https://www.accessdata.fda.gov/drugsatfda_docs/label/2013/019151s012lbl.pdf.

64. Betapace AF® [package insert on the Internet]. Wayne: Bayer HealthCare Pharmaceuticals; 2011 [Accessed 18 Nov 2019]. Available from: https://www.accessdata.fda.gov/drugsatfda_docs/label/2011/021151s010lbl.pdf.

65. Eliquis® [package insert on the Internet]. Princeton: Bristol-Myers Squibb; 2019 [Accessed 18 Nov 2019]. Available from: https://packageinserts.bms.com/pi/pi_eliquis.pdf.

66. Savaysa® [package insert on the Internet]. Tokyo: Daiichi Sankyo; 2019 [Accessed 18 Nov 2019]. Available from: https://dsi.com/prescribing-information-portlet/getPIContent?productName=Savaysa&inline=true.

67. Pradaxa® [package insert on the Internet]. Ridgefield: Boehringer Ingelheim Pharmaceuticals; 2018 [Accessed 18 Nov 2019]. Available from: https://docs.boehringer-ingelheim.com/Prescribing%20Information/PIs/Pradaxa/Pradaxa.pdf.

68. Lovenox® [package insert on the Internet]. Bridgewater: Sanofi-Aventis U.S.; 2018 [Accessed 18 Nov 2019]. Available from: http://products.sanofi.us/Lovenox/Lovenox.pdf.

69. Xarelto® [package insert on the Internet]. Gurabo: Janssen Ortho; 2019 [Accessed 18 Nov 2019]. Available from: http://www.janssenlabels.com/package-insert/product-monograph/prescribing-information/XARELTO-pi.pdf.

70. Glucotrol® [package insert on the Internet]. New York: Pfizer; 2008 [Accessed 18 Nov 2019]. Available from: https://www.accessdata.fda.gov/drugsatfda_docs/label/2008/017783s019lbl.pdf.

71. Diabeta® [package insert on the Internet]. Bridgewater: Sanofi-Aventis U.S.; 2009 [Accessed 18 Nov 2019]. Available from: https://www.accessdata.fda.gov/drugsatfda_docs/label/2009/017532s030lbl.pdf.

72. Glynase® Prestab® [package insert on the Internet]. New York: Pfizer; 2017 [Accessed 18 Nov 2019]. Available from: http://labeling.pfizer.com/ShowLabeling.aspx?format=PDF&id=597.

73. Glucophage® [package insert on the Internet]. Princeton: Bristol-Myers Squibb; 2018 [Accessed 18 Nov 2019]. Available from: https://packageinserts.bms.com/pi/pi_glucophage.pdf.

74. Invokana® [package insert on the Internet]. Titusville: Janssen Pharmaceuticals; 2019 [Accessed 18 Nov 2019]. Available from: http://www.janssenlabels.com/package-insert/product-monograph/prescribing-information/INVOKANA-pi.pdf.

75. Farxiga® [package insert on the Internet]. Princeton: Bristol-Myers Squibb; 2014 [Accessed 18 Nov 2019]. Available from: https://www.accessdata.fda.gov/drugsatfda_docs/label/2014/202293s003lbl.pdf.

76. Jardiance® [package insert on the Internet]. Ridgefield: Boehringer Ingelheim Pharmaceuticals; 2018 [Accessed 18 Nov 2019]. Available from: https://docs.boehringer-ingelheim.com/Prescribing%20Information/PIs/Jardiance/jardiance.pdf.

77. Tradjenta® [package insert on the Internet]. Ridgefield: Boehringer Ingelheim Pharmaceuticals; 2019 [Accessed 18 Nov 2019]. Available from: https://docs.boehringer-ingelheim.com/Prescribing%20Information/PIs/Tradjenta/Tradjenta.pdf?DMW_FORMAT=pdf.

78. Onglyza® [package insert on the Internet]. Princeton: Bristol-Myers Squibb; 2009 [Accessed 18 Nov 2019]. Available from: https://www.accessdata.fda.gov/drugsatfda_docs/label/2009/022350lbl.pdf.

79. Januvia® [package insert on the Internet]. Whitehouse Station: Merck & Co.; 2019 [Accessed 18 Nov 2019]. Available from: https://www.merck.com/product/usa/pi_circulars/j/januvia/januvia_pi.pdf.

80. Briviact® [package insert on the Internet]. Smyrna: UCB; 2018 [Accessed 18 Nov 2019]. Available from: https://www.briviact.com/briviact-PI.pdf.

81. Aptiom® [package insert on the Internet]. Marlborough: Sunovion Pharmaceuticals; 2019 [Accessed 18 Nov 2019]. Available from: http://www.aptiom.com/Aptiom-Prescribing-Information.pdf.

82. Felbatol® [package insert on the Internet]. Somerset: MEDA Pharmaceuticals; 2011 [Accessed 18 Nov 2019]. Available from: https://www.accessdata.fda.gov/drugsatfda_docs/label/2012/020189s027lbl.pdf.

83. Neurontin® [package insert on the Internet]. New York: Pfizer; 2017 [Accessed 18 Nov 2019]. Available from: https://www.accessdata.fda.gov/drugsatfda_docs/label/2017/02023 5s064_020882s047_021129s046lbl.pdf.
84. Vimpat® [package insert on the Internet]. Smyrna: UCB; 2019 [Accessed 18 Nov 2019]. Available from: https://www.vimpat.com/vimpat-prescribing-information.pdf.
85. Keppra® [package insert on the Internet]. Smyrna: UCB; 2009 [Accessed 18 Nov 2019]. Available from: https://www.accessdata.fda.gov/drugsatfda_docs/label/2009/021035s07 8s080,021505s021s024lbl.pdf.
86. Fycompa® [package insert on the Internet]. Woodcliff Lake: Eisai; 2019 [Accessed 18 Nov 2019]. Available from: https://www.fycompa.com/-/media/Files/Fycompa/Fycompa_ Prescribing_Information.pdf.
87. Lyrica® [package insert on the Internet]. New York: Pfizer; 2019 [Accessed 18 Nov 2019]. Available from: http://labeling.pfizer.com/ShowLabeling.aspx?id=561.
88. Mysoline® [package insert on the Internet]. Aliso Viejo: Valeant; 2009 [Accessed 18 Nov 2019]. Available from: https://www.accessdata.fda.gov/drugsatfda_docs/ label/2009/009170s036lbl.pdf.
89. Banzel® [package insert on the Internet]. Woodcliff Lake: Eisai; 2015 [Accessed 18 Nov 2019]. Available from: https://www.banzel.com/~/media/Files/BanzelPatient/BanzelPI.pdf.
90. Diacomit® [package insert on the Internet]. Beauvais: Biocodex; 2018 [Accessed 18 Nov 2019]. Available from: https://www.diacomit.com/pdf/PI-Diacomit-2018.pdf.
91. Topamax® [package insert on the Internet]. Gurabo: Janssen Ortho; 2009 [Accessed 18 Nov 2019]. Available from: https://www.accessdata.fda.gov/drugsatfda_docs/ label/2012/020844s041lbl.pdf.
92. Sabril® [package insert on the Internet]. Cincinnati: Patheon; 2019 [Accessed 18 Nov 2019]. Available from: https://www.lundbeck.com/upload/us/files/pdf/Products/ Sabril_PI_US_EN.pdf.
93. Zonisamide [package insert on the Internet]. Morgantown: Mylan Pharmaceuticals; 2019 [Accessed 18 Nov 2019]. Available from: https://www.mylan.com/en/products/ product-catalog/product-profile-page?id=f20980fe-83f4-4da0-b9da-23c75f6e848c.
94. Allopurinol [package insert on the Internet]. Morgantown: Mylan Pharmaceuticals; 2019 [Accessed 18 Nov 2019]. Available from: https://dailymed.nlm.nih.gov/dailymed/drugInfo. cfm?setid=bdbf5ad4-86f2-4e9c-a51a-fb0c7220c480.
95. Gloperba® [package insert on the Internet]. Ferndale: Ferndale Laboratories; 2019 [Accessed 18 Nov 2019]. Available from: https://www.accessdata.fda.gov/drugsatfda_docs/ label/2019/210942s000lbl.pdf.
96. Reglan® [package insert on the Internet]. Baudette: ANI Pharmaceuticals; 2017 [Accessed 18 Nov 2019]. Available from: https://www.accessdata.fda.gov/drugsatfda_docs/ label/2017/017854s062lbl.pdf.
97. Cimetidine [package insert on the Internet]. Pulaski: AvKARE; 2016 [Accessed 18 Nov 2019]. Available from: https://dailymed.nlm.nih.gov/dailymed/lookup. cfm?setid=17c827aa-682c-919e-3595-c1aee9ebb341.
98. Pepcid® [package insert on the Internet]. Whitehouse Station: Merck & Co.; 2011 [Accessed 18 Nov 2019]. Available from: https://www.accessdata.fda.gov/drugsatfda_docs/ label/2011/019462s037lbl.pdf.
99. Axid® [package insert on the Internet]. Liberty Corner: Reliant Pharmaceuticals; 2004 [Accessed 18 Nov 2019]. Available from: https://www.accessdata.fda.gov/drugsatfda_docs/ label/2005/21494s001lbl.pdf.
100. Zantac® [package insert on the Internet]. Research Triangle Park: GlaxoSmithKline; 2009 [Accessed 18 Nov 2019]. Available from: https://www.accessdata.fda.gov/drugsatfda_docs/ label/2009/018703s068,019675s035,020251s019lbl.pdf.

Chapter 22
Use of Iodinated and Gadolinium-Containing Contrast Media in CKD

T. Conor McKee and Colette Shaw

Introduction

Contrast media are chemical substances used in medical X-ray, magnetic resonance imaging (MRI), computed tomography (CT), angiography, and ultrasound imaging. Contrast enhances and improves the quality of imaging enabling the radiologist to provide an accurate diagnosis. It can help delineate structures such as tumors, abscesses, and blood vessels making them more conspicuous to the interpreter (Case 1). While contrast is not always necessary (Case 2), it is often helpful and, in some cases, required. As the aging population grows, so too does the complexity of disease; this has led to increased demand for contrast-enhanced diagnostic studies. As with any medication, there are possible adverse effects that must be weighed against the potential benefit. In this chapter the issues surrounding the administration of intravenous contrast as it relates to patients with chronic renal dysfunction will be discussed. Iodine-containing contrast media and gadolinium-based contrast media have specific risks associated with their use in patients with chronic kidney disease (CKD) that will be addressed separately. Finally alternative non-nephrotoxic imaging options, e.g., contrast-enhanced ultrasound (CEUS), will be reviewed.

T. C. McKee · C. Shaw (✉)
Department of Radiology, Thomas Jefferson University Hospital, Philadelphia, PA, USA
e-mail: timothy.mckee@jefferson.edu; colette.shaw@jefferson.edu

© Springer Nature Switzerland AG 2022
J. McCauley et al. (eds.), *Approaches to Chronic Kidney Disease*,
https://doi.org/10.1007/978-3-030-83082-3_22

Iodinated Contrast

Contrast-Induced Nephropathy

> Contrast-induced nephropathy is defined as acute kidney injury that occurs within 48 hours after the administration of iodinated contrast that cannot be attributed to other causes.

Iodinated intravenous contrast used in CT studies and many interventional procedures is generally a safe medication with a relatively low rate of adverse events, particularly when using the nonionic contrast agents that are now standard of care [1–3]. The most common adverse reaction to contrast media is an allergic-type reaction. Symptoms can range from mild (focal urticaria, pruritis, mild nausea) to severe, life-threatening reactions resulting in hypotension and hypoxia. Nephrotoxicity associated with iodinated contrast material results in the phenomenon known as contrast-induced nephropathy (CIN) (Fig. 22.1). There is much debate in the literature over the prevalence of CIN as acute kidney injury (AKI) directly attributable to contrast is extremely difficult to distinguish from AKI due to other comorbid factors [4–6]. Despite this, there is agreement from both the American College of Radiology and Kidney Disease Improving Global Outcomes (KDIGO) that CIN is a true albeit rare entity [7, 8]. The incidence of CIN in the nonemergent, outpatient setting has been reported at <1%, even in patients with mild baseline chronic renal disease [9]. The incidence was found to be much higher in patients receiving intravenous contrast in the emergency department, perhaps due to the poorer clinical status of the patients [10]. The diagnosis of AKI was defined by the Acute Kidney Injury Network (AKIN) in 2007 and has been recently used to diagnose CIN. Acute kidney injury in this circumstance is diagnosed if one of the following occurs within 48 hours of exposure to the nephrotoxic agent (iodinated contrast):

1. Absolute serum creatinine increase $\geq$0.3 mg/dL.
2. A percentage increase in serum creatinine $\geq$50% ($\geq$1.5-fold above baseline).
3. Urine output reduced to $\leq$0.5 mg/kg/hour for at least 6 hours.

Diagnosis based on these criteria is not specific to CIN; AKI due to any cause can fulfill these criteria. CIN is present when the decline in renal function occurs without another reasonable explanation. The serum creatinine will usually peak at about day 4 and return to baseline 7 to 10 days post-contrast administration. Permanent renal dysfunction is uncommon. In hospitalized patients, other comorbidities can often obscure the diagnosis.

The exact mechanism of nephrotoxicity is not well understood, but there have been many proposed theories such as medullary vasoconstriction and hypoxia, direct cytotoxicity to renal tubules, and the release of vasoconstrictive mediators [11–14]. The true pathophysiology is likely multifactorial.

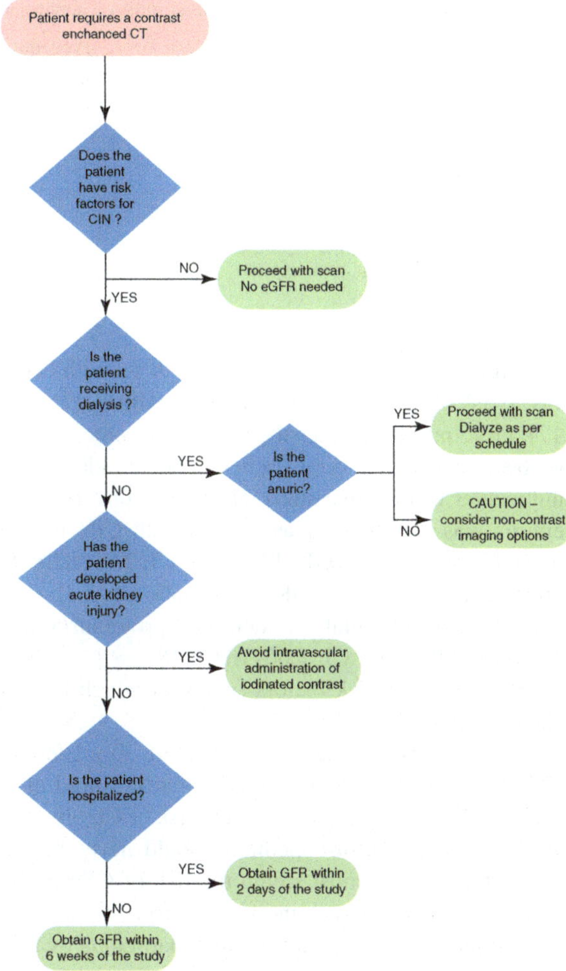

Fig. 22.1 Flowchart: screening and prevention of contrast-induced nephropathy (CIN)

Who Is at Risk for CIN?

The incidence of contrast-induced nephropathy is higher among patients with CKD and increases with the severity of renal dysfunction.

While many aspects of CIN are avidly debated in the literature, it seems clear that the most significant underlying risk factor is preexisting renal dysfunction [15–17]. There is no determined threshold, creatinine, or eGFR, at which there is risk of CIN although one study has shown low osmolar CT contrast material to be a risk factor in patients with a stable eGFR <30 ml/min/1.73m^2. The same study also

Table 22.1 Potential risk factors for contrast-induced nephropathy

Patient-related risk factors	Procedure-related risk factors
Pre-existing renal dysfunction	Route of administration–arterial > venous
Diabetes mellitus	Intracardiac procedures
Advanced age	
Congestive heart failure	
Multiple myeloma	
Dehydration	
Nephrotoxic drugs, e.g., nonsteroidal anti-inflammatory drugs	

showed a trend toward significance in those with eGFR <45 ml/min/1.73m^2. There was no risk of nephrotoxicity in patients with eGFR of greater than 45 ml/min/1.73m^2 [17]. Proteinuria increases the risk further among patients with reduced eGFR and has been shown in several studies to be an independent risk factor for CIN. In one multicenter prospective study of patients undergoing cardiac catheterization, proteinuria was significantly associated with CIN in patients with eGFR 30–44 ml/min/1.73 m^2 ($n = 239$) (OR, 12.1; 95% CI: 2.81–82.8; $P = 0.0006$) and eGFR<30 ml/min/1.73 m^2 ($n = 122$) (OR, 17.4; 95% CI: 3.32–321; $P = 0.0001$). Multivariate logistic regression analysis identified proteinuria as an independent predictor of CIN (OR, 4.09; 95% CI: 1.66–10.0) [18].

Other potential risk factors (many of which have not been robustly tested) are listed in Table 22.1.

Some centers have adopted eGFR of 30 mL/min/1.73 m^2 as the threshold for CIN; however, there is no agreed-upon threshold of serum creatinine elevation or eGFR declination beyond which the risk of CIN is considered so great that intravascular iodinated contrast medium should never be administered. The decision to administer contrast must weigh the risk of CIN against the benefit of making the correct diagnosis for each individual case.

Patients undergoing arteriography particularly cardiac angiography are at higher risk of CIN than intravenous procedures or contrast-enhanced diagnostic scans [19, 20]. This may be explained by the fact that the contrast administration is arterial and suprarenal, the dose to the kidneys is more concentrated, and catheter manipulation may predispose the patient to atheroembolic events. The relationship between dose and toxicity for intracardiac iodinated contrast medium is directly proportional [21]. The data relating to intravenous contrast dosing and toxicity is inconclusive. As a result, the American College of Radiology (ACR) does not recommend a threshold dose of contrast volume beyond which no further contrast should be administered in a 24-hour period, nor does it suggest withholding contrast in patients who have received contrast in the preceding 24 hours [8].

Screening

Screening is needed to identify "at-risk" patients.

Renal function is not always known, and certain patients should be screened prior to contrast administration to mitigate the risk of CIN (Table 22.2). Choyke et al. designed a questionnaire consisting of six simple questions to be answered by patients prior to their radiologic study. A negative response to all six questions predicted a serum creatinine <1.7 (the cutoff used at their institution), in 99% of patients [22]. The six questions were as follows:

1. Have you ever been told you have renal problems?
2. Have you ever been told you have protein in your urine?
3. Do you have high blood pressure?
4. Do you have diabetes mellitus?
5. Do you have gout?
6. Have you ever had kidney surgery?

The results of the Choyke questionnaire have been further validated using rapid point of care creatinine testing [23]. Similarly, the European Society of Urogenital Radiology (ESUR) recommends evaluation for the same underlying conditions and the additional clinical history of other, recently administered nephrotoxic drugs [24]. Additionally, the American College of Radiology recommends screening all patients over 60 years of age [8].

All at-risk patients should have a baseline serum creatinine (with or without estimated GFR) obtained prior to administration of contrast. The maximum time interval for the bloodwork varies by institution. Many will accept 30 days for outpatients.

Table 22.2 ACR suggested indications for renal function assessment prior to administration of iodinated contrast medium

Indications for renal function assessment
Age > 60

History of renal disease, including:
    Dialysis
    Kidney transplant
    Single kidney
    Renal cancer
    Renal surgery

History of hypertension requiring medical therapy
History of diabetes mellitus
Metformin or metformin-containing drug combinations

Prevention

> Prevent CIN in those at risk by avoiding iodinated contrast or pre-treat with intravenous volume expansion if contrast administration is necessary.

The most effective strategy for preventing CIN is to avoid contrast administration in the first place. This fact should serve as a reminder to evaluate the risk-benefit of the contrast and to determine if another study that does not require iodinated contrast material could answer the clinical question. Common alternative radiologic studies not requiring iodinated contrast are discussed below. Communication with the radiologist is critical in these cases to plan the study that presents the least amount of risk while providing the clinical information needed. There are times, however, in which the benefit of the contrast administration outweighs the risk of withholding contrast. In these situations, prevention of CIN is paramount.

Intravenous hydration with isotonic fluids has been shown to decrease the risk of CIN, although this is not a practical approach for outpatient studies [25]. The ideal regimen has not been elucidated; however, a study showing benefit of administered isotonic saline for a total of 24 hours, beginning 12 hours before the administration of contrast. Patients receiving intravenous hydration had a lower rate of acute kidney injury compared to patients with unrestricted oral intake [26]. Another study comparing isotonic saline with 0.45 percent saline, administered over a similar time course, found acute kidney injury to be lower in the isotonic saline group [27]. Other strategies for the prevention of CIN including pretreatment with sodium bicarbonate [28–30] or N-acetylcysteine (NAC) [31–33] have had mixed results in the literature. Both have had studies advocating their routine use while others have shown no benefit.

At present, both the KDOQI, and the American College of Radiology recommend intravascular volume expansion to reduce the risk of CIN, noting that this is only feasible in the inpatient setting. The ACR recommends isotonic solution while the KDOQI recommends either isotonic sodium chloride or sodium bicarbonate solutions for hydration. The ACR considers the evidence for sodium bicarbonate and NAC insufficient and, thus, cannot recommend these agents to prevent CIN. Conversely, the KDOQI recommends using oral NAC together with intravenous isotonic fluids in patients at increased risk of CIN with level 2D evidence [7, 8].

Dialysis

Patients with anuria and end-stage renal disease already routinely receiving hemodialysis treatments are not at risk for CIN as the kidneys have no residual function. Contrast can be given to these patients without risk of further renal damage, and dialysis can be maintained on the current schedule. There is no indication for additional dialysis sessions [34]. Patients who undergo hemodialysis and still make some urine are at risk for CIN and loss of their residual kidney function should they receive an iodinated contrast medium. Residual renal function in patients on dialysis, particularly those on peritoneal dialysis, is important for volume balance and toxin removal [35, 36]. All attempts should be made to preserve any remaining renal function.

Most low-osmolality iodinated contrast media are readily cleared by dialysis. In general there is no need for urgent dialysis after intravascular iodinated contrast medium administration [34]. Prophylactic hemodialysis in patients with reduced renal function does not diminish the incidence of CIN. A recent consensus statement from the ACR and National Kidney Foundation advised against initiating or changing the schedule for acute dialysis or continuous renal replacement therapy solely based on the administration of iodinated contrast media irrespective of residual renal function [37].

There is also a concern that patients undergoing dialysis who receive intravascular iodinated contrast could become fluid overloaded. This is attributed to the increased osmotic load of the contrast leading to expansion of the intravascular space. In these patients, radiologists and operators should be using low osmolality or iso-osmolality contrast media and using as low a dose as reasonably achievable.

Metformin

Metformin is absolutely contraindicated in patients with eGFR < 30 ml/min and should be avoided in patients with eGFR 30–45 ml/min [38]. If the eGFR falls below 45 ml/min in a patient on metformin, the drug should be held at or prior to iodinated contrast administration and withheld for 48 hours subsequent to the contrast exposure. The drug should be restarted only after the renal function has been rechecked and found to be unchanged from baseline [8].

Metformin is an orally administered medication used for the treatment of non-insulin-dependent diabetes mellitus. Although metformin itself is not a nephrotoxic medication, it is predominantly renally excreted. In patients with renal insufficiency, metformin can accumulate in the blood and lead to one of the most significant complications of metformin use – lactic acidosis [39]. Mortality in cases of metformin-associated lactic acidosis has historically been reported as high as 50% but a more recent study reported that since the year 2000 the mortality has been closer to 25% [40]. Iodinated contrast is not known to interact with metformin but the potential for CIN resulting in subsequent lactic acidosis warrants caution in patients at risk. There is considerable variation in the recommendations from international societies concerning the management of patients taking metformin who are also receiving iodinated contrast material [41].

In patients taking metformin who have chronic kidney disease or are undergoing arterial catheter studies that might result in emboli (atheromatous or other) to the renal arteries, the ACR recommends holding metformin at the time of or prior to the procedure and withheld for 48 hours subsequent to the procedure. The drug should be restarted only after renal function has been rechecked and found to be unchanged from baseline [8].

Metformin does not need to be discontinued prior to injection with clinical doses of gadolinium-based contrast agents.

Gadolinium-Based Contrast

Gadolinium-based contrast agents are primarily used for contrast enhancement in MRI. The incidence of adverse events associated with gadolinium-based contrast agents administered at clinical doses ranges from 0.07 to 2.4%. Most reactions are mild and physiologic. There is no cross-reactivity with iodinated contrast media.

Unlike iodinated contrast, gadolinium is not nephrotoxic; however, caution must still be exercised in patients with either acute kidney injury or advanced chronic kidney disease. The primary concern with gadolinium-based contrast is the development of nephrogenic systemic fibrosis (NSF). NSF was first described in 2000 in a paper by Cowper et al. and identified 15 patients, all receiving dialysis treatments, who developed extensive hardening and thickening of the skin [42]. The condition can be debilitating and can result in permanent disability. It would later be determined that the condition was not limited to the skin and could involve the lungs, heart, liver, and muscles. Subsequent papers linked exposure to gadolinium-based contrast agents to the development of NSF [43, 44]. Although advanced CKD (stage IV or V) or acute renal failure is necessary for the development of NSF, the disease does not affect every patient with kidney disease. The exact mechanism is unknown, and the low number of confirmed cases limits the ability to fully study the disease. Other potential risk factors include metabolic acidosis, elevated iron, calcium, and/or phosphate levels, high-dose erythropoietin, immunosuppression, vasculopathy, infection, or inflammatory conditions. It should be noted that the vast majority of cases of NSF occurred with the use of older, nonionic-linear agents. The newer class of macrocyclic agents has been associated with fewer cases of NSF [45].

Screening for chronic kidney disease prior to outpatient studies can be performed using the Choyke questionnaire, the same as that used for iodinated contrast. The six-question form effectively identifies patients with eGFR <30 ml/min/1.73 m^2, those most at risk for NSF [46]. Unlike iodinated contrast, which is safe to use in anuric patients receiving hemodialysis, gadolinium-based agents should be used with extreme caution in these patients, and the newer, macrocyclic agents should be used when possible. If no other alternative study is adequate and a gadolinium-based agent must be used, the free gadolinium can be removed by hemodialysis. In patients with stage six CKD, three consecutive dialysis treatments clear over 98% of the agent, limiting but not eliminating the risk of NSF [47]. Since hemodialysis does not remove free gadolinium from the tissues, its use in preventing and treating NSF has not been established.

What Is the Alternative?

> Ultrasound contrast agents are not nephrotoxic and can be used safely in patients with chronic kidney disease.

For high-risk cases, a risk-benefit assessment should be performed. Radiologists with the appropriate clinical information may be able to make the diagnosis with non-contrast CT or MRI. MRI studies can be protocoled to include noncontrast sequences that may provide the additional information to clench the diagnosis, e.g., time of flight sequences and diffusion-weighted sequences. For focused exams contrast-enhanced ultrasound (CEUS) may be considered. The latter involves the use of microbubbles administered intravenously to assess blood flow and tissue perfusion. Microbubble contrast agents are not nephrotoxic and may be used in patients with any level of renal function. CEUS can be used to assess tissue structure and evaluate blood volume and perfusion in an organ or area of interest and characterize a lesion. In the United States, ultrasound contrast agents are approved for echocardiography and hepatic ultrasonography. CEUS in the kidney is performed off-label in some centers (Case 3).

Summary

Contrast-induced nephropathy and nephrogenic systemic fibrosis are very rare but serious conditions, both associated with the use of contrast media. One is a nephropathy, the other a systemic disease. The mechanism underlying these complications is poorly understood, and the diagnosis is often challenging. Patients with advanced kidney disease (stage 4 and 5) are among those at greatest risk. Prior to ordering contrast-enhanced CT or MRI, patients should be screened for risk factors. The most effective way to prevent these complications in "at-risk" patients is to avoid contrast. Alternative imaging modalities should be considered. Patient education and aggressive management of modifiable risk factors including withholding other nephrotoxic drugs optimize blood-glucose levels and treatment of hypertension and ensure adequate intravascular hydration pre- and post-contrast administration all play an important role in reducing the risk in these patients. Close collaboration with the radiologist is necessary to ensure a diagnosis can be made with the appropriate level of risk.

Case 1
A 38-year-old male with a renal mass is evaluated with multiphase CT of the abdomen including noncontrast and post-contrast (Fig. 22.2). In this case the contrast

allows for better visualization of the tumor and differentiates it from the surrounding renal parenchyma.

Case 2

A 55-year-old male with hematuria is evaluated with multiphase CT of the abdomen including noncontrast and delayed phase (Fig. 22.3). In this case a noncontrast CT illustrates the pathology best.

Case 3

A 61-year-old male with hypertension-related chronic kidney disease stage 4 (eGFR 17 ml/min) was evaluated for renal transplant. The patient had not yet commenced dialysis therapy and continued to make urine. A noncontrast CT abdomen identified a 2.2 cm solid mass in the lower pole of the left kidney. The absence of macroscopic fat was suggestive of a renal cell carcinoma rather than a benign entity, e.g., angiomyolipoma. In the setting of severe CKD, the patient underwent a CEUS of the lesion. Findings were suspicious for a renal cell carcinoma (Fig. 22.4). The patient

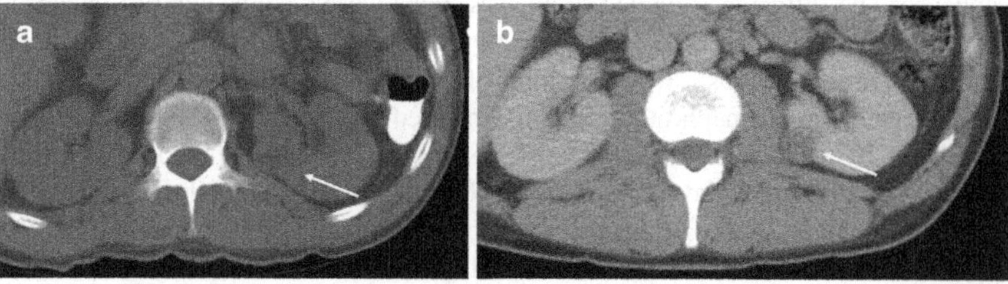

Fig. 22.2 Noncontrast (**a**) and post-contrast (**b**) axial CT images. The post-contrast image demonstrates a 1.5 cm partially exophytic cortical mass arising from the posterior and medial aspect of the left kidney (*arrow*). The mass is mildly enhancing but is hypodense compared to the surrounding renal parenchyma. The finding is suspicious for renal cell carcinoma

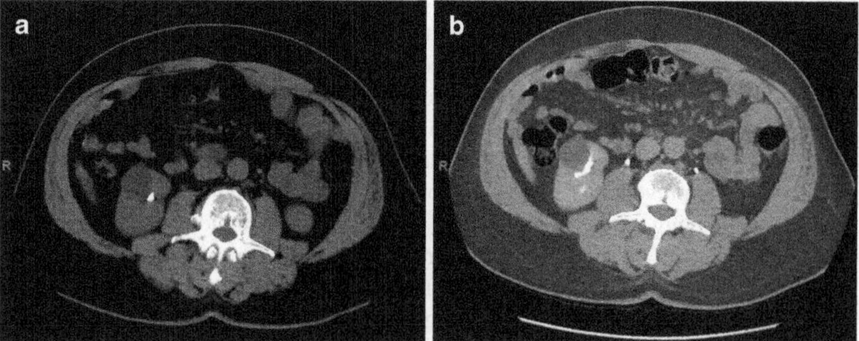

Fig. 22.3 Noncontrast axial CT image (**a**) demonstrates a large stone in the right collecting system. The lack of contrast allows the stone to be easily differentiated from the surrounding structures. The delayed phase CT (**b**) demonstrates contrast being excreted by the kidney into the collecting system. The contrast is similar density to the kidney stone and therefore, obscures the pathology

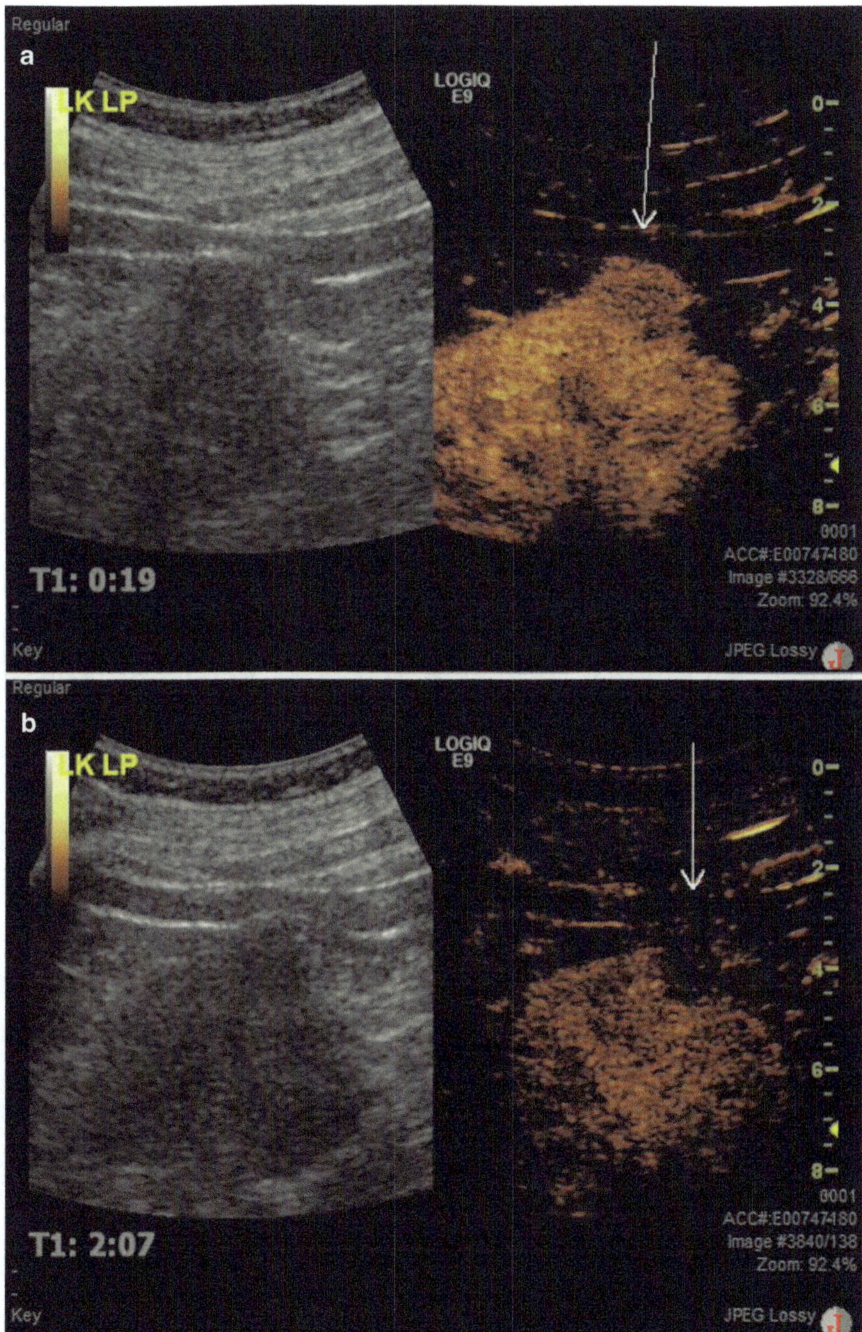

Fig. 22.4 *Gray* scale (*left*) and contrast-enhanced (*right*) ultrasound of the left kidney demonstrate 2.2 cm exophytic mass that enhances but to a lesser degree than the renal parenchyma (**a**) and rapidly washes out (**b**). Findings are highly suspicious for a renal cell carcinoma

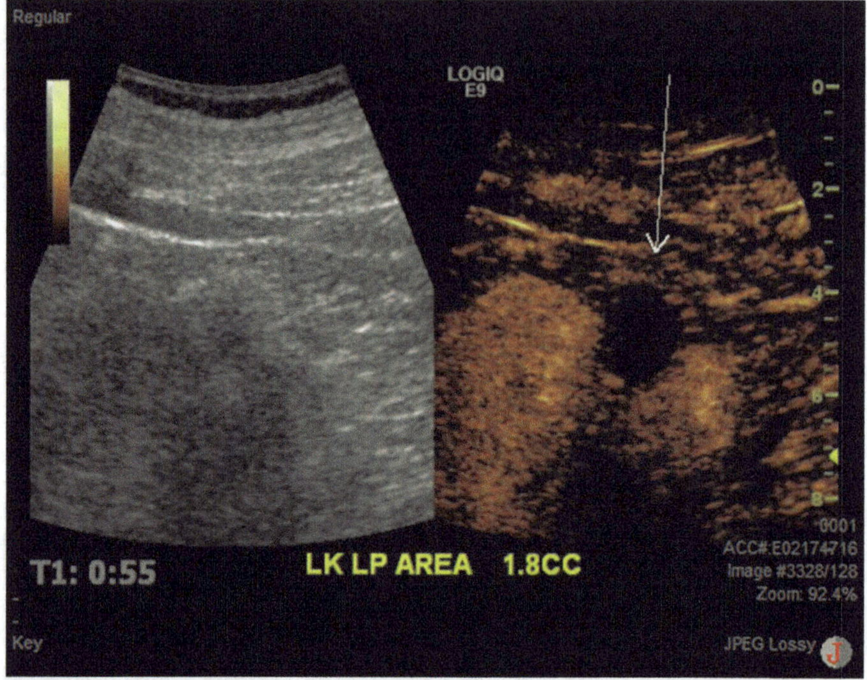

Fig. 22.5 *Gray* scale (*left*) and contrast-enhanced (*right*) ultrasound demonstrates decreased size (1.8 cm from 2.2 cm) of the left lower pole renal mass. Following administration of contrast, there was no internal enhancement, consistent with complete ablation

underwent percutaneous biopsy and microwave ablation. The histopathological diagnosis was papillary renal cell carcinoma. Eighteen months post-ablation, the treated lesion was evaluated with CEUS (Fig. 22.5). The patient was listed for transplant.

References

1. Katayama H, Yamaguchi K, Kozuka T, Takashima T, Seez P, Matsuura K. Adverse reactions to ionic and nonionic contrast media. A report from the Japanese Committee on the Safety of Contrast Media. Radiology. 1990;175(3):621–8.
2. Cochran ST, Bomyea K, Sayre JW. Trends in adverse events after IV administration of contrast media. AJR Am J Roentgenol. 2001;176(6):1385–8.
3. Mortelé KJ, Oliva MR, Ondategui S, Ros PR, Silverman SG. Universal use of nonionic iodinated contrast medium for CT: evaluation of safety in a large urban teaching hospital. AJR Am J Roentgenol. 2005;184(1):31–4.
4. Davenport MS, Cohan RH, Ellis JH. Contrast media controversies in 2015: imaging patients with renal impairment or risk of contrast reaction. AJR Am J Roentgenol. 2015;204(6):1174–81.

5. Mcdonald RJ, Mcdonald JS, Bida JP, et al. Intravenous contrast material-induced nephropathy: causal or coincident phenomenon? Radiology. 2013;267(1):106–18.
6. Mcdonald JS, Mcdonald RJ, Carter RE, Katzberg RW, Kallmes DF, Williamson EE. Risk of intravenous contrast material-mediated acute kidney injury: a propensity score-matched study stratified by baseline-estimated glomerular filtration rate. Radiology. 2014;271(1):65–73.
7. Kidney Disease Improving Global Outcomes. KDIGO Clinical Practice Guideline for Acute Kidney Injury. https://kdigo.org/wp-content/uploads/2016/10/KDIGO-2012-AKI-Guideline-English.pdf. Published March 2012. Accessed 7 Jan 2020.
8. ACR Committee on Drugs and Contrast Media. ACR manual on contrast media. https://www.acr.org/Quality-Safety/Resources/Contrast-Manual. Published June 2018. Accessed 23 Jan 2020.
9. Weisbord SD, Mor MK, Resnick AL, Hartwig KC, Palevsky PM, Fine MJ. Incidence and outcomes of contrast-induced AKI following computed tomography. Clin J Am Soc Nephrol. 2008;3(5):1274–81.
10. Mitchell AM, Jones AE, Tumlin JA, Kline JA. Incidence of contrast-induced nephropathy after contrast-enhanced computed tomography in the outpatient setting. Clin J Am Soc Nephrol. 2010;5(1):4–9.
11. Heyman SN, Brezis M, Epstein FH, Spokes K, Silva P, Rosen S. Early renal medullary hypoxic injury from radiocontrast and indomethacin. Kidney Int. 1991;40(4):632–42.
12. Sendeski M, Patzak A, Pallone TL, Cao C, Persson AE, Persson PB. Iodixanol, constriction of medullary descending vasa recta, and risk for contrast medium-induced nephropathy. Radiology. 2009;251(3):697–704.
13. Liss P, Nygren A, Erikson U, Ulfendahl HR. Injection of low and iso-osmolar contrast medium decreases oxygen tension in the renal medulla. Kidney Int. 1998;53(3):698–702.
14. Quintavalle C, Brenca M, De micco F, et al. In vivo and in vitro assessment of pathways involved in contrast media-induced renal cells apoptosis. Cell Death Dis. 2011;2:e155.
15. Rudnick MR, Goldfarb S, Wexler L, et al. Nephrotoxicity of ionic and nonionic contrast media in 1196 patients: a randomized trial. The Iohexol Cooperative Study. Kidney Int. 1995;47(1):254–61.
16. Davenport MS, Khalatbari S, Dillman JR, Cohan RH, Caoili EM, Ellis JH. Contrast material-induced nephrotoxicity and intravenous low-osmolality iodinated contrast material. Radiology. 2013;267(1):94–105.
17. Davenport MS, Khalatbari S, Cohan RH, Dillman JR, Myles JD, Ellis JH. Contrast material-induced nephrotoxicity and intravenous low-osmolality iodinated contrast material: risk stratification by using estimated glomerular filtration rate. Radiology. 2013;268(3):719–28.
18. Saito Y, Watanabe M, Aonuma K, et al. Proteinuria and reduced estimated glomerular filtration rate are independent risk factors for contrast-induced nephropathy after cardiac catheterization. Circ J. 2015;79(7):1624–30.
19. Davenport MS, Cohan RH, Khalatbari S, Ellis JH. The challenges in assessing contrast-induced nephropathy: where are we now? AJR Am J Roentgenol. 2014;202(4):784–9.
20. Kooiman J, Seth M, Share D, Dixon S, Gurm HS. The association between contrast dose and renal complications post PCI across the continuum of procedural estimated risk. PLoS One. 2014;9(3):e90233.
21. Katzberg RW, Newhouse JH. Intravenous contrast medium-induced nephrotoxicity: is the medical risk really as great as we have come to believe? Radiology. 2010;256(1):21–8.
22. Choyke PL, Cady J, Depollar SL, Austin H. Determination of serum creatinine prior to iodinated contrast media: is it necessary in all patients? Tech Urol. 1998;4(2):65–9.
23. Too CW, Ng WY, Tan CC, Mahmood MI, Tay KH. Screening for impaired renal function in outpatients before iodinated contrast injection: comparing the Choyke questionnaire with a rapid point-of-care-test. Eur J Radiol. 2015;84(7):1227–31.
24. Thomsen HS, Morcos SK. In which patients should serum creatinine be measured before iodinated contrast medium administration? Eur Radiol. 2005;15(4):749–54.

25. Barrett BJ, Parfrey PS. Prevention of nephrotoxicity induced by radiocontrast agents. N Engl J Med. 1994;331(21):1449–50.
26. Trivedi HS, Moore H, Nasr S, et al. A randomized prospective trial to assess the role of saline hydration on the development of contrast nephrotoxicity. Nephron Clin Pract. 2003;93(1):C29–34.
27. Mueller C, Buerkle G, Buettner HJ, et al. Prevention of contrast media-associated nephropathy: randomized comparison of 2 hydration regimens in 1620 patients undergoing coronary angioplasty. Arch Intern Med. 2002;162(3):329–36.
28. Merten GJ, Burgess WP, Gray LV, et al. Prevention of contrast-induced nephropathy with sodium bicarbonate: a randomized controlled trial. JAMA. 2004;291(19):2328–34.
29. Brar SS, Shen AY, Jorgensen MB, et al. Sodium bicarbonate vs sodium chloride for the prevention of contrast medium-induced nephropathy in patients undergoing coronary angiography: a randomized trial. JAMA. 2008;300(9):1038–46.
30. Navaneethan SD, Singh S, Appasamy S, Wing RE, Sehgal AR. Sodium bicarbonate therapy for prevention of contrast-induced nephropathy: a systematic review and meta-analysis. Am J Kidney Dis. 2009;53(4):617–27.
31. Marenzi G, Assanelli E, Marana I, et al. N-acetylcysteine and contrast-induced nephropathy in primary angioplasty. N Engl J Med. 2006;354(26):2773–82.
32. Kshirsagar AV, Poole C, Mottl A, et al. N-acetylcysteine for the prevention of radiocontrast induced nephropathy: a meta-analysis of prospective controlled trials. J Am Soc Nephrol. 2004;15(3):761–9.
33. Loomba RS, Shah PH, Aggarwal S, Arora RR. Role of N-acetylcysteine to prevent contrast-induced nephropathy: a meta-analysis. Am J Ther. 2016;23(1):e172–83.
34. Younathan CM, Kaude JV, Cook MD, Shaw GS, Peterson JC. Dialysis is not indicated immediately after administration of nonionic contrast agents in patients with end-stage renal disease treated by maintenance dialysis. AJR Am J Roentgenol. 1994;163(4):969–71.
35. Wang AY, Lai KN. The importance of residual renal function in dialysis patients. Kidney Int. 2006;69(10):1726–32.
36. Bargman JM, Golper TA. The importance of residual renal function for patients on dialysis. Nephrol Dial Transplant. 2005;20(4):671–3.
37. Davenport MS, Perazella MA, Yee J, et al. Use of intravenous iodinated contrast media in patients with kidney disease: consensus statements from the American College of Radiology and the National Kidney Foundation. Radiology. 2020;294(3):660–8.
38. US Food and Drug Administration, Silver Spring, MD. FDA Drug Safety Communication: FDA revises warnings regarding use of the diabetes medicine metformin in certain patients with reduced kidney function. 2016. http://www.fda.gov/downloads/Drugs/DrugSafety/UCM494140.pdf.
39. Bailey CJ, Turner RC. Metformin. N Engl J Med. 1996;334(9):574–9.
40. Kajbaf F, Lalau JD. Mortality rate in so-called "metformin-associated lactic acidosis": a review of the data since the 1960s. Pharmacoepidemiol Drug Saf. 2014;23(11):1123–7.
41. Goergen SK, Rumbold G, Compton G, Harris C. Systematic review of current guidelines, and their evidence base, on risk of lactic acidosis after administration of contrast medium for patients receiving metformin. Radiology. 2010;254(1):261–9.
42. Cowper SE, Robin HS, Steinberg SM, Su LD, Gupta S, Leboit PE. Scleromyxoedema-like cutaneous diseases in renal-dialysis patients. Lancet. 2000;356(9234):1000–1.
43. Marckmann P, Skov L, Rossen K, et al. Nephrogenic systemic fibrosis: suspected causative role of gadodiamide used for contrast-enhanced magnetic resonance imaging. J Am Soc Nephrol. 2006;17(9):2359–62.
44. Grobner T. Gadolinium--a specific trigger for the development of nephrogenic fibrosing dermopathy and nephrogenic systemic fibrosis? Nephrol Dial Transplant. 2006;21(4):1104–8.
45. Attari H, Cao Y, Elmholdt TR, Zhao Y, Prince MR. A systematic review of 639 patients with biopsy-confirmed nephrogenic systemic fibrosis. Radiology. 2019;292(2):376–86.

46. Sena BF, Stern JP, Pandharipande PV, et al. Screening patients to assess renal function before administering gadolinium chelates: assessment of the Choyke questionnaire. AJR Am J Roentgenol. 2010;195(2):424–8.
47. Saitoh T, Hayasaka K, Tanaka Y, et al. Dialyzability of gadodiamide in hemodialysis patients. Radiat Med. 2006;24:445–51.

Chapter 23
Preparation for Renal Replacement Therapy

Hannah Roni Troutman

End-stage renal disease (ESRD) has a high mortality rate; about a quarter of patients who start dialysis are no longer alive after 1 year. This rate is even higher in patients who start dialysis urgently, without a permanent access in place, and patients over the age of 75 [1–3]. Thus, advance preparation for renal replacement therapy (RRT) is crucial to mitigate mortality risk and treatment-related complications. In order to prepare for RRT, patients need to be referred to nephrology earlier rather than later and preferably greater than 1 year prior to initiation of RRT. It is also important to recognize patients with rapid progression of chronic kidney disease (CKD) and patients with a high risk of ESRD. Rapid progression is defined as a persistent decline in estimated glomerular filtration rate (eGFR) of more than 5 ml/min/1.73 m^2 per year [4]. Elevated risk of ESRD can be predicted by validated risk prediction tools. There is a four-variable kidney failure risk equation that has been studied which includes: age, gender, eGFR, urine albumin to creatinine ratio, and region (North America or non-North America). The eight-variable kidney failure risk equation includes the aforementioned plus the following: serum bicarbonate, serum albumin, serum calcium, and serum phosphorus [5, 6].

Progressive CKD should be managed in a multidisciplinary care setting. This includes dialysis modality education, dietary counseling, vascular or peritoneal access surgery evaluation, and referral for kidney transplant evaluation. Additionally, ethical, psychological, and social care plays a key role in the dialysis modality decision. Ideally, dialysis modality education should begin when patients reach CKD stage 4 (eGFR < 30 ml/min/1.73 m^2). Home dialysis modalities include home hemodialysis (HHD) and peritoneal dialysis (PD). In-center modalities include daytime and nocturnal hemodialysis. Observational studies suggest that patients who

H. R. Troutman (✉)
Department of Nephrology, Thomas Jefferson University, Sidney Kimmel Medical College, Philadelphia, PA, USA
e-mail: hannah.troutman@jefferson.edu

© Springer Nature Switzerland AG 2022
J. McCauley et al. (eds.), *Approaches to Chronic Kidney Disease*,
https://doi.org/10.1007/978-3-030-83082-3_23

"

undergo structured dialysis modality education are more likely to choose a home modality [7]. Initial survival benefit has been observed with peritoneal dialysis, but after several years on dialysis, survival is similar between modalities. This has been demonstrated in studies from the USA, Canada, Northern Europe, Australia, and New Zealand [1, 8–10]. Shared decision-making among patients and providers should be central to the management discussions. Patients should be referred for kidney transplant evaluation when eGFR $\leq$ 20 ml/min/1.73 m^2, the threshold for being placed on the waiting list [4]. If living donors are not available, patients may need to wait for several years to receive a deceased donor transplant given the supply and demand mismatch. Although initial postoperative mortality is higher in the first few months post-kidney transplant, long-term mortality rates are much improved in patients who undergo kidney transplant compared to patients who remain on chronic dialysis [11].

Modality education should assist the patient in determining a "life plan" that acknowledges the potential need for more than one modality over the course of a lifetime. Dialysis modality choice should reflect the goal of quality and quantity of life. It is important to recognize that the dialysis plan must continually adapt to changes in a patient's clinical course [12]. If a patient is struggling with one dialysis modality, consideration of a change in modality is appropriate. Additionally, the "surprise" question "would the nephrologist be surprised if the patient died in the next year" has been shown to accurately identify patients at high risk of early mortality with dialysis [13]. It is important to recognize patients with limited ability to gain any benefit from renal replacement therapy due to a significant burden of comorbid conditions. Patients who are chronic or recent nursing home residents demonstrate a significant decline in functional status within the 3 months just prior to initiating dialysis and will continue on a downward trajectory several months after initiation of dialysis [14]. Patients over the age of 75 with an unplanned start on dialysis have a significantly higher mortality compared to a planned start on dialysis [3]. The presence of significant physical limitations, cognitive decline, and overall frailty prior to initiation of dialysis are associated with the worst outcomes, including the highest mortality with renal replacement therapy [15]. These parameters should help guide the decision whether to pursue dialysis or not.

Conservative management is the alternative if and when patients with ESRD elect not to initiate or continue dialysis. According to the Kidney Disease: Improving Global Outcomes (KDIGO) international evidence-based guidelines, a comprehensive conservative management program should include several protocols. Patients who elect to forgo or stop dialysis need assistance with control of the symptoms of kidney failure and should be referred for palliative care support. Interventions can be made to assist with the control of pain and uremic symptoms like constipation, myoclonus, hypervolemia, nausea, vomiting, and delirium. Patients, families, and caregivers may also benefit from psychological services and spiritual or religious support coordinated by a palliative care team. Patients should be enrolled in hospice care either at home or in an inpatient setting. Ideally, bereavement support should be made available to families and caregivers after a patient's death [4]. Patients should be encouraged to discuss their decision regarding dialysis with family and caregivers in advance of complete kidney failure. Uremia may interfere with a patient's ability to effectively communicate decisions including consent for dialysis and associated procedures. Advanced directives should be created and reviewed in geriatric patients with advanced CKD to alleviate any ambiguity regarding ESRD management decisions [16]. Patients may elect to pursue hospice for another terminal illness, but remain on dialysis for preexisting ESRD. However, it is important for healthcare providers to maintain ongoing conversations with patients and families about changes in prognosis and whether continuing dialysis remains appropriate or not.

Initiation of dialysis is suggested at the GFR range of 5–10 ml/min/1.73 m^2 but may be initiated earlier if clinical symptoms dictate it. An earlier start on long-term dialysis with a GFR above 10 ml/min/m^2 is not recommended unless patients are symptomatic [4]. Patients typically develop profound uremic symptoms when the GFR is less than or equal to 10 ml/min/1.73 m^2. These symptoms may include anorexia, dysgeusia, nausea, vomiting, fatigue, pruritus, sleep disturbances, and mild cognitive impairment. However, the presence of uremic pericarditis, pleuritis, muscle twitching, hiccups, asterixis, and encephalopathy are absolute indications for initiation of renal replacement therapy [4, 17]. Volume overload and/or uncontrolled hypertension refractory to medical therapy, progressive malnutrition refractory to dietary intervention, and persistent acid-base/electrolyte abnormalities are also common indications to initiate dialysis [4, 17]. Patients with GFR $\leq$ to 5 ml/min/1.73 m^2 should be initiated on dialysis regardless of the presence/absence of symptoms given the difficulty in management with medical therapy alone [4].

Hemodialysis prescription includes the length of time, frequency of sessions, dialyzer, blood and dialysate flow rates, and dialysate solution composition. The hemodialysis apparatus consists of the dialyzer, dialysate solution, tubing for the transport of blood and dialysate, and the dialysis machine. The dialyzer is essentially the "artificial kidney;" the location of solute and water removal. It is most commonly composed of porous hollow fibers within a polyurethane shell. These fibers act as a semipermeable membrane for solutes and water to flow between blood and dialysate, which occurs in both directions. The fibers may be composed of unmodified cellulose, cellulose polymer, cellulosynthetic, and non-cellulose synthetic membranes. Biocompatible synthetic membranes have a lower likelihood of inflammatory reactions with blood. Removal of solutes from the blood occurs via diffusive and convective transport within the dialyzer. Blood and dialysate have different concentrations and flow in opposite directions within the dialyzer at different flow rates; thus, diffusion occurs down a concentration gradient, similar to the countercurrent mechanism within the nephron. Solute transport is also affected by the dialyzer membrane surface area, thickness, and size of pores as well as the molecular size of the solute. Smaller solutes move from blood to dialysate more quickly by diffusion. Larger solutes move from blood to dialysate more slowly along with fluid by convective transport. Ultrafiltration, the removal of water (without solute) from the blood, occurs via hydrostatic pressure applied to the blood by the dialysis machine. Water flows from high-pressure environment in the blood through the membrane to the low-pressure environment in the dialyzer. This transmembrane

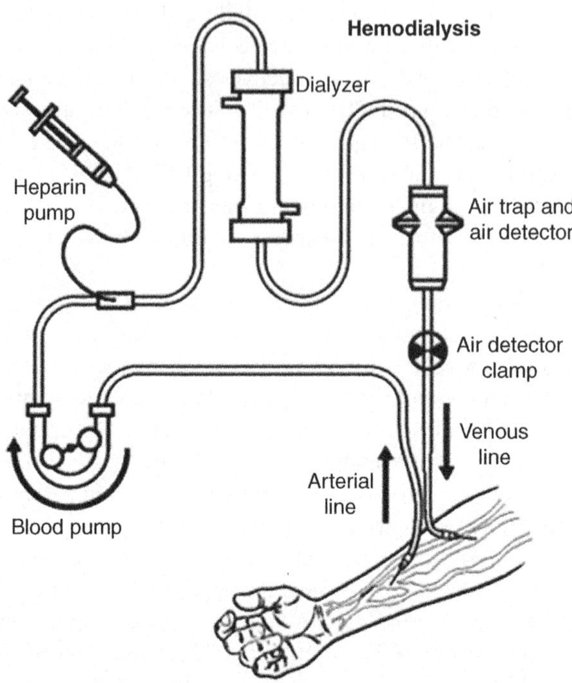

Fig. 23.1 Pathway of a patient's blood from arteriovenous access through the dialysis apparatus and back to patient. (With permissions from Pal [18])

pressure is set to match an individual patient's volume removal goal over the time course of a dialysis session. Synthetic tubing transports blood from the patient's dialysis access to the dialyzer and the back to the patient after leaving the dialyzer (Fig. 23.1). Dialysate solution contains water that must be purified to eliminate the risk of toxicities and infections. Reverse osmosis may be combined with deionization to purify water. Additionally, carbon filtration of water is used to remove chlorine and ammonia, which may be present in a municipal water supply and are not removed by reverse osmosis. Dialysate solution also contains sodium, potassium, calcium, magnesium, chloride, and glucose, and the buffer used most commonly is bicarbonate. The dialysis machine has a blood pump used to set the blood flow rate, followed by an air trap/detector to prevent air embolism. The machine also monitors venous pressures within the circuit as well as the dialysate temperature and urea clearance. The use of heparin or other anticoagulants to prevent blood clotting in the dialysis circuit is patient dependent [17]. The patient's blood pressure is also monitored at repeated intervals throughout treatment. Figure 23.2 demonstrates the entire dialysis circuit as described above.

Hemodialysis may be performed at home by the patient and caregivers or outside the home at an outpatient unit (also called "in-center" dialysis) by technicians and nurses. Home hemodialysis is performed more frequently, and sessions may be shorter compared to the typical in-center schedule of 3 days per week for 3–4 hours

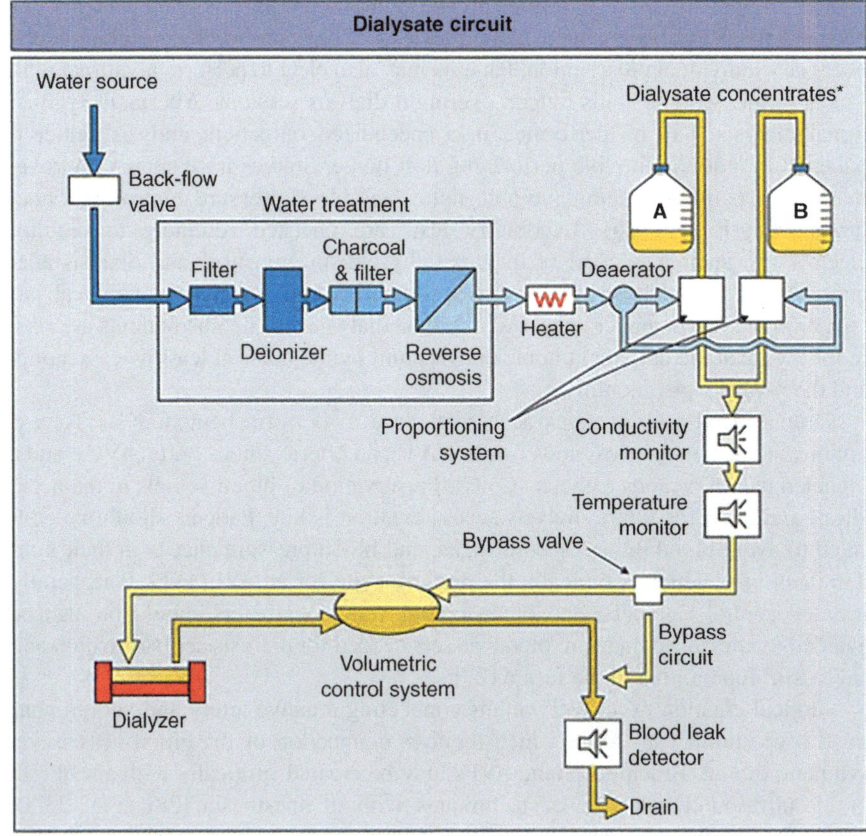

Fig. 23.2 Hemodialysis circuit. (With permissions from Ahmad [19])

each session. The "typical" in-center schedule is based on the HEMO study which showed similar mortality rates between standard dose and high dose based on clearance targets [20]. Subsequent studies have demonstrated that home hemodialysis provides better patient outcomes, including patient survival and quality of life as well as hypertension control with fewer antihypertensive medications compared with in-center hemodialysis [21, 22]. A United States Renal Data System (USRDS) database study showed that patients on home hemodialysis had a lower unadjusted risk of death compared with patients dialyzing in-center [23]. Studies from Europe, Australia, and New Zealand also indicate improved survival with home hemodialysis compared to in-center hemodialysis [24]. It is recommended that patients have a partner at home to assist with home hemodialysis and/or be available in case of emergency. Patients and partners undergo intensive daily training at an outpatient home dialysis unit with a hemodialysis nurse, who is supervised by a nephrologist. When a patient, nurse, and physician are comfortable with access cannulation and operating the dialysis equipment, then the home hemodialysis nurse travels to the patient's home to assist in setting up the home hemodialysis environment. The patient typically performs home hemodialysis 4–7 days per week depending on the necessary individual prescription. Patients may also elect to perform nocturnal dialysis at home, which entails longer, overnight dialysis sessions. Alternatively, nocturnal dialysis may be performed in a specialized outpatient dialysis center if patients are not comfortable performing it at home. Studies have shown improvements in hyperphosphatemia, volume status, and blood pressure control with nocturnal dialysis [25, 26]. Laboratory tests are checked routinely to monitor electrolytes, anemia, secondary hyperparathyroidism, nutrition, and dialysis adequacy for all hemodialysis patients. In-center patients are typically seen by a physician or physician extender once a week at the dialysis unit. Home patients are seen in follow-up at the outpatient home dialysis unit by the nurse at least twice a month and the nephrologist monthly.

Patients need arteriovenous access in place to perform hemodialysis. Access options include an arteriovenous fistula (AVF), an arteriovenous graft (AVG), and a tunneled central venous catheter (CVC). Preservation of blood vessels in the neck, chest, and arms for future dialysis access creation is key. Patients should be educated to avoid blood draws, needle sticks, and blood pressure checks in their non-dominant arm, which is typically the preferred site for an AVF/AVG. Peripherally inserted central catheters, and other central venous catheters should be also be avoided to alleviate damage to blood vessels needed for dialysis access creation and successful functioning in the future [27].

Surgical creation of an AVF entails connecting a native artery and vein in contrast to creation of an AVG, which requires connection of the blood vessels via synthetic tubing. Brachiocephalic AVFs may be created surgically with anesthesia or by ultrasound/endovascular techniques without anesthesia [28] (Fig. 23.3). Brachiobasilic fistulas and AVG creation require open surgical procedures with a regional nerve block or general anesthesia (Fig. 23.4). Patients with AVFs have the lowest risk of access failure and infectious complications; however, there is a risk of

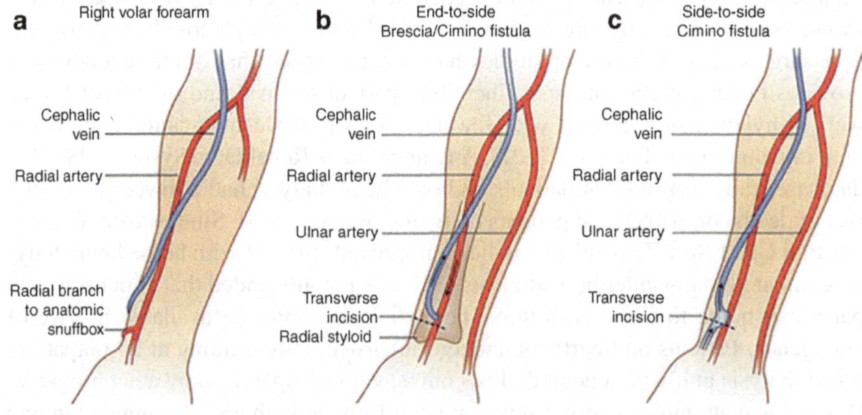

Fig. 23.3 Brachiocephalic arteriovenous fistulas. (With permissions from Marshalleck [29])

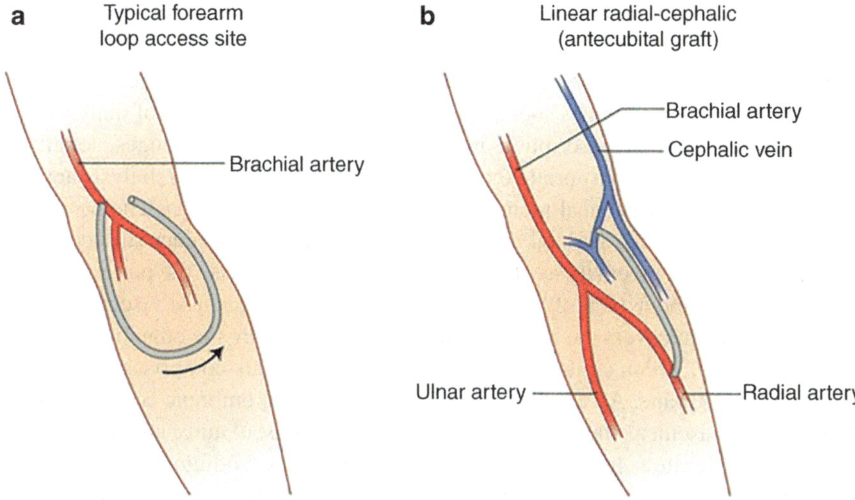

Fig. 23.4 Arteriovenous grafts. (With permissions from Marshalleck [29])

non-maturation, which requires subsequent access placement. Access thrombosis occurs more frequently in AVGs compared to AVFs. It is crucial that all potential access options available within the constraints of an individual patient's anatomy are explored prior to access creation in an attempt to ensure the longevity of the access. Patients should be made aware of the possibility of additional access creation in the future should the original access fail. Ideally, an AVF/AVG should be in place and ready to use prior to starting dialysis, to avoid the use of a CVC.

Patients with CVCs demonstrate a higher mortality risk compared to patients with AVFs/AVGs. Although the placement of a CVC does not require surgery, this type of access has the highest risk of complications, thus it is the least desirable [9]. CVC complications are often mechanical, but also include: low blood flow/thrombosis, damage to central veins, and infections. Mechanical complications include extruded cuffs, cracked lumens, and accidental dislodgement, which necessitate catheter removal and replacement. Infectious complications include exit site/tunnel infections and bloodstream infections [30]. Exit site and tunnel infections may present with erythema, pain, and swelling near the site of the catheter. Systemic symptoms indicating bacteremia often include fever and chills; patients may also demonstrate hemodynamic changes a during dialysis session. Infections are treated with systemic antibiotics. However, this may not successfully eradicate bacteria from a biofilm that can develop within the lumen of a catheter. Thus, patients require catheter change over a guidewire and/or complete catheter removal depending on the virulence and persistence of the organism. Bacteremia may lead to metastatic infections such as endocarditis, osteomyelitis, epidural abscess, and septic joints; all of which are associated with a high mortality [31]. Prophylactic use of topical antibiotics at catheter exit sites has been shown to decrease rates of bacteremia. Patients require adequate and repetitive education about proper hygiene and routine care of dialysis access to limit the risk of infection [32, 33]. Higher rates of death, cardiovascular events, and infections have been observed in patients who initiate dialysis with a CVC, rather than an AVF/AVG. Thus, every effort should be made to refer for vascular access placement as soon as possible prior to the initiation of dialysis.

Peritoneal dialysis prescription includes the number of exchanges, length of dwells, and choice of appropriate dialysate solution. The peritoneal dialysis apparatus consists of the peritoneal membrane and the dialysate solution. The peritoneal membrane includes the parietal and visceral peritoneum. The inner surface of the abdominal and pelvic cavity as well as the diaphragm comprise the parietal peritoneum, which is about 10% of the entire peritoneal membrane. The visceral portion of the peritoneum covers the intra-abdominal organs forming the omentum and visceral mesentery, which connects to loops of the bowel. This comprises 90% of the peritoneal membrane. At a cellular level, the peritoneal membrane contains mesothelial cells, basement membrane, interstitium, microvasculature, and lymphatics. Peritoneal dialysate solution is composed of electrolytes (sodium, potassium, calcium, and magnesium), a racemic mixture of D and L lactate as the buffer, and glucose or a glucose polymer as the osmotic agent. Solute transport occurs by diffusion. Factors affecting the transport of solutes include surface area and permeability of the PD membrane, dialysate flow, concentration gradients, and time. The molecular weight of solutes also affects the transport, which slows as weight increases. Ultrafiltration occurs via an osmotic gradient between blood and dialysate but is also affected by the transmembrane hydrostatic and oncotic pressure. Glucose leads to rapid ultrafiltration that decreases with time as glucose is absorbed in contrast with glucose polymers that permit constant but slower ultrafiltration without being absorbed. Solvent drag or convective transport may occur as well when solutes travel with fluid during ultrafiltration. Patients who are considered "slow transporters" have a "tighter" peritoneal membrane which permits glucose to diffuse out of the cavity more slowly, maintaining the osmotic gradient longer, allowing more ultrafiltration to occur. Patients who are considered "fast transporters" have a "leakier" peritoneal membrane which permits glucose to diffuse out of the cavity more quickly. This leads to a loss of the osmotic gradient and thus, less ultrafiltration occurs. It is also important to recognize that despite the goal of ultrafiltration with dialysis, absorption of fluid occurs continuously via the lymphatics. This absorption may be augmented by increased intra-abdominal pressure from regular activities of daily living. This is one reason that diligent preservation of residual renal function is crucial to aid in the maintenance of volume control in these patients [34, 35].

Continuous ambulatory peritoneal dialysis (CAPD) consists of multiple manual daytime exchanges with shorter dwell times and a longer overnight dwell (Fig. 23.5). Automated peritoneal dialysis (APD) consists of using a cycler machine that performs multiple nighttime exchanges with shorter dwell times. The last fill remains in the peritoneal cavity for prolonged daytime dwell. Alternatively, patients may perform a mid-day manual exchange, if necessary for additional solute clearance [34]. PD prescription should be modified to suit an individual patient's peritoneal membrane characteristics. This is determined by a peritoneal equilibration test (PET) performed 1 month after starting PD, which demonstrates the peritoneal

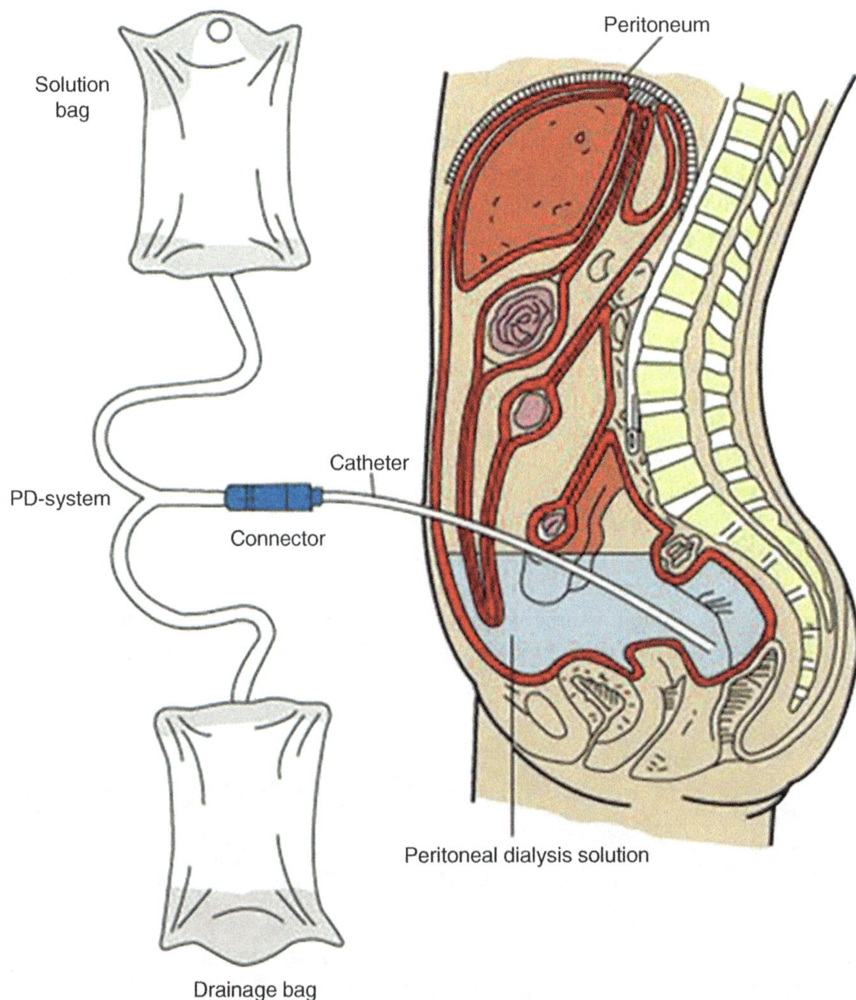

Fig. 23.5 CAPD apparatus. (With permissions from: Findlay and Isles [36])

membrane's rate of solute clearance and ultrafiltration [34, 37]. Patients may then be classified either as a "fast" or a "slow" transporter, thus affecting the length of dwells, number of exchanges, and content of dialysate fluid. PD prescription should also be modified based on a patient's residual renal function, which is determined by a 24-hour urine collection. Residual renal function assists with volume control, and thus, efforts should be made to preserve it. Urine output may be maximized with the use of loop diuretics. Studies have demonstrated similar patient outcomes in terms of mortality and risk of complications between CAPD and APD [38]. Patients undergo intensive daily training at an outpatient home dialysis unit with a peritoneal dialysis nurse, who is supervised by a nephrologist. When a patient, nurse, and physician are comfortable with the patient's ability to perform dialysis, then the peritoneal dialysis nurse travels to the patient's home to assist in setting up the peritoneal dialysis environment. Laboratory tests are checked routinely to monitor electrolytes, anemia, secondary hyperparathyroidism, nutrition, and dialysis adequacy. The patient is seen in follow-up at the outpatient PD unit by the nurse at least twice a month and the nephrologist monthly. Ideal candidates for PD include patients who have the desire, adequate residual renal function, minimal/lack of prior abdominal surgeries, adequate cognitive/physical ability, and a suitable home environment to store supplies. However, patients can dialyze successfully on PD with assistance from a caregiver at home even if cognitive or physical limitations exist [34].

Peritoneal dialysis requires the placement of a peritoneal dialysis catheter in the abdomen. This can be done by open or laparoscopic surgery and usually takes about 2 weeks to heal (Fig. 23.6). Urgent start PD may be an option in patients with newly diagnosed ESRD in need of dialysis, but without an absolute indication for emergency dialysis. This allows adequate time for the access to heal and may alleviate the need for a temporary hemodialysis catheter [34]. Percutaneous fluoroscopy-guided peritoneal catheter placement by interventional radiologists or nephrologists has been performed, but this technique is associated with higher rates of the late leak [40]. It is possible for surgeons to tunnel the catheter under the skin at the time of insertion so that the surgical site heals in advance of needing to start dialysis.

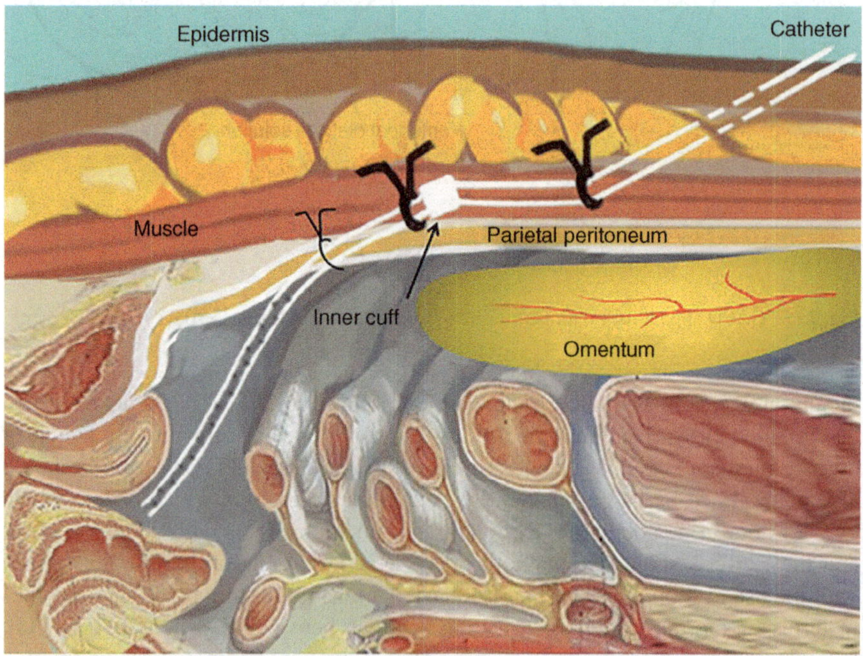

Fig. 23.6 Placement of peritoneal dialysis catheter. (With permissions from: Li et al. [39])

Tunneling the catheter under the skin at the time of insertion allows the catheter to be ready when needed without having to perform exit-site care and eliminates the risk of exit-site infection prior to catheter use. Once it is time to initiate dialysis, the surgeon can externalize the catheter with a skin incision creating an exit site [34]. This is typically located in the abdomen, but occasionally it may be in the chest due to a patient's body habitus. Catheters should be flushed with dialysate once a week to ensure patency until dialysis commences.

PD catheters require proper monitoring and care including routine exit site cleaning and topical antibiotic application for infectious prophylaxis. Patients are advised not to submerge PD catheter in water to avoid unnecessary risk of infection. Infectious complications include exit site or tunnel infection and peritonitis. Symptoms may include abdominal or back pain, bloating, fever, chills, erythema at the catheter exit site, and cloudy or bloody PD fluid. Infections often can be diagnosed clinically, but confirmation of organism with gram stain and culture of the exit site and/or PD fluid should be done to guide treatment. Exit site infection can usually be treated with systemic antibiotics alone. Tunnel infections typically require catheter removal and replacement. Peritonitis may be treated with intraperitoneal, intravenous, or oral antibiotics depending on the organism. Fungal peritonitis necessitates the removal of the PD catheter in addition to treatment with antifungal agents. Relapsing peritonitis is defined as recurrent infection with the same organism 4 weeks after completion of the antibiotic course. This should raise suspicion for the possibility of tunnel infection or intra-abdominal abscess [34, 35].

Noninfectious PD catheter complications include outflow failure, peri-catheter leak, catheter cuff extrusion, intestinal perforation, and bleeding. Outflow failure may be due to blockade due to high stool burden/constipation, malposition of the catheter tip, catheter kinking, intraluminal occlusion by thrombosis, and extraluminal occlusion by omentum or adhesions. Various types of hernias may develop including incisional (catheter site or other), ventral, umbilical, or inguinal hernias. Patients may also develop hypoalbuminemia due to the loss of albumin via the peritoneal membrane. Weight gain, hyperglycemia, and hypertriglyceridemia are also possible in the setting of increased caloric uptake from the dialysate solution [34, 35]. Thus, in diabetic patients, it is important to consider adjustments to medication regimen as needed for adequate glucose control.

Early referral to nephrology is necessary for patients who need to prepare for renal replacement therapy. Adequate time is needed to discuss whether dialysis is desired or appropriate. Patients benefit from dialysis modality education to assist in decision-making prior to initiation of dialysis. Uremia may interfere with cognitive function, thus advanced directives and communication of wishes with family and caregivers should be encouraged in advance of complete kidney failure. Referral for dialysis access evaluation and placement of access should occur prior to initiation of dialysis. Patients who are educated and play an active role in their treatment choices achieve better outcomes on dialysis [17]. Alternatively, early referral to nephrology also helps determine which patients will not gain any benefit from dialysis and assist with conservative management of ESRD, allowing patients to have dignity at the end of their lives.

References

1. United States Renal Data System. USRDS annual data report: epidemiology of kidney disease in the United States. Bethesda: National Institutes of Health, National Institute of Diabetes and Digestive and Kidney Diseases; 2018.
2. Foote C, Kotwal S, Gallagher M, Cass A, Brown M, Jardine M. Survival outcomes of supportive care versus dialysis therapies for elderly patients with end-stage kidney disease: a systematic review and meta-analysis. Nephrology (Carlton). 2016;21(3):241–53.
3. Roy D, Chowdhury AR, Pande S, Kam JW. Evaluation of unplanned dialysis as a predictor of mortality in elderly dialysis patients: a retrospective data analysis. BMC Nephrol. 2017;18:364.
4. Kidney Disease: Improving Global Outcomes. 2012 clinical practice guideline for the evaluation and management of chronic kidney disease. Kidney Int Suppl. 2013;3(1):5–14.
5. Tangri N, Stevens LA, Griffith J, Tighiouart H, Djurdjev O, Naimark D, et al. A predictive model for progression of chronic kidney disease to kidney failure. JAMA. 2011;305(15):1553–9.
6. Tangri N, Grams ME, Levey AS, Coresh K, Appel LJ, Astor BC, et al. Multinational assessment of accuracy of equations for predicting risk of kidney failure: a meta-analysis. JAMA. 2016;315(2):164–74.
7. Devoe DJ, Wong B, James MT, Ravani P, Oliver MJ, Barnieh L, et al. Patient education and peritoneal dialysis modality selection: a systematic review and meta-analysis. Am J Kidney Dis. 2016;68(3):422.
8. Fenton SS, Schaubel DE, Desmeules M, Morrison HI, Mao Y, Copleston P, et al. Hemodialysis versus peritoneal dialysis: a comparison of adjusted mortality rates. Am J Kidney Dis. 1997;30(3):334–42.
9. Liem YS, Wong JB, Hunink MG, de Charro FT, Winkelmayer WC. Comparison of hemodialysis and peritoneal dialysis survival in the Netherlands. Kidney Int. 2007;71(2):153–8.
10. McDonald SP, Marshall MR, Johnson DW, Polinghorne KR. Relationship between dialysis modality and mortality. J Am Soc Nephrol. 2009;20(1):155–63.
11. Wolfe RA, Ashby VB, Milford EL, Ojo AO, Ettenger RE, Agodoa LY, et al. Comparison of mortality in all patients on dialysis awaiting transplantation, and recipients of a first cadaveric transplant. N Engl J Med. 1999;341(23):1725–30.
12. Lok CE, Davidson I. Optimal choice of dialysis access for chronic kidney disease patients: developing a life plan for dialysis access. Semin Nephrol. 2012;32(6):530–7.
13. Moss AH, Ganjoo J, Sharma S, Gansor J, Senft S, Weaner B, et al. Utility of the "surprise" questions to identify dialysis patients with high mortality. Clin J Am Soc Nephrol. 2008;3(5):1379–84.
14. Tamura MK, Covinsky KE, Chertow GM, Yaffe K, Landefeld CS, McCulloch CE. Functional status of elderly adults before and after initiation of dialysis. N Engl J Med. 2009;361:1539–47.
15. Kallenberg MH, Kleinveld HA, Dekker FW, van Munster BC, Rabelink TJ, van Buren M, et al. Functional and cognitive impairment, frailty, and adverse health outcomes in older patients reaching ESRD-A systematic review. Clin J Am Soc Nephrol. 2016;11(9):1624–39.
16. Holley JL. Advance care planning in CKD/ESRD: an evolving process. Clin J Am Soc Nephrol. 2012;7(6):1033–8.
17. Yeun JY, Ornt DB, Depner TA. Hemodialysis. In: Taal MW, Chertow GM, Marsden PA, Skorecki K, Yu ASL, Brenner BM, editors. Brenner & rector's the kidney. 9th ed. Philadelphia: Elsevier; 2012. p. 2295–325.
18. Pal S. The kidney and its artificial replacement. In: Design of artificial human joints & organs. Boston: Springer; 2014.
19. Ahmad S. Hemodialysis technique. In: Manual of clinical dialysis. Boston: Springer; 2009.
20. Eknoyan G, Beck GJ, Cheung AK, Daugirdas JT, Greene T, Kusek JW, et al. Effect of dialysis dose and membrane flux in maintenance hemodialysis. N Engl J Med. 2002;347(25):2010–9.
21. Finkelstein FO, Finkelstein SH, Wuerth D, Shirani S, Troidle L. Effects of home hemodialysis on health-related quality of life measures. Semin Dial. 2007;20(3):265–8.

22. McGregor DO, Buttimore AL, Lynn KL, Nicholis MG, Jardine DLA. Comparative study of blood pressure control with short in-center versus long home hemodialysis. Blood Purif. 2001;19(3):293–300.

23. Woods JD, Port FK, Stannard D, Blagg CR, Held PJ. Comparison of mortality with home hemodialysis and center hemodialysis: a national study. Kidney Int. 1996;49(5):1464–70.

24. Marshall MR, Hawley CM, Kerr PG, Polkinghorne KR, Marshall RJ, Agar JW, et al. Home hemodialysis and mortality risk in Australian and New Zealand populations. Am J Kidney Dis. 2011;58(5):782–93.

25. Rocco MV, Lockridge RS Jr, Beck GJ, Eggers PW, Gassman JJ, Greene T, et al. The effects of frequent nocturnal home hemodialysis: the frequent hemodialysis network nocturnal trial. Kidney Int. 2011;80(10):1080–91.

26. Daugirdas JT, Chertow GM, Larive B, Pierratos A, Greene T, Ayus JC, et al. Effects of frequent hemodialysis on measures of CKD mineral and bone disorder. J Am Soc Nephrol. 2012;23(4):727–38.

27. Hoggard J, Saad T, Schon D, Vesely TM, Royer T. Guidelines for venous access in patients with chronic kidney disease. A position statement from the American Society of Diagnostic and Interventional Nephrology, Clinical Practice Committee and the Association for Vascular Access. Semin Dial. 2008;21(2):186–91.

28. Hull JE, Jennings WC, Cooper RI, Waheed U, Schaefer ME, Narayan R. The pivotal multi-center trial of ultrasound-guided percutaneous arteriovenous fistula creation for hemodialysis access. J Vasc Interv Radiol. 2018;29(2):149–58.

29. Marshalleck FE. Hemodialysis graft and fistula access and intervention. In: Temple M, Marshalleck F, editors. Pediatric interventional radiology. New York: Springer; 2014.

30. Poinen K, Quinn RR, Clarke A, Ravani P, Hiremath S, Miller LM, et al. Complications from tunneled hemodialysis catheters:a Canadian observational cohort study. Am J Kidney Dis. 2019;73(4):467–75.

31. Allon M. Dialysis catheter-related bacteremia: treatment and prophylaxis. Am J Kidney Dis. 2004;44(5):779–91.

32. Arhuidese IJ, Orandi BJ, Nejim B, Malas M. Utilization, patency, and complications associated with vascular access for hemodialysis in the United States. J Vasc Surg. 2018;68(4):1166–74.

33. Ravani P, Palmer SC, Oliver MJ, Quinn RR, MacRae JM, Tai DJ, et al. Associations between hemodialysis access type and clinical outcomes: a systematic review. J Am Soc Nephrol. 2013;24(3):465–73.

34. Teitelbaum I, Burkart J. Peritoneal dialysis. Am J Kidney Dis. 2003;42(5):1082–96.

35. Correa-Rotter R, Cueto-Manzano A, Khanna R. Peritoneal dialysis. In: Taal MW, Chertow GM, Marsden PA, Skorecki K, Yu ASL, Brenner BM, editors. Brenner & rector's the kidney. 9th ed. Philadelphia: Elsevier; 2012. p. 2347–60.

36. Findlay M, Isles C. Peritoneal dialysis. In: Clinical companion in nephrology. Cham: Springer; 2015.

37. Pannekeet MM, Imholz AL, Struijk DG, Koomen GC, Langedijk MJ, Schouten N, et al. The standard peritoneal permeability analysis: a tool for the assessment of peritoneal permeability characteristics in CAPD patients. Kidney Int. 1995;48(3):866–75.

38. Rabindranath KS, Adams J, Ali TZ, MacLeod AM, Vale L, Cody J, et al. Continuous ambulatory peritoneal dialysis versus automated peritoneal dialysis for end-stage renal disease. Cochrane Database Syst Rev. 2007;2:CD006515.

39. Li Y, Zhu Y, Liang Z, Zheng X, Zhang H, Zhu W. A Simple modified open peritoneal dialysis catheter insertion procedure reduces the need for secondary surgery. Int Urol Nephrol. 2019;51(4):729–36.

40. Moon JY, Song S, Jung KH, Park M, Lee SH, Ihm CG, et al. Fluoroscopically guided peritoneal dialysis catheter placement: long-term results from a single center. Perit Dial Int. 2008;28(2):163–9.

Chapter 24
Preemptive Kidney Transplant: An Alternative to Dialysis

Goni Katz-Greenberg and Pooja Singh

Introduction

There are two available options for renal replacement therapy (RRT) – chronic dialysis (either hemodialysis or peritoneal dialysis) and kidney transplantation.

Kidney transplantation is the treatment of choice for patients with ESRD. Compared with dialysis, kidney transplantation is associated with improved patient survival, improved quality of life, and lower costs [1, 2].

According to the United States Renal Data System (USRDS) on 12/31/2017, there were 746,557 individuals with ESRD living in the United States. Of these, 69.8% were on chronic dialysis, and 29.9% had a functioning kidney allograft. This represents more than a 90% increase in ESRD prevalence since 2000 and is the result of increasing incident cases but also of longer survival among patients with ESRD [3].

Prior to the 1970s, both dialysis and kidney transplantations were of limited utility in the United States and the world at large. There were only a few dialysis facilities available, and patients had to undergo substantial screening prior to treatment initiation. Kidney transplantation was its in infancy, with the first successful transplant performed in 1954 between identical twins by Dr. Joseph Murray [4]. This was followed by an increase in the number of kidney transplantations done in the United States in the 1960s with the introduction of the first immunosuppression regimen with mercaptopurine (6-MP), radiation, and corticosteroids, which made it possible to use non-immunologic identical deceased donors [5]. One of the major government

G. Katz-Greenberg (✉)
Division of Nephrology, Department of Medicine, Duke University School of Medicine, Durham, NC, USA
e-mail: goni.katzgreenberg@duke.edu

P. Singh
Division of Nephrology, Department of Medicine, Thomas Jefferson University Hospital, Philadelphia, PA, USA
e-mail: goni.katzgreenberg@duke.edu; pooja.singh@jefferson.edu

© Springer Nature Switzerland AG 2022
J. McCauley et al. (eds.), *Approaches to Chronic Kidney Disease*,
https://doi.org/10.1007/978-3-030-83082-3_24

legislations in the United States, which increased prevalence of both chronic dialysis and kidney transplantation, was the passage of Medicare End Stage Renal Disease Program in 1972. This program enabled any patient with ESRD to qualify for Medicare regardless of their age and has since saved the lives of hundreds of thousands of patients. This program was broadened in 1978 to cover the cost of posttransplant care from 1 to 3 years [6]. A factor which led to an improvement in transplant outcome was the emergent of a new immunosuppressive medication, cyclosporine, which was first of its class of calcineurin inhibitors. With its use, acute rejection rates dropped below 50%, and 1-year graft survival exceeded 85%. As the number of kidney transplantations continued to increase, more data emerged establishing kidney transplantation as the treatment of choice for patients with ESRD with improved patient and allograft survival, better quality of life, and reduced costs compared to chronic dialysis [7, 8]. Further progress included the development and broad use of additional medications, for both induction (i.e., anti-thymocyte globulin and basiliximab), and for maintenance (i.e., tacrolimus and sirolimus), further improving 1-year graft survival rates to more than 90%, with lower rejection rates.

The most prevalent type of kidney transplantation, accounting for about two thirds, is deceased donor kidney transplantation (DDKT), with living donor kidney transplantations (LDKT) accounting for the remaining third [9]. LDKT have been proven superior to DDKT, with a 6-month and 10-year all-cause graft failure only 1.4% and 34.1%, respectively. While the number of DDKTs has increased in recent decades, the number of LDKT has initially remained stable [10], with less than 6000 kidney transplants yearly, until 2017, when it has started to steadily rise to 6184 LDKT in 2017, 6850 LDKT in 2018, and 7370 LDKT in 2019 [9].

Another differentiating factor between types of transplantations is timing. The timing of transplantation can be either after the patient was initiated on chronic dialysis, which is the majority of cases, or prior to dialysis initiation, which is referred to as preemptive kidney transplantation (PKT). PKT have been proven superior to transplantation done after patients are on chronic dialysis, with PKT recipients having a 5–10% better 5-year survival benefit [11, 12]. Timing of the kidney transplant is strongly influenced by recipient circumstance, with PKT showing both a survival advantage and a financial advantage.

For patients to be considered for a PKT, they must first be referred to a transplant center and undergo a thorough evaluation. Late referral may reduce the chance of patient to undergo a PKT, as they will not have sufficient time to complete the work-up.

The continuous severe organ shortage is a major limiting factor for the number of kidney transplantations performed annually. In 2017, there were 20,945 kidney transplantations preformed in the United States. While this number represents a small but steady increase in the number of kidney transplantations, the gap between the number who receive a kidney transplantation to those on the waiting list remains significant with 75,745 dialysis patients on the kidney transplant wait list as of December 31, 2017 [13].

Prior to 2014, patients received a transplant based on the time spent on the waiting list. This led to ethnic and socioeconomic disparities in access to transplantations as certain groups, such as African Americans and Hispanics, were not referred

Table 24.1 Donor variables included in KDPI donor calculation [14]

Demographics	Medical history	Death related
Age	History of hypertension	Cause of death
Height	History of diabetes	DCD donor
Weight	HCV status	
Ethnicity/race		

to transplant centers as much as their White counterparts, thereby having less access to the kidney transplant waiting list [11].

In 2014, the new kidney allocation system (KAS) was introduced with the goals of increasing the longevity-matching by using a new allocation tool – Kidney Donor Profile Index (KDPI). The KDPI looks at multiple donor factors and translates them into a single number (percentage) which correlates to the likelihood of graft failure following a DDKT (Table 24.1). Allocation advantage was given on a sliding scale to patients who had increased level of sensitization, thereby increasing availability of organs to patients with the highest calculated panel-reactive antibody (CPRA) and taking in account the time patients spent on dialysis prior to being referred for transplantation as part of their wait time for a kidney transplant [15].

Several studies following the new KAS have shown that the new allocation system has improved some of long-standing disparities in listing; however, equity of access to kidney transplantation, in general, and to PKT remains an issue even post implementation of the new kidney allocation system (KAS) in 2014 [16].

This is also true in regard to access to LDKT, as not all patients have the same access to LDKT. In fact, according to the OPTN/SRTR 2017 annual report, only 12.5% of LDKT in 2017 were performed in black recipients, while 32.6% of candidates in 2017 were black. In contrast, 65.9% of transplant recipients of living donation were white, though they made up only 36.2% of the waiting list.

Renal Replacement Therapies

There are two main modalities of renal replacement therapy once patients reach ESRD – dialysis (either hemodialysis or peritoneal dialysis) and kidney transplantation.

A minority of patients may have significant comorbidities which preclude them from benefiting from any form of RRT or may opt to not pursue any. Initiation of chronic dialysis is a complex decision which should be made jointly by the patient, their family, and the physician. In fact, this is one of the five performance criteria of the choosing wisely initiative in nephrology [17].

As medical professionals, the goal is that all patients with chronic kidney disease, stage 3 and above, regardless of the etiology of their chronic kidney disease (CKD), would establish care under a nephrologist. This would not only enhance medical care but would allow a thorough discussion about the different renal replacement modalities available and more importantly, kidney transplantation.

However, many patients are seen for the first time by a nephrologist only upon diagnosis of ESRD. In fact, based on USRDS annual data report, in 2017 33.4% of incident ESRD patients received little to no pre-ESRD nephrology care [13].

Late referral to a nephrologist is associated with higher morbidity and worse long-term outcomes [18]. Not surprisingly, when patients are referred late in the disease course, they experience worse access to transplantation in general, and especially to PKT, as they will not have sufficient time to undergo a timely transplant evaluation [19].

Dialysis Initiation

Nephrologists use a combination laboratory and clinical parameters to assess the need for initiation of dialysis. These include estimated glomerular filtration rate (eGFR) value, and the presence of one or more signs or symptoms attributable to kidney failure (uremia, pericarditis, anorexia, medically resistant acid-base or electrolyte abnormalities, reduced energy level, weight loss with no other potential explanation, intractable pruritus, or bleeding) or an inability to control volume status or blood pressure.

When dialysis initiation is done without proper preparation, these patients are at high risk for 90 days mortality from coronary artery disease and access-related issues such as sepsis.

Even if patients do have pre-ESRD care, the overall survival of patients on chronic hemodialysis is 78% at 1 year, 57% at 3 years, and only 42% at 5 years [13].

This amplifies the importance of pre-ESRD care, including early referral to a kidney transplantation center. When patients are referred and evaluated for PKT, the complications noted above can be avoided. Once a patient manifests early uremic symptoms and signs, the transplant team with patient and family can move forward with the PKT, especially if a live donor who completed the work-up is available.

Referrals and Kidney Transplantations

In the United States, a patient can be listed actively on the waiting list once their GFR is 20 ml/min/1.73 m^2 or lower. However, if we take into account the thorough evaluation and battery of tests as part of the work-up that these patients need to undergo before being listed, it is important to refer them to a transplant center earlier rather than later.

Optimally, once a patient reach CKD stage 4 and seems to be progressing, a referral to a kidney transplant center should be made [20].

Once referred, patient will undergo extensive work-up which is based on their different comorbidities, as well as the specific center's protocols. Following the work-up, most centers will discuss the patients in a multidisciplinary forum which can include nephrologist, transplant surgeons, coordinators, social workers, financial coordinators, and dieticians. In addition, other consultants are involved in the process, as necessitated by the patient's specific comorbidities.

There are few absolute contraindications for kidney transplantations which are listed in Table 24.2. Other relative contraindications such as BMI cutoff, or length of follow-up time after treatment of a malignancy, are mainly derived from expert opinion and can be adopted by the different transplant centers. There is no consensus on the exclusion of potential recipients based on age, and there is evidence showing survival benefit following a kidney transplant even in advanced age. Most centers will evaluate potential candidates based on their medical status, rather than chronological age.

Following the evaluation, if suitable, patient would be listed for a transplant on the deceased donor waiting list.

The median waiting time on the deceased donor waiting list in the United States is 3.9 years and greatly depends on the geographic location where the patient is listed [21]. Approximately a third of transplant candidates will die waiting for a kidney transplantation or will be removed from the waiting list if they become too sick to undergo the surgery [10].

Unfortunately, only 14% patients with incidence ESRD will be placed on the waiting list or receive a kidney within a year of being diagnosed with ESRD [22].

Another preferred option for kidney transplant is a living donor kidney transplant (LDKT), which has been shown in multiple studies to be associated with better patient and allograft survival.

After more than a decade of decline in the number of LDKT, their numbers increased in 2017 and 2018. However, LDKT still represent a small part of total transplants [23]. Transplant centers should educate patients and their families about the benefits of LDKT and encourage patients to explore the possibility of living donation.

Kidney transplantations are not only associated with better outcomes, with decreased morbidity and mortality compared to dialysis, but they also have a significant financial advantage. Based on USRDS data, in 2017 the total Medicare expenditure per ESRD person was 91,795 for hemodialysis, 78,159 for peritoneal dialysis, and 35,817 for kidney transplant (all costs in US dollars) [13].

Table 24.2 Absolute contraindications for kidney transplantation

Active infection
Active malignancy
Active substance abuse
Chronic illness/comorbidity with a life expectancy of under 1 year
Uncontrolled psychosis

Preemptive Kidney Transplantation

Preemptive kidney transplantation refers to transplantation prior to dialysis initiation.

Whether from a deceased donor, or from a living donor, PKT has shown a benefit in allograft survival.

The advantages of PKT include lack of exposure to dialysis, avoidance of dialysis-related morbidity and mortality, and avoidance of access issues and related complications [24]. Finally, from a financial standpoint, Medicare expenditure on dialysis patients is 2.5 times the expenditure on transplant patients per year.

In an Internet survey sent to US-based nephrologists, 71% of 460 analyzed responses (of 5901 surveys sent), stated that PKT is the best form of therapy for patients nearing ESRD. However, about a quarter of responders also mentioned that nephrologists and mainly dialysis centers lose revenue when patients are referred to PKT [21].

Unfortunately, many times patients are first seen by a nephrologist when in an already very advanced stage of CKD, which does not allow enough time for referral, work-up, listing, and subsequent PKT, prior to patients requiring initiation of dialysis.

The length of dialysis exposure has been adversely linked to worse allograft and patient outcomes following a kidney transplant. This is one of the major advantages of PKT, where patients are spared dialysis exposure [25].

Given the organ shortage, and prolonged waiting time on the deceased donor waiting list, most patients will experience a period of dialysis pretransplant, even if listed preemptively. However, these patients will likely have a substantial less time on dialysis, thereby maintaining some of the survival benefit associated with PKT [26].

Patients who receive a DDKT following a prolonged exposure to dialysis have increased graft loss and mortality than patients who undergo PKT or early DDKT (i.e., listed preemptively).

There have been many hypotheses surrounding the allograft survival benefit seen in PKT. In a large retrospective study of 40,000 kidney transplant recipients, of which 27% of living donor transplants were done preemptively (2999) and 10% of deceased donor transplants were preemptive (2967), the authors concluded that the allograft survival benefit stems from patient selection or reduced burden of complications and comorbidities associated with uremia and dialysis [27].

In the year prior to the implementation of KAS, 942 (8.7%) of the total number of deceased donor kidney transplantation were done preemptively. In the first year after KAS, this number dropped to 631 (5.7%) of total number. This decrease is probably related to the large number of patients on the waiting list getting credit for time on dialysis prior to being referred for transplantation. On a following report from King et al. [16] summarizing the pre-KAS period from 2000 to 2013 and the post-KAS period from 2015 to 2018, the rate of preemptive deceased donor kidney transplantation rose slightly from 9.0 to 9.8% of the total number of transplantations.

While some believe that PKT can benefit any patient, others believe some patient groups may not be able to reap the benefits associated with PKT [24–26]. While superior outcomes with a first PKT are well-known, not much is known about patients getting a repeat KT preemptively (i.e., once their allograft is close to failing). Although previous reports have not shown an advantage for this patient population, a recently published multicenter French cohort study showed better graft survival in a second preemptive transplant as well. Furthermore, the beneficial effect was more pronounced in the deceased donor PKT subset, compared to living donor PKT [28].

Timing of Preemptive Transplantation

It has long been proven that long wait times on dialysis adversely affect graft and patient survival posttransplant [29]. However, there remains a controversy regarding optimal time of a PKT. Some believe that PKT done too early precludes maximizing the use of the native kidney function [30] and expose the recipients to the risks of the operation and subsequent immunosuppressive regimens prematurely [31]. On the other hand, restoration of kidney function may slow cardiovascular progression, associated with advanced CKD, thereby decreasing cardiovascular associated morbidity and mortality. In their study spanning 15 years, Grams et al. [32] found a strong trend toward "early" PKT (eGFR > 15 ml/min/1.73m^2) over "late" (eGFR < 10 ml/min/1.73m^2). In 19,471 PKT recipients between 1995 and 2009, eGFR was 9.2 ml/min/1.73 m^2 in 1995 and 13.8 ml/min/1.73 m^2 in 2009 (p < 0.001). Furthermore, 9.2% of PKT were transplanted in 1995 with eGFR > 15 ml/min/1.73 m^2, whereas this proportion rose to 34.7% in 2009. A more striking increase was also shown with PKT performed in recipients with eGFR > 10 ml/min/1.73 m^2, 30.0% in 1995 to 72.4% in 2009. Analysis of transplantation outcomes in this cohort of patients did not demonstrate any advantage of "early" PKT compared to "late" PKT in terms of graft function and survival and patient survival.

This trend for "early" PKT is probably driven by the overall data pointing to the benefits of PKT as compared to transplantation after dialysis initiation. PKT was reported to have better outcomes in patients and graft survival, better quality of life, and lower overall cost [30, 33]. These results combined with the "Kidney First Initiative from 2012" positioned PKT as the optimal renal replacement therapy for ESRD [24, 34, 35]. However, the optimal timing for PKT remains an open question. "Early" PKTs can result in transplantation of patients who probably have enough residual renal function to maintain them for a period of time without dialysis or a kidney transplantation. Furthermore, allocating a deceased donor allograft for "early" PKT may deprive this allograft from a recipient on dialysis who is on the waiting list whose need for transplantation is not debatable. The residual kidney function in "early" PKT not only can sustain the patients for a longer period of time without transplantation, but it may decline with PKT [31, 36].

The benefits of PKT are well established; however, an important question remains of whether these benefits can be maintained in patients who are transplanted only after short period of dialysis. If the advantages are maintained even after a short course of dialysis, one can argue that initiation of dialysis is a more defined and justified time point for deciding on transplantation. In a large observational study, of 121,853 DDKT performed between 1995 to 2011, 10,992 received a PKT and 14,428 received an early (within 1 year of initiation of dialysis) kidney transplantation. Although no difference was observed in patient survival, graft survival was better in the PKT recipients (early recipients had 23% high risk of graft loss compared to PKT, $p < 0.001$) [37].

Practical and Policy Considerations of Preemptive Kidney Transplantation

The clear benefits of kidney transplantation, on the one hand, and the critical shortage of organs, on the other hand, are the basis for an ongoing ethical and policy discussions for creating an allocation system with the right balance between utility and justice. The kidney allocation system evolved over the last few years from a "justice" concept where time on the waiting list was the main determining factor and as such promotes equity in kidney allocation, to the new KAS which adopted a more "utility" concept in which 20% of the best allograft are allocated to the 20% of recipients with the higher chance of survival post transplantation. The new KAS implemented also a "justice" element by granting time waiting to the length of ESRD before the time point of listing for transplantation. This approach was aimed to address some of the disparities in access to nephrology care and transplantation waiting list especially between certain ethnic groups.

The challenges of maintaining and improving an allocation system that addresses both justice and utility are mounting when assessing the concept and practice of PKT, especially when addressing PKT in the contest of deceased donor transplantation.

Access to Preemptive Deceased Donor Kidney Transplantation

Only about a quarter of the patients on dialysis therapy are listed for kidney transplantation and of those only about 20% are being transplanted yearly.

The OPTN Final Rule [38] called for initiatives to increase organ availability and to improve the utility and fairness of the allocation system. In December of 2014, after years of comprehensive deliberations the new kidney allocation system (KAS) was implemented [39] with the goals of better utilization of a scare resource, increasing access to transplantation, improving outcomes, and reducing disparities in access to transplantation.

With the new KAS striking a modified balance between utility and equity by prioritizing recipients with the best probability of survival, PKT seems as an attractive undertaking due to its agreed upon benefits compared to transplantation on dialysis. The positive potential of PKT was clearly recognized in the Healthy People 2020 initiative of the DHHS in which objective CKD-13.2 is "Increase the proportion of patients who receive a preemptive transplant at the start of ESRD" [40]. The obvious question to be asked at this time is whether the new KAS provided a system which increases the number of the PKT and the access to PKT and decreases the different disparities of those who are receiving PKT.

In a large observational study of 121,853 first time adult DDKT recipients done before the implementation of KAS (1995–2011), PKT was performed in 10,992 (9%) recipients. Within these patients, disparity in receiving PKT was clearly demonstrated. African American compared to Caucasians had a lower likelihood of PKT. Also, older patients, females, having private insurance, were all associated with higher chance to receive PKT [37]. Race disparity in access to health care may have been one of the reasons for the lower probability of African American to receive PKT. One can therefore conclude that PKT is a reflection for overall a better access to health care: early diagnosis of ESRD, early listing, and overall better care. The better chance for older patients to receive PKT underscore this notion as these older patients are covered by Medicare which provide an easier and direct access to health care.

Immediately following the implementation of the new KAS, there was a decline in deceased donor PKT. This was an expected decline, as patients were given prioritization for any pre-listing time on dialysis [41, 42].

Does the new KAS increase the number of PKT and reduces known access disparities? Actually, the answer to both of these is probably negative. Another large observation study [16] compared the data related to PKT before and after the implementation of the new KAS. PKT was performed in 10,045 (9%) recipients of total DDKT performed in 111,153 recipients before the new KAS (2000–2013) and in 3603 (10%) of a total of DDKT performed in 36,584 recipients after the new KAS (2015–2018). The mild increase in proportion of patients receiving PKT was mainly attributed to increase rate of PKT among white recipients. Furthermore, adjusted comparative analysis revealed persistence disparities in access to PKT. Non-white, younger patients, males, lower education, and nonprivate insurance all had a lower probability of having PKT. These observations in the PKT population contrast with the finding that racial disparities in DDKT on dialysis were reduced after the implementation of KAS [43]. In addition, in the era of the new KAS, the median waiting time on the list for PKT was increased probably due to the points given to patients on dialysis, which translates to time since dialysis initiation, even if were not listed at that time.

Further future system changes are required to increase access for PKT and to decreased existing disparities. Changes in healthcare system may have a positive impact on PKT as shown with the implementation of the Medicaid expansion under the Affordable Care Act, which resulted in increase in PKT [44]. Education of patients, caregivers, and healthcare policy makers should improve understanding and managing of ESRD with early referral to nephrology facilities with expertise in the care of these patients and with awareness of the positive potential of PKT.

In the new KAS era high proportion of recipients with EPTS < 20% receive PKT compared to non-preemptive recipients, and the use of kidneys with KDPI > 85% was lower in the PKT compared to the non-preemptive [16]. These findings support the goal of higher utility of a scared resource by implementing PKT as a preferred option of kidney transplantation in a recipient with a better chance to benefit from a higher quality organ. Hence, PKT may be the best option to achieve some of the main goals of the new KAS by improving the utility and the outcomes of kidney transplantation. However, the data regarding PKT in the new KAS era is disappointing as no increase in the number of PKT performed and persisting disparities were evident. Therefore, an important medical and policy question should be raised at this time. Should the new KAS be modified going forward to give priority for PKT? It seems clear that increasing the number of PKT and increasing the access to PKT to all patients is a goal reflected well with the Kidney First, Healthy People 2020, and Trump administration initiatives and seems justified based on the accumulative data of the benefits of PKT as compared to transplantation on dialysis. The possibility of granting priority for PKT should be discussed thoroughly within the transplantation community and policy makers. The ethical justification for such a change should also be discussed and considered. In essence the ethical principle related to this issue is the "principle of double effect" [45] which assesses the balance of doing something good (PKT) versus doing something bad (depriving patient on dialysis from a potential donor). As discussed above the new KAS moved on the ethical axis more toward utility than equity and introducing a priority for PKT would move at the same direction. If priority is considered, a strict and clear set of rules defining who is listed for PKT and when is a mandatory requirement to assure equity and fairness among patients. The degree of priority as related to other factors determining priority on the transplantation waiting list should be a subject of deliberations and agreement. If implemented the goal of increasing the number of PKT will hopefully be achieved with improvement in transplantation outcomes and reduction in overall cost for the care of these patients.

Living Donor PKT

LDKT are associated with a shorter wait time to transplantation and superior outcomes. As previously discussed, after years in which the numbers of LDKT remained stable, there has been a positive increase in the last couple of years. However, only a third of living donor transplants in the United States are performed preemptively, and this proportion has not changed in over 15 years. When looking at the characteristics of recipients of LDKT, similar disparities in access to care and race are seen, and LD PKT recipients are more likely to be white, female, older, and more educated and hold private insurance [16]. The timing considerations of PKT in living donation should be the same as in DD to assure appropriate use of a precious "gift" and avoid pre-matured risks for the living donor and the recipient. In the contest of nonrelated living donor and using the chain living donor transplantation, adherence to the appropriate principles of determining the need and timing for PKT would preserve the integrity of the system and allows for maximal utilization of living donation and PKT.

On July 10, 2019, President Donald J. Trump issued a presidential executive order on advancing American kidney health. Several sections of this order are aimed to improve access and numbers of kidney transplantations – doubling the organs available for transplant by 2030, remove financial barriers to living organ donation, and setting a benchmark that 80% of patients with incidence ESRD in 2025 should be on either home dialysis or receiving a kidney transplant [46]. Only time will tell how these new provisions will change the landscape of kidney transplantation in the United States, but the hopes is that one major benefit will be that living donors will not face the financial burden that may be associated with donation, such as missing work, traveling expenses, childcare expenses, etc. Hopefully this order will help increase the number of LDKT in the United States and thereby also increase the number of PKT, resulting in improved morbidity and mortality for our patients.

Future Perspectives

Longer time is required to assess how the kidney allocation system, introduced just over 5 years ago would affect the landscape of preemptive transplantation long term. This is also true in regard to the effects of the executive order on PKT.

Looking into the future, the potential of the successful development of kidney xenotransplantation, with the possibility of almost unlimited supply of kidney xenografts, may make preemptive kidney transplantation the treatment of choice for patients with CKD stage 5 [47], with chronic dialysis becoming a part of medical history.

Disclaimers The data and analyses reported in the 2017 and 2018 Annual Data Report of the US Organ Procurement and Transplantation Network and the Scientific Registry of Transplant Recipients have been supplied by the United Network for Organ Sharing and the Hennepin Healthcare Research Institute under contract with HHS/HRSA. The authors alone are responsible for reporting and interpreting these data; the views expressed herein are those of the authors and not necessarily those of the US government.

References

1. Wolfe RA, Ashby VB, Milford EL, et al. Comparison of mortality in all patients on dialysis, patients on dialysis awaiting transplantation, and recipients of a first cadaveric transplant. N Engl J Med. 1999;341(23):1725–30. http://content.nejm.org/cgi/content/abstract/341/23/1725. https://doi.org/10.1056/NEJM199912023412303.
2. Friedewald JJ, Reese PP. The kidney-first initiative: what is the current status of preemptive transplantation? Adv Chronic Kidney Dis. 2012;19(4):252–6. https://www.clinicalkey.es/playcontent/1-s2.0-S1548559512000961. https://doi.org/10.1053/j.ackd.2012.05.001.

3. United States Renal Data System. 2019 annual data report: epidemiology of kidney disease in the United States; executive summary; Bethesda, National Institutes of Health, National Institute of Diabetes and Digestive and Kidney Diseases. 2018;8(10):1–64.

4. Knepper MA, Feature Editor. Milestones in nephrology. J Am Soc Nephrol. 2001;12:201–4.

5. Starzl TE. History of clinical transplantation. World J Surg. 2000;24(7):759–82. https://www.ncbi.nlm.nih.gov/pubmed/10833242. https://doi.org/10.1007/s002680010124.

6. Eggers PW. Medicare's end stage renal disease program. Health Care Financ Rev. 2000;Fall;22(1):55–60. PMCID: PMC4194691.

7. Tonelli M, Wiebe N, Knoll G, et al. Systematic review: kidney transplantation compared with dialysis in clinically relevant outcomes. Am J Transplant. 2011;11(10):2093–109. https://onlinelibrary.wiley.com/doi/abs/10.1111/j.1600-6143.2011.03686.x. https://doi.org/10.1111/j.1600-6143.2011.03686.x.

8. Andreas L, Paul K, Nancy P, Hans K, Beryl F, Cindy W, Norman M. A study of the quality of life and cost utility of renal transplantation. Kidney Int. 1996;50:235–42.

9. Https://Optn.transplant.hrsa.gov/data/view-data-reports/national-data/. Accessed 1 Mar 2020.

10. Hart A, Smith JM, Skeans MA, et al. OPTN:SRTR 2017 annual data report kidney. Am J Transplant. 2019;19:1–106.

11. Unsal MG, Yilmaz M, Sezer T, et al. Comparison of preemptive kidney transplantation with nonpreemptive kidney transplantation in a single center: a follow-up study. Transplant Proc. 2015;47(5):1385–7. https://www.clinicalkey.es/playcontent/1-s2.0-S0041134515003644. https://doi.org/10.1016/j.transproceed.2015.04.039.

12. Sayin B, Colak T, Tutal E, Sezer S. Comparison of preemptive kidney transplant recipients with nonpreemptive kidney recipients in single center: 5 years of follow-up. Int J Nephrol Renov Dis. 2013;6:95–9. https://www.ncbi.nlm.nih.gov/pubmed/23761978. https://doi.org/10.2147/IJNRD.S42042.

13. Saran R, Robinson B, Abbott KC, et al. US renal data system 2019 annual data report: epidemiology of kidney disease in the United States. Am J Kidney Dis. 2019;73(3):A7–8. https://doi.org/10.1053/j.ajkd.2019.01.001.

14. Https://Optn.transplant.hrsa.gov/resources/allocation-calculators/kdpi-calculator/. Accessed 1 Mar 2020.

15. Israni AK, Salkowski N, Gustafson S, et al. New national allocation policy for deceased donor kidneys in the United States and possible effect on patient outcomes. J Am Soc Nephrol. 2014;25(8):1842–8. https://www.ncbi.nlm.nih.gov/pubmed/24833128. https://doi.org/10.1681/ASN.2013070784.

16. King KL, Husain SA, Jin Z, Brennan C, Mohan S. Trends in disparities in preemptive kidney transplantation in the United States. Clin J Am Soc Nephrol. 2019;14(10):1500–11. https://www.ncbi.nlm.nih.gov/pubmed/31413065. https://doi.org/10.2215/CJN.03140319.

17. American Academy of Family Physicians. Five things physicians and patients should question. J Okla State Med Assoc. 2012;105(9):370. https://www.ncbi.nlm.nih.gov/pubmed/23155846.

18. Vassalotti JA, Centor R, Turner BJ, Greer RC, Choi M, Sequist TD. Practical approach to detection and management of chronic kidney disease for the primary care clinician. Am J Med. 2016;129(2):153. https://search.proquest.com/docview/1767329311.

19. Cass A, Cunningham J, et al. Late referral to a nephrologist reduces access to renal transplantation. Am J Kidney Dis. 2003;42(5):1043–9.

20. Https://Optn.transplant.hrsa.gov/resources/guidance/educational-guidance-on-patient-referral-to-kidney-transplantation/. Accessed 1 Mar 2020.

21. Cohen JB, Shults J, Goldberg DS, Abt PL, Sawinski DL, Reese PP. Kidney allograft offers: predictors of turndown and the impact of late organ acceptance on allograft survival. Am J Transplant. 2018;18(2):391–401. https://onlinelibrary.wiley.com/doi/abs/10.1111/ajt.14449. https://doi.org/10.1111/ajt.14449.

22. Gander JC, Zhang X, Ross K, et al. Association between dialysis facility ownership and access to kidney transplantation. JAMA. 2019;322(10):957–73. https://www.ncbi.nlm.nih.gov/pubmed/31503308. https://doi.org/10.1001/jama.2019.12803.

23. Hart A, Smith JM, Skeans MA, et al. OPTN/SRTR 2018 annual data report: kidney. Am J Transplant. 2020;20(s1):20–130. https://onlinelibrary.wiley.com/doi/abs/10.1111/ajt.15672. https://doi.org/10.1111/ajt.15672.

24. Kallab S, Bassil N, Esposito L, Cardeau-Desangles I, Rostaing L, Kamar N. Indications for and barriers to preemptive kidney transplantation: a review. Transplant Proc. 2010;42(3):782–4. https://www.clinicalkey.es/playcontent/1-s2.0-S0041134510002460. https://doi.org/10.1016/j.transproceed.2010.02.031.

25. Haller MC, Kainz A, Baer H, Oberbauer R. Dialysis vintage and outcomes after kidney transplantation: a retrospective cohort study. Clin J Am Soc Nephrol. 2017;12(1):122–30. https://www.ncbi.nlm.nih.gov/pubmed/27895135. https://doi.org/10.2215/CJN.04120416.

26. Harhay MN, Harhay MO, Ranganna K, et al. Association of the kidney allocation system with dialysis exposure before deceased donor kidney transplantation by preemptive wait-listing status. Clin Transpl. 2018;32:1–12.

27. Gill JS, Tonelli M, Johnson N, Pereira BJG. Why do preemptive kidney transplant recipients have an allograft survival advantage? Transplantation. 2004;78(6):873–9. https://www.ncbi.nlm.nih.gov/pubmed/15385807. https://doi.org/10.1097/01.TP.0000130204.80781.68.

28. Girerd S, Girerd N, Duarte K, et al. Preemptive second kidney transplantation is associated with better graft survival compared with non-preemptive second transplantation: a multicenter French 2000–2014 cohort study. Transpl Int. 2018;31(4):408–23. https://onlinelibrary.wiley.com/doi/abs/10.1111/tri.13105. https://doi.org/10.1111/tri.13105.

29. Meier-Kriesche H, Port FK, Ojo AO, et al. Effect of waiting time on renal transplant outcome. Kidney Int. 2000;58(3):1311–7. https://www.sciencedirect.com/science/article/pii/S0085253815472229. https://doi.org/10.1046/j.1523-1755.2000.00287.x.

30. Kasiske BL, Snyder JJ, Matas AJ, Ellison MD, Gill JS, Kausz AT. Preemptive kidney transplantation: the advantage and the advantaged. J Am Soc Nephrol. 2002;13(5):1358–64. https://www.ncbi.nlm.nih.gov/pubmed/11961024. https://doi.org/10.1097/01.ASN.0000013295.11876.C9.

31. Akkina SK, Connaire JJ, Snyder JJ, Matas AJ, Kasiske BL. Earlier is not necessarily better in preemptive kidney transplantation. Am J Transplant. 2013;8:575–82.

32. Grams ME, Massie AB, Coresh J, Segev DL. Trends in the timing of preemptive kidney transplantation. J Am Soc Nephrol. 2011;22(9):1615–20. https://doi.org/10.1681/ASN.2011010023.

33. Mange KC, Joffe MM, Feldman HI. Effect of the use or nonuse of long-term dialysis on the subsequent survival of renal transplants from living donors. N Engl J Med. 2001;344(10):726–31. http://content.nejm.org/cgi/content/abstract/344/10/726. https://doi.org/10.1056/NEJM200103083441004.

34. Davis C. Preemptive transplantation and the transplant first initiative. Curr Opin Nephrol Hypertens. 2010;19(6):592–7. https://www.ncbi.nlm.nih.gov/pubmed/20827196. https://doi.org/10.1097/MNH.0b013e32833e04f5.

35. Yoo SW, Kwon OJ, Kang CM. Preemptive living-donor renal transplantation: outcome and clinical advantages. Transplant Proc. 2009;41(1):117–20. https://www.clinicalkey.es/playcontent/1-s2.0-S0041134508015741. https://doi.org/10.1016/j.transproceed.2008.09.063.

36. Ishani A, Ibrahim HN, Gilbertson D, Collins AJ. The impact of residual renal function on graft and patient survival rates in recipients of preemptive renal transplants. Am J Kidney Dis. 2003;42(6):1275–82. https://www.sciencedirect.com/science/article/pii/S027263860301117X. https://doi.org/10.1053/j.ajkd.2003.08.030.

37. Grams ME, Chen BP-H, Coresh J, Segev DL. Preemptive deceased donor kidney transplantation: considerations of equity and utility. Clin J Am Soc Nephrol. 2013;8(4):575–82. http://cjasn.asnjournals.org/content/8/4/575.abstract. https://doi.org/10.2215/CJN.05310512.

38. Policy, Committee on Organ Procurement and Transplantation, Medicine Io. Organ procurement and transplantation. Washington, DC: National Academies Press; 2000. https://www.nap.edu/9628. https://doi.org/10.17226/9628.

39. Friedewald JJ, Samana CJ, Kasiske BL, et al. The kidney allocation system. Surg Clin North Am. 2013;93(6):1395–406. https://www.clinicalkey.es/playcontent/1-s2.0-S0039610913001321. https://doi.org/10.1016/j.suc.2013.08.007.

40. Https://Www.healthypeople.gov/2020/topics-objectives/topic/chronic-kidney-disease/objectives.
41. Stewart DE, Klassen DK. Early experience with the new kidney allocation system: a perspective from UNOS. Clin J Am Soc Nephrol. 2017;12(12):2063–5. https://www.ncbi.nlm.nih.gov/pubmed/29162594. https://doi.org/10.2215/CJN.06380617.
42. Massie AB, Luo X, Lonze BE, et al. Early changes in kidney distribution under the new allocation system. J Am Soc Nephrol. 2016;27(8):2495–501. https://www.ncbi.nlm.nih.gov/pubmed/26677865. https://doi.org/10.1681/ASN.2015080934.
43. Melanson TA, Hockenberry JM, Plantinga L, et al. New kidney allocation system associated with increased rates of transplants among black and hispanic patients. Health Aff (Project Hope). 2017;36(6):1078–85. https://www.ncbi.nlm.nih.gov/pubmed/28583967. https://doi.org/10.1377/hlthaff.2016.1625.
44. Harhay MN, McKenna RM, Boyle SM, et al. Association between medicaid expansion under the affordable care act and preemptive listings for kidney transplantation. Clin J Am Soc Nephrol. 2018;13(7):1069–78. https://www.ncbi.nlm.nih.gov/pubmed/29929999. https://doi.org/10.2215/CJN.00100118.
45. Petrini C. Preemptive kidney transplantation: an ethical challenge for organ allocation policies. Clin Ter. 2017;168(3):192–3.
46. Https://Www.whitehouse.gov/presidential-actions/executive-order-advancing-american-kidney-health/.
47. Cooper DKC, Hara H, Iwase H, et al. Clinical pig kidney xenotransplantation: how close are we? J Am Soc Nephrol. 2020;31(1):12–21. https://www.ncbi.nlm.nih.gov/pubmed/31792154. https://doi.org/10.1681/ASN.2019070651.

Index

Made in the USA
Monee, IL
07 July 2026

56550262R00256